The Penn Center Guide
to Bioethics

Vardit Ravitsky, PhD, is faculty at the Department of Medical Ethics and a senior fellow at the Center for Bioethics at the University of Pennsylvania. Previously, she was a postdoctoral fellow at the Department of Clinical Bioethics at the National Institute of Health and at the Social and Behavioral Research Branch of the National Human Genome Research Institute (NHGRI). Born and raised in Jerusalem, she received her BA in philosophy from the Sorbonne University in Paris, her MA in philosophy from the University of New Mexico, and her PhD in philosophy with a focus in bioethics from Bar Ilan University in Israel. Ravitsky worked as a researcher for the Gertner Institute for Health Policy Research and as a consultant for Genome Canada on ethical, economic, environmental, legal, and social implications of genomics research. Her main research interests include ethical aspects of human genetics and reproduction, end of life, research ethics, and the ways in which culture shapes health policy. Her work in these areas has been published in journals such as the *American Journal of Bioethics* and the *British Medical Journal.*

Autumn Fiester, PhD, is a senior fellow at the Center for Bioethics. She is also the director of Graduate Studies in the Department of Medical Ethics, which is home to the UPenn Master of Bioethics Program, the largest, and one of the most prestigious, graduate programs in bioethics in the United States. Fiester began her graduate training at Harvard University, where she received an AM in sociology. She completed her PhD in moral philosophy from the University of Pennsylvania in 2002. Since coming to the Center for Bioethics, her research interests have included ethics of animal biotechnology, clinical professionalism, and moral theory. Fiester has worked with both national and international projects in the field of animal biotechnology, having recently completed a European Union–sponsored project on the ethics of human-animal chimeras. Her work has been published in leading bioethics journals, including the *American Journal of Bioethics* and the *Hastings Center Report.*

Arthur L. Caplan, PhD, is the Emmanuel and Robert Hart Professor of Bioethics, chair of the Department of Medical Ethics and the director of the Center for Bioethics at the University of Pennsylvania in Philadelphia. He is the author or editor of 25 books and over 500 papers in refereed journals of medicine, science, philosophy, bioethics, and health policy. Caplan is the recipient of many awards and honors including the McGovern Medal of the American Medical Writers Association, Person of the Year—2001 from *USA Today,* and he was named one of the 50 most influential people in American health care by *Modern Health Care* magazine and one of the 10 most influential people in America in biotechnology by the *National Journal.* He holds six honorary degrees from colleges and medical schools. He is a fellow of the Hastings Center, the New York Academy of Medicine, the College of Physicians of Philadelphia, and the American Association for the Advancement of Science.

The Penn Center Guide to Bioethics

Vardit Ravitsky, PhD,
Autumn Fiester, PhD, and
Arthur L. Caplan, PhD

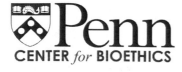

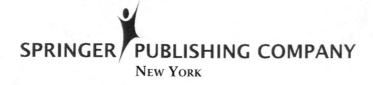

SPRINGER PUBLISHING COMPANY
New York

Springer Publishing Company, LLC
11 West 42nd Street
New York, NY 10036
www.springerpub.com

Acquisitions Editor: Philip Laughlin
Project Manager: Julia Rosen
Cover Design: Mimi Flow
Composition: Apex CoVantage, LLC

Ebook ISBN: 978–0–8261–1731–1

10 11 / 5 4 3 2

Library of Congress Cataloging-in-Publication Data

The Penn Center guide to bioethics / Arthur L. Caplan, Autumn Fiester, and Vardit Ravitsky, editors.
        p. cm.
   Includes bibliographical references and index.
   ISBN 978-0-8261-1522-5 (alk. paper)
  1. Bioethics.   I. Caplan, Arthur L.   II. Fiester, Autumn.   III. Ravitsky, Vardit.   IV. Penn Center (University of Pennsylvania)
   QH332.P46   2009
   174'.957—dc22   2009000148

Printed in the United States of America by Hamilton Printing.

Contents

PART I

PART II

PART III

Contributors

Peter L. Abt, MD
Department of Surgery
Hospital of the University of
    Pennsylvania
Children's Hospital of Philadelphia

Mark B. Adams, PhD
Department of History and
    Sociology of Science
University of Pennsylvania

Anita L. Allen, JD, PhD
Henry R. Silverman Professor
    of Law
Professor of Philosophy
University of Pennsylvania Law
    School

Robert Baker, PhD
Director & Professor of Bioethics
The Union Graduate College-
    Mount Sinai School of
    Medicine Bioethics Program
William D. Williams Professor of
    Philosophy, Union College

Visiting Scholar
Center for Bioethics
University of Pennsylvania

H. Jorge Baluarte, MD
Professor of Pediatrics
Medical Director, Renal
    Transplant Program
The Children's Hospital of
    Philadelphia

**Jill M. Baren, MD, MBE, ГАСЕР,
    FAAP**
Associate Professor of Emergency
    Medicine and Pediatrics
University of Pennsylvania
    School of Medicine
Attending Physician, Department
    of Emergency Medicine
Hospital of the University of
    Pennsylvania and Division
    of Emergency Medicine,
    Department of Pediatrics
The Children's Hospital of
    Philadelphia

Frances R. Batzer, MD, MBE
Professor of Obstetrics and
  Gynecology
Thomas Jefferson University
Philadelphia, PA

Ronald Bayer, PhD
Professor, Center for the History
  and Ethics of Public Health
Department of Sociomedical
  Sciences
Mailman School of Public
  Health
Columbia University, New York

Edward J. Bergman, JD
Center for Bioethics, University
  of Pennsylvania
Department of Legal Studies
  and Business Ethics, Wharton
  School of Business
University of Pennsylvania

Michael B. Blank, PhD
Associate Professor of Psychology
  in Psychiatry
Associate Professor of Nursing
Senior Fellow at the Leonard
  Davis Institute of Health
  Economics
University of Pennsylvania

Roy D. Bloom, MD
Associate Professor of
  Medicine
Medical Director, Kidney and
  Pancreas Transplant Program
University of Pennsylvania

Debra A. Budiani-Saberi, PhD
Executive Director
Coalition for Organ-Failure
  Solutions (COFS)
Visiting Research Associate

Center for Bioethics
University of Pennsylvania

Arthur L. Caplan, PhD
Emmanuel and Robert Hart
  Professor of Bioethics
Director, Center for Bioethics
University of Pennsylvania

James Colgrove, PhD, MPH
Center for the History and Ethics
  of Public Health
Department of Sociomedical
  Sciences
Mailman School of Public Health
Columbia University, New York

Amy M. Corcoran, MD
Assistant Professor of Clinical
  Medicine
Division of Geriatrics
University of Pennsylvania
  School of Medicine

**Curtis R. Coughlin II, MS,
  CGC**
Section of Biochemical
  Genetics
Children's Hospital of
  Philadelphia

Mahnu Davar, JD, MBE
Attorney
FDA & Healthcare Group
Arnold & Porter, LLP
Washington, DC

Horace M. DeLisser, MD
Associate Professor of Medicine
Pulmonary, Allergy and Critical
  Care Division
University of Pennsylvania
  School of Medicine

David J. Doukas, MD
William Ray Moore Endowed
  Chair of Family Medicine and
  Medical Humanism
Director, Division of Medical
  Humanism and Ethics,
Department of Family and
  Geriatric Medicine,
University of Louisville
Louisville, KY

Marlene Eisenberg, PhD
Director, Penn HIV Prevention
  Trials Network Quality
  Assurance
HIV Prevention Research Division
University of Pennsylvania

Bernice S. Elger, MD, PhD, MA
Adjunct Professor
Center for Legal Medicine (health
  law and human rights)
University of Geneva, Switzerland

Susan S. Ellenberg, PhD
Professor of Biostatistics
Associate Director for Clinical
  Research
Senior Scholar, Center for Clinical
  Epidemiology and Biostatistics
University of Pennsylvania
  School of Medicine

Martha J. Farah, PhD
Walter H. Annenberg Professor in
  Natural Sciences
Director, Center for Cognitive
  Neuroscience
University of Pennsylvania

Thomas W. Faust, MD, MBE
Associate Professor of Clinical
  Medicine
Division of Gastroenterology

Department of Internal Medicine
The University of Pennsylvania
  School of Medicine

Eric A. Feldman, JD, PhD
Professor of Law, University of
  Pennsylvania Law School
Visiting Professor of Law,
  Stanford Law School

Chris Feudtner, MD, PhD, MPH
Steven D. Handler Endowed
  Chair of Medical Ethics
Director, Department of Medical
  Ethics
The Children's Hospital of
  Philadelphia

Robert I. Field, JD, MPH, PhD
Chair, Department of Health
  Policy and Public Health
Professor of Health Policy
University of the Sciences in
  Philadelphia

Autumn Fiester, PhD
Senior Fellow, Center for
  Bioethics
Director, Graduate Studies
Department of Medical Ethics
University of Pennsylvania
  School of Medicine

Barry R. Furrow, JD
Professor of Law and Director,
  the Health Law Program
Earle Mack School of Law
Drexel University,
  Philadelphia, PA

Joanne Godley, MD, MPH, MBE
Associate Fellow, Center for
  Bioethics
University of Pennsylvania

Judah L. Goldberg, MD, MBE
Department of Emergency
    Medicine
New York Hospital Queens,
    Queens, NY

Cynthia Green, MSS, LSW
Program Manager/Social
    Worker
Division of Nephrology
The Children's Hospital of
    Philadelphia

Mark Greene, BVSc, PhD
Department of Philosophy
University of Delaware
Newark, DE

**Scott D. Halpern, MD, PhD,
    MBE**
Division of Pulmonary and
    Critical Care Medicine
Center for Clinical Epidemiology
    and Biostatistics
Center for Bioethics
University of Pennsylvania
    School of Medicine

Steven D. Handler, MD, MBE
Endowed Chair and Associate
    Director of Pediatric
    Otolaryngology
The Children's Hospital of
    Philadelphia
Professor of Otolaryngology:
    Head and Neck Surgery
University of Pennsylvania
    School of Medicine

Stephen S. Hanson, PhD
Department of Philosophy
Department of Family and
    Geriatric Medicine
University of Louisville, KY

Jan Jaeger, PhD
Center for Bioethics
University of Pennsylvania

Nora L. Jones, PhD
Senior Fellow
Center for Bioethics
University of Pennsylvania

Bernard S. Kaplan, MB, BCh
Director of Pediatric
    Nephrology
Laffey-Connolly Professor of
    Pediatric Nephrology
The Children's Hospital of
    Philadelphia

Jennifer M. Kapo, MD
Assistant Professor of Clinical
    Medicine
Department of Medicine,
    Division of Geriatrics
Senior Fellow, Center for
    Bioethics
University of Pennsylvania
Medical Director, Palliative Care
    Services
Philadelphia Veteran's Medical
    Center
Philadelphia, PA

Georgios Karnakis, MD
Research Fellow, Yale Fertility
    Center
Yale University, New Haven,
    CT

William R. LaFleur, PhD
E. Dale Saunders Professor in
    Japanese Studies
Department of East Asian
    Languages and Civilizations
University of Pennsylvania

Stephen E. Lammers, PhD
Department of Religious Studies
Lafayette College
Easton, PA

Donald W. Light, PhD
Senior Fellow, Center for Bioethics
University of Pennsylvania
Professor, Department of
    Psychiatry
University of Medicine and
    Dentistry of New Jersey
Newark, NJ

Holly Fernandez Lynch, JD, MBE
Associate, Pharmaceuticals and
    Biotechnology Group
Hogan & Hartson, LLP
Washington DC

David C. Magnus, PhD
Stanford Center for Biomedical
    Ethics
School of Medicine
Stanford University
Stanford, CA

**Margaret M. Mahon, PhD, RN,
    FAAN**
College of Health and Human
    Services
George Mason University
Fairfax, VA
Associate Fellow
Center for Bioethics
University of Pennsylvania

Marisa P. Marcin, JD
Center for Bioethics
University of Pennsylvania

Thomas A. Marino, PhD
Professor of Anatomy and Cell
    Biology

Temple University School of
    Medicine
Philadelphia, PA
Adjunct Professor, School of
    Nursing
Associate Fellow, Center for
    Bioethics
University of Pennsylvania

**Luigi Mastroianni, Jr., MD,
    MBE**
The William Goodell Emeritus
    Professor of Obstetrics and
    Gynecology
University of Pennsylvania
    School of Medicine

James J. McCartney, PhD
Associate Professor
Department of Philosophy
Villanova University
Villanova, PA

Jon F. Merz, MBA, JD, PhD
Department of Medical Ethics
University of Pennsylvania
    School of Medicine

Kevin E. C. Meyers, MB, BCh
Pediatric Nephrologist
Department of Pediatrics
Associate Professor of Pediatrics
The Children's Hospital of
    Philadelphia and
The University of Pennsylvania

Victoria A. Miller, PhD
Center for Research Integrity
The Children's Hospital of
    Philadelphia
Department of Anesthesiology
    and Critical Care
University of Pennsylvania
    School of Medicine

Perry B. Molinoff, MD
Professor of Pharmacology
Department of Pharmacology
Senior Fellow, Center for Bioethics
University of Pennsylvania

Jonathan D. Moreno, PhD
David and Lyn Silfen University
  Professor of Ethics
Department of Medical Ethics
Department of the History and
  Sociology of Science
University of Pennsylvania

Wynne Morrison, MD
Department of Anesthesiology
  and Critical Care
The Children's Hospital of
  Philadelphia
University of Pennsylvania
  School of Medicine

David Munson, MD
Associate Medical Director,
  Pediatric Advanced Care Team
Associate Medical Director,
  Newborn/Infant Intensive
  Care Unit
The Children's Hospital of
  Philadelphia

Robert M. Nelson, MD, PhD
Center for Research Integrity
Children's Hospital of
  Philadelphia
Department of Anesthesiology
  and Critical Care
University of Pennsylvania
  School of Medicine

Alisa A. Padon, MBE
Center for Bioethics
Office of Regulatory Affairs
University of Pennsylvania

**Pasquale Patrizio, MD, MBE,
  HCLD**
Associate Professor of Medicine
Pulmonary, Allergy and Critical
  Care Division
University of Pennsylvania
  School of Medicine

David Perlman, PhD
President and Founder, E4–
  Eclipse Ethics Education
  Enterprises, LLC
Senior Lecturer, Penn School of
  Nursing
Associate Fellow, Center for
  Bioethics
University of Pennsylvania

Michael S. Peroski
Student, Allegheny College,
  Allegheny, PA
Student, Oxford University, UK
Former Penn Bioethics intern

Vardit Ravitsky, PhD
Center for Bioethics
University of Pennsylvania

Barbara K. Redman, PhD, MBE
Dean and Professor, Wayne State
  University College of Nursing
Detroit, MI
Visiting Scholar, Center for
  Bioethics
University of Pennsylvania

Peter P. Reese, MD, MSCE
Renal Electrolyte and
  Hypertension Division
University of Pennsylvania

Angelique M. Reitsma, MD, MA
Associate Fellow
Center for Bioethics
University of Pennsylvania

William W. Reynolds, PhD
School of Social and Behavioral
    Sciences
The Richard Stockton College of
    New Jersey
Pomona, NJ

Jennifer L. Rosato, JD
Earle Mack School of Law
Drexel University
Philadelphia, PA

Theodore W. Ruger, JD
Professor of Law
University of Pennsylvania Law
    School

Pamela Sankar, PhD
Associate Professor of Bioethics,
    Department of Medical Ethics
Senior Fellow, Center for
    Bioethics
University of Pennsylvania
    School of Medicine

Carol Schilling, PhD
Visiting Scholar
Center for Bioethics and
    Department of Medical Ethics
University of Pennsylvania

Susan Schneider, PhD
Assistant Professor
Department of Philosophy
Center for Cognitive
    Neuroscience and Institute for
    Cognitive Science
University of Pennsylvania

Jason L. Schwartz, MBE, AM
Center for Bioethics
Department of History and
    Sociology of Science
University of Pennsylvania

Dominic Sisti, MBE
Center for Bioethics, University
    of Pennsylvania
Department of Philosophy,
    Michigan State University
East Lansing, MI

Michael J. Smith, MD, MSCE
Assistant Professor of
    Pediatrics
University of Louisville School of
    Medicine
Louisville, KY

Roberta M. Snow, PhD
Professor of Management
Management Department
West Chester University
West Chester, PA

John Timpane, PhD
Editor/Writer, *Philadelphia
    Inquirer*

Connie M. Ulrich, PhD, RN
Assistant Professor of Bioethics
    and Nursing
Senior Fellow, Center for
    Bioethics
Senior Fellow, Leonard Davis
    Institute of Economics
University of Pennsylvania

Raluca Vrabie, MD
Fellow, Department of
    Gastroenterology
Hospital of the University of
    Pennsylvania

Debra Wiegand, PhD, MBE, RN
Assistant Professor, School of
    Nursing
University of Maryland
Baltimore, MD

Gerald I. Wolpe, Rabbi, DD
Senior Fellow Emeritus
Center for Bioethics
University of Pennsylvania

Paul Root Wolpe, PhD
Asa Griggs Candler Professor of
    Bioethics
Director, Center for Ethics
Emory University
Atlanta, GA

Michael Yudell, PhD, MPH
Assistant Professor, Department
    of Community Health and
    Prevention
School of Public Health

Drexel University
Philadelphia, PA

**Mindy B. Zeitzer, PhD(c), MBE,
    CRNP**
University of Pennsylvania
    School of Nursing
Ruth L. Kirschstein NRSA
    Predoctoral Fellow

Diana Zuckerman, PhD
President, National Research
    Center for Women &
    Families
Associate Fellow, Center for
    Bioethics
University of Pennsylvania

Preface

AUTUMN FIESTER

The *Penn Center Guide to Bioethics* is a collection that represents the "Penn way" of doing bioethics. The University of Pennsylvania's Center for Bioethics takes a distinct approach to the field of bioethics, reflected in the issues we address, the integration of the empirical and the normative, the educational programs we offer, and the level of engagement we have with both the public and the stakeholders in the controversies of bioethics.

The Penn Center for Bioethics is recognized as one of the global leaders in the field of bioethics. Since its founding in 1994, under the leadership of Arthur Caplan, the Penn Center has sought to tackle the traditional issues of bioethics as well as the emerging issues, helping to shape the academic and public discourse on the challenging questions generated by new technologies and medical advances.

The field of bioethics came into being decades ago because of ethical quandaries such as abortion, withdrawal of life support, and human research subjects protection, and the Penn Center includes these important issues in its research agenda. However, as both the life and medical sciences have experienced unprecedented growth and progress, a host of new ethical issues have emerged, and the Penn Center seeks to navigate these uncharted ethical terrains as well.

The Penn Center closely follows the latest technical and medical advances to map out and help resolve the issues raised by cutting-edge research. The Penn Center has an eye out for the ethical quandaries that are on the horizon so that public debate can have a head start in grappling with emerging ethical issues involved in areas such as neuroethics, biobanking, genetic screening, nanoethics, bioterrorism, and animal biotechnology—to name just a few.

The Penn Center is known for innovative, multidisciplinary scholarship that draws on the expertise of disciplines as diverse as social science, philosophy, theology, law, public policy, business, and clinical training. The Penn Center was one of the first bioethics centers to emphasize and produce empiricized bioethics, using the methods and approaches of empirical inquiry to shed light on bioethical issues. The *Penn Guide* effectively reveals this diversity in discipline and method.

The *Penn Guide* also reflects the center's pioneering approach of integrating bioethics scholarship with practical application, not merely in clinical medicine but in the realms of public policy, public debate, and industry. The Penn Center has always viewed its mission as the marriage of theory and practice: the center is not an armchair institution, generating publications by scholars to be read merely by other scholars. That approach has its place in the academy. But the Penn Center strives to play an active role in policy, education, consultation, and public debate because bioethics is not just academic—bioethical dilemmas confront all of us, at one time or another, in either our personal or professional lives.

The Penn Center fosters public discourse, from our unique High School Bioethics Program to our consultations with medical institutes, advocacy organizations, and industry, as well as the many public lectures Penn faculty and fellows deliver. The Penn Center intentionally uses print, electronic, and other broadcast media to put bioethical issues on the public's agenda.

This commitment to assisting individuals who are on the frontlines of bioethics can be seen in our renowned Master of Bioethics Program, founded in 1997. The Penn Master of Bioethics Program is designed for professionals who work in areas that put them at the center of bioethical conflict. Our students come from the fields of medicine, nursing, veterinary medicine, dentistry, law, public health, the pharmaceutical and biotech industries, clergy, and government. Our mission is to give professionals the tools they need to address the bioethical issues that arise in their workplace.

The *Penn Guide* mirrors the style and commitment of the Penn Center for Bioethics, and we hope it will promote these important debates.

Introduction

VARDIT RAVITSKY

Although it is coming of age, bioethics is still a relatively young field of inquiry. It constantly searches for appropriate methodologies and conceptual tools and frequently embraces complex multidisciplinary approaches. It is exciting and challenging, embedded in cultural and political contexts and always in touch with cutting-edge scientific progress. Bioethicists think, write, and advise, contributing perspectives that benefit patients, research participants, communities, professionals, policy makers, and the public at large.

The Center for Bioethics at the University of Pennsylvania has been a leading hub in American bioethics for over a decade. *The Penn Center Guide to Bioethics* features the diverse bioethics expertise of scholars around the university, as well as the contributions of those who have been associated with the center in the past years.

Contributors to this volume were asked to provide an overview of their area of study that would be accessible for professionals and lay readers alike. At the same time, the editors invited authors to speak in their own voices and express their own perceptions of how their field has evolved, where it stands today, and where they believe it is heading. We encouraged them to maintain a distinctive style that reflects not only their own disciplinary background, but also their unique personal viewpoints. Rather than adopting a *neutral* stance, chapters are intended to engage the reader by provoking thought and critical reaction.

Many of the contributors are senior researchers who have established themselves as academic authorities in their respective fields. Others are more junior bioethicists who show great promise to become the leading scholars of the future, representing the next generation that will shape bioethics in the coming years.

Each chapter offers some historical background and an overview of the relevant issues, but also a focus on certain arguments—of the authors' choosing—within the general topic. The *Penn Guide* allows any reader, coming from any background, to appreciate the context and the scope of each subject while obtaining a more nuanced and sophisticated analysis of some specific aspects.

These diverse voices complement each other at times, and diverge at others. The interplay of perspectives offers the reader a rounded view of the vibrant world of bioethics as it unfolds. The *Penn Guide* thus captures a snapshot of present-day bioethics through the lens of the research carried out in a leading university and by those associated with it. It does not aspire to be a comprehensive collection representing every aspect of the field. Considering the broad scope of bioethics today, this would have been impossible. Rather, the *Penn Guide* is meant to provide a rich and integrated overview, allowing the reader to appreciate classical topics as well as a sample of recent developments.

In this volume, you will find:

- both classical topics in clinical bioethics—such as confidentiality, advance directives, and medical futility—and emerging issues, such as nonprofessional caregiving;
- a focus on long established practices, such as nursing, as well as an exploration of new ones, such as mediation;
- elaboration of well-established areas in research ethics—such as informed consent and placebo control trials—as well as new areas, such as innovative surgery or how race, gender, and age play a role in inclusion and exclusion of participants in clinical trials;
- reflections on centuries-old issues, such as eugenics, but also new ones, such as privacy of thought in the age of brain imaging;
- a discussion of established technologies, such as prenatal genetic testing and in vitro fertilization, and more recent ones, such as pre-implantation genetic diagnosis and the cloning of animals; and
- an examination of familiar bioethical topics in public health, such as quarantine and vaccination, but also emerging issues in this field, such as national security or nonprofit organizations.

The outcome is a book that offers a rich and colorful tapestry of current viewpoints, set in a myriad of tones and styles, mirroring the diversity of a field in which new challenges emerge daily.

* * *

A brief look at the history and evolution of bioethics sheds light on the *Penn Guide* and what it has to offer. Bioethics has come a long way since its inception in the 1960s. Born in response to violations of human rights in biomedical research, its initial focus was the protection of individuals. Indeed, one of its most successful endeavors has been the establishment of principles and mechanisms for protecting research subjects, particularly by developing the concept of *informed consent.* The core ethical principle underlying this focus has been *autonomy,* the right of every individual to self-determination as a patient and as a subject within health care and research systems that were growing in size and complexity.

Bioethics' focus on autonomy also meant that it pushed toward a shift in the physician-patient relationship, from a paternalistic model to a more contractual one. It promoted the empowerment of patients and obliged professionals to acknowledge patients' rights to decide for themselves what is in their best interest, including their right to refuse treatment and to make end-of-life decisions.

For the first couple of decades, bioethicists' intellectual energy was thus invested mostly in the realm of *negative rights,* rights to be protected from unwarranted intrusion and to be left alone to exercise one's autonomy. One important aspect of the evolution of bioethics is the shifting of its attention toward *positive rights,* rights that impose obligations on others not just to refrain from action, but rather to provide certain benefits, such as the right to health care or the right to be included in research. Such rights create obligations on the part of society, and their implementation can be costly. They therefore entail an ethical discourse that goes far beyond the focus on autonomy, to include considerations such as distributive justice, allocation of resources, and priority setting.

As bioethics evolved, these considerations began to take center stage, and a growing number of bioethicists started to tackle complex and politically charged issues such as the right to health care and strategies for rationing. Their work reveals the progress that bioethics has been making in realizing that the protection of autonomy is not sufficient when many Americans, as free and informed as they may be, have no access to health care and are denied benefits that privileged individuals take for granted. Furthermore, this work expands the scope of bioethical discourse from the traditional focus on Western democracies to a global perspective. It embraces a discussion of the needs of the poor in developing countries and does not shy away from advocacy.

This shift is evident in the content of the *Penn Guide.* Some chapters structure their ethical discussion around principles such as autonomy, while others expand the discussion to include these more recent debates, such as access to health care, fair pricing of medicines for the poor, and the rights of minorities to be included in research.

A second aspect of the evolution of bioethics is reflected in the growing attention dedicated not just to individuals but also to the interests and perspectives of communities, cultures, and societies. For example, the rapidly growing area of *public health ethics* is focused on the tension—and the appropriate balance—between respecting the rights of individuals and the interests of the public. When these two perspectives clash, intriguing bioethical challenges emerge. Bioethicists have begun to describe and analyze these issues, and to propose ethical frameworks for addressing them.

Some of the *Penn Guide*'s chapters reflect this development. Authors outline possible frameworks for public health ethics, discuss a *code of ethics for public health,* and even demonstrate how bioethical analysis plays out in specific cases encountered by practitioners on the ground. They explain when practices such as isolation and quarantine, which limit the freedom of individuals, can be ethically justified as a public health measure. They also explore diverse issues such as mandating vaccination of health care workers, which is crucial for the protection of vulnerable patient populations but may violate the rights of individual workers, or tobacco taxes that are designed to discourage smokers in order to promote public health but have an adverse economic impact on the poor.

Moreover, chapters in various sections of the *Penn Guide* address bioethical concerns on a social, not just an individual, level. Genetic research, for example, benefits individuals in many ways, and its ethical implications for individuals have been discussed extensively in the bioethical literature. However, genetic research gradually reveals information about genetic differences between populations that has the potential to harm certain populations by strengthening misconceptions about race. This raises questions about the *social* consequences of conducting such research and whether it should be pursued in the first place. The *Penn Guide* explores the possible expansion of research ethics from its classical concern for the protection of *individuals* to include questions about what type of research can benefit or harm *society* and whether it should be supported or discouraged.

A third aspect of the evolution of bioethics is related to the ethical challenges raised by new technologies. Bioethics initially focused on the ethical implications of new technologies such as mechanical ventilation, artificial nutrition and hydration, and organ transplantation at the end of life, as well as in vitro fertilization and prenatal genetic testing in the beginning of life. Bioethics has traditionally applied theories and principles, developing new conceptual tools and methodologies that were necessary for the analysis of such issues.

As bioethics evolves into a more mature discipline, the ethical, legal, and social implications of biotechnology are becoming an even greater focus of its work. Bioethicists debate among themselves about the need to develop new specialized subdisciplines to address new types of technologies. For example, advances in brain imaging raise new and fascinating ethical questions, but do we need new conceptual tools to address them? Do we need *neuroethics, genethics,* and *nanoethics* as offshoots of *bioethics?* The *Penn Guide* tackles these issues and offers the unique perspectives of leading scholars in the relevant fields.

Finally, the evolution of bioethics has brought the field to a point in which it requires specific training and expertise and allows for a spectrum of possible careers, from traditional academic positions all the way to consultant positions for government or industry. This development brought to the forefront the need for bioethicists to be accountable and aware of their own potential biases and conflicts of interest. Rather than relying solely on personal integrity, bioethics as a discipline is now conscious of the need for a more formalized mechanism, *a code of ethics for bioethics.* This recent debate is depicted in a few chapters of the *Penn Guide* that allow the reader a glimpse into this internal discourse that will shape the future of the discipline.

* * *

I would like to express my gratitude to Andrea Spence-Aizenberg for her help with the manuscript and to Philip Laughlin for valuable editorial advice. I would like to thank my husband, Shane, and my children, Ellan, Liad, and Lyanne, for their support throughout this complex project and for interesting discussions of various chapters of the *Penn Guide* around the dinner table.

Part I

Bioethics: Birth, Evolution, and Context

The Birth and Evolution of Bioethics

Arthur L. Caplan

THE ORIGINS OF bioethics are hard to pinpoint but not, as is often the case in trying to pinpoint when something began, as a result of the obscuring effects of the mists of time. Bioethics is still very young—the mist is not all that dense. Indeed, bioethics is so young that some of those present at its birth are still with us.

A few of the founders have taken pen in hand and given us their thoughts about the field's origins (Jonsen, 1998; Macklin, 1987). Others from outside the field have offered their analysis of bioethics' origins (Fox & Swazey, 2008; Rothman, 1991; Stevens, 2000). Still, there is no obvious consensus in these works about when bioethics began. The battle over the field's origins is not so much a fight about who did what to get things going and when, but rather whether one dates the origins to a particular institution, scandal, or issue.

THE ORIGINS OF BIOETHICS

SOME DATE THE field to the founding of the first think tank devoted to the subject, the Hastings Center. The center began, somewhat inauspiciously in terms of long-term financial security, in the Hastings-on-Hudson, New York, home of the Columbia University psychiatrist Willard Gaylin in partnership with Gaylin's neighbor, the philosophically trained writer and editor Daniel Callahan, in 1969.

Those who doubt any claim about the existence of anything until it is confirmed lean toward 1971 as the date of origin for bioethics. In that year, Hastings was joined by the Joseph and Rose Kennedy Institute of Ethics at Georgetown University. Unlike the Hastings Center, the Kennedy Institute was explicitly organized around religious perspectives on bioethical issues. Hastings tended to operate with groups of scholars from different disciplines addressing problems. Kennedy followed a more traditional model of individuals pursuing their particular scholarly projects and interests.

There are those who see the field as beginning much earlier. Some point to the creation of the renal dialysis so-called life and death selection committee in Seattle, Washington in 1961 (Jonsen, 1998). This committee commands attention because it was one of the first efforts to ration access to a life-preserving therapy by a committee of physicians and lay persons explicitly charged with making ethical rather than purely medical decisions. But, while the committee was a watershed in how America thought about distributing scarce resources, it did not really give birth to a field of scholarship and inquiry.

A few go back to the trial of Nazi doctors for their role in horrific experiments in the concentration camps (Annas, 2005). The Nuremburg Code, which resulted from this trial and subsequently was modified into what became the World Medical Association's 1964 Declaration of Helsinki, is seen as a key foundational document that grounded bioethics in a human rights framework.

Still others see bioethics as having its birth date in the Tuskegee scandal, when the whistle was first blown in 1971 on a study of the impact of syphilis on poor Black men in rural Alabama that had begun in 1932. An effective treatment for syphilis, penicillin, was well-established and widely available by the late 1940s, but the study continued for 30 more years, fueled by a powerful current of racism until the whole sordid tale was presented to Congress at a series of hearings held by a young Senator Edward Kennedy in 1973.

And a few see bioethics as having its roots far back in the medical ethics thinking done in earlier centuries by such giants of the philosophy of medicine as Robert Koch, Claude Bernard, William Osler, and even Maimonides. However, the work of these men is better understood as contributing to the creation of the ethics of the medical profession rather than the contemporary field of bioethics. The norms that ought to guide medicine as expressed in professional medical ethics are neither sufficient nor equivalent to the field of bioethics, which examines the problems and dilemmas arising from the health and life sciences for patients and the public as well as for professionals.

Bioethics, in my view, began in response to scandal and uncertainty. As much as the field should have begun in the aftermath of the Holocaust and the prominent role played by medicine and science in both horrific mass murder and awful human experimentation, it did not (Caplan, 2005a). Human rights thinking may have begun then (Annas, 2005), but bioethics as a field did not. Few Americans wrote about ethical problems in medicine or medical research in the 1950s and 1960s. The Nuremburg Code was seen as requisite for Nazis and other ideological lunatics, not for researchers working in the United States, Britain, or Western Europe.

Scandal surrounding the abuse of subjects in various research studies—as exemplified in the classic paper of Henry Beecher, MD (Beecher, 1966) and the Tuskegee experiment—made it clear that American researchers were more than capable of treating subjects in unethical ways. Emerging technologies such as ventilators, heart-lung machines, transplants, and kidney dialysis raised in the late 1960s new and profound questions about who should be granted access to expensive treatments and when they could be withheld, withdrawn, or denied (Caplan, 1993). Such technologies created uncertainty and posed new challenges to clinicians. This combination of scandals in research and uncertainty about managing new and expensive therapies combined to set the stage for the birth of bioethics. The Hastings Center and the Kennedy Institute of Ethics were conceived in the midst of scandal and flourished in an environment of a medical profession eager for help.

THE DEVELOPMENT OF BIOETHICS

BIOETHICS BEGAN AS a field, not a discipline. No single theory or outlook defined bioethics as would be the case for most disciplines. All voices, creeds, and types of expertise were welcome to engage in formulating answers to questions of research ethics and managing therapies. It was problems that held inquiries together and created the field of bioethics, rather than a particular mode of analysis, a set of theoretical views, or a set of disciplinary tools. But that quickly changed.

It proved very difficult to do bioethics in public in anything approximating a religious voice. While theologians were drawn to bioethics in the 1970s in large numbers and from many creeds, it quickly became clear that to command the attention of scientists and physicians, as well as policy-makers, a more secular language was required. Philosophy, emerging out of decades of mainly futile wrangling about meta-ethical issues, was more than happy to oblige, and medicine was happy to utilize its science-friendly worldview (Toulmin, 1973).

As bioethics began to grow, it was philosophical analysis and language that became the primary spoken tongue of the field. This period lasted about 10 years. At that time, in the 1980s, both lawyers and physicians began to assert more authority over bioethical discourse. As bioethics began to move away from its peripheral status outside American universities to centers and programs within them, academic medical centers became the home of choice. The culture of academic medicine—grant-driven, pragmatic, publication-oriented, and clinically focused—came to reshape bioethics from a field where people talked philosophy into a discipline where communicating with physicians was essential.

Since that time bioethics has rapidly evolved to become a discipline. Noninitiates who lack formal training in bioethics are not as welcome. Having a graduate degree of some sort in bioethics has become a bit of a credentialing requirement for someone to be taken seriously in matters bioethical. The pressure to conform to the mandates and norms of academic medicine has grown stronger, with much talk of the impact factor of journals, empirical and quantitative studies of bioethical issues, and research ethics compliance. There is even growing attention to the so-called ethics of bioethics and to potential conflicts of interest bioethicists may find themselves struggling with, which parallels the larger crisis of confidence in the integrity of the medical profession.

The public, media, and public officials in the economically developed world have grown somewhat accustomed to showing some deference to bioethical practitioners on a wide range of subjects, even if there is still discomfort about the concept of nonreligious ethical experts or, in some more secular quarters, any ethics expert, no matter how secular they may sound. Commissions and blue ribbon panels are now common. And bioethics has become international with programs, centers, and practitioners scattered around the globe.

CONCLUSION

HAVING GROWN INTO a feisty young adult, bioethics is now both eager to work with powerful social institutions and governments (Caplan, 2005b) and at the same time is more than willing to get down on the ground and wrestle over its appropriate focus, techniques, methods, and value-stance. Born in troubled times, bioethics continues to be a cultural flashpoint where disagreements run deep, the stakes continue to be high, and the voices and sources of authority are diverse.

What is uncertain is whether the discipline of bioethics, which now has its own canon, textbooks, encyclopedias, legal landmarks, legislative triumphs, associations, degree programs, tenured positions, chairs, handbooks, and, yes, guides, will continue to enmesh itself with academic medicine or take a turn back toward the humanities, law, or public policy. It is also unclear whether pressures to cover cost will lead to the emergence of professional requirements including licensure for those working in clinical settings and stronger efforts to form consulting and educational programs in the research area. It is clear that what began as a response to American research scandals and an explosion of technology into American medicine has grown into a far different entity with entirely new challenges, pressures and opportunities.

REFERENCES

Annas, G. J. (2005). *American bioethics: Crossing human rights and health law boundaries*. New York: Oxford University Press.

Beecher, H. K. (1966). Ethics and clinical research. *New England Journal of Medicine, 274*(24), 1354–1360.

Caplan, A. L. (1993). What bioethics brought to the public. *Hastings Center Report, 23*(6), 14–15.

Caplan, A. L. (2005a). Too hard to face. *Journal of the American Academy of Psychiatry and the Law, 33*(3), 394–400.

Caplan, A. L. (2005b). Who lost China?: A foreshadowing of today's ideological disputes in bioethics. *Hastings Center Report, 23*, 12–13.

Fox, R. C., & Swazey, J. (2008). *Observing bioethics*. New York: Oxford University Press.

Jonsen, A. R. (1998). *The birth of bioethics*. New York: Oxford University Press.

Macklin, R. (1987). *Mortal choices*. New York: Pantheon.

Rothman, D. J. (1991). *Strangers at the bedside*. New York: Basic Books.

Stevens, M. L. T. (2000). *Bioethics in America*. Baltimore, MD: Johns Hopkins University Press.

Toulmin, S. (1973). How medicine saved the life of ethics. *Perspectives in Biology and Medicine, 25*, 736–750.

The Ethics of Bioethics

ROBERT BAKER

U NTIL RECENTLY, FEW bioethicists took the ethics of bioethics seriously—if they gave it any thought at all.[1] Over the last decade, North American bioethicists—or, at least those who belong
to the American Society for Bioethics and Humanities (ASBH) and the
Canadian Bioethics Society (CBS)—began to favor a code of ethics for
bioethics. A recent survey found ASBH members favoring such a code
by a margin of 3.6 to 1 (Baker, Pearlman, Taylor, & Kipnis, 2006, p. 9).
This chapter discusses the events that led most American bioethicists
to change their view on the need for an ethics for bioethicists.

THE CHARLESTON AND TORONTO INCIDENTS AND THE SOLIPSISTIC CONCEPTION OF BIOETHICS

AMERICAN AND CANADIAN bioethicists' changed attitude toward an ethics of bioethics can be traced to events that unfolded
in Charleston, South Carolina and Toronto, Ontario in the late 1990s.
Although separated by climate and a national boundary, bioethicists
in both cities found their jobs in jeopardy because their employers
expected them to act in ways contrary to their own sense of professional propriety. In Toronto, a bioethicist who questioned a decision
by a hospital ethics committee wanted to discuss it publicly. Initially,
the employing medical center denied the bioethicist permission to

discuss the issue publicly. Although the medical center eventually relented, permitting public discussion of its decision-making, during contract renewal negotiations the bioethicist's supervisor admonished the bioethicist "not to cause problems in the future." In Charleston, the director of a bioethics program was initially denied a promotion after testifying, under subpoena, that the employing medical center's "policy [of incarcerating noncompliant, pregnant, drug-addicted Medicaid patients] fail[ed] to meet the institution's norms or standards that have to do with informed consent…[because] the risk of…arrest and incarceration was not made clear to the patients up front" (American Association of University Professors, 1999; Antommaria, 2004, p. W24).

Both medical centers believed that the bioethicists had failed to act as loyal employees, mindful of the need to speak and act in public forums in ways that protect the interests of the medical centers that employ them. The bioethicists, on the other hand, believed that they had responsibilities that overrode their institutional loyalties. Within 2 years, both bioethicists had sought new employment. The Charleston bioethicist had no choice, since the medical center declined to fund the bioethics program, which was consequently disbanded. The Toronto bioethicist left voluntarily, unable to accept the conditions implicitly demanded by the employing medical center. The underlying problem in both cases lay in the conflicting beliefs about responsibilities of bioethicists.

In 1997, when these incidents began to unfold, no official document endorsed by any bioethics society addressed the issue of the correlative rights and responsibilities of bioethicists and the institutions employing them. A year later, in 1998, the ASBH published a consensus statement, *Core Competencies for Bioethics Consultation* (Society for Health and Human Values—Society for Bioethics Consultation Task Force on Standards for Bioethics Consultation, 1998, hereafter, *CC*), that forthrightly recognized that "conflicts of interest" can arise because "ethics consultants are employed by a health care institution [and their] jobs are dependent on the good will of an institution." *CC*'s approach was to recommend that bioethicists negotiate their prerogatives "proactively with the…institution," and urged institutions to "foster a climate [in which ethicists] can carry out their work with integrity…free of concerns about job security, reprisals, undue political pressure" (*CC*, 5.2). *CC* warned, however, that ethicists, "giving advice or otherwise acting against an institution's perceived financial, public relations or other interest may pose potential harms to ethics consultants' personal interests." If a "conflict of interest…puts ethics consultants in the position of shading an opinion to avoid personal risk, [they] should either take the risk or withdraw from the case" (*CC*, 5.1.4).

CC was thus advising bioethicists to let their conscience be their guide and to quit if their employers required them to act unconscionably. The Charleston and Toronto bioethicists had acted in precisely this way, which apparently was the conventional wisdom of the day. Following this wisdom, however, had left the employing medical centers unapologetically aggrieved and the bioethicists feeling martyred and actually (albeit temporarily) unemployed. By any account, the outcome was unsatisfactory. If the field was to flourish, an alternative was needed.

BREAKING THE SOLIPSISTIC MODEL: THE NEED FOR A COLLABORATIVE ETHICS OF BIOETHICS

THE IDEA OF an ethics of bioethics can appear paradoxical. If one cannot trust ethicists to be ethical, who can one trust? Moreover, if ethicists do not know what is ethical, they lack a raison d'être;[2] if they know what is ethical but cannot be trusted to act ethically, they are self-evidently not in any position to advise others on acting ethically. Thus, if bioethics makes sense as a field, it seems senseless to ponder the ethics of bioethics.

The notion of the ethics of bioethics only appears paradoxical, oxymoronic, or self-evidently redundant if one presupposes that the bioethicist functions in a social vacuum in which only the bioethicist's personal beliefs and willingness to act are relevant.[3] The events in Charleston and Toronto, however, demonstrate what should have been obvious: bioethicists do not exist or function in their own solipsistic world, and they typically function in communal environments—hospitals, medical centers, universities—in which they hold others accountable and are held accountable to others.

By the end of the 20th century, bioethics had matured beyond a set of abstruse personal reflections on ethics, biomedicine, and health care to become a multidisciplinary field of practice. No longer the domain of philosophers and theologians and a few sympathetic researchers and clinicians, this multidisciplinary field draws half of its members from clinical areas and the remainder from the humanities/philosophy, the biomedical and social sciences, and religion/theology (Baker et al., 2006, Table 2.3). Pooling their expertise, bioethicists perform an array of administrative, advisory, and educational functions. They consult, evaluate, facilitate, mediate, research, and support people, organizations, and society as they deal with ethical issues in the biological and health related fields. To cite but one example, bioethicists serve on Hospital Ethics Committees, Institutional Animal Care and Use Committees,

Institutional Review Boards or Research Ethics Boards (familiarly referred by their acronyms: HECs, IACUCs, IRBs, and REBs; Baker et al., 2006, Table 2.5). Over two-thirds of bioethicists in the ASBH perform these functions as part of their written job descriptions; one-fifth receive external compensation (Baker et al., 2006, Table 2.6).

Bioethics, as practiced, is not a solipsistic activity; it is not primarily about the sense of propriety that an individual intuitively believes to be correct. Bioethicists are compensated for complex institutional and social activities touching on socially volatile areas. Their practices are subject to assessment and scrutiny by other professionals, by the media, by the public at large, and—as the Charleston and Toronto cases attest—by employers. Fields providing expertise in less volatile areas, from archeologists and beauticians to yacht designers and zoo keepers, offer codes of ethics to provide employers, media, the public, practitioners, and newcomers to their fields with considered statements of their shared understanding of the appropriate ways to practice. Bioethics is unique and, as the Charleston and Toronto cases indicate, uniquely vulnerable because its practices are bereft of the considered collaborative reflection and because its members lack the organizational protections afforded by a code of ethics.

Personal certitude and commitment, however deeply felt, is no substitute for a consensus arising from collaborative reflection on the practices of a field. Moreover, as the Charleston and Toronto incidents attest, in the absence of any publicly articulated standards, bioethicists have no reason to expect employing institutions to accept an individual's sense of moral propriety as authoritative. If bioethicists are to hold their practices to the same standards of public accountability that they demand of their colleagues in the health care fields—and that these professionals demand of themselves—bioethics organizations need to develop codes of ethics for bioethicists.

CC offered the first code of ethics, if not for bioethicists, at least for the clinical ethics consultation. Unlike the rest of the *CC* report, however, the code was almost never cited in the literature and had little impact on the field. No bioethics organization moved forward to endorse the code; more surprisingly, the authors of the code never sought any organizational imprimatur, perhaps because a solipsistic conception of the ethics of bioethics seems to permeate the code. *CC* repeatedly envisions the bioethicist as an isolated solo practitioner whose only guide is personal conviction—left unmentioned is the notion that bioethicists have *professional* as opposed to *personal* obligations. Thus *CC* notes that individual ethicists may give "advice…against an institution's perceived…interest" which "may pose potential harms to ethics consultants' *personal* interests" (*CC*, 5.1.4, emphasis added). It is, moreover, said to be the ethicist's *personal* responsibility not to "shad[e] an opinion to avoid personal risk" and the individual ethicist's personal responsibility to "either take the risk or withdraw from the case" (*CC*, 5.1.4). The ethicist is envisioned as a solo practitioner, not as a member of a profession, accountable to others for responsibilities delineated by their role as bioethicists.

It is ironic, but perhaps not surprising, that *CC*, the first code of ethics for clinical ethicists, portrays reflection on the responsibilities of bioethicists in terms of personal belief rather than professional responsibility. *CC* reflected the field as it functioned in 1997. At the time, and even today, collaborative reflections on the ethics of bioethical practices were largely absent from the literature. Suppose, for example, that the Toronto bioethicist had turned to the bioethics literature for ethical guidance. A December 3, 2007, *PubMed* search for "hospital, ethics, committees, confidentiality," yielded 70 references; searching for "hospital ethics committee publishing" yielded 13 additional references. Yet although many publications by bioethicists discuss the decisions of hospital ethics committees, none addresses the extent to which decisions of hospital ethics committees are to be considered confidential. By contrast, a December 3, 2007, *PubMed* search of "physicians confidentiality" yielded 2,915 citations on physicians' obligations of confidentiality.

One reason for the disparity is the influence of the solipsistic model: bioethicists still believe that decisions about the propriety of their practices are personal matters; physicians, however, accept that they belong to a profession and have professional responsibilities. Medical societies, in striking contrast to bioethical societies, thus offer detailed statements on physicians' professional responsibilities in specific circumstances. These statements serve as the impetus for most discussions of physicians' obligations of confidentiality in the literature. For example, the first five articles cited in the December 3 search on physicians' responsibility focus on statements by such organizations as the American Academy of Pediatrics Committee on Bioethics (Fallat & Glover, 2007), the American Heart Association and the Emergency Nurses Association (Critchell & Marik, 2007), and the World Health Organization (Ferrario et al., 2007). Presumably, were bioethics societies to issue statements on the ethics of bioethical practices, these statements too would generate a rich literature on the ethics of bioethics.

BIOETHICS, SCANDAL, AND THE NEED FOR A CODE OF ETHICS TO ASSERT PROFESSIONALISM

IN THE OPENING years of the 21st century, bioethicists began to appreciate the need for a code of ethics for reasons that differ from the problems with employing institutions that led to the Charleston and Toronto incidents. Bioethics was conceived and born in the United States circa 1960–1970,[4] during a period of political and religious liberalism. The Kennedy-Johnson (and even Nixon) administrations' liberal domestic policies and Vatican Council II (1962–1965) shielded the infant field from conservative political and religious criticism (Baker, 2005b). As the 21st century dawned, Vatican II's influence waned, and conservative Catholics joined with evangelicals and neoconservative politicians to challenge secular bioethics over such issues as the propriety of embryonic stem cell research and the discontinuation of artificial nutrition and hydration—the traditional abortion/euthanasia debates in nontraditional guise.

While these issues played out, commentators from the left and right blended their disparate voices in a chorus of disparaging criticism. The left condemned bioethics as antidemocratic elitism, a secular priesthood who, the right chimed in, abused philosophy to trespass on the traditional social authority of law, medicine, and religion (Shalit, 1997; Siegler, 1999; Smith, 2000). With the election and re-election of the Bush administration (2000–2008), a conservative Catholic-evangelical-neoconservative alliance ascended to power, which the White House used to remove bioethicists and scientists critical of its bioethical policies from government posts.[5]

On another front, critics on the left disparaged bioethics, charging that prestige, power, and money had tempted bioethicists to abandon their watchdog role (Evans, 2001; Stevens, 2000). Public policy and professional journals joined the fray (Elliot, 2001a, 2001b; Sharpe, 2002). To quote the striking prose of one major critic, "If bioethicists have gained any credibility in the public eye, it rests on the perception that they have no financial interest in the objects of their scrutiny.... The problem with ethics consultants is that they look like watchdogs but can be used like show dogs" (Elliot, 2001a). As this critique gained resonance, bioethicists who consulted with biotech and pharmaceutical companies were pilloried in such publications as *US News and World Report* ("And Now Ethics for Sale: Bioethicists and Big Bucks," Boyce, 2001) and the *New York Times* ("Bioethicists Find Themselves the Ones Being Scrutinized," Stolberg, 2001).

Yet the bioethicists criticized for consulting with the biotech and pharmaceutical industry thought of themselves as serving the public interest by offering ethical advice to those most in need of it, even as they themselves had to resist pressure to serve as mere show dogs (Perlman, 2005). As in the Charleston and Toronto incidents, everyone felt aggrieved if anyone challenged their personal testimony about the conscientiousness of their conduct. In the absence of any publicly accepted standard of conduct, what defense could anyone offer except to rehearse one's personal belief in one's own integrity?

BIOETHICS ORGANIZATIONS RESPOND

SLOWLY AND UNSTEADILY, bioethics organizations began to respond. In 1998, the bioethicist at the center of the Charleston incident was elected president of ASBH and discussed the incident in her presidential address, "Speaking Truth to Power." In the same year, the CBS responded to the Toronto case by forming an Ad Hoc Working Group on Employment Standards (MacDonald et al., 2000). By 2002, the ASBH had revised its bylaws to permit it to take "positions relat[ing] to academic freedom and professionalism in bioethics." Also in 2002, a joint ASBH and the American Society of Law, Medicine and Ethics (ASLME) task force published voluntary guidelines, *Bioethics Consultation in the Private Sector,* in the *Hastings Center Report* (Brody et al., 2002).

Reformers in both the ASBH and the CBS continued to press for more action. A panel titled "The Public Face of Bioethics: Watchdog or Show Dog"[6] and a workshop titled "Codes of Ethics"[7] were featured at the 2002 ASBH national conference. The CBS Working Group on Employment Standards issued a *Draft Model Code of Ethics for Bioethics* that was published on the CBS Web site.[8] This code asserts a "national standard for ethical conduct in bioethics" because the "social role" that bioethicists play "implies" that they have "fiduciary responsibilities" as "those to whom the public looks for guidance." Despite this language, the *Draft Model Code* retains a lingering solipsism since bioethical obligations are formulated as a personal pledge that, "I will conduct myself in a professional manner" (MacDonald, 2003).[9] Bioethicists personally commit themselves to eleven obligations: professional integrity, humility, confidentiality, disclosure and recusal, nonauthoritarianism, nonexploitation, professional honor, advancing the field, and integrity in conditions of personal employment and in the employment of others (MacDonald, 2002). Although flawed by lingering solipsism, the draft model Canadian code remains the only code of ethics that enjoys the imprimatur of a bioethics society.

South of the Canadian border, official ASBH action on a code of ethics stalled for 2 years, until Steve Miles, a founding member, resigned publicly. Miles decried the ASBH's "reluctan[ce] or [in]abil[ity] to act on behalf of the threatened academic interests of its members" and its "failure to articulate…standards of conduct of bioethicists" (Miles, 2004; for response see Board of Directors, 2004). Shortly thereafter, the ASBH formed a Task Force on Ethics Standards and made the ethics of bioethics the subject of a spring conference where attendees discussed a draft code of ethics for bioethicists (Baker, 2005a). The issue gained additional momentum as ASBH president Arthur Derse urged "Ethics Standards for Bioethicists" (Derse, 2005) and as an ASBH task force endorsed a code of ethics at the ASBH's 2005 annual meeting. At the same meeting, a panel on the ethics of bioethics ended with the organizer, an ageing civil rights protestor, singing "Uncoded," a version of Johnny Cash's tune "I've Been Everywhere,"[10] to chide board members about the ASBH's dilatory attitude toward a code of ethics.

After the meeting, the ASBH board commissioned the Advisory Committee on Ethics Standards (ACES) to survey members about developing an official code of ethics. The ACES committee found that the members supported a code of ethics for bioethicists by a ratio of 3.6 to 1, with 305 of the respondents favoring a code and only 84 opposed (Baker et al., 2006, Table 3.1). Three quarters of the ASBH's members believe that the code should focus broadly on issues relevant to everyone in the field rather than on some narrow area, such as clinical ethics. Members also thought that a code would be most useful to those newly entering the field (Baker et al., 2006, Table 3.3).

Not surprisingly, the issues that the respondents to the ASBH survey thought that a code should address were those that had historically proved vexatious (see parenthetical comments in the following list). About 90% of the respondents believe a code should address:

- Identifying and disclosing conflicts or interest (scandal headlines),
- confidentiality and obligations to disclose (Charleston-Toronto issues),
- reporting serious misconduct (Charleston-Toronto issues),
- improper pressures by employer/supervisors (Charleston-Toronto issues), and
- ascribing (co)authorship and crediting contributors to published work.

Seventy percent or more thought that a code ought to address the following two issues:

- Presenting incomplete characterizations of complex issues in public venues (the Terri Schiavo case) and
- obligations to report problems to employers, supervisors (Baker et al., 2006, Table 3.4).

Members submitted 88 narratives of incidents raising ethical issues about the practice of bioethics (Baker et al., 2006, Section 5). The wealth of cases makes clear that once bioethicists contemplate the ethics of their practices, a host of issues surface.

CONCLUSION

As this chapter is written, the ASBH Board of Directors is contemplating how best to develop a code of ethics. Code development is a watershed moment in the maturation of a field. The ACES survey found that ASBH members desire a code of ethics to protect their autonomy and integrity and to delineate their values and responsibilities to new entrants. As the Charleston and Toronto incidents established, an effective code must go beyond a statement of principles to provide guidance on the specific issues affecting members and their employing institutions. The challenge is thus to design a transparent, participatory code-development process for a professional society representing a multidisciplinary field that will culminate in a viable code with sufficient specificity to effectively serve the interests of bioethicists, employing institutions, and the public.

NOTES

1. When the Canadian bioethicist Benjamin Freedman proposed a code of ethics for clinical ethicists at a 1986 conference (Freedman, 1989), his suggestion was met with that overly polite condescension that decent people reserve for well-meaning but utterly insane ideas. Everyone changed the subject (Baker, 2007).

2. Some bioethicists are uncomfortable accepting claims of expertise (Parens, 2005; for a response, see Nelson, 2007).

3. Some bioethicists idealize moral solipsism as a virtue (Elliott, 2007).

4. Some scholars date the birth of the bioethics earlier (Jonsen, 1998) or ascribe European origins (Campbell, 2000; Moreno, 2004). I date bioethics from the first appearance of bioethical discourse—including the term *bioethics* itself in 1971—which occurred in American publications during the 1970s. I also distinguish between bioethics and traditional medical ethics. Medical ethics is the self-regulatory ethics of medical professionals, governing their own conduct and their relations with their peers, their profession, their patients, and the public. *Bioethics,* as I use the term, is a multidisciplinary field/discourse addressing ethical issues in the biomedical sciences, as well as in health care, *without privileging* physicians' or scientists' conceptions/discourse.

5. To cite but two examples, in December 2002 the Bush administration removed, Thomas Murray, president and CEO of the Hastings Center, from the Biological Response Modifiers Advisory Committee (Brickley, 2002); in March 2004, it fired scientist Elizabeth Blackburn from the President's Council on Bioethics. Murray and Blackburn were critics of the administration's stem cell policy (Associated Press, 2004; Meslin, 2004—for a defense of the council, see Elliott, 2004; for a general overview, see Mooney, 2005).

6. Panelists: Francois Baylis, Lisa Eckenwiler, and Virginia Ashby Sharp.

7. Organized by Robert Baker with Arthur Derse, Glenn McGee, and Matthew Wynia.

8. The name "Draft Model" was chosen because the double modifier would make "less contentious than a formal code of ethics" (C. MacDonald, personal communication, March 22, 2005).

9. "I thought that it is an important aspect of codes that they are personal. I wanted people to swear to code—also—I didn't want the code to sound like a list of orders—here is what I expect of myself as a professional in this role" (MacDonald, 2003).

10. Adopted by R. Baker from Geoff Mack's song "I've Been Everywhere."

> Codes are everywhere, man
> Codes are in rulebooks bare, man
> Codes are in the internet air, man
> Everyone's got their share, man
>
> [List of 38 fields, accountants to zoo keepers, with codes of ethics]
>
> Codes are everywhere, man
> But in bioethics the cupboard's bare, man
> They are nowhere, man
> They haven't done their share, man
> For Pete's sake....
> What a pity
> Cause codes are everywhere, man
> Codes are everywhere

REFERENCES

American Academy of Pediatrics, Committee on Bioethics, Fallat, M. E., & Glover, J. (2007). Professionalism in pediatrics: Statement of principles. *Pediatrics, 120*(4), 895–897.

American Association of University Professors. (1999). Medical University of South Carolina administration backs down. *Academe Online, 85*(4), 6.

Antommaria, A. (2004). A Gower maneuver: The American Society for Bioethics and Humanities' resolution of the taking stands debate. *The American Journal of Bioethics, 4*(1), W24.

Associated Press. (2004, March 19). *Scientists rally around stem cell advocate fired by Bush.* Retrieved December 26, 2007, from http://www.usatoday.com/news/science/2004-03-19-fired-bioethicist_x.htm

Baker, R. (2005a). A draft model aggregated code of ethics for bioethicists. *American Journal of Bioethics, 5*(5), 33–41.

Baker, R. (2005b). Getting agreement: How bioethics got started. *The Hastings Center Report, 35*(3), 50–51.

Baker, R. (2007). A history of codes of ethics for bioethicists. In L. Eckenweiler & F. Cohen (Eds.), *The ethics of bioethics: Mapping the moral landscape* (pp. 24–42). Baltimore, MD: Johns Hopkins University Press.

Baker, R., Pearlman, R., Taylor, H., & Kipnis, K. (2006). *Report and recommendations of the ASBH Advisory Committee on Ethics Standards.* Retrieved December 8, 2007, from http://www.asbh.org/membership/protected/pdfs/acesrprt.pdf

Board of Directors, American Society for Bioethics and Humanities. (2004, May 12). *To members of the American Society for Bioethics and Humanities: Issues raised by Steven Miles letter of resignation from ASBH.* Retrieved October 1, 2005 (no longer accessible), from www.asbh.org/news/Letter%20to%20Members%200504.pdf

Boyce, N. (2001, July 30). And now ethics for sale: Bioethicists and big bucks. *US News and World Report.* Retrieved December 26, 2007, from http://www.mindfully.org/GE/GE2/Bioethicists-For-Sale.htm

Brickley, P. (2002, December 30). Panel politics unresolved: Concerns continue over US advisory panels' new make-up. *The Scientist.* Retrieved December 26, 2007, from http://www.biomedcentral.com/news/20021230/05/

Brody, B., Dubler, N., Blustein, J., Caplan, A., Kahn, J. P., Kass, N., et al. (2002). Bioethics consultation in the private sector. *Hastings Center Report, 32*(3), 14–20 (CPS).

Campbell, A. V. (2000). "My country tis of thee"—the myopia of American bioethics. *Medicine, Health Care and Philosophy, 3,* 195–198.

Critchell, C. D., & Marik, P. E. (2007). Should family members be present during cardiopulmonary resuscitation? *American Journal of Hospice and Palliative Care Medicine, 24*(4), 311–317.

Derse, A. (2005). Ethics standards for bioethicists. *ASBH Exchange, 3*(8), 2.

Elliott, C. (2001a, September 24). Pharma buys a conscience. *The American Prospect, 12*(17). Retrieved December 26, 2007, from http://www.prospect.org/web/page.ww?section=root&name=ViewPrint&articleId=5904

Elliott, C. (2001b). Throwing a bone to the watchdog. *Hastings Center Report, 31*(2), 19–21.

Elliott, C. (2004, March 9). Beyond politics: Why have bioethicists focused on the President's Council's dismissals and ignored its remarkable work? *Slate.* Retrieved December 26, 2007, http://www.tc.umn.edu/~ellio023/otherworks.shtml

Elliott, C. (2007). The tyranny of expertise. In L. Eckenweiler & F. Cohen (Eds.), *The ethics of bioethics: Mapping the moral landscape* (pp. 43–46). Baltimore, MD: Johns Hopkins University Press.

Evans, J. H. (2001). *Playing God? Human genetic engineering and the rationalization of public bioethical debate, 1959–1995.* Chicago: University of Chicago Press.

Ferrario, M. M., Apostoli, P., Bertazzi, P. A., Cesana, G., Mosconi, G., & Riboldi, L. (2007). Occupational medicine faces new health challenges: The example of alcohol dependence. *Medicina del Lavoro, 98*(6), 443–445.

Freedman, B. (1989). Bringing codes to Newcastle. In B. Hoffmaster, B. Freed-man, & G. Fraser (Eds.), *Clinical ethics: Theory and practice* (pp. 125–130). Clifton, NJ: Humana Press.

Jonsen, A. (1998). *The birth of bioethics*. New York: Oxford University Press.

MacDonald, C. (2003). *Draft model code of ethics for bioethics.* Retrieved November 13, 2008, from http://www.bioethics.ca/draftcode.pdf

MacDonald, C., Coughlin, M., Harrison, C., Lynch, A., Murphy, P., Rowell, M., et al. (2000). *Working conditions for bioethics in Canada* (v. 8.0). Retrieved December 27, 2007, http://www.bioethics.ca/publications-ang.html

Meslin, E. (2004). The president's council: Fair and balanced? *Hastings Center Report, 34*(2), 6–8.

Miles, S. (2004, March 31). *To the Board and Officers of the American Society for Bioethics and Humanities: An open letter of resignation from the society.* Retrieved October 1, 2005 (no longer accessible) http://www.asbh.org/news/Miles_letter%200304.pdf

Mooney, C. (2005) *The republican war on science*. New York: Basic Books.

Moreno, J. D. (2004). Bioethics imperialism. *ASBH Exchange, 7*(3), 2.

Nelson, J. (2007). Trusting bioethicists. In L. Eckenweiler & F. Cohen (Eds.), *The ethics of bioethics: Mapping the moral landscape* (pp. 47–55). Baltimore, MD: Johns Hopkins University Press.

Parens, E. (2005). A good label is hard to find. *Hastings Center Report, 35* (inside front cover).

Perlman, D. (2005). Bioethics in industry settings: One situation where a code for bioethics would help. *The American Journal of Bioethics, 5*(5), 62–64.

Shalit, R. (1997, April 28). When we were philosopher kings. *New Republic.* Retrieved December 26, 2007, from http://catholiceducation.org/articles/medical_ethics/me0008.html

Sharpe, V. A. (2002). Science, bioethics and the public interest: On the need for transparency. *Hastings Center Report, 32*(3), 23–26.

Siegler, M. (1999). Medical ethics a medical matter. In R. Baker, A. Caplan, L. Emanuel, & S. Latham (Eds.) *The American medical ethics revolution* (pp. 171–179). Baltimore, MD: Johns Hopkins University Press.

Smith, W. J. (2000). *Culture of death: The assault on medical ethics in America*. San Francisco: Encounter Books.

Society for Health and Human Values—Society for Bioethics Consultation Task Force on Standards for Bioethics Consultation. (1998). *Core competencies for ethics consultation.* Glenville, IL: American Society for Bioethics and Humanities.

Stevens, M. L. T. (2000). *Bioethics in America: Origins and cultural politics*. Baltimore, MD: The Johns Hopkins University Press.

Stolberg, S. G. (2001, August 2). Bioethicists find themselves the ones being scrutinized. *New York Times.* Retrieved December 26, 2007, from http://query.nytimes.com/gst/fullpage.html?res=9C07E3DF143CF931A3575BC0A9679C8B63

3

The Independence Principle in Bioethics

DAVID PERLMAN

THIS CHAPTER DISCUSSES the independence principle in the corporate setting as a way to mitigate conflicts of interest that arise in issues related to the ethics of bioethics. As topics of bioethical inquiry, the ethics of bioethics and the ethics of bioethicists are not new. In the early years of bioethics in the 1970s and 1980s (called *applied ethics* then), when a variety of professionals began to be asked to provide ethical advice on specific cases in health care, one concern focused on the qualifications, methods, roles, and authority of the so-called health care ethics consultant. Canadian bioethicist Benjamin Freedman even proposed a code of ethics to govern health care ethics consulting in 1989 (Freedman, 1989). According to contemporary reports, it was not well received but, in retrospect, it should be considered ahead of its time. The debate surrounding the ethics of bioethicists continued into the 1990s, culminating in 1998 when the newly enshrined American Society for Bioethics and Humanities (ASBH) endorsed a report of recommended core competencies for health care ethics consulting. Since that time, the focus on the ethics of bioethics has shifted from health care ethics consultants providing ethical advice in health facilities, on institutional review boards (IRBs), or on government policy bodies. Recent revelations that bioethicists have started to receive consulting fees from industry sparked renewed interest in the topic of the ethics of bioethicists and how those arrangements might impinge on the public perception of bioethics as a field. This chapter highlights the recent debate on the topic of the ethics of bioethics and ends by considering several examples of the independence principle from corporate ethics consulting as a means to manage potential conflicts of interest in bioethics.

BIOETHICS CONSULTING FOR INDUSTRY

THERE IS A burgeoning interest and literature on the topic of bioethics consulting for industry. Bioethics' traditional consulting focus has been on bedside clinical ethics consultation (ASBH, 1998) or bioethicists who work on advisory, policy, or review bodies such as commissions, professional associations, government boards, and IRBs. There are many books, articles, and presentations on these topics, and chapter 12 in this volume provides an excellent overview of these issues.[1] In the last few years, however, the traditional focus on ethics consulting has shifted. Reports in the peer-reviewed literature, the lay press, and bioethics conference presentations about bioethicists' consulting for industry has caused a furor about conflict of interests and the ethics of bioethicists.[2] One commentator even expressed it as a "crisis in bioethics" and wondered if bioethics has a soul (Miles, 2003). As a response to the publicity and disclosure of bioethicists' consulting relationships, several articles and conference presentations have been offered to suggest that such consulting arrangements might undermine individual bioethicists' integrity and that of bioethics as a profession or vocation (Baylis, 2000, 2004; Brody et al., 2002; Callahan, 2001; Elliott, 2001a, 2001b).

DANGERS AND OPPORTUNITIES IN BIOETHICS CONSULTING FOR INDUSTRY

I AM SYMPATHETIC to the claims that authors make regarding the potential threats to the integrity of individual bioethicists and bioethics as a field that consulting for industry can present. I have gone on record as suggesting that employment or consulting opportunities for bioethicists in or with industry have both dangers and opportunities associated with them (Perlman, 2005, 2007; Perlman, MacDonald, Cohen, & Philips, 2004). Briefly, some of the opportunities include the following: (a) an opportunity to educate executives on ethical decision-making; (b) practical opportunities to bring frequently

theoretical considerations of ethical analysis to practical business decisions; (c) illustrating the importance of not divorcing ethics from business decisions; (d) interesting employment, research, and publication
opportunities for the individual bioethicist; (e) opportunities to place
students in internships and other practical learning experiences; and
(f) learning about the newest developments in biotechnology.

On the other hand, these opportunities can represent significant
dangers to the individual bioethicist or the field as a whole: (a) lack of
public scrutiny of ethical decision-making processes or outcomes by
the individual ethicist;[3] (b) the appearance of ethical endorsement of
protocols, products, or decisions with questionable or disastrous outcomes for the public, research subjects, shareholders, or employees of the
company—a danger that Carl Elliott has called being an ethical "show
dog" (Elliott, 2004); (c) lack of freedom to publish or speak about the
topics discussed at company meetings, unless specifically negotiated
and included in consulting agreements; and (d) inability or lack of willingness to report to regulatory oversight bodies or serve as a whistleblower, when justified, for fear of retaliation in the form of lawsuits,
termination or nonrenewal of current contracts, or denial of future
consulting work.

HISTORICAL CONTEXT

I WOULD LIKE to argue that we should focus on the opportunities
inherent in such forms of employment or consultation, as long as
efforts have been made to limit the dangers. There are several mechanisms to do so. Disclosure of such relationships (in presentations,
publications, and other public venues) has been posited as a minimal
requirement (Brody et al., 2002). Some bioethicists argue that disclosure is not enough; what is required is independence (Donaldson,
2001a, 2001b; Perlman, 2001; see also chapter 25 in this book). Others
argue that these two (and other) professional values—honest disclosure and independence—should be enshrined in a code of ethics for
bioethicists. The strongest proponents of this latter argument suggest
that recent revelations about the employment conditions of several
prominent bioethicists lead inextricably to the need for a code of ethics, both to protect individual bioethicists and to secure the integrity
of the field. A brief survey of this history, while not linked to consulting or employment in industry settings, will serve the purpose of making the connection to that topic clearer.

The recent history of employment conditions in U.S. bioethics came
to public attention when bioethicist Mary Faith Marshall detailed the
dangers associated with testifying against her institution's interests in

Ferguson v. The City of Charleston et al. (2001) at the 1999 ASBH incoming president's address. Immediately following her address, at the ASBH business meeting, several members proposed that ASBH form a task force to investigate whether it could change its bylaws to take stands on substantive issues involving the professional integrity and academic freedom of its members. In the years since Mary Faith Marshall's case, several additional whistleblower cases have been reported in the bioethics literature.[4] The results of such cases have been multifold. Mary Faith Marshall's case, in particular, galvanized support to investigate the working conditions of U.S. bioethicists and develop a code of ethics for such bioethicists. Vociferous debate at several ASBH meetings on whether the Society should take stands on substantive professional and societal ethical issues sparked interest in a spring 2005 conference, held in Albany, New York on the ethics of bioethics (http://www.ethics. bioethics.net), from which the most definitive collection (Eckenwiler & Cohn, 2007) and review (chapter 2 in this volume) to date on the subject of the ethics of bioethics were produced.

Notably, Eckenwiler and Cohn's book lacks a dedicated article or argument for or against the ethics of bioethicists consulting for or seeking employment in industry. That history has a different evolution, but it has one focal point with the formation of a Task Force on Bioethics Consultation for the Private Sector and its report (Brody et al., 2002). The report endorses complete disclosure as a key feature of ethical accountability for those wishing to offer ethics consultations to industry.

MOVING BEYOND DISCLOSURE: THE INDEPENDENCE PRINCIPLE

MUCH OF THE literature on conflicts of interests argues for disclosure as one, and frequently the primary or sole, means of managing conflicts. The same argument could be extrapolated to conflicts inherent in ethics consulting relationships, except that such conflicts will likely be broader than mere financial conflicts of interests. Ethicists may have particular moral commitments to certain theories, principles, approaches, or methodologies that might pose conflicts in the types or outcomes of consultations they offer. Certainly, disclosure of such conflicts is a necessary but perhaps insufficient condition to maintain one's intellectual honesty and integrity in ethics consultation. Nevertheless, like other authors (Sharpe, 2002), I believe that in certain cases, disclosure is not enough. Bioethicists should strive for greater transparency. In this chapter, I wish to suggest that one form of greater transparency can be captured by the term *independence*. Independence should be characterized by firewalls, separation of interests (financial, professional, or other), or moral impartiality (Perlman, 2001b) toward the client for whom one is consulting and their reasons for seeking ethics consultation.

As a beginning point for the inquiry into the concept of independence, I wondered to what extent my own personal employment experiences might represent illustrative examples. Soon after completing my doctoral degree, I began working as a consultant, employed by PricewaterhouseCoopers LLP (PwC), a large auditing firm. The group I worked with provided advice on research ethics and compliance to clients in industry, academia, and government, and was in a separate division of the firm that conducted financial and valuation audits of such organizations. Nevertheless, in such a large firm, there were times when this protective firewall—separation of auditing of client's financial statements and consulting for those same clients—came into conflict. In these situations, the potential for financial, professional, and advisory conflicts of interest were huge, and the firm had a dedicated Independence Office that ensured compliance with independence rules prohibiting consulting for audit clients or potential clients or employees holding financial interests in audit clients for whom consulting services were being offered (American Institute of Certified Public Accountants [AICPA], 1988).

My first encounter with the firm's Independence Office, which required a review of my professional and financial interests before hire, followed by in-depth training on the independence requirements, helped me formulate a rough, initial hypothesis about how my employment situation might be extrapolated to ethical considerations in bioethics consulting. Fortuitously, this connection was crystallized in a series of articles that appeared in the *Hastings Center Report* (2001, vol. 31, no. 2) soon after I started working. This one issue of the *Report* focused on the role of business in bioethics and the conflicts of interest inherent in such relationships. One of the frequently repeated worries of providing ethics consulting services for industry was the independence of (a) the advice, (b) the ethicist doing the advising, and (c) the motivations of the organization requesting the advice.

In one article, Thomas Donaldson, a business ethicist at Penn's Wharton School of Business, made the argument that bioethics consulting should be similar to the sort of business ethics or management consulting in which business school professors and others, like myself at the time, engage. Donaldson's explicit use of the term *independence* in his article made an immediate connection to my own employment conditions at PwC. In some cases, the independence review required at PwC and other auditing firms might require an employee to dispose of significant financial ties (frequently at a financial loss to the employee) before being employed or working with a particular client. The independence review, much like the conflicts review an attorney must conduct before taking on a new client, was before hire, before each individual engagement, and required that the employee keep his or her independence profile updated with relevant financial and other information in order to proactively manage any potential conflicts of interests in the business development process.

CAN THERE BE INDEPENDENCE IN BIOETHICS?

AFTER READING THE articles from the *Hastings Center Report* and reflecting on my own consulting experience at PwC, several questions occurred to me regarding the independence principle and its possible relevance to bioethics consulting: (a) Is or can the advice an ethics consultant provides ever be truly independent of motivations such as fame, money, or moral, social, or personal commitments; (b) What are the motivations of the organization requesting the advice—legitimization, moral concern, patient or subject protection, or, as Carl Elliott (2001b) wondered, "window dressing"; and (c) What is the format of the consultation process (a lone ethics advisor versus an ethicist serving on an advisory board) and who controls the work products from such consultations?

Fortunately, I wasn't the only one wondering about such topics or encountering such issues. My research into the topic of independence provided several examples that were already present or emerging in bioethics. As was already mentioned, a first and most noticeable example was the Task Force on Bioethics Consultation in the Private Sector and its report, whose recommendations are an attempt to ensure the independence of bioethics advice and the bioethics consultant (Brody et al., 2002). Second, around the same time, Penn's Center for Bioethics came under fire for accepting fees from industry (most notably from Pfizer to investigate the influence of gifts to health care providers). In response, the Center published a policy on how external support would be handled (http://www.bioethics.upenn.edu:16080/resources/?pageId=4). Third, several quasi-governmental science organizations (National Academy of Sciences, National Regulatory Council, Institute of Medicine, and the Office of Technology Assessment) had published reports on issues of bioethical import and required independence in investigating, reporting, and making recommendations on such topics.

In the area of responsible conduct of research, the authorship and sponsorship of research guidelines produced by the International

Council of Medical Journal Editors is an example of independence in several senses. First, the development and promulgation of the guidelines represents collaboration between the medical publishing enterprise, and in this way, represents a consensus viewpoint on the ethics of authorship and publication. Second, the guidelines require disclosure of conflicts of interest as the minimum ethical condition of publication and peer review.

In the area of human research subject protections, several examples of independence are of note. The first is AbioMed's AbioCor Independent Patient Advisory Council (IPAC; Morreim, 2004a, 2004b).[5] The second example involved the use of an independent external review committee to investigate instances of serious breaches of research ethics (e.g., the Johns Hopkins External Review Committee [Hellman, Cassel, Stock, Wood, & Zapol, 2001]). Third, recent voluntary efforts to inspect and offer a stamp of approval for institutions' research-protection programs represents yet additional examples of independence. The two agencies that initiated these accreditation programs were independent partnerships between major research stakeholders.[6] The last example of independence in human research protections pertains to IRBs. Regulations prohibit IRB members with conflicting interests from voting on or discussing research proposals. Moreover, there is an emerging and critical literature in bioethics on ensuring independence of IRBs, including how IRBs should be institutionally structured and composed so as to avoid the issue of so-called IRB shopping by investigators when one IRB rejects one of their projects (Lemmons & Freedman, 2000). Although independence is encouraged in how institutions choose to structure, staff, and implement IRBs and human research protection programs, most are far from truly independent. Those who serve on the IRB or provide research oversight are, with the exception of the unaffiliated members on the IRB, paid employees of the institution. It is a case of the foxes watching the hen house, and this type of structure can pose significant conflicts of interest to the institution, the IRB members, and research oversight staff in institutions that lack a culture of integrity and ethics. Another example in the research ethics context is the Data Safety Monitoring Board (see chapter 12 of this volume).

In all of these examples, the concept of independence was stressed as a recognized mechanism to mitigate conflicts of interests. Perhaps, I hypothesized, if independence could be formally operationalized in the bioethics consulting context, much like the independence review required at PwC, some of the problems with conflicts of interests could be avoided or at least minimized. True independence in bioethics might require disclosure of financial interests and contracts that individual bioethicists have or plan to have with industry to an independent group for review. Interestingly, many of the conclusions the

Task Force on Bioethics Consultation in the Private Sector reached concurred with the analysis of applying independence to my own bioethics consulting employment situations. In those situations, independence was a necessary component of ethical accountability. As such, the Task Force on Bioethics Consultation in the Private Sector report and recommendations represented an excellent, initial analysis of independence requirements in consulting for industry.

After I left PwC, I took a position directly in industry, providing advisory educational services on issues related to bioethics, business ethics, and the responsible conduct of research at GlaxoSmithKline (Perlman, 2005). In this new setting, the issue of independence and integrity took on new meaning for me, as I grappled with providing advice in an environment where independence was not possible. I was an employee of the organization to whom I was providing advice. The conclusion I reached was that in those situations where independence is not possible—such as when a bioethicist seeks employment in industry or in settings where political pressure may be applied to the bioethicist—it is imperative for a bioethicist interested in upholding his or her own individual integrity and that of the field, to have a code of ethics to provide support and recourse should the bioethicist's recommendations or work be subject to challenge by the organization.

SPEAKING TRUTH TO POWER WHEN INDEPENDENCE IS IMPOSSIBLE: A CODE OF ETHICS CAN HELP

FREEDMAN'S (1989) AND Baylis' (2000) work on the topic of how clinical bioethicists should handle threats to their professional integrity in the performance of their duties encouraged bioethicists to speak truth to power even if that meant significant pressure from those in power at the institution would be brought against a bioethicist. It was more important to speak the truth than to worry about one's continued employment. Excellent advice, but my most recent experience has shown that Freedman's advice is easier said than done. According to Baylis, Freedman encouraged bioethicists to "keep a quit letter in your desk" (Baylis, 2000, p. 37). Imagine my own surprise when, upon my first week of starting my position as director of the Human Research Ethics Program (HREP) at the New Jersey Department of Health and Senior Services (NJDHSS), I was informed of the need to submit an undated but signed letter of resignation. I was assured that all unclassified, non–civil service employees at the department were required to submit such letters when there was a change in administration in the

State (at that time, Gov. Jon Corzine succeeded Acting Gov. Richard Cody). To me, this was Freedman's advice turned on its head.

Unlike most employees in State agencies, who enjoy civil service protection, my job was unclassified, so if I heeded Freedman's advice to speak truth to power, and if it was not received well by my superiors, it wouldn't be necessary for me to break out my own quit letter—they already had a signed and undated one! To me, this represented a huge potential conflict, one that was a quantum leap beyond the one I wrote about when employed in the pharmaceutical industry and advocated for a code of ethics for bioethicists working in industry (Perlman, 2005). That peer response to the question of whether there should be a code of ethics for bioethicists concluded that, for bioethicists who work in industry, where there is no professional protection and little professional support, a minimal code might help prevent or minimize threats against speaking truth to power. When confronted with such situations, rather than rely on arguments from one's own personal morality, it would help to say that no professional bioethicist would do or not do whatever was in question. Other professions have such codes of ethics, and, if bioethics wants to be considered a profession, it will need one, too, I argued.

The need to have a code of ethics or at least some professional standards was made more urgent and necessary when I viewed my potentially tenuous employment in New Jersey. I was working in an inherently political environment, trying to protect research subjects and their identifiable private information (in the form of the numerous amounts of data that a public health agency collects) from unauthorized research uses.[7] There was significant pressure on HREP to view certain projects as public health practice rather than research so as to avoid the perceived hassles of IRB review and oversight. There's a great deal at stake in determining whether an activity is research or public health practice—time, money, and other important and scarce resources. If an activity is wrongly deemed to be research, IRB review is required. IRB review takes additional time, money, and other resources. As a very influential public health guidance document put the dilemma: When public health activities are misclassified as research, "public health authorities [must] engage in time-consuming reviews through governmental or private sector IRBs. In some cases, the mere assessment by an IRB, even when expedited, may thwart an activity to the detriment of the public's health. In other cases, the IRB may require additional protections for persons viewed as human research subjects that defeat public health objectives in principle or design, or for lack of funding" (Hodge & Gostin, 2004, p. 21). The second horn of the dilemma is the converse of the first: "Conversely, public health research that is misclassified as practice may allow governmental health authorities to collect and analyze sensitive health data in possible violation of health information privacy interests, or interact with human subjects without complete adherence to research protections to the detriment of the individual participants" (Hodge & Gostin, 2004, p. 21).

The possibility of conflicts was compounded when the decision was made to constitute an IRB at the department during my tenure there. There was always the possibility of political pressure on the IRB and its members to make decisions that might have little to do with the protection of subjects or good ethical practices, despite efforts to shelter the IRB from such machinations. As my presentation at the 2006 ASBH meeting indicated, because of the fact that there was no code of ethics for me to look to for support against such potential threats, meant that I relied on the clinical ethics skills I learned during my doctorate and fellowship training to convince those in power of the need for the IRB to operate with independence. I found that the best approach was to build skills in having difficult conversations (Stone, Patton, & Heen, 1999). The thrust of Stone et al.'s book was to know that when having a difficult conversation, people's personal and professional identities are frequently tied to their work products. What is required are good listening and communication skills, especially the ability to build trust and speak truth to power in a way that preserves trust. The most challenging situations required maintaining a precarious but necessary balance between *compliance* and *colleague*. The problem, to put it succinctly, was that I had to be viewed as someone trustworthy by researchers and the senior leadership at my department, but I also had to uphold the ethical and regulatory standards from the Belmont Report and the Federal regulations for the protection of human subjects. Frequently, the two were diametrically opposed, and without any form of external bioethics guidance in the form of a code of ethics, the obvious choice was to weigh on the side of ethics and regulations. Siding with ethics and regulations and speaking truth to power, especially without the support of a code of ethics, can have drastic consequences (Perlman, 2008). For this reason, bioethics needs a code of ethics, and soon.

CONCLUSION

I AM ALWAYS astounded how a fresh set of eyes can yield new perspectives on difficult situations. Interestingly, it was a colleague at NJDHSS,[8] unaffiliated with the IRB and HREP, who suggested that what would have prevented the difficulties mentioned above (and by extrapolation, the same difficulties of any IRB oversight program at any institution) was independence. My colleague suggested that those who provide oversight to researchers should be federal employees, under the aegis and imprimatur of the Department of Health and Human Services' Office for Human Research Protections or the Food and Drug Administration's Office of Good Clinical Practices. The institution would have a contract to protect human subjects called a federalwide assurance or FWA. Moreover, the same institution would be required to provide the oversight program's salaries and support in order to have the privilege to conduct human subjects research. To my knowledge, this proposed form of independence for the ethical oversight of research is not part of any of the recent proposals to revamp the system for protection of research subjects in the United States (Emanuel et al., 2004). Based on my experience, it should be, and, as I have tried to show in this chapter, the general principle of independence might represent one way to overcome conflicts of interest in a wealth of bioethical situations. Therefore, not only should bioethicists strive to make their consulting arrangements independent and more transparent, but the concept of independence should be incorporated into the debate on development of a code of ethics for bioethicists.

NOTES

1. The American Society for Bioethics and Humanities (ASBH)-American Society of Law, Medicine and Ethics (ASLME)–sponsored Task Force on Bioethics Consultation in the Private Sector (Brody et al., 2002) contains a bibliography of several examples of these forms of consultation.

2. Some notable examples include: (a) former Penn professor Glenn McGee's well-publicized resignation from the ethics board at Advanced Cell Technologies (Green et al., 2002); (b) E. Haavi Morreim's service as chair of artificial heart manufacturer AbioMed's Independent Patient Advocacy Committee (IPAC; Morreim, 2004a, 2004b) and two Penn bioethicists, David Casarett and Sheldon Zink, serving as patient advocates for recipients of AbioMed's experimental artificial heart (Wilson, 2003); and (c) Laurie Zoloth's role on Geron's ethics board (Geron Ethics Advisory Board, 1999).

3. An argument could be made that traditionally structured formal or informal ethics consultation in other nonpublic settings (e.g., IRBs and bedside clinical ethics consultations) confront this danger as well (Brody et al., 2002). Nevertheless, as many bioethicists have chosen to do, one way to overcome it is to publish or publicly speak about the issues, decisions, and processes used to reach them (Brody et al., 2002; Morreim, 2004a, 2004b; Perlman, 2001a, 2005).

4. Francoise Baylis (2004) summarizes the case of Dr. Nancy Olivieri in her article "The Olivieri Debacle: Where Were the Heroes of Bioethics." Carl

Elliott (2001a) summarizes the case of Dr. David Healy in his article "Pharma Buys a Conscience."

5. The IPAC had an interesting, independent structure that bears greater analysis but is beyond the scope of the present chapter. AbioCor established a blind trust for its IPAC, then selected a chairperson from the research ethics community to administer the IPAC, the blind trust, and to set policy, guidelines, recommendations, and implementation of protections for subject recruitment for the company's artificial heart.

6. The Association for the Accreditation of Human Research Protection Programs (AAHRPP) and the (now defunct) Partnership for Human Research Protection (PHRP) at the National Committee for Quality Assurance (NCQA).

7. I should note that New Jersey labor law provides some protection under the New Jersey Conscientious Employment Protection Act (2007).

8. P. Bost, personal communication, March, 2008.

REFERENCES

American Institute of Certified Public Accountants. (1988). *AICPA professional code of ethics, section 101, independence*. Retrieved May 1, 2008, from http://www.aicpa.org/about/code/et_101.html#et_101

American Society for Bioethics and Humanities. (1998). *Core competencies for health care ethics consultation*. Glenview, IL: Author.

Baylis, F. (2000). Heroes in bioethics. *Hastings Center Report, 30*(3), 34–39.

Baylis, F. (2004). The Olivieri debacle: Where were the heroes of bioethics? *Journal of Medical Ethics, 30,* 44–49.

Brody B., Dubler, N., Blustein, J., Caplan, A. C., Kahn, J. P., Kass, N., et al. (2002). Bioethics consultation in the private sector. *Hastings Center Report, 32*(3), 14–20.

Callahan, D. (2001). Doing good and doing well. *Hastings Center Report, 3*(12), 19–21.

Donaldson, T. (2001). The business ethics of bioethics consulting. *Hastings Center Report, 3*(12), 12–14.

Eckenwiler, L. A., & Cohn, F. G. (2007). *The ethics of bioethics: Mapping the moral landscape*. Baltimore, MD: Johns Hopkins University Press.

Elliott, C. (2001a). Pharma buys a conscience. *The American Prospect, 12*(17), 16–20.

Elliott, C. (2001b). Throwing a bone to the watchdog. *Hastings Center Report, 31*(2), 9–12.

Elliott C. (2004). Six problems with Pharma-funded bioethics. *Studies in the History and Philosophy of Biology and Biological Sciences, 35,* 135–139.

Emanuel, E. J., Wood, A., Fleischman, A., Bowen, A., Getz, K. A., Grady, C., et al. (2004). Oversight of human participants research: Identifying problems to evaluate reform proposals. *Annals of Intern Medicine, 141,* 282–291.

Ferguson v. the City of Charleston. (2001). 532 U.S. 67.

Freedman, B. (1989). Bringing codes to Newcastle. In B. Hoffmaster, B. Freedman, & G. Fraser (Eds), *Clinical ethics: Theory and practice* (pp. 125–139). Clifton, NJ: Humana Press.

Geron Ethics Advisory Board. (1999). Research with human embryonic stem cells: Ethical considerations *Hastings Center Report, 19*(2), 31–36.

Green, R. M., DeVries, K. O., Bernstein, J., Goodman, K. W., Kaufman, R., Kiessling, A. A., et al. (2002). Overseeing research on therapeutic cloning: A private ethics board responds to its critics. *Hastings Center Report, 32*(3), 27–33.

Hellman, S., Cassel, C., Stock, C., Wood, A. & Zapol, W. (2001). *Report of Johns Hopkins University External Review Committee.* Retrieved January 1, 2008, from http://www.hopkinsmedicine.org/external.pdf

Hodge, J. G., & Gostin, L. O. (2004). *Public health practice vs. research: A report for public health practitioners including cases and guidance for making decisions.* Council of State and Territorial Epidemiologists. Retrieved January 27, 2007, from http://www.cste.org/pdffiles/newpdffiles/CSTEPHResRpt HodgeFinal.5.24.04.pdf

Lemmens, T., & Freedman, B. (2000). Ethics review for sale?: Conflict of interest and commercial research review boards. *Milbank Quarterly, 78*(4), 547–584.

Miles, S. (2003). Does American bioethics have a soul? *ASBH Exchange, 7*(2), 10.

Morreim, E. H. (2004a). By any other name: The many iterations of "patient advocate" in clinical research. *IRB: Ethics and Human Research, 26*(6), 1–8.

Morreim, E. H. (2004b). High-profile research and the media: The case of the AbioCor artificial heart. *Hastings Center Report, 34*(1), 11–24.

New Jersey Conscientious Employment Protection Act, N.J.S.A. 34:19-1 (2007).

Perlman, D. J. (2001a, October). *The independence principle and its implications for clinical and research ethics consulting.* Presented at 4th Annual American Society for Bioethics and Humanities Meeting, Nashville, TN.

Perlman, D. J. (2001b). *Mediation and ethics consultation: Towards a new understanding of impartiality.* Retrieved from http://www.abanet.org/dispute/ perlman2001.pdf and http://www.mediate.com/articles/perlman.cfm

Perlman, D. J. (2005). Bioethics in industry settings: One situation where a code for bioethicists would help. *American Journal of Bioethics, 5*(5), 62–64.

Perlman, D. J. (2007). *Danger and opportunity: Bioethic(ist)s and the pharmaceutical industry.* Ursinus College, Collegeville, PA.

Perlman, D. J. (2008). Speaking truth to power: Another reason why bioethics needs a code of ethics. *ASBH Exchange, 11*(3), 3.

Perlman, D. J., MacDonald, C., Cohen, G., & Philips, T. (2004, October). *Danger and opportunity: A panel discussion on bioethics in industry.* 6th Annual American Society for Bioethics and Humanities Meeting, Philadelphia, PA.

Sharpe, V. A. (2002). Science, bioethics, and the public interest: On the need for transparency. *Hastings Center Report, 32*(2), 23–26.

Stone, D., Patton, B., & Heen, S. (1999). *Difficult conversations: How to discuss what matters most*. New York: Penguin Books.

Wilson, R. (2003). Penn anthropologist fights subpoenas for field notes regarding artificial-heart surgery she observed. *The Chronicle of Higher Education*. Retrieved January 1, 2008, from http://chronicle.com/daily/2003/03/2003030504n.htm

4

Health Law and Bioethics

Barry R. Furrow

HEALTH LAW HAS grown from the topic of an occasional seminar to a new legal industry. Law school courses are proliferating as new casebooks pour from the publishers' presses. Major law firms now have health law sections, and boutique health law firms are also common in many cities. At the same time, bioethics has become a major field, promising ethical analyses on topics ranging from medical treatments to scientific research, with some hospitals hiring bioethicists to provide oversight on human subjects research and end-of-life issues.

Traditional bioethics has applied ethical analysis to the morality of medical treatments, technological innovations, and general conflicts in the doctor-patient relationship (Jonsen, 1998). The categories of problems that typically have led to major subdivisions of bioethics are human subject research, genetics, organ transplantation, death and dying, and reproduction (Jonsen, 1998). More recently, bioethics has expanded its concerns to ethical questions that arise in the intersections of life sciences, biotechnology, medicine, politics, law, philosophy, theology, and more.

Health law, by contrast, is the legal domain that addresses health care delivery, and the health care industry, in all of its component parts: providers, insurers, patients, drug companies, and researchers. Health law represents a specialized legal response to the increased complexity of relationships in the health care field and the intense fragmentation of the U.S. health care delivery system. Health care delivery is an unruly domain, characterized by the lack of a comprehensive national health policy and an untidy morass of state and federal regulatory schemes. Lawyers represent various constituencies in this health care system, from injured patients to physician groups trying to work out agreements with large insurers, and from drug manufacturers to pharmacies to universities conducting human subjects research.

The relationship between health law and bioethics is dynamic, given the substantial overlap of legal and ethical concerns in most areas mentioned. Bioethics often asks fundamental questions early in the emergence of a problem area, dealing as it does with providing guidance to behavior and analyses of problems, not binding rules backed by the threat of monetary or other sanctions. The philosophical definitions and analyses of bioethics contribute core concepts and values that may be imported into legal rules, case law, and statutory obligations. As the troublesome problems move into the judicial and legislative arenas, courts and policy makers often draw on bioethical principles while also aggressively developing their own sophisticated frameworks, as in fiduciary law and constitutional death and dying jurisprudence, that redefine these bioethical principles.

THE SCOPE OF BIOETHICS

THREE SUBSTANTIVE PRINCIPLES generally have informed bioethics debates: autonomy, beneficence, and social justice (Beauchamp & Childress, 2001). The principle of autonomy declares that each person is in control of his own person, including his body and mind. This principle, in its purest form, presumes that no other person or social institution ought to intervene to overcome a person's desires, whether or not those desires are right from any external perspective. If Furrow wants to die, then Furrow is entitled to die without health care assistance. The tort doctrine of informed consent, the federal rules on human subject research and subject consent, and the death and dying debates are all grounded in this principle of autonomy.

The principle of beneficence declares that what is best for each person should be accomplished. The principle incorporates both the negative obligation of nonmaleficence ("primum non nocere"—"first of all, do no harm"—the foundation of the Hippocratic oath) and the positive obligation to do that which is good. Thus, a physician is obliged, under the principle of beneficence, to provide the highest quality medical care for each of his patients that he can within the patient's resource limits.

When a person does not desire what others determine to be in his interest, the principles of autonomy and beneficence conflict. For example, if we treat the continued life of a healthy person to be in that person's interest, the values of autonomy and beneficence become inconsistent when a healthy competent adult decides to take his own life. As a general matter, most courts now appear to recognize the principle of autonomy as the first principle of medical ethics. Living will legislation and case law acknowledge the right of competent adults to make their own decisions about declining medically valuable health care.

The principle of beneficence is generally applied by courts and bioethics scholars when autonomy is impossible to apply, as where the patient is a newborn infant or an incompetent elderly patient. The principles can be reshaped by legislative enactments, by prevailing judicial philosophies, and by the emergence of other competing principles. Bioethics is not static, reflecting, as does the law, changes in the environment of health care.

Courts, when confronted with hard health care conflicts, look at both the traditions of the common law and the traditions of ethics and medicine. Judicial decisions have also often formed the basis for new ethical and medical approaches. Consider the debates over appropriate ethical policy in determining when life support systems should be initiated or discontinued and whether physicians should be permitted to aid in the death of a patient. These death and dying controversies involve lawyers as much as bioethics scholars. The power of the hospital to revive patients through the use of tools of CPR—a tool developed in the 1960s for resuscitation of patients if done immediately upon a patient's distress—spawned an interest in the new field of bioethics in the 1960s (Committee on CPR of the Division of Medical Sciences, National Academy of Sciences—National Research Council, 1966). Patients began to fear being kept alive against their wishes, as a byproduct of the normal use of CPR on everyone in the hospital who experienced cardio-pulmonary distress. Fears about control over death and dying began to be expressed by patients and ethicists, and litigation followed, from the *Quinlan* case to *Brother Fox* (*In re Quinlan*, 1976; *In re Eichner*, 1980).[1] Task forces discussed these issues at both the state and the national levels, as ethicists participated in setting the agenda and developing analytical frameworks; lawyers began to handle cases on behalf of patients, not only for malpractice claims but in termination of life cases like that of Karen Ann Quinlan and Nancy Cruzan (*Cruzan v. Director*, 1990).

Public debates on these issues, and many other ethical/legal issues, have centered on the judicial and legislative resolution of these problem areas, drawing on ethical sources of formal principles and legal considerations of process and tools. The law does not always look to ethics for potential methods of analysis but instead often usurps ethics in the debates. We give our courts and judges the authority to resolve them and have confidence that they will do so in a coherent and fair manner.

My concern in this chapter is with the more primary analysis of the role and obligations of providers—both physicians and institutions like hospitals—and the interface between bioethics and health law as health care services are delivered to patients.

THE DOCTOR-PATIENT RELATIONSHIP: THE FIDUCIARY EXTENSION

THE HISTORICAL EVOLUTION of both bioethics and health law starts with a central focus on the physician-patient relationship. The ethical analysis came first, with early discussions of physician obligations in Greek and other ancient cultures. The core definition of the role of the physician is at the heart of bioethics. The notion of the physician as a fiduciary with obligations to protect vulnerable patients pervades both ethical and legal discussions of professional obligations (Percival, 1803). The physician is motivated by classic ethical virtues of beneficence and nonmaleficence, in part in response to the vulnerability of patients and to a physician's superior knowledge and skill imparted by medical training. The courts have nipped and tucked at the edges of the provider-patient relationship, developing legal doctrines in malpractice cases, with informed consent doctrine as an important development. Judicially developed general legal and ethical principles govern the dyadic relationship of a sole practitioner and patient. The law surrounding the physician-patient relationship is treated in Furrow et al. (2001). What are the doctor's obligations to patients? Under what circumstances is a doctor responsible to patients for his errors?

Consider the case of Bonnie Rauch, an elderly woman who broke her elbow—an injury repairable through surgery (*Rauch v. Mike-Mayer,* 2001). The risks of such surgery were, however, very high for Bonnie because she was elderly and was taking a wide variety of medications for heart and other medical problems, medications that would complicate any surgery. The ethical principle of nonmaleficence would dictate that the doctor not operate. This principle in a minimalist way is incorporated into liability standards of care, practice guidelines, and other practice-limiting rules of modern medical practice. Beneficence assumes that the doctor does what is best for the patient. Respect for patient autonomy further requires that the patient be informed of the benefits, risks, and alternatives to a medical procedure. Decision-making is shared, so that even if the standard of care is to perform the operation, the patient can say no. Bonnie's example represents the operation of both nonmaleficence and autonomy—ethical principles at the core of U.S. contract law, settled in the tort doctrine of informed consent, and built into more complex decision-making processes in hospitals and other institutions. In Bonnie's case, the surgeon operated, she died, and the court in a tort suit held that the doctor's actions were negligent and that the hospital also should have prevented the surgery in such a high-risk case.

Once the physician-patient relationship is established, the law imposes a higher level of duty on physicians than normal contract law would require for arm's-length transactions. The terms of the contract are largely fixed in advance of any bargaining, by standard or customary practices that the physician must follow at the risk of liability for malpractice. We impute to both the physician and the patient standard intentions and reasonable expectations (Goodin, 1985, pp. 63, 64–65).

Second, professional ethics imposes fiduciary obligations on physicians in a variety of ways. Courts draw on these fiduciary obligations, looking outside the parameters of contract law analysis in judging the obligations of a physician to treat a patient. The courts stress that the physician's obligation to his patient, while having its origins in contract, is governed also by fiduciary obligations and other public considerations "inseparable from the nature and exercise of his calling" (*Norton v. Hamilton*, 1955).

Third, professionals are constrained in their ability to withdraw from their contracts by case law defining patient abandonment. A doctor who withdraws from the physician-patient relationship before a cure is achieved or the patient is transferred to the care of another may be liable for abandonment (*Cole v. Marshall Medical Center*, 2007; *Payton v. Weaver*, 1982).

A fiduciary obligation in medicine means that the physician focuses exclusively on the patient's health; the patient assumes the doctor's single-minded devotion to him; and the doctor-patient relationship is expected to be free of conflict.[2] One ethicist defines a health care fiduciary as "someone who commits to becoming and remaining scientifically and clinically competent, acts primarily to protect and promote the interests of the patient and keeps self-interest systematically secondary, and maintains and passes on medicine as a public trust for current and future physicians and patients" (McCullough, 2006, p. 3). Medical ethicists frequently speak of the doctor's special duties in relation to the patient, often characterizing the doctor as a special friend to the patient, connected by bond of loyalty normally subsumed within the meaning of friendship. It is a strong agency relationship in which we trust the physician as our agent to look out for our best interests. Hans Jonas describes this duty owed by the physician to a patient as a "sacred trust," an intense obligation to ignore social and other concerns that interfere with the care of the specific patient:

> In the course of treatment, the physician is obligated to the patient and no one else. He is not the agent of society, nor of the interests of medical science, nor of the patient's family, nor of his co-sufferers, or future sufferers from the same disease. The patient alone counts when he is under the physician's care.... The physician is bound not to let any other interest interfere with that of the patient in being cured. But manifestly more sublime norms than contractual ones are involved. We may speak of a sacred trust; strictly by its terms, the doctor is, as it were, alone with his patient and God. (Jonas, 1969, p. 238)

The patient, lacking equality in the relationship, is, in Judge Spottswood Robinson's phrase, "well nigh abject" in his ignorance of medicine and uncertainty about treatment (*Canterbury v. Spence*, 1972). The law, acknowledging this inequality, and not completely trusting physician ethics and objectivity, has created legal frameworks to equalize the relationship and empower the patient. The doctrine of informed consent is one such example, but disclosure obligations stretch beyond informed consent to include disclosure of possible economic conflicts of interest and even personal shortcomings of the physician independent of treatment risks, such as inexperience.[3] Preserving, justifying, and enhancing trust is the fundamental goal of much of medical ethics and a major objective in health care law and public policy (Hall, 2002). We don't completely trust our doctors because of situational pressures that may at times corrupt or at least tempt them: doctors work for economic and other gains, as we all do; they are weak at times, prey to needs and pressures not aligned with those of their patients; and they are under tremendous pressures from patients, insurers, their own needs, other doctors, and drug companies. Conflicts of interest run through the physician-patient relationship. One function of legal rules is to manage or reduce these conflicts of interest.

INSTITUTIONS AND THE PROBLEM OF FIDUCIARY OBLIGATION

L ET US USE another case example. Consider the case of *Esquivel v. Watters*, a 2007 Kansas case. Michelle Esquivel learned she was pregnant and got obstetric counseling from the Ark City Clinic. A clinic worker gave Michelle a certificate from South Central Kansas Regional Medical Center (SCKRMC) for a free gender-determination sonogram, and Michelle went to get her free sonogram on November 15, 2001. She had signed a consent form that said the sonogram was only to determine the fetus's sex and that "this procedure is not to determine any fetal abnormality or any other complication of pregnancy and is not considered a diagnostic examination for any medical purpose other than to attempt to determine the sex of my unborn baby." She waived any right to sue. The technician who performed the sonogram noted that Michelle's baby's bowel was outside of his body, a condition known as gastroschisis, but he did not inform Michelle because he was not a doctor. He could not confirm the gender. He did take sonogram pictures, which he sent to a radiologist at the Ark City Clinic. In the court's words, "[t]he radiologist refused to look at them because the sonogram was only for gender determination and not for diagnosis." He also reported the problem to Dr. Watters, Michelle's obstetrician, but did not send any pictures nor a written report. Confusion then reigned, with Watters failing to make notes in the chart, but with his nurse trying to reach Michelle many times over the phone. Finally Watters saw Michelle, but having made no notes on the chart, he forgot to discuss the problem with her.

In February, Michelle became ill and went to SCKRMC for treatment. Her son Jadon was born by emergency caesarean section the next day. Neither Michelle nor Jesse (her husband) nor the medical staff who delivered Jadon were aware that Jadon had gastroschisis until he was born. Jadon's bowel had been dead for weeks before his birth, and so he was sent home with parents to die, which he did 2 weeks later. Michelle then sued.

The district court and the appellate court both held that "SCKRMC's undertaking was limited to performing a sonogram to determine the gender of Michelle's baby, which it did in a non-negligent manner. Having performed the sonogram in a careful manner, no further duty was owed to Michelle, and there was no obligation to inform her about anything other than Jadon's gender." The court was troubled by the boundary between law and ethics in this case. Can the law recognize a duty to inform, in spite of the clear limits set on the sonogram's purpose and acknowledgement by the patient? In the court's words:

> Our analysis of this essential element of Michelle and Jesse's causes of action is a rather disheartening exercise. As a society we expect of ourselves a certain level of looking out for the welfare of others. This is an attribute which society encourages rather than discourages. We would expect this urge to be particularly strong in the hearts of those who choose to enter the medical and health care community. However, the transition from a societal expectation to a legal duty is often determined by public policy considerations which are not within the purview of an intermediate appellate court such as ours. Consequently, we turn to the case law for guidance.

Their reading of the law was conservative. Absent a doctor-patient relationship here, the court found that the hospital owed no duty to Michelle. It contended that a hospital-patient relationship is not a fiduciary one, unlike a doctor-patient relationship. The court also suggested that there was an ethical duty on the hospital to properly disclose the information to Michelle, but it was not a legal duty enforceable by the courts. At this boundary between ethics and law, there is much to quarrel about. Once the problem with the fetus was recognized, we surely expect the provider to meet a standard of organizational competence sufficient to make a note to remind him at the patient's next office visit. More importantly, we expect the hospital and clinic to inform the patient, although they may have no further obligations to take action. The free sonogram was a promotional scheme of the hospital to attract patients, and one could argue that they had created some form of relationship in such a case (McCullough, 1999).

Here is a transitional case, where marketing inducements may create a duty to warn a patient about an unexpected problem. Other courts have observed that fiduciary analysis applies to hospital agency law, and a hospital may be responsible for the negligence of its independent contractors as a fiduciary for its patients. Managed care liability rules are also grounded on fiduciary obligations of honest dealing with insurance policyholders; an insurance company may have a fiduciary relationship with those who choose to become members of that health maintenance organization (e.g., *Pagarigan v. Aetna U.S. Healthcare of California, Inc.*, 2005). Here we see courts taking the measure of the new world of hospitals as they incorporate all the corporate marketing tricks of the for-profit world. And the courts are suspicious, finding an ethical grounding in health care that may entangle hospitals if they dash people's expectations about how they should be treated by hospitals.

JUSTICE AND THE INSTITUTIONAL PROVIDER–PATIENT RELATIONSHIP

LET US USE another case to state the larger ethical problem of social justice in terms of access to necessary health care. We have seen health care get more expensive, insurance coverage shrink, and hospitals pursue aggressive bill collection techniques. Should our institutional providers be treated just like other providers, such as car dealers? In *Muse v. Charter Hospital of Winston-Salem, Inc*, a 1995 decision, a physician treating Joe Muse, a depressed and suicidal teenager, was faced with a limit on insurance coverage for the boy's treatment in the hospital. Convincing evidence was presented (and believed by the jury) that Charter Hospital of Winston-Salem, Inc. had a policy or practice that required physicians to discharge patients when their insurance expired, and, in the court's words, "this policy interfered with the exercise of the medical judgment of Joe's treating physician." Muse, while in the hospital, had auditory hallucinations, suicidal and homicidal thoughts, and major depression. As his insurance coverage limits approached, his doctor decided he needed a blood test to determine the proper dosage for an antidepressant drug. The blood test was scheduled the day after Joe's insurance was to expire. Joe's doctor asked for a 2-day extension. The parents signed a note to pay for the extra 2 days, but the test results did not come back until 3 days later, and Joe was discharged the day before and referred to an outpatient therapist. After a short trip with his parents, Joe killed himself. The court, in reviewing the jury verdict for the plaintiffs on appeal, found strongly for the doctor. They wrote: "[I]t seems axiomatic that the hospital has the duty not to institute policies or practices which interfere with the doctor's medical judgment. We hold that pursuant to the reasonable person standard, Charter Hospital had a duty not to institute a policy or practice which required that patients be discharged when their insurance expired and which interfered with the medical judgment of Dr. Barnhill."

Here we have a strong judicial assertion of the primacy of physician's clinical judgment, trumping institutional resource limits, at least in an exceptional case where a patient's life is arguably at risk. Perhaps it is little more than an observation of a duty to rescue in extreme cases, requiring absorption of costs in rare, life-threatening contexts.[4] The courts are testing the limits of institutional refusals to treat by social justice benchmarks. The decision is troubling, and illustrates the limitations of judicial analysis at times. Courts must resolve the case before them, and they rarely subject the case to the kind of intense analysis that a bioethicist might. Nor do they take into account the complexity of resource limitations and other constraints under which health care providers may operate.

CONCLUSION

THERE ARE HUNDREDS of examples in case law and legislation of the cross-pollination of health law and bioethics. Much of bioethical work goes on behind the scenes, in ethics committees and institutional review boards, as ethical principles are used to navigate difficult personal situations. The law, triggered by one of the actors in a conflict, will step in when conflicts burst out of the privacy of institutions, when outcomes are bad, families are torn apart, and patients are at risk in conflict situations. And when courts take on these tough cases in the overlap of health law and ethics, they draw on existing ethical analyses but also move into the legal domain that must also recognize rules of evidence, constraints of due process, and issues of institutional competence. Law and bioethics may often have an uncomfortable relationship but also a rich and productive one.

NOTES

1. A patient in a persistent vegetative state "has no health, and, in the true sense, no life, for the State to protect"), modified in *In re Storar* (1981).

2. The language of fiduciary law is often used to describe special obligations that one person owes to another. Justice Cardozo writes, "Many forms of conduct permissible in a workaday world for those acting at arm's length, are forbidden to those bound by fiduciary ties. A trustee is held to something stricter than the morals of the market place. Not honesty alone, but the punctilio of an honor the most sensitive, is then the standard of behavior" (*Meinhard v. Salmon*, 1928).

3. For an instance of the obligation of a surgeon to disclose inexperience with a dangerous procedure, see, for example, *Johnson v. Kokemoor* (1996).

4. The problem with judicial pronouncements is that they are not always so limiting in their language and interpretation. The early *Wickline* decision (*Wickline v. State of California,* 1986) had held in a more nuanced decision that a physician has to at least understand reimbursement constraints and be willing to push until their limits are reached.

REFERENCES

Beauchamp, T. L., & Childress, J. E. (2001). *Principles of biomedical ethics* (5th ed). New York: Oxford University Press.

Canterbury v. Spence, 464 F.2d 772 (1972).

Cole v. Marshall Medical Center, 2007 WL 1576391 (Cal.App. 3 Dist., 2007).

Committee on CPR of the Division of Medical Sciences, National Academy of Sciences—National Research Council. (1966). Cardiopulmonary resuscitation. *Journal of the American Medical Association, 198,* 138–145, 372–379.

Cruzan v. Director, Missouri Department of Health, 497 U.S. 261 (1990).

Esquivel v. Watters, 154 P.3d 1184, 2007 WL 1041762 (Court of Appeals of Kansas, 2007).

Furrow, B. R., Greaney, T., Johnson, S., Jost, T. S., & Schwartz, R. (2001). *Health law* (2nd ed). St. Paul, MN: West Publishing Co.

Goodin, R. (1985). *Protecting the vulnerable*. Chicago: University of Chicago Press.

Hall, M. (2002). Law, medicine, and trust. *Stanford Law Review, 55,* 463, 470–471.

In re Eichner, 73 App. Div. 2d 431, 465, 426 N.Y.S. 2d 517, 543 (1980).

In re Quinlan, 70 N.J. 10, 355 A.2d 647 (S.C. N.J. 1976).

In re Storar, 52 N.Y. 2d 363, 420 N.E. 2d 64 (1981).

Johnson v. Kokemoor, 199 Wis. 2d 615, 545 N.W.2d 495 (S.C. Wis. 1996)

Jonas, H. (1969). Ethical aspects of experimentation with human subjects. *Daedalus, 98*(2), 219–247.

Jonsen, A. R. (1998). *The birth of bioethics.* New York: Oxford University Press.

McCullough, L. (2006, September). *A primer on bioethics* (2nd ed.). American College of Physician Executives. Retrieved November 13, 2008, from http://net.acpe.org/InterAct/Ethics/BioethicsPrimer.pdf

McCullough, L. B. (1999). A basic concept in the clinical ethics of managed care: Physicians and institutions as economically disciplined co-fiduciaries of a population of patients. *Journal of Medicine and Philosophy, 24,* 77–97.

Meinhard v. Salmon, 249 N.Y. 458, 164 N.E. 545, 546 (1928).

Muse v. Charter Hospital of Winston-Salem, Inc, 117 N. C.App. 468, 452 S.E.2d 589 (Court of Appeals of North Carolina, 1995).

Norton v. Hamilton, 92 Ga.App. 727, 89 S.E.2d 809, 812 (1955).

Pagarigan v. Aetna U.S. Healthcare of California, Inc., 2005 WL 2742807 (California Court of Appeal, 2005).

Payton v. Weaver, 131 Cal.App.3d 38, 182 Cal.Rptr. 225 (Cal.App., 1982).

Percival T. (1803). *Medical ethics, or a code of institutes and precepts, adapted to the professional conduct of physicians and surgeons.* London: Johnson & Bickerstaff.

Rauch v. Mike-Mayer, 783 A.2d 815 (Sup. Ct. Pa. 2001).

Wickline v. State of California, 192 Cal. App. 3d 1630, 239 Cal Rptr 810 (2d Dist. 1986).

5

Bioethics:
The Citizen View
and Its Perils

JOHN TIMPANE

A S I WRITE this chapter, I am trying to cool down from an exchange with a reader of an editorial I recently wrote ("Vaccinations and Autism," 2008).

Editorials are statements of opinion. They set forth an argument. They take a stand and seek impact in the public forum. At the *Philadelphia Inquirer,* editorials are unsigned and traditionally carry with them the institutional credit of the paper.

My editorial argued that, especially in light of a raft of new studies, small and large, there was still no solid reason to believe in a link between vaccination and the perceived rise of autism rates in the United States. I tried to be careful. I limited the discussion to the government-mandated vaccines common to nearly all U.S. children. (The regnant myth is that the rising number of mandated childhood vaccinations is directly tied to the 10-fold rise in the rates of diagnosis of autism in U.S. children since the 1980s.) I tried to be compassionate (compassion is what I feel) toward parents and families of autistic children: autism can be a terrible misfortune, an occasion for thankless labor and suffering. Alas, no one knows why the autism rates are rising. That rise may be in part factitious, a result of increased awareness and changing diagnostic criteria and methods. It is understandable that people search for answers, but in this case, science doesn't have them yet; genetic links seem like a good guess, but a guess is all they are at the moment.

I got swamped. Letter writers told me I had not checked my facts. I was told I was in bed with the science-industrial-governmental complex. I responded by referring to studies I trusted and admired; my studies were seen and raised with Web sites galore (full of bad information wrongly understood). As a colleague put it, I was "called everything but a child of God."

Reader response—lively, engaged—is one of the best things about my job. Since I write many science-related editorials, I have fielded many objections and objurgations about many bioethical issues: stem-cell research; end-of-life management; reproductive technologies; genetic manipulation of people, food products, and farm animals; evolution and religion; and global warming. My profession has allowed me to get a good, long glimpse of how citizens view bioethics.

Most people see bioethics as a set of political issues—matters of public policy they can vote up or down. They do not see them primarily as scientific issues because, to them, science is somewhat of a hermetically sealed-off realm, poorly explained, and none too responsive. Yes, these are outdated clichés about science; that doesn't matter. Many people see bioethical issues either as intensely personal matters—if the issues touch their own lives—or already politicized and partisanized matters (that is, issues for debate between the political parties), much the same as nonscientific policy issues. Bioethical issues get thrown in the ring and batted around as part of the rough-and-tumble of the democratic process in this country.

Since 1975, that process has become increasingly polarized, more so (or so we say) than before. Advances in science—especially advances on the horizon that promise to challenge or revise certain widely held beliefs—often are portrayed as threats, as zero-sum, all-or-nothing, last-ditch battles over principle. Instantly they are recruited into the struggle between those two incredibly wealthy, powerful, loud, pushy, and tedious private clubs, the Republican Party and the Democratic Party, abetted by a newly empowered popular media. Who's left behind in the bioethics debate? Scientists who actually know something about the science. They need to claim themselves a place at the table.

For the main drivers of its political debate, U.S. society, as mentioned, is saddled with these two private clubs, with little constitutional standing (they are hardly mentioned in the Constitution, and, outside of the outdated Electoral College, they play no role in the architecture of government) but almost all the money and all the airtime. Each hoovers up whatever shards of ideas or events it can and turns them into planks in a platform. (An especially prominent and hilarious example is a February 2007 David Brooks column in the *New York Times,* in which that well-known conservative tried to recruit epigenetics as evidence supporting the wisdom of a conservative worldview [Brooks, 2007].¹) Americans now define themselves as Republican or Democratic, as conservative or liberal, partly by where they stand on reproductive technology, stem-cell research, and evolution. Assisting in the partisanization of bioethics, a huge, new, democratic, and almost completely irresponsible array of popular media have arisen in the past 20 years. Pop media, especially the blog world, are largely free from rules of demonstration or standards of authority, free also of the consequences of being wrong (no bloggers ever fire themselves for running mistaken material); they are also, sadly, permanent (once something appears, it can be replicated endlessly throughout the virtual cosmos).

These (no longer new) pop media allow anyone who can self-publish to crown themselves experts. In that sense, the rise of the blog hasn't been great for science: bloggers regularly arrogate to themselves the role of assessors and adjudicators of science fact and debate. One of my favorites in this regard in Glenn Reynolds, who in his influential blog *Instapundit* regularly selects fringe-science reports that question supposedly left-wing science views (http://www.instapundit.com). On global warming, he often posts material suggesting (wrongly) that the sun is the real culprit. When news comes of any so-called progress in stem-cell research—and by this Reynolds means progress that obviates the *need* for human embryonic stem-cell research—he gives it his personal stamp of approval, as on 9:34 A.M. on February 11, 2008: "MORE NEWS ON induced pluripotent stem cells. I'm very happy to see such rapid progress." I am pained to point out that he links the reader to Fight Aging!, an unkempt clearinghouse of articles on almost *any* research with a shred of connection to human aging. There are no rules of reference in the blogosphere. We get 2nd-, 3rd-, and 12th-hand references constantly, at a very high rate of iterative decay, since, very often, each referrer gets it a little bit wrong. Reynolds is a law professor with a bent toward the ethics of technology, but he uses his blog about as responsibly as most bloggers do. Bad habits of the blogosphere cross back over into the fixed-print media. Writers here, too, perhaps to compete with the runaway self-ordination of the Web writers, increasingly drape over their own shoulders the mantle of instant expertise. Thus Joan Didion, writing in *The New York Review of Books,* darkly questioned the agreement of neurologists that Terri Schiavo was in a persistent vegetative state (PVS; Didion, 2005). Nat Hentoff of the *Village Voice* felt he could write that Schiavo "is not brain-dead or comatose"—PVS is *not* an observation of either of these states, by the way—"and breathes naturally on her own. Although brain-damaged, she is not in a persistent vegetative state, according to an increasing number of radiologists and neurologists" (Hentoff, 2005). Hentoff, very blogger-like, waves a general hand at the old "increasing numbers" canard, a favorite of Web writers too busy to perform actual research, or so distrustful of the science community that they assume that, even if a preponderance of scientists agree on a point, such agreement doesn't necessarily mean much. Such are the virtues that render these media ideal for the perpetuation of misinformation, subtle misrepresentation, often for the sake of being provocative, and also for implacable, inaccessible insistence in the face of countervailing evidence. That, in turn, makes them prime material for manipulation by the parties. So when we say that people see bioethics as primarily political issues, we must keep in mind all the new ways people get (and in millions of cases, generate their own versions of) scientific or scientistic information.

The state of global warming…the plight of the polar bear (both supposedly exposed as myths by John Stossel of the ABC show *20/20* [Stossel, 2007],[2] and thus, I might add, partisanized)…"test-tube babies" (a phrase that persists even though there never have been any[3])…end-of-life issues (Schnieder & Lin, 2005)…the age of the earth…evidence for evolution…stem-cell research…genetic screening (which has existed for years for diseases having a readily available treatment, as with Phenylketonuria (PKU) screening—but pop media treat it as if it is a widely available means of selecting or aborting offspring on the basis of traits such as sexual orientation or eye color[4])…the vaccine-autism debate…food products made from cloned or genetically modified plants or animals (the clever and misleading label "Frankenfood" has been with us since 1992[5])…many people feel they can determine your party from your stances on these issues. Science doesn't decide. Science is the last thing to be consulted.

At the edges, the rigid partisanship of it all can break down, which is encouraging. After all, isn't green living at least potentially a conservative stance? And can't liberals be profoundly troubled by abortion? Still, to me there is no doubt that science, or rather the image of science purveyed by the parties for their own purposes, has been rendered forever political—and so has bioethics. It's understandable: science is enabling human beings, and will continue to enable them, to do things that raise profound and controversial ethical issues. Debate on those issues is trampled by the far stronger partisan debate, with its knack for deforming anything of value. I especially regret the way personal beliefs about the cosmos are now a shuttlecock for such contention, thoroughly partisanized thanks to shrill conservative Christian thinkers and members of the self-described brights movement and atheists who assert their right to be nasty in the name of science—doing themselves and their argument a bad disservice.

It's too late to ask: Is this good? Bad? Ask instead: What is the process of which bioethics are now a part? And what role can scientists take in that process?

The process is that of coming to public judgment.

As political theorist Daniel Yankelovich (1991) recognizes in his book by that title, this process is only intermittently rational. Politics, after all, concerns not what logic dictates, but rather what people want. Its main engine is not reason but rhetoric, the art of persuasion. Rationalists, therefore, stand to be incredibly frustrated if they look to politics for wholly rational outcomes. Like theorists such as Jürgen Habermas, Yankelovich reminds us that scientific and technological demands need not be—and probably won't be—the first needs served in any single public judgment. Yankelovich sees the science/technology complex as one of the elites with which citizens must contend in the process of making public decisions. He insists that citizens, while they can consult these elites to make up their minds, ultimately must bypass these elites and come to decisions on behalf of the greater commonalty.

This is a process on behalf of all and necessarily must be engaged in as such. Remember, we wouldn't be having such bioethical ferment if these questions were only academic. They are not. They are questions such as "Is X [selection of embryos for desired traits? stem-cell research? creation of embryonic chimeras with both human and non-human genetic material?,[6] etc.] something we wish to allow? Should it be legal? Should government regulate it? Do we want it?" These are not questions of science. If scientists wish to join the debate (and I beg them to), they must think apart from science.

So here are a few thoughts about what happens, or should happen, with bioethics in the public sphere.

DEMOCRACY DOES NOT COME UP WITH SOLUTIONS; IT COMES UP WITH DECISIONS REGARDING THE HANDLING OF ISSUES AND PROBLEMS

TOO MANY OF us—and as a journalist, I belong to the class of worst offenders—write the word *solutions,* when we should be writing *negotiations.* Society is likely to change its mind, and often. We may try one way of doing things and decide to take a different direction ("Science Raises Questions," 2003). To some extent, this may be what is happening with abortion—and I say this with all the hedges, caveats, and uncertainties I can acknowledge. It does seem as though one side of the debate is listening more to the other side. In the 1970s, it was common to hear or read those who swore that all abortions are equally defensible; as of 2008, such chin-out advocacy is rarely seen. Indeed, it seems dated: such language is stamped with a different time and place. Fewer people still would *hinge* the notion of women's rights on absolutely unquestionable rights to abort. Social attitudes have very much changed, however, regarding other reproductive technologies. When in-vitro fertilization first succeeded, it was hailed with ambivalence. Today, it is accepted by all but a minority of Americans. In my editorial on the 25th anniversary of Louise Brown, the first person whose conception took place outside the mother's body, I reminded readers that "true to human nature, we largely have sidestepped the grand cultural conversation we should be having about" the bioethics of reproduction ("Science Raises Questions," 2003, A5). Looking back, however, I realize that sometimes inaction is a form of action. In vitro fertilization is legal, gives birth to 20,000 people a year in the United States, has given birth to more than 1 million people who would not otherwise exist—in my book, that constitutes acceptance. So once again, with feeling: democracy is not a solution-machine but a means of negotiation. Often this process is case-to-case, in a very Aristotelian fashion. The process is never complete, never done.

THE WAY THIS SOCIETY COMES TO HANDLE BIOETHICAL ISSUES WILL BE NEITHER CONSERVATIVE NOR LIBERAL

OUR FUTURE NEGOTIATIONS with our bioethical challenges will likely discomfit, perplex, and even enrage people of all political persuasions. It is written nowhere that one particular side has to win. That, above all, is what both the scientific community and citizenry need to see. In the United States, the right was discomfited by the pragmatic solution to the Terri Schiavo affair;[7] the left by the Bush stem-cell funding policy; the right by the final decision of Judge John E. Jones III in the 2005 case of *Kitzmiller et al. vs. Dover School Board et al.,* striking down a school board rule directing teachers to read a misleading statement on evolution before teaching it; the left by genetic research (and medical marketing!) that questioned the leftward motto that race is nothing but a social construct; both right and left by the 2008 FDA decision to allow animal-based food to be processed from cloned sources; the left by Bush administration policies that tightened oversight of the National Science Foundation and other science organizations that use federal money.

The best we can hope for—and it is much—is that the process by which we arrive at those solutions will be as democratic as possible, and that it will include more scientists and well-informed citizens.

The science community is not a monolith of one political or moral set of values. Scientists span the spectrum of political persuasion, and they will line up all over the place on the issues. Scientists themselves will come out on either political side, as we see today in the partisanized climate change debate, in which scientists tussle in public, just like TV talk show hosts, who are too delighted to watch them. An apparent consensus may emerge at times—but too many scientists write as though they think that's enough. No: all it means is one more endorsement. The next challenge is to sell that point of view in the marketplace of ideas and elect people who will ensure it becomes policy.

SCIENTISTS AND NONSCIENTISTS ALIKE WHO ARE CONCERNED ABOUT BIOETHICS MUST, AT SOME POINT, STOP THINKING LIKE SCIENTISTS AND START THINKING LIKE CITIZENS

JUST AS SOCIETY must get smarter about science, scientists must get smarter about democracy, and shoulder the holsters of debate, persuasion, and advocacy. They are faced with an incredible task: to step across from the elite to the public. Battles cannot be won simply with superior fact—that is not how this process works, and anyone who thinks it does is a steer galloping toward the slaughterhouse. Scientists must first be good scientists—and then, if they wish to join the debate about ethical issues, they must learn to love the assembly of coalitions, the patient, repeated, public advocacy of ideas in the people's language. They have to forget the politics of prestige and aggression in their own realm and face the job of bringing nonscientists into the democratic ring with them.[8] Bioethical issues cannot be solved by precept, as groups ranging from Planned Parenthood ("reproductive rights for every man and woman") to the President's Council on Bioethics (constantly warning us against using human beings "as means to an end," when our society already does, in transfusions and transplants, by the millions each year) seem to think. Bioethical issues can, however, be made accessible by excellent communication, willingness to engage straight-across with a range of viewpoints (including those who don't know much about science and probably never will), and savvy politics.

In a moment, I will address communications. But I wish to stress again the savvy politics part. What do successful groups do in the public sphere? They find out what other groups are likely to be affected by the policies they wish to enshrine. They reach out to them. They explain to them how the things they advocate will help them. It doesn't have to be a perfect fit, but it does have to motivate these groups to vote for those policies. In the stem-cell debate, for example, savvy scientists could have made much more of their constituency among seniors. Scientists wishing to advance genetically modified food sources could make much better political allies in the hugely powerful agricultural industry.

THE SCIENCES IN THE UNITED STATES SHOULD CONTINUE THE REVOLUTION IN SCIENCE COMMUNICATION THAT BEGAN IN THE 1980S—AND MUST NOT STOP

As a person who has written about the sciences for more than 30 years, I celebrate this revolution. Young scientists today take communications courses from the moment they start to study science; more than ever, the young scientist is trained to be a communicator. As a whole, the U.S. science community is much better at making itself understood than it was 30 years ago. That improvement must continue.

Most blogs purporting to be about science and society turn out to be hopelessly ill-informed. When science blogs are valuable, it is because their proprietors and contributors both (a) know science and (b) know how to argue in the democratic forum. So, yes, scientists should run more of these blogs—but, unless they are also very comfortable and effective in the public forum, they should team up with writers who *are* comfortable there. One site I especially like is *DNA Today* (http://www.dnalc.org/ddnalc/dna_today/), a project of the Cold Spring Harbor Laboratory, in which two scientists, Micklos and Jan Witkowski, review recent research in DNA and genetics in an accessible but well-informed videoblog. Another is *Frontal Cortex* (http://scienceblogs.com/cortex/), whose proprietor is Jonah Lehrer, a contributing editor of *Seed* magazine. A third is the *Center for Science Writings* blog out of the Stevens Institute of Technology, ably managed by author and educator John Horgan (http://www.stevens.edu/csw/cgi-bin/index.php). The great Internet challenge is to set up a canon of trustworthy Web sources for news, debate, and discussion of science and science ethics. That will be a huge, collaborative effort—not just to create the venues, but also to get out the word that these are the most trustworthy.

Scientists are appearing more and more as part of our political deliberations. For the purposes of which I speak here, however, this revolution is just beginning and has to keep going. Indeed, we should train scientists not only to be able to explain science well (and we're doing that), but also how to advocate forcefully and knowledgeably in the public arena.

MORE OF OUR POLITICAL REPRESENTATIVES OF ALL PARTIES SHOULD HAVE EXPERIENCE AS WORKING SCIENTISTS

THAT MEANS MORE former research scientists in both houses of Congress. For several years, U.S. Senator Bill Frist of Tennessee was presented as the Congressional spokesman for science, but, with great respect to him and his very august career as a surgeon, it's important that we have more than that—something more like the research career of Rush Holt, representative for New Jersey's 12th Congressional District. Representative Holt was assistant director of the Princeton Plasma Physics Laboratory from 1989 to 1998, after which he ran for the House and won. Many people point out the double sadness that he is one of only a dozen PhDs in Congress, and the only Quaker. More to the point, he has been both a working scientist and a working representative; he actually knows both fields professionally. So does Republican representative Vern Ehlers of Michigan, and Democratic representative Nancy Boyda of Kansas. Needed are people who can straddle the two realms, people with experience as working scientists and as public representatives; American society can do better than to furnish fewer than a handful of such people in the House and none at all in the Senate.

Knowing more science can't guarantee that anybody will be a better public servant; nothing can. If a larger number of public servants have science backgrounds, however, it may become harder and harder for those servants, and the Congress as a whole, to ignore the claims—and the political might—of science. It takes a great deal of work to demarginalize a marginalized group, and that is exactly the work facing those who care about bioethics.

KEEP IMPROVING SCIENCE JOURNALISM

SCIENCE JOURNALISM ON the news side has had a Renaissance since the 1970s, when people first realized it had to improve. I am less persuaded by the state of op-eds on science subjects, which strike me as either too credulous, too eagerly consuming partisanized science or conspiring to create it, or just wrong. In print, online, on our TVs and iPods and computers, let there be more discussion that can (a) communicate the science, (b) speculate on what it means, and (c) look ahead to practical outcomes and applications in a calm and informed way. Those are what should drive the debate.

Practical wisdom—what the Greeks called *sophrosyne*—is the hoped-for outcome of the democratic debate. Like science itself, it need be neither Republican nor Democratic. If scientists and citizens well informed about bioethics do not accept the challenge to engage in vigorous, conspicuous, constant, deliberative democracy, other parties, as has happened all too often in the last 30 years, will own the issues, drive the debate, and secure or prevent the decisions. And that strikes me as neither practical nor wise.

NOTES

1. I was so entertained by Brooks's column that I ran a gentle rebuttal (Timpane, 2007).

2. The title, "Man vs. Nature," is, as many such titles are, wholly misleading. Climate change, to whatever degree it may exist, reflects the use of nature by human beings, not some age-old struggle between opponents. Stossel's title also implies that somehow nature is posed against us, that it won't give us what we're looking for—when we exist firmly within nature and express all its laws. It's everything we've got. Industrialization is a triumph of both humanity and nature.

3. We find the Associated Press leading with the phrase in an article from March 2002: "Infertile couples shouldn't be deterred by new studies that show test-tube babies have double the risk of birth defects and tend to be smaller than usual, researchers said." And we can trust pop media to say almost anything to grab a few eyes, as in Lisa Habib (2006). The first half of Habib's title, "Test Tube Babies," trots out the fallacious phrase, then pulls it back in after the colon with the more generalized "assisted reproduction." This move, as far as I am concerned, is a kind of lie, a tacit pretense that one may fairly equate the two. One should not and cannot.

4. Good ethical overviews were available comparatively early, as in David Devore (1992). As for the energetic effort by politicized advocates to "get out in front of" the issue, see remarks by O. Carter Snead (2005), general counsel to President Bush's Council on Bioethics, in remarks posted on the Web site for the Center for Genetics and Society. The effort to "get out in front" of an "issue" is a clear sign that some groups already see it as a partisan issue.

5. Coined—at least, as a label for genetically modified foods—in a June 2, 1992, letter to the editor of the *New York Times* by Paul Lewis of Newton Center, MA. He was referring to genetically altered tomatoes: "Ever since Mary Shelley's baron rolled his improved human out of the lab, scientists have been bringing just such good things to life. If they want to sell us Frankenfood, perhaps it's time to gather the villagers, light some torches and head to the castle" (http://www.wordspy.com/words/Frankenfood.asp).

6. This practice is illegal, as of this writing, in the United States, but a research team in the United Kingdom was recently granted a license to create a human-bovine embryo with only a slight amount of bovine genetic material (http://www.telegraph.co.uk/core/Content/displayPrintable.jhtml;jsessi onid=I4WJBDOR35YFVQFIQMGCFFOAVCBQUIV0?xml=/news/2008/01/17/ neggs217.xml&site=5&page=0).

7. The Terri Schiavo case *appeared* to pit the forces of Christian conservatism against the forces of scientific liberalism. While the bioethical issues were real, as were the passions of those who disagreed, the media (I now believe) misreported the case from the start. In the end, it was brought to a close through a pragmatic legal decision that had little to do with the ethics of the matter.

I have rather unexciting news about the Schiavo case: state law held, and state law won. Michael Schiavo made his decision, and Terri Schiavo died. The spectacular wheeling of the great machineries of Congress and the President, in an effort to block the disconnection of the feeding tube…the hectoring of Randall Terry, founder of Operation Rescue, that there would be "hell to pay" for lawmakers if they did not find a way to prevent the removal of the tube…all failed. It was traumatic, and often viscerally tedious…and that is what democracy looks like.

One might say: But this is not an answer to an ethical dilemma. Not in ethical terms, it isn't: agreed. In pragmatic, policy terms, however, it did answer the case of Terri Schiavo. Some accept the way it turned out; some don't. This is—and believe me, I'm not comfortable with it either—the nature of negotiations in a democracy. They often hold at bay inherent conflicts, deny gorillas in the room, fail to resolve the supposedly real question—in favor of an ending. Far too often, people (especially in the academy) speak as if negotiations in the public sphere proceed on principle. Not a whole lot, they don't. Best be prepared for the way they really do proceed.

8. For the importance of prestige in science, see John Timpane (1995). What was truly disheartening about the way the belief versus nonbelief debate, joined by Daniel Dennett (2006), Richard Dawkins (2006), John Allen Paulos (2007), and too many fundamentalist Christian advocates to name, is how each side came to think of itself as entitled to a shrill, exclusivist rhetoric. When they seemed to be aware (sadly intermittently) of this huge rhetorical mistake (and it is a terrible beginner's error, especially if they wish to persuade people), they justified their tone in exactly the same way as their putative religious opponents did: by claiming their point of view had been marginalized. These were people all too accustomed to the way science discussions sometimes proceed (through hectoring and other lovely means). It's not that I either agree or disagree with their arguments. My only advice, to any scientists willing to engage in truly democratic deliberative debate: don't do what these writers did.

REFERENCES

Brooks, D. (2007, February 18). Human nature redux. *New York Times*. Retrieved August 22, 2008, from http://select.nytimes.com/2007/02/18/opinion/18brooks.html?_r=1&scp=2&sq=Brooks+epigenetic&st=nyt&oref=slogin

Dawkins, R. (2006). *The god delusion*. New York: Houghton Mifflin.

Dennett, D. (2006). *Breaking the spell: Religion as a natural phenomenon*. New York: Viking.

Devore, D. (1992). *Genetic screening and ethics: An overview*. Woodrow Wilson Biology Institute. Retrieved June 29, 2008, from http://www.woodrow. org/teachers/bi/1992/gen_screen1.html

Didion, J. (2005, June 9). The case of Theresa Schiavo, *New York Review of Books*. Retrieved August 22, 2008, from http://www.nybooks.com/articles/18050

Habib, L. (2006, June 22). Test tube babies: 3 million born by assisted reproduction. *FoxNews.com*. Retrieved July 17, 2008, from http://www.foxnews. com/story/0,2933,200631,00.html

Hentoff, N. (2005, March 25). Terri Schiavo: Judicial murder. *Village Voice*. Retrieved July 24, 2008, from http://www.villagevoice.com/news/0513, hentoff,62489,6.html

Kitzmiller et al. vs. Dover School Board et al. (2005). *Decision of the court*. Retrieved August 22, 2008, from http://www.pamd.uscourts.gov/kitz miller/kitzmiller_342.pdf

Paulos, J. A. (2007). *Irreligion: A mathematician explains why the arguments for God just don't add up*. New York: Hill and Wang.

Schnieder, B., & Lin, C. (2005, March 25). Schnieder: Schiavo case "'being made very political." [Transcript.] *On the Scene*. CNN. Retrieved May 20, 2008, from http://www.cnn.com/2005/ALLPOLITICS/03/25/schneider/index. html

Science raises questions: In-vitro fertilization begot more than just babies. *Philadelphia Inquirer*, August 2, 2003.

Snead O. C. (2005). *Roberts v. the future: Genetic screening and the future of personal autonomy*. Retrieved May 12, 2008, from http://geneticsandsoci ety.org/article.php?id=1700

Stossel, J. (2007, October 19). Man vs. nature. *20/20*, ABC. Retrieved December 16, 2007, from http://abcnews.go.com/2020/Stossel/story?id=3751219&page=1

Timpane, J. (1995). How to convince a reluctant scientist. *Scientific American*, *272*(1), 104.

Timpane, J. (2007, February 22). Sure, we're machines—but such machines! *Philadelphia Inquirer*, A15.

Vaccinations and autism: No link exists. (2008, February 9). *Philadelphia Inquirer*, A8.

Yankelovich, D. (1991). *Coming to public judgment: Making democracy work in a complex world*. Syracuse, NY: Syracuse University Press.

6

Health and Disease: Conceptual Perspectives and Ethical Implications

DOMINIC SISTI

THE CONCEPTS OF health and disease are fundamental to conversations about biomedical ethics. When bioethicists talk about end of life care, biomedical research, quality of life, or resource allocation, the words *health* and *disease* are bandied about. It is usually taken for granted that there exists a shared understanding of their meanings. Indeed, at first glance, the meanings of health and disease seem self-evident: health is the absence of disease, while disease is a biological abnormality or malfunction. Perhaps, one might also say that health includes a positive dimension, such as in the World Health Organization's (WHO) definition of "health" as "a state of complete physical, mental and social well-being and not merely the absence of disease or infirmity" (WHO, 1981).

If only things were this simple. Notwithstanding the ease with which we talk about health and disease, these interrelated concepts are philosophically complex and exceptionally ambiguous. If asked, most people would find it difficult to settle on a simple statement about how we should define health and disease. Most people will agree that breast cancer and HIV/AIDS should count as diseases. Others might raise their eyebrows when asked about attention deficit hyperactivity disorder (ADHD) or restless leg syndrome.

Why the ambivalence? Are the concepts of health and disease so amorphous that they are completely subjective? Is it possible to determine biological standards and an objective method for determining what constitutes health and disease? Should the concept of disease be limited to biological abnormalities or deviations in species-typical functioning? And, if so, what *is* normal? These questions suggest that the concepts of health and disease are moving targets—as they pass in and out of our conceptual sights they become impossible to pin down.

This chapter has two goals. First, it presents in very broad strokes some of the recent philosophical work that has sought to define more clearly the concepts of health and disease. We will see a basic tension resulting from an epistemic question concerning the role of values: is our knowledge and classification of disease value-free and biologically based or is it value-laden and socially constructed? Second, it argues that a more robust philosophical understanding of the concepts of health and disease is necessary for several ethically important purposes. The way in which we understand the concepts of health and disease will have important implications in addressing ethical issues arising at the bedside and in the corporate boardroom, from the laboratory to the floor of Congress. Ultimately, bioethical analysis will be impoverished without a robust philosophical understanding of the concepts of health and disease.

THE CENTRAL PHILOSOPHICAL DEBATE

CONTEMPORARY PHILOSOPHICAL PERSPECTIVES about the concepts of health and disease generally fall into one of two categories: naturalism and normativism. Naturalists argue that health and disease can be understood and described in natural or biological terms, while normativists claim that health and disease are value-laden concepts that reflect social ideals and norms.

THE NATURALIST PERSPECTIVE

BOORSE IS THE most often cited and paradigmatic of the naturalists. Boorse claims that the concept of disease is grounded in the "value-free" and "autonomous framework of medical theory, a body of doctrine that describes the functioning of a healthy body [and] classifies various deviations from such functioning as diseases" (Boorse, 1981,

61

*Health and
Disease:
Conceptual
Perspectives
and Ethical
Implications*

p. 550). Boorse describes how organ systems function according to the way in which evolution has designed them to work and argues that deviations or deficiencies in this function constitute a disease. For Boorse and other naturalists, the concept of health is value-free. To describe an individual as healthy is to assess an individual's function in comparison to the rest of his or her species. Thus, species-typical functioning grounds the naturalists' concepts of health and disease. Health is defined as the capacity of an organism to achieve evolutionarily determined goals (i.e., survive, reproduce, enhance fitness through kin selection, etc.). Thus, one of the attractive features of Boorse's theory is that it dovetails nicely with evolutionary theory (Nordenfelt, 2007).

THE NORMATIVIST PERSPECTIVE

AS WE MIGHT expect, some scholars in philosophy, sociology, and history of medicine have been skeptical about Boorse's theory. Despite his account, the history of medicine is rife with examples of value-laden conceptualizations of disease, leading many people to the normativist perspective: namely, that the concept of disease is inextricably entwined with sociopolitical power and ideology. For an obvious example we need only recall drapetomania, the antebellum pseudodisease characterized by Dr. Samuel Cartwright as the tendency of slaves to run away (Cartwright, 2004). Similarly, examinations into the medicalization of premenstrual syndrome, menopause, masturbation, attention deficit disorder, and so-called child abuse syndrome reveal the role of social and political values and, more importantly, of the power of the medical professions to determine what counts as normal or pathological (Conrad, 2004; Engelhardt, 1974; McCrea, 2004; Pfohl, 1977; Richardson, 2004).

Naturalists would object by claiming that drapetomania and similar historical examples do not provide evidence that disease is a value-laden concept; rather, these are cases in which the correct objective concept of disease was simply misapplied. Ironically, these diseases might support the naturalist position, since our recognition of pseudo-diseases seems to reflect an objective set of criteria that expose the absurdity of examples like drapetomania.

In any case, an ongoing debate between normativism and naturalism continues and is most obvious in psychiatry. Early on, Foucault's genealogical analysis of madness exposed the power and social dynamics from which particular forms of mental illness were objectified (Foucault, 1965). Szasz's decades-long refusal to accept mental illness as anything but a myth licensing clinicians to intervene to adjust nonconformist behavior is an example of strong normativism or social constructionism in psychiatry (Szasz, 1960, 1961).

Engelhardt offers a moderate normative analysis, which clearly rec-ognizes the roles played by social values, religion, and law in construct-ing medical realities such as diseases (Engelhardt, 1996). Other forms of normativism take a different tack by describing diseases in terms of disorders in the integrity of the body or mind that inhibit so-called prudential functions (i.e., those things that matter to attaining pru-dential values such as the avoidance of pain, death, and security) or that diminish a person's ability to achieve vital goals (Margolis, 1981; Nordenfelt, 2007).

More recently, feminist philosophers have expressed deep suspi-cions about the medicalization of various aspects of women's lived ex-periences. Sherwin (1992) argues that the concepts of health and disease emerge from a power structure that is both insidiously and outwardly sexist. In the cases of menopause and premenstrual syndrome (PMS), supposedly natural female deference is disrupted by hormonal imbal-ances. In cases of personality disorders, such as borderline or histrionic, we find marked deficiencies in the functional status of a stable, rational, and unified concept of the self as idealized by Kant and other Enlight-enment philosophers (Wirth-Cauchon, 2001). The assumption that the female self is unstable has served as the basis for the invention of other mental illnesses like kleptomania by offering a way to explain deviant behavior by well-to-do middle-class women (Abelson, 1989). The upshot, feminist philosophers argue, is that psychiatric categories place women in a double bind, where attaining health is only possible through def-erence to (male) authority and a medical diagnosis is bestowed upon those women who do not conform (Frye, 1983; Sherwin, 1992).

Along similar lines, disability scholars have clarified the distinction between the social and biological models of disability—a distinction that is the analog of the normativist-naturalist split in philosophy of medicine. Activist scholars reject purely naturalistic accounts of dis-ability, claiming instead that disability is a social construction that marginalizes people whose bodies or minds do not meet the stan-dards of the status quo. They claim the biomedical model of disability is so pervasive it has led to what Amundson calls the standard view: the idea that being disabled is a biological deficiency that is obviously bad for one's quality of life (Amundson, 2005). This view is also en-trenched in philosophical literature on quality of life and, as we will see, drives the prioritization of social and health policy. Interestingly, however, empirical evidence has exposed the paralogism of the stan-dard view: disabled people feel their quality of life is only slightly less than nondisabled people, and it is much higher than what nondisabled people would have ever guessed (Amundson, 2005, pp. 102–105). This revelation lends credence to the social constructionists' call for accom-modation and acceptance of the full range of human ability.

63

*Health and
Disease:
Conceptual
Perspectives
and Ethical
Implications*

MODERATE OR HYBRID POSITIONS

BETWEEN THE NORMATIVIST and naturalist positions lies an ensemble of moderate or hybrid positions. Wakefield has developed a moderate form of naturalism in his hybrid account of disorder, particularly in relation to mental illness. He tries, in his own ambitious words, "to construct a more adequate analysis and to resolve the fact/value debate" vis-à-vis the concepts of health and disease (Wakefield, 1992, p. 374). To do this, Wakefield offers his two-part concept of harmful dysfunction used to determine a disorder. He begins by describing function in a very specific medical sense. He states, "Function and dysfunction in the medical sense refer, in the first instance, not to the quality of a person's performance in a given environment but to whether mechanisms within the person are performing or failing to perform functions they were designed to perform" (Wakefield, 2000, p. 20). In much the same way as Boorse, Wakefield claims that biological functions are completely value neutral, while the degree to which these dysfunctions are harmful include normative and value-based judgments. Once a dysfunction is considered harmful, it is called a disorder. In other words, healthy cells, tissues, organs, and systems perform a function determined by evolution, which when disrupted and determined to be harmful, can be described as a disorder.

To bridge the gap between normativism and naturalism, Caplan argues that we can apply a set of very general criteria to determine whether a bodily or psychological state counts as a disease (Caplan, 2004). His criteria require that we consider whether the particular state causes suffering, determine its root cause, provide evidence of structural change (macro- or microscopic), and observe clinical symptoms and impairment in function or behavior. Caplan claims that, in the end, any analysis of health and disease turn on these basic criteria, and thus the conceptual dichotomy between normativism and naturalism can be reconciled.

In contrast, Ereshefsky (n.d.) claims that no consensus can be reached because normativism, naturalism, and hybrid models are all ultimately incoherent and the current debate is not productive. He suggests jettisoning the normativism-naturalism distinction altogether and looks instead to so-called state descriptions (objective physiological measurements) and normative claims (a claim that the state is good or bad for a person). Instead of defining health and disease in naturalistic or normative terms, state descriptions and normative claims provide more conceptual promise because they pinpoint the phenomena in question and provide an account of whether it is valuable or not.

From this brief conceptual overview of health and disease we can see that a continuum of philosophical positions exists and that the concepts are not as self-evident as might be first imagined. Let us now consider why and how continued philosophical analysis of the concepts of health and disease is ethically important.

THE BIOETHICAL IMPLICATIONS OF THE CONCEPTS OF HEALTH AND DISEASE

W E SHOULD NOW ask: what's at stake in the philosophical debate about the concepts of health and disease? Does a deeper analysis of these fundamental concepts provide us with anything other than more questions to answer? Can we not go on with our current concepts in hand, muddling through debates about disease categories on an ad hoc basis? It is certainly true that medicine is not the only discipline "saddled with fuzzy-edge concepts" (Caplan, 2004, p. 124). Legal theorists, for example, continue to debate basic concepts of jurisprudence and political philosophy. But just as there are sometimes profound consequences when philosophical concepts are brought to bear in constitutional law, there are similarly far-reaching effects when the concepts of health and disease are critically examined or when they are haphazardly overlooked for the sake of expedience. There are at least three ethically important and interdependent reasons to continue (and to intensify) the philosophical analysis of the concepts of health and disease.

First, conceptual clarification is necessary to determine social roles and appropriate accommodations for sick or disabled people. As Parsons (1951) described, one function of medicine in society is to sanction certain forms of deviant behavior as provisionally acceptable, as they carry with them new roles and responsibilities for the patient. This is to say, when a person is deemed to be sick, they are relieved of certain social responsibilities while they take on new responsibilities (e.g., comply with a treatment plan to get better). Thus, it is necessary to know what counts as a disease before a person can take on the sick role and societal resources can be deployed on behalf of that person. This point is obvious when we consider debates concerning worker disability and remuneration, insurance coverage and entitlement packages, or reasonable accommodations for the mentally ill or disabled.

This first concern grades into our second: a clearer understanding of the concepts of health and disease is necessary to appropriately demarcate the boundaries between so-called problems of life and legitimate medical problems. It is true that there is no bright line here; both kinds of problems commingle. But without critical analysis of which problems are which and how important social institutions are related to and influenced by medicine, we run the risk of medical experts

65

*Health and
Disease:
Conceptual
Perspectives
and Ethical
Implications*

exerting too much power over what some would argue are essentially lifestyle choices or individual idiosyncrasies. This concern is what ultimately lies behind many of the aforementioned normativist theories.

Third, health care allocation decisions demand a clear understanding of what counts as disease, what our ideal of health is and what ideal we as a society ought to be striving toward. We can see how differing perspectives on the concept of disease result in very different models of just allocation of health care resources. For example, Daniels's Rawlsian model of health care justice relies on the naturalist core of species-typical functioning (Daniels, 1985). For Daniels, "the central function of healthcare is to maintain normal functioning" such that equality of opportunity is safeguarded (Daniels, 2001, p. 2). Thus, policy recommendations that presuppose this kind of biological objectivity would allow for coverage of growth hormone in short children, where there is biological abnormality, but not in short children who are otherwise normal.

Clearly, such a model will meet with a variety of objections such as the question of determining the root cause of short stature (i.e., ought not pedigree be as important as an endocrine abnormality?). Likewise, another objection turns on the fact that disease-centric models of medical coverage miss the point. Short stature diminishes opportunity, no matter its cause, so a coherent policy must aim to correct this potential injustice. In contrast, a more positive account of health—similar to the WHO definition—would demand much more of governments and health care providers. The basic point here is that different theories of health will yield very different policy results.

Indeed, the conceptual pastiche of the meanings of health and disease is evident across the fragmented world of contemporary health care. When a physician worries about the quality of life outcomes of a particular medical intervention, she employs a particular ideal of health. When a pharmaceutical detailer pitches a new erectile dysfunction remedy, he relies on a specific standard of normalcy. When a patient-to-be crafts an advance directive refusing life-sustaining treatment, she envisions a subjective state of intolerable unhealthiness. When politicians attempt to formulate policies around mental health care parity, they either question or endorse the legitimacy of particular disease categories. In each context, the concepts of health and disease might be employed in very different ways for very different purposes.

CONCLUSION

WE SEE THAT the concepts of health and disease are as ethically fraught as they are conceptually slippery. Moreover, as our knowledge about the biological bases of physical and mental illnesses grows, our concepts of disease and health will continue to shift. Likewise, as the line between treatment and enhancement continues to blur, our notions about what is normal and healthy and what is abnormal and unhealthy will continue to become muddled. Thus, continuing to examine the complexities of the concepts of health and disease is an imperative for bioethics if we are to make any ethical sense of coming issues. As Pellegrino (2004) has suggested, "clarification of medicine's basic concepts is as much a moral as an intellectual obligation...confusion about the nature of health and disease is ultimately confusion about the concept of medicine itself" (p. xii).

REFERENCES

Abelson, E. S. (1989). The invention of kleptomania. *Signs, 15*(1), 123–143.

Amundson, R. (2005). Disability, ideology, and quality of life: A bias in biomedical ethics. In D. T. Wasserman, R. S. Wachbroit, & J. E. Bickenbach (Eds.), *Quality of life and human difference* (pp. 101–124). New York: Cambridge University Press.

Boorse, C. (1981). On the distinction between disease and illness. In A. L. Caplan, H. T. Engelhardt, & J. J. McCartney (Eds.), *Concepts of health and disease: Interdisciplinary perspectives* (pp. 545–560). Reading, MA: Addison-Wesley.

Caplan, A. L. (2004). The "unnaturalness" of aging—Give me reason to live!" In A. L. Caplan, J. J. McCartney, & D. A. Sisti (Eds.), *Health, disease, and illness: Concepts in medicine* (pp. 117–127). Washington, DC: Georgetown University Press.

Cartwright, S. (2004). Report on the diseases and physical peculiarities of the negro race. In A. L. Caplan, J. J. McCartney, & D. A. Sisti (Eds.), *Health, disease, and illness: Concepts in medicine* (pp. 28–39). Washington, DC: Georgetown University Press.

Conrad, P. (2004). The discovery of hyperkinesis: Notes on the medicalization of deviant behavior. In A. L. Caplan, J. J. McCartney, & D. A. Sisti (Eds.), *Health, disease, and illness: Concepts in medicine* (pp. 153–162). Washington, DC: Georgetown University Press.

Daniels, N. (1985). *Just health care*. New York: Cambridge University Press.

Daniels, N. (2001). Justice, health, and healthcare. *American Journal of Bioethics, 1*(2), 2–16.

Engelhardt, H. T. (1974). The disease of masturbation: Values and the concept of disease. *Bulletin of the History of Medicine, 48*(2), 234–248.

Engelhardt, H. T. (1996). *The foundations of bioethics* (2nd ed.). New York: Oxford University Press.

Ereshefsky, M. (n.d.). *Defining "health" and "disease."* Retrieved January 2008, from http://www.ucalgary.ca/~ereshefs/

67

*Health and
Disease:
Conceptual
Perspectives
and Ethical
Implications*

Foucault, M. (1965). *Madness and civilization: A history of insanity in the age of reason*. New York: Random House.

Frye, M. (1983). *The politics of reality: Essays in feminist theory*. Freedom, CA: Crossing Press.

Margolis, J. (1981). The concept of disease. In A. L Caplan, H. T. Engelhardt, & J. J. McCartney (Eds.), *Concepts of health and disease: Interdisciplinary perspectives* (pp. 561–578). Reading, MA: Addison-Wesley.

McCrea, F. (2004). The politics of menopause: The discovery of a "deficiency" disease. In A. L. Caplan, J. J. McCartney, & D. A. Sisti (Eds.), *Health, disease, and illness: Concepts in medicine* (pp. 187–200). Washington, DC: Georgetown University Press.

Nordenfelt, L. (2007). The concepts of health and illness revisited. *Medicine, Health Care and Philosophy, 10*, 5–10.

Parsons, T. (1951). *The social system*. New York: Free Press.

Pellegrino, E. (2004). Foreword: Renewing medicine's basic concepts. In A. L. Caplan, J. J. McCartney, & D. A. Sisti (Eds.) *Health, disease, and illness: Concepts in medicine* (pp. xi–xiv). Washington, DC: Georgetown University Press.

Pfohl, S. J. (1977). The "discovery" of child abuse. *Social Problems, 24*(3), 310–323.

Richardson, J. (2004). The premenstrual syndrome: A brief history. In A. L. Caplan, J. J. McCartney, & D. A. Sisti (Eds.), *Health, disease, and illness: Concepts in medicine* (pp. 176–186). Washington, DC: Georgetown University Press.

Sherwin, S. (1992). *No longer patient: Feminist ethics and health care*. Philadelphia: Temple University Press.

Szasz, T. (1960). The myth of mental illness. *American Psychologist, 15*, 113–118.

Szasz, T. (1961). *The myth of mental illness: Foundations of a theory of personal conduct*. New York: Paul B. Hoeber.

Wakefield, J. C. (1992). The concept of mental disorder: On the boundary between biological facts and social values. *American Psychologist, 47*(3), 373–388.

Wakefield, J. C. (2000). Aristotle as sociobiologist: The "function of a human being argument, black box essentialism, and the concept of mental disorder." *Philosophy, Psychiatry, and Psychology, 7*(1), 17–44.

Wirth-Cauchon, J. (2001). *Women and borderline personality disorder: Symptoms and stories*. New Brunswick, NJ: Rutgers University Press.

World Health Organization. (1981). Constitution of the World Health Organization. In A. L Caplan, H. T. Engelhardt, & J. J. McCartney (Eds.), *Concepts of health and disease: Interdisciplinary perspectives* (pp. 83–84). Reading, MA: Addison-Wesley.

Part II

Emerging Issues: Neuroethics and Nanoethics

7

Neuroethics

Martha J. Farah

THE INTELLECTUAL SCOPE of neuroethics is broad, intersecting with many fields. There are familiar bioethical issues, which pertain to the brain as well as other organ systems and for which the existing bioethics literature offers helpful guidance. There are also issues that arise uniquely in connection with the brain, because it is the organ of the mind, and which are responsible for the coining of a new term, *neuroethics*. Both types of issues will be reviewed in this chapter. The second set of issues, which are unique to neuroethics, include the social and ethical implications of brain imaging, psychopharmacology, brain stimulation, and brain-machine interfaces, as well as the ways in which our advancing understanding of mind-brain relations calls into question basic assumptions about what it means to be a person.

FAMILIAR BIOETHICAL ISSUES IN NEUROETHICS

THE ISSUES TO be reviewed in this section involve neuroscience, but the ethical issues are not fundamentally different from those arising in other branches of life science. That is, although the brain is central to these issues, from an ethical perspective its role is not substantially different from that played by other organ systems in analogous situations. A few examples will be reviewed here.

The development of predictive tests for incurable neurodegenerative diseases has raised ethical concerns. For example, research on vulnerability to Alzheimer's disease, mechanisms of disease onset, and treatment response relies in part on functional neuroimaging, especially positron emission tomography (PET) scanning, to measure brain function more sensitively than is possible with the more conventional behavioral tests of clinical dementia research. Almost inevitably, this research has revealed neuroimaging correlates of incipient Alzheimer's disease, which in some cases may herald the clinical onset several years in advance. With the enthusiastic backing of PET scanner manufacturers, the medical community has been encouraged to consider the use of this method as a diagnostic test to be used for differential diagnosis of patients already showing signs of cognitive decline. In 2004 the U.S. government agreed to provide Medicare reimbursement for such scans under specific circumstances.

No one has yet proposed scanning seemingly healthy elderly individuals to predict future disease or mental status, but one can imagine numerous motivations for doing so. For insurance companies, personnel departments, and even the individual him- or herself, prediction of Alzheimer's disease would allow for more rational planning for the future. Of course, this added planning capability comes at a price. The knowledge that one is bound to develop Alzheimer's disease is a terrible burden, particularly because there is no cure. Although this dilemma results from recent advances in neuroscience, relevant ethical analyses have been developed by bioethicists working on the implications of genetic testing (Bell, 1998). The main ethical concerns, including privacy rights (should your insurance company or boss know the test results?) and quality of life concerns (what are the effects on patient well-being of knowing versus not knowing?) are common to genetic and neuroimaging-based prediction.

Another important ethical issue is the safety of newly developed research methods in neuroscience. One such method is transcranial magnetic stimulation (TMS), which alters brain function using powerful magnetic fields. It is noninvasive in the sense that the magnet remains outside the head, but the magnetic fields pass through the skull and other tissue and induce electrical currents in cortical tissue. For some applications a single pulse (onset followed by offset of magnetic field) is used, but more commonly repetitive pulses are used (rTMS). The effects of TMS vary according to where the field is focused, its strength, and its pulse frequency and can either increase or decrease cortical activity near the stimulation site as well as in other brain regions to which the stimulated area projects.

The ability to target specific brain areas for temporary activation or deactivation makes TMS a valuable research tool, and cognitive neuroscientists have embraced it. The impressive ability of TMS to bring about scientifically informative brain changes raises the question: What other kinds of brain changes does it cause? Concern about the side effects of TMS, especially rTMS, has accompanied its use from the start. We now know that high-frequency, high-intensity rTMS can provoke seizures, even in people with no seizure history, although guidelines developed in the 1990s have largely eliminated this phenomenon (Wassermann, 1997). Is TMS safe enough to be used therapeutically? Is it safe enough to be used as a research method with healthy people who have nothing to gain from the procedure? Is short-term safety a sufficient criterion, or are long-term follow-up studies needed? And who should decide? These are important ethical questions about TMS of the human brain, but they are not substantially different from the kinds of questions we would ask about any new biomedical research method for studying any aspect of human physiology.

A more widely used application of magnetism in neuroscience is functional magnetic resonance imaging (fMRI). This has been the workhorse of cognitive neuroscience research since the 1990s, thanks to its ability to measure brain activity with a useful degree of spatial and temporal resolution, without the need for radioactive tracers or injected contrast media. Most current research involves placing the human subject in a magnetic field of strength 1.5 or 3 Tesla (i.e., units measuring magnetic flux density), and all indications are that this is safe. Until recently, technical limitations prevented the use of stronger fields; they could be created only across spaces too small to accommodate a human head. However, it is now possible to scan humans at 7 Tesla and higher.

Strong static magnetic fields can affect blood pressure, cardiac function, and neural activity. In addition, image acquisition with MRI involves exposure to varying magnetic fields and radio frequency fields, which pose risks that range from activation of nerves and muscles to heating of tissue. Subjects in high-field scanners sometimes report seeing lights as a result of induced currents in their retina and/or optic nerve. Although safety studies have suggested that such effects are benign, little is known about the long-term effects of these newer and more powerful scanning protocols.

As with TMS, high-field MRI raises important questions about the risks to which we put human research subjects. How thoroughly should such methods be tested for safety before they are used in research with humans? Who should decide? These are important ethical questions that must be addressed as researchers push the envelope of brain fMRI, but they are not substantially different from questions regarding the safety of new methods for studying any other part of the body. Although high-field scanning is mainly of interest in the study of brain function, as opposed to other body parts, the ethical issues it poses are not fundamentally different from the ethical issues surrounding any new scientific method with potential risks and benefits used in the study of any organ system.

Another ethical issue that arises in connection with fMRI concerns brain abnormalities found by chance in the course of research scanning. fMRI studies generally include a nonfunctional scan of brain structure, to enable localization of the brain activity revealed by fMRI relative to the anatomy of each research subject. The structural scans are of sufficient sensitivity and resolution that anatomical abnormalities and signs of disease will often show up. This raises the question of what researchers should do with these so-called incidental findings. One recent survey found that most researchers had encountered incidental findings, and in a small fraction of these cases the findings led to diagnoses of tumors and other serious neurological conditions (Illes et al., 2004). There is currently no generally accepted procedure for dealing with incidental findings from research scans, or even general agreement on the ethical obligations of the researcher to the subject in these cases. However, the ethical issues raised by incidental findings from brain scans are not fundamentally different from those that would be raised by imaging other organ systems. Indeed, one of the most relevant legal precedents does not come from imaging at all but from testing of blood lead levels. In 2001 a Maryland state appeals court decided that researchers studying the effects of lead abatement should have notified families of children with dangerously high levels of lead in their blood. At stake is the legal and moral obligation of researchers to inform their subjects when a serious medical condition is discovered but not anything specific to brains per se.

The issues just reviewed are the most commonly discussed neuroethical issues that have extensive precedents in bioethics, but they are not the only ones. Most bioethical issues have some intersection with neuroscience. For example, some of the most sought-after applications of stem cell research involve neurological diseases such as Alzheimer's and Parkinson's disease (Goldman, 2005). Future genetic technologies for selecting or altering the traits of a child are likely to include mental traits such as intelligence and personality, which are functions of the brain, as well as other physical traits (Chapman & Frankel, 2003). Arguments for and against abortion have relied on information about fetal brain function (Jones, 2004). Issues of drug industry marketing, regulation, and safety are nowhere more relevant than with drugs for neuropsychiatric illness (Antonuccio, Danton, & McClanahan, 2003), as the chronic nature of such illnesses make treatments more profitable and questions of long-term safety more pressing.

UNIQUELY NEUROETHICAL ISSUES

IN CONTRAST TO the neuroethical issues just reviewed, some ethical issues involving the brain arise specifically because the brain is the organ of the mind. Of course, to say that these neuroethical issues are unique to neuroethics is to invite all good critical readers to begin searching their memory for precedents in mainstream bioethics, and nothing is entirely without precedent if one describes the issues abstractly enough! All I wish to do is emphasize that some neuroethical issues are *relatively* novel and emerge *primarily* because of the very special status of the brain, compared to other organs, in human life.

The issues that fall into this general category include those raised by advances in functional neuroimaging, psychopharmacology, and other ways of modifying brain function. Also included are challenges to our concepts of personhood posed by our growing understanding of the neural bases of behavior, personality, consciousness, and states of spiritual transcendence.

BRAIN IMAGING

THE MAIN CONCERN to be discussed here is not with safety or incidental findings, but with privacy of thought. Unlike imaging other bodily organs, imaging the brain reveals information about the mind. Researchers have found neuroimaging correlates of individual differences in personality and intelligence, which could eventually be applied outside the research lab, for example by employers and marketers. Methods such as fMRI are being adapted for lie detection and behavior prediction, which has attracted attention and funding from the intelligence community and criminal justice agencies. These trends raise new questions about whether, when, and how to ensure the privacy of one's own mind.

One of the most widely discussed new applications of functional neuroimaging is based on correlations between brain activity and intentional deception (e.g., Wolpe, Foster, & Langleben, 2005). Most experts believe that fMRI-based lie detection is not feasible in real-world situations, although a number of different research groups have identified fMRI correlates of intentional deception in laboratory tasks. Among the brain areas most reliably activated in association with lying are the anterior cingulate cortex, which is also typically involved in tasks that evoke cognitive conflict, and prefrontal areas important for holding task contexts in working memory and retrieving long-term memories. This makes sense, in that deception requires making responses that conflict with what the liar knows to be true, and may also require holding the fabricated version of the truth in working memory or retrieving it from long-term memory. Whether deception has a specific brain signature, distinct from other effortful processes involving cognitive conflict and memory, remains to be determined. Nevertheless, two companies have been formed to offer fMRI-based lie detection commercially, Cephos and No Lie MRI.

Brain imaging can also be used to measure correlates of people's desire for certain products, an application that has been called "neuromarketing" (Kenning, Plassman, & Ahlert, 2007). To the extent that neuroimaging can measure unconscious motivation to buy, it provides a valuable new kind of information for marketers.

The use of brain imaging to read mental states has been greatly enhanced by the application of pattern classification techniques developed in a branch of computer science known as machine learning. Conventional image analysis involves spatial smoothing, that is, averaging the signal strength measured in nearby voxels (three-dimensional pixels) to obtain a more reliable measure of the overall level of activity in a region. An alternative approach is to analyze the pattern of variability across voxels in the unsmoothed image. Although some of that variability is noise, some of it is the result of activity in different groups of neurons, and as such it bears information about the state of the brain (Haynes & Rees, 2006).

Brain imaging can also provide information about more enduring mental traits, an application that is in many ways analogous to genetic information. Like genotyping, so-called brainotyping can reveal information about mental health vulnerabilities and predilection for violent crime. Unconscious racial attitudes are manifest in brain activation. Sexual preferences can in principle be determined based on the finding that sexual attraction and even the attempt to suppress feelings of attraction have neuroimaging correlates. A growing body of literature has investigated the neural correlates of personality using brain imaging, including extraversion and neuroticism, risk-aversion, pessimism, persistence, and empathy, and functional imaging correlates have also been found for various aspects of intelligence (Farah, Smith, Gawuga, Lindsell, & Foster, in press).

These capabilities of brain imaging, actual and potential, raise a number of ethical issues. The most obvious concern involves privacy. For example, employers, marketers, and the government all have a strong interest in knowing the abilities, personality, truthfulness, and other mental contents of certain people. This raises the question of whether, when, and how to ensure the privacy of our own minds.

Another ethical problem is that brain scans are often viewed as more accurate and objective than in fact they are (Weisberg, Keil, Goodstein, Rawson, & Gray, 2008). Many layers of signal processing, statistical analysis, and interpretation separate imaged brain activity from the psychological traits and states inferred from it. There is a danger that the public (including judges and juries, employers, insurers, etc.) will ignore these complexities and treat brain images as a kind of indisputable truth.

PSYCHOPHARMACOLOGY

A MONG THE NEW capabilities of neuroscience considered here is the ability to alter people's minds by altering their brain function. Psychopharmacology is the most common method for achieving altered mental function, and it is usually used as therapy for individuals with neuropsychiatric illness. However, it can also be used to change or enhance normal people's cognitive abilities and moods.

Two main cognitive systems have been targeted for pharmacological enhancement: attention and memory. Stimulant drugs such as methyphenidate (Ritalin) and amphetamine (Aderall) improve the attention of people with attention deficit hyperactivity disorder (ADHD) and can also enhance attention in healthy people (Farah et al., 2004). Although these medications are ostensibly prescribed mainly for the treatment of ADHD, surveys suggest that many healthy individuals are using them for enhancement. Prescription stimulants are currently widely used by college students, many of whom obtain it from friends or campus dealers as a recreational drug and study aid (McCabe, Knight, Teter, & Wechsler, 2005).

A huge research effort is now being directed to the development of memory-boosting drugs. The candidate drugs target various stages in the molecular cascade that underlies memory formation, including the initial induction of long-term potentiation and the later stages of memory consolidation. Although this research is aimed at finding treatments for dementia, there is reason to believe that some of the products under development would enhance normal memory as well, particularly in middle and old age, when a degree of increased forgetfulness is normal (Farah et al., 2004).

The weakening of unwanted memories is another type of memory treatment, under development for posttraumatic stress disorder that may cross over to enhancement of healthy individuals. It could conceivably be used psychologically, for example, by soldiers going into battle or rescue workers in a disaster situation (Kolber, 2006).

Peter Kramer first drew society's attention to the growing use of psychopharmacology for enhancing mood. In his book *Listening to Prozac* (1993) he recounted the stories of patients whose depressions were successfully treated with Prozac but who chose to continue taking the drug. They were free of depression, or well, but on the drug they were "better than well." Although Prozac and other SSRI (selective serotonin reuptake inhibitor) antidepressants are not happy pills, they do seem to attenuate negative affect—for example, by reducing the subjectively experienced "hassle factor of life. They also seem to have a subtle but positive influence on the quality of people's social interactions (Knutson et al., 1998).

The ethical issues surrounding enhancement can be grouped into three general categories. The first is safety. Side effects and unintended consequences are a concern with all medications and procedures, but in comparison to other comparably elective treatments such as cosmetic surgery, neuroscience-based enhancement involves intervening in a far more complex system. We are therefore at greater risk of unanticipated problems when we tinker. In addition, drug safety testing does not routinely address long-term use, and relatively little evidence is available on long-term use by healthy subjects.

The second category of ethical issue is social: How will the lives of all individuals, including those who choose not to enhance, be influenced by living in a society with widespread enhancement? In competitive situations such as SAT testing, we may end up needing the equivalent of the regulations surrounding performance-enhancing drugs at sports events. Even in everyday work and school contexts, enhancement is likely to touch all of us. The freedom not to enhance may be difficult to maintain in a society where one's competition is using enhancement to improve attention, memory, or the ability to withstand unsettling experiences. Workers might find themselves pressured to enhance mood by a boss who prefers a cheery workplace. Treatments or enhancements that influence mood or motivation could also conceivably be used for social control. Conversely, barriers such as cost will prevent some people who would like to enhance from doing so. This could exacerbate the disadvantages already faced by people of low socioeconomic status in education and employment.

The third category of ethical issues is more abstract, in that it concerns our values and our sense of self. We generally view self-improvement as a laudable goal. At the same time, improving our natural endowments for traits such as attention span runs the risk of commodifying those traits. We generally encourage innovations that save time and effort, because they enable us to be more productive and to direct our efforts toward potentially more worthy goals. However, when we improve our productivity by taking a pill, there is the concern that we may be undermining the value and dignity of hard work, medicalizing human effort, and pathologizing a normal attention span. Perhaps even more than cognitive enhancement, mood enhancement raises questions about personal identity and authenticity. If we fall in love with some-one who is on Prozac and then find she is difficult and temperamental off the drug, do we conclude we don't love her after all? Then who was it we loved?

BRAIN STIMULATION AND BRAIN PROSTHESES

TWO LINES OF neuroscience research are paving the way for the possibility of electronic brain enhancement. The first is research on brain stimulation, either by implanted electrodes or transcranially, from outside the head. These methods are capable of affecting mood and cognition, and in the future may gain wider use for those purposes in healthy individuals as well as those with neuropsychiatric illness.

As mentioned earlier, TMS involves stimulation of small areas of the brain by magnetic fields generated outside the head. In recent years it has moved from lab to clinic as a means of treating depression (Loo & Mitchell, 2005). It is also being explored with healthy subjects as a means to alter mood and boost creativity, although its efficacy for these pur-poses has not been well established. Transcranial direct current stimu-lation (DCS) is also being explored as a means of modulating brain function. Both types of transcranial stimulation have been shown to en-hance the cognitive performance of normal healthy people in laboratory tasks (Fregni et al., 2005; Kirschen, Davis-Ratner, Jerde, Schraedley-Desmond, & Desmond, 2006). More invasive methods of brain stimu-lation with implanted electrodes are currently last-resort treatments for Parkinson's disease, epilepsy, depression, and obsessive-compulsive disorder. Because they are capable of improving mood and cognitive function in at least some cases, they may eventually gain wider use for those purposes.

The second line of research is on brain-machine interfaces (BMIs). Here the goals are primarily to enable information from the world to be transduced into neural activity and to enable neural activity to be transduced into information that is externally useful for communica-tion or robotic control. Some BMIs are already in clinical use. The most common BMI is the cochlear implant, which transduces sound waves into electrical patterns that can be sensed by auditory neurons in order to restore hearing in some deaf individuals. Systems that take informa-tion in the opposite direction, from brain to world, have been used clinically with paralyzed patients. These systems typically use features of the patient's electroencephalograph (EEG), recorded noninvasively from electrodes on the scalp, to convey simple commands, although some humans have participated in research trials with neural implants (Hochberg et al., 2006).

The full potential of BMIs has only begun to be explored, primarily in research with nonhuman subjects. Memory augmentation, as well as perceptual and motor prostheses, is under study. In addition to the formidable technical challenges of interfacing silicon with sufficient numbers of neurons with sufficient precision and reliability, fundamental scientific problems remain. For example, to converse with the brain we must speak its language. One of the goals of BMI research is to better understand the neural coding of information.

Research on electronic brain enhancement conjures up frightening scenarios involving mind control and new breeds of cyborg. The dominant role of the American military in funding the most cutting edge research in this area does little to allay these worries (Hoag, 2003). In the short term, however, the ethical concerns here are similar to those raised by the pharmacological enhancements discussed previously in this chapter: safety, social effects, and philosophical conundrums involving personhood. Of course, the irreversible nature of some of the nonpharmacological interventions exacerbates these problems. In the long term, humanity may indeed find itself transformed by the incorporation of new technology into our nervous systems (see chapter 9 in this volume).

BRAINS AND PERSONS

KNOWLEDGE OF BRAIN function raises another type of neuroethical issue, forcing us to reexamine our understanding of ourselves as moral agents and spiritual beings. The idea that behavior is determined is hard to reconcile with the intuitive notions of free will and moral agency. Although many people believe that, in principle, human behavior is the physical result of a causally determined chain of biophysical events, most of us also put that aside when making moral judgments. We don't say "but he had no choice—the laws of physics made him do it!" However, as the neuroscience of decision-making and impulse control begins to offer a more detailed and specific account of the physical processes leading to irresponsible or criminal behavior, the amoral deterministic viewpoint will probably gain a stronger hold on our intuitions. Whereas the laws of physics are a little too vague and general to displace the concept of personal responsibility in our minds, our moral judgments might well be moved by a demonstration of subtle damage to prefrontal inhibitory mechanisms wrought by, for example, past drug abuse or childhood neglect. This has already happened to an extent with the so-called disease model of drug abuse (Morse, 2000).

In addition to our assumption that persons have moral agency, our intuitive understanding of persons includes the ideas that they have an essence that persists over time, that they are categorically either alive or dead, and that they have a nonmaterial dimension such as a spirit or soul. Yet none of these fits with the idea that a person is his or her brain (Farah & Heberlein, 2007). As physical objects, brains can and do change in countless ways in response to injury, disease, drugs, and even normal life experience. There is a continuum of levels of brain function between life and death. Finally, as neuroscience reveals progressively more about the physical mechanisms of personality, character, and even sense of spirituality, there is little about a human being left to attribute to an immaterial soul.

CONCLUSION

THE LANDSCAPE OF bioethical issues has changed over the last decade, with the arrival of a large and diverse set of new issues related to neuroscience. These issues include problems with clear precedents in the bioethics, requiring that the solutions to these precedents be adapted and generalized, and they include some more novel problems that arise only in connection with the brain because it is the organ of the mind. These latter problems have the potential for wide social impact, far beyond the health care system or laboratory. Brain enhancement and brain imaging can affect our professional lives, the ways we educate our children, the legal system, and even our understanding of what it means to be a person.

REFERENCES

Antonuccio, D. O., Danton, W. G., & McClanahan, T. M. (2003). Psychology in the prescription era: Building a firewall between marketing and science. *American Psychologist, 58*(12), 1028–1043.

Bell, J. (1998). The new genetics in clinical practice. *British Medical Journal, 316,* 618–620.

Chapman, A. R., & Frankel, M. S. (2003). *Designing our descendants: The promises and perils of genetic modifications.* Baltimore, MD: Johns Hopkins University Press.

Farah, M. J., & Heberlein, A. S. (2007). Personhood and neuroscience: Naturalizing or nihilating? *American Journal of Bioethics—Neuroscience, 7,* 37–48.

Farah, M. J., Illes, J., Cook-Deegan, R., Gardner, H., Kandel, E., King, P., et al. (2004). Neurocognitive enhancement: What can we do? What should we do? *Nature Reviews Neuroscience, 5,* 421–425.

Farah, M. J., Smith, M. E., Gawuga, C., Lindsell, D., & Foster, D. (in press). Brain imaging and brain privacy: A realistic concern? *Journal of Cognitive Neuroscience*.

Fregni, F., Boggio, P. S., Nitsche, M., Bermpohl, F. Antal, F. A., Feredoes, E., et al. (2005). Anodal transcranial direct current stimulation of prefrontal cortex enhances working memory. *Experimental Brain Research, 166,* 23–30.

Goldman, S. (2005). Stem and progenitor cell-based therapy of the human central nervous system. *Nature Biotechnology, 23,* 862–871.

Haynes, J. D., & Rees, G. (2006). Decoding mental states from brain activity in humans. *Nature Reviews Neuroscience, 7*(7), 523–534.

Hoag, H. (2003). Neuroengineering: Remote control. *Nature, 423,* 796–798.

Hochberg, L. R., Serruya, M. D., Friehs, G. M., Mukand, J. A., Saleh, M., Caplan, M., et al. (2006). Neuronal ensemble control of prosthetic devices by a human with tetraplegia. *Nature, 442*(7099), 164–171.

Illes, J., Kirschen, M. P., Edwards. E., Stanford, L. R., Bandettini, P., Cho, M. K., et al. (2004). Incidental findings in brain imaging research. *Science, 311,* 783–784.

Jones, D. G. (2004). The emergence of persons. In M. Jeeves (Ed.), *From cells to souls—and beyond* (pp. 11–33). Grand Rapids, MI: William B. Eerdmans.

Kenning, P., Plassman, H., & Ahlert, D. (2007). Applications of functional magnetic resonance imaging for market research. *Qualitative Market Research: An International Journal, 10*(2), 135–152.

Kirschen, M. P., Davis-Ratner, M. S., Jerde, T. E., Schraedley-Desmond, P., & Desmond, J. E. (2006). Enhancement of phonological memory following transcranial magnetic stimulation (TMS). *Behavioral Neurology, 17*(3–4), 187.

Knutson, B., Wolkowitz, O. M., Cole, S. W., Chan, T., Moore, E. A., Johnson, R. C., et al. (1998). Selective alteration of personality and social behavior by serotonergic intervention. *American Journal of Psychiatry, 155,* 373–379.

Kolber, A. J. (2006). Therapeutic forgetting: The legal and ethical implications of memory dampening. *Vanderbilt Law Review, 59*(5), 1559–1615.

Kramer, P. D. (1993). *Listening to Prozac.* London: Penguin Books.

Loo, C., & Mitchell, P. (2005). A review of the efficacy of transcranial magnetic stimulation (TMS) treatment for depression, and current and future strategies to optimize efficacy. *Journal of Affective Disorders, 88*(3), 255–267.

McCabe, S. E., Knight, J. R., Teter, C. J., & Wechsler, H. (2005). Non-medical use of prescription stimulants among US college students: Prevalence and correlates from a national survey. *Addiction, 100*(1), 96–106.

Morse, S. J. (2000). Hooked on hype: Addiction and responsibility. *Law and Philosophy, 19,* 3–49.

Wassermann, E. M. (1997). Risk and safety of repetitive transcranial magnetic stimulation: Report and suggested guidelines from the International Workshop on the Safety of Repetitive Transcranial Magnetic Stimulation,

June 5–7, 1996. *Electroencephalography and Clinical Neurophysiology, 108,* 1–16.

Weisberg, D. S., Keil, F. C., Goodstein, J., Rawson, E., & Gray, J. R. (2008). The seductive allure of neuroscience explanations. *Journal of Cognitive Neuroscience, 20,* 470–477.

Wolpe, P. R., Foster, K. R., & Langleben, D. D. (2005). Emerging neurotechnologies for lie-detection: Promises and perils. *The American Journal of Bioethics, 5*(2), 39.

8

Is My Mind Mine? Neuroethics and Brain Imaging

PAUL ROOT WOLPE

NEW ETHICAL CHALLENGES can come from many different directions. In bioethics, ethical challenges can arise because of new forms of health care provision, such as managed care; new diseases, such as AIDS; or changing social attitudes, such as those toward sex reassignment surgery. Often, though, the impetus for new ethical challenges in bioethics is new technologies. The advent of dialysis brought new considerations of scarcity and allocation. Artificial ventilation prolonged dying and created new questions about sustaining life at all cost. Genetic technology challenged human limits in manipulating the plasms and molecules of life. And now neurotechnologies have begun changing our ability to understand and manipulate the human brain, raising a host of new questions about what it means to be human, whether and how we should alter human neurological functioning, and who should have access to the inner workings of our minds.

It is the last question that is the topic of this chapter. Because of the recent development of a new set of technologies, we are faced with a thorny set of new ethical questions.

Throughout history, the human mind and its inner workings have been humanity's one impenetrable refuge. No one could see what I was thinking, could feel what I was feeling. Any communication between me and the outside world took place through my peripheral nervous system—through language, through expression, even through the quickening of the heart and the flushing of the skin. Any inner thought, any subjective component of the brain, any aspect of that part of human cogitation that we think of as "mind" was the privileged domain of my individual functioning, unless I chose (consciously or unconsciously, intentionally or unintentionally) to reveal it. And the way I revealed it was through the impulses I sent to my peripheral nervous system.

What was not accessible was the brain itself. Its inner workings were so obscure that for most of history, human beings had little idea of what the brain actually did, never mind how it did it. Uncommunicated thoughts, feelings, ideas, and memories were considered to be accessible only to the individual who had them and, in some cultures, to God. The brain could not itself reveal anything; inside the skull it was inaccessible, and after death it was inert. One exception might have been phrenology, the idea that by measuring the shape of the cranium one could infer the relative sizes of areas of the brain that were believed to correlate with human traits such as intelligence, lustfulness, prudence, or wit. (Sir Francis Gall, the inventor of phrenology was, incidentally, one of the first to believe that the brain was the source of all mental activity.) Even phrenology, however, claimed to be able to detect people's general personality traits only, not the content of their thoughts.

Aside from phrenology and craniometry, which correlated intelligence and other desirable human faculties with the size of one's skull, there was no way to use the brain itself to understand anything about the individual who owned it. And, needless to say, both phrenology and craniometry were discredited by the early 20th century. The brain and its workings remained a mystery, generally inaccessible. And the content of the brain was to be inferred, not experienced, by the scientists and researchers who were trying to understand its workings.

But now that has changed. The first wave of technologies that can peer directly into the skull is here. And in a very short time, these technologies have advanced to the point where they raise some crucial questions that would have seemed fantastic only a short time ago: Who should have access to my thoughts? What are my rights to the workings of my brain? How should technologies that can peer into the brain be used? Can the state or the court demand that a scan expose my innermost thoughts, or is my mind mine?

THE TECHNOLOGY

A GROWING NUMBER of studies have shown that it is possible, using brain imaging, to determine certain kinds of subjective mental experiences. The most common technology used for these studies is fMRI (functional magnetic resonance imaging); in fact, it is not an exaggeration to say that fMRI is the most important internal imaging technology since X-rays. Images created by fMRI represent hemodynamic changes in the brain associated with brain activity. Neurons themselves cannot store energy in any quantity, so when they are firing, energy must be brought in through increased oxygen transfer from the blood. Blood-oxygen-level dependent, or BOLD fMRI, exploits the difference in the magnetic properties of oxygenated and deoxygenated blood, and so gives a map of the areas of the brain that are being used more actively in, for example, a situation at rest versus one where the subject is performing a task. The temporal resolution of fMRI is on the order of 100 milliseconds and the spatial resolution is of 1–2 millimeters, which is much greater than that of other kinds of brain imaging technologies, such as PET (positron emission tomography) and SPECT (single photon emission computed tomography) scanning. As spatial specificity increases with magnetic field strength, and as the next generation of scanners have stronger magnetic fields, optimize magnetic pulse sequencing, and use new techniques such as parallel imaging, the resolution of fMRI will only increase with time (though some of the limitations are due to the functional organization of the brain itself) (see Logothetis, 2008, for an important critique of fMRI study methods).

In addition to its spatiotemporal resolution, fMRI is a good tool for brain research because it is noninvasive—it does not require injecting dyes or tracers in the subject—and it allows the researcher to image the entire brain as the subject engages in tasks. Despite claims to the contrary, however, this ability in no sense allows fMRI to read minds. Still, by being able to identify the areas of the brain that are active during various tasks, we can learn more about what is going on in people's minds than one might guess.

MIND READING

A NUMBER OF studies have demonstrated that, when used creatively, fMRI can tell us something about what is going on in people's brains and thought processes that we would otherwise have no way of knowing.

For example, using fMRI, Kamitani and Tong (2005) could look at a subject's brain and decode which of eight orientations of stripes (e.g., horizontal, vertical, diagonal) a subject had been looking at. Similarly, Haxby et al. (2001) found distinct brain patterns when subjects looked at objects such as faces, cats, man-made objects, and nonsense pictures. In research studies such as these, identification is made by first mapping how the brain responds selectively to those kinds of stimuli, then matching the map to the stimuli later in the research setting. But research has started going even further; Kay, Naselaris, Prenger, and Gallant (2008) have begun to show that by identifying the areas of the brain that respond to space, orientation, and spatial frequency, it soon may be possible to determine what a subject is seeing without previous measurements of brain activity based on those stimuli.

However, the studies are not simply about what people have seen. In her now well-known study, Phelps et al. (2000) showed that White males' cultural evaluation of race correlated with activation of the amygdala, thought to be involved with emotional learning. In that study, researchers showed that White subjects' unconscious attitudes toward race (determined through written questionnaires that contain hidden racial bias scales) correlated with activation of the amygdala when the subjects viewed pictures of unfamiliar Black faces; those who demonstrated greater racial bias on the questionnaire also tended to have more amygdala activation when they looked at Black faces they did not know. Other researchers are looking for correlations between brain function and personality traits, such as Canli's (2004) study showing that test measures of traits such as extroversion and neuroticism are correlated with individual differences in brain activations of specific regions when the subjects were exposed to stimuli such as pictures with different affective content. While it is too early to read too much into such studies, they suggest that at some point we may be able to learn things about people—such as their level of racial bias or their personality traits—by looking directly at their brains.

More recent research seems to show that we can not only (sometimes) tell what people are thinking, but what they are intending. In an important study by Haynes et al. (2007), subjects were given two numbers and told to decide whether or not to add or subtract them, keeping the decision to themselves. A few seconds later, they were shown answers and pointed to either the sum or the difference, according to what they had decided to do. Researchers imaged the brains of the subjects during the interval between their decision and their choice of the number, which revealed what they had decided, and found that they could predict, based on brain patterns in the prefrontal cortex, which way the subject had decided to go. The ability to predict intention, instead of what a person may be thinking about, raises the bar even higher. While this initial research can only predict someone's intention in a particular task executed seconds later, the implications are profound; imagine how desirable it would be for security, forensic, military, or intelligence agencies to be able to predict someone's intentions!

Other examples might be equally attractive to such agencies. Studies have determined the specific areas of the brain used in reading.

The research suggests that we may be able to flash words in various languages in front of a subject and tell whether or not they can read any particular language and even, perhaps, understand it (imagine how much intelligence agencies would want to know whether a suspected spy could read a foreign language, for example; Haller, Klarhoefer, Schwarzbach, Radue, & Indefrey, 2007, Price & Mechelli, 2005). A great deal of work has been done on trying to understand the neural basis of criminal behavior, especially violent behavior. While most of it focuses on structural, not functional, differences between violent offenders and others, so many studies have found correlations between violent offenses and brain dysfunction that a review by Bufkin and Luttrell (2005) concludes: "The consistency with which prefrontal disruption occurs across studies, each of which investigated participants with different types of violent behaviors, suggests that prefrontal dysfunction may underlie a predisposition to violence" (p. 181). One can imagine the temptation of turning that around, of screening children and trying to predict who might be a criminal later by the state of their prefrontal cortex.

Perhaps the most current and controversial technology is the use of brain imaging for lie detection (Wolpe, Foster, & Langleben, 2005). A number of studies have suggested that brain imaging technologies might be an effective technology for determining whether a subject is trying to deceive an investigator, though the application of the research to the real world is still controversial (see, for example, Langleben, 2008). The government has been very interested in developing a reliable lie detection device, and evidence suggests that there are covert efforts by government agencies to work on the technology, including brain imaging for lie detection (Foster, Wolpe, & Caplan, 2003). In the public realm, two companies have already been incorporated to offer brain-imaging lie-detection services to the public, Cephos and No Lie MRI.

Brain imaging research is also being used to try and determine public behaviors such as consumer behaviors and voting patterns. The booming field of neuromarketing tries to determine consumer behavior by looking at the brains of consumers as they think about products or look at advertising (Lee, Brodericka, & Chamberlain, 2007). Neuroscience and brain imaging have also been used to try to determine voters preferences, and a book by Drew Westen (2007), *The Political Brain: The Role of Emotion in Deciding the Fate of the Nation,* which drew on such research, has been credited with playing a prominent role in democratic strategy in the 2008 U.S. presidential election.

Before moving on to the ethical implications of these studies, it is important to emphasize that these studies are in no sense conclusive. Critics have pointed out that many of these studies infer a particular mental state (for example, anxiety) from the activation of a particular brain region (such as the amygdala; Logothetis, 2008; Miller, 2008) and suffer from other methodological problems as well (e.g., see the debate between Haynes, 2008, and Sip, Roepstorff, McGregor, & Frith, 2008). Still, the literature on these technologies is growing rapidly, and some are already moving into the public realm. An examination of the ethical implications of brain imaging and personal privacy is therefore warranted.

ETHICAL CHALLENGES

As long as brain-imaging studies remain in laboratories and academic settings, the ethical issues are not that much different than those arising in the context of other new technologies (though there are a few exceptions; see, for example, Illes et al., 2006, for the problem of finding unanticipated brain tumors and other abnormalities in routine brain imaging studies). The real challenge involves the use of these technologies in military, security, and intelligence settings; in courtrooms and criminal law; and in the public realm, such as by employers. When even scholars have been accused by critics of over-interpreting results (Logothetis, 2008; Miller, 2008), one wonders how rigorous the interpretation will be when this sophisticated technology moves into the public realm.

The first concern is that the technology will be used prematurely. Most studies in the literature are preliminary and suggestive rather than replicated and reliable. Take lie detection, for example. The bulk of published research uses small numbers of subjects, primarily drawn from college and graduate students (who know it is an exercise), and often tests them in unrealistic ways. The technology has not been reliably tested on people with psychopathologies, on con men or others who lie for a living, or on the desperate or those in fear of their lives or freedom. The effects of potential countermeasures against the technology have not been rigorously studied. More fundamentally, we know far too little about the underlying brain mechanisms of deception to have any confidence in what these tests are detecting—or in what they are missing.

In the longer term, the greater threat may be to our personal freedoms. Brain imaging challenges us with a new form of invasion of privacy, potentially stripping a person of the right to refuse to divulge information, the right to say no (Wolpe et al., 2005). The use of brain imaging in jurisprudence raises a host of legal and constitutional questions about such things as definitions of search and seizure, due process, privacy rights, and self-incrimination (Greely & Illes, 2007; Stoller & Wolpe, 2007). At the present time, at least, a patient must co-operate for brain imaging to be used effectively. In the future, how-ever, it is possible that the technology might advance to the point that we can use it coercively, or even covertly. What limits will we set to the right of others to access the workings of our brains, our innermost thoughts, those areas of self that we think of as uniquely personal?

The transitioning of brain imaging from a research technology in the academy to a tool in public life raises a number of practical ques-tions. Who should have access to brain imaging, and under what cir-cumstances? Should courts be able to order a defendant to undergo imaging? Should an employer be allowed to use imaging to screen em-ployees? If a parent comes home and finds the car dented, should he be able to drag his two teenage children to No Lie MRI to try and deter-mine which one loses her allowance?

Who will supervise and oversee such uses of brain imaging? Who will train the technicians, assure quality control, take responsibility for mistakes? What about the problems of false positives and false negatives—how much faith should we put in a lie detection technol-ogy if a person's life or freedom is on the line?

CONCLUSION

AS GENETIC TECHNOLOGIES have become more sophisti-cated and available, ethicists and others have worried about who would have access to genetic information. A person's genetic profile, the argument goes, is a fundamental aspect of their sense of identity, and merits protection. In response, genetic privacy legislation has been passed on the state and federal level. It is now generally accepted that we all have a right to the privacy of our DNA, which is seen, rightly or wrongly, as fundamental to a sense of selfhood and identity.

How much more so is that true for our brains! As Donald Kennedy (2003), former editor of *Science,* put it: "I don't want my insurance com-pany to know my genome. But as for my 'brainome,' I don't want any-body to know it for any purpose whatsoever. It is way too close to who I am."

If the right to privacy means anything, it must include my right to protect the innermost musings of my brain. For the first time in his-tory, that right is being threatened. How we solve the problem of brain imaging's ability to peer into the seat of our souls is one of the thorni-est bioethical issues of the 21st century.

REFERENCES

Bufkin, J. L., & Luttrell, V. R. (2005). Neuroimaging studies of aggressive and violent behavior: Current findings and implications for criminology and criminal justice. *Trauma, Violence, and Abuse, 6*(2), 176–191.

Canli, T. (2004). Functional brain mapping of extraversion and neuroticism: Learning from individual differences in emotion processing. *Journal of Personality, 72*(6), 1105–1132.

Foster, K. R., Wolpe, P. R., & Caplan, A. (2003). Bioethics and the brain. *IEEE Spectrum,* June, 34–39.

Greely, H. T., & Illes, J. (2007). Neuroscience-based lie detection: The urgent need for regulation. *American Journal of Law and Medicine, 33*(2–3), 377–431.

Haller, S., Klarhoefer, M., Schwarzbach, J., Radue, E. W., & Indefrey, P. (2007). Spatial and temporal analysis of fMRI data on word and sentence reading. *European Journal of Neuroscience, 26*(7), 2074–2084.

Haxby, J. V., Gobbini, M. I., Furey, M. L., Ishai, A., Schouten, J. L., & Pietrini, P. (2001). Distributed and overlapping representations of faces and objects in ventral temporal cortex. *Science, 293*(5539), 2425–2430.

Haynes, J. (2008). Detecting deception from neuroimaging signals—a data-driven perspective. *Trends in Cognitive Science, 12*(4), 126–127.

Haynes, J., Sakai, K., Rees, G., Gilbert, S., Frith, C., & Passingham, R. (2007). Reading hidden intentions in the human brain. *Current Biology, 17*(4), 323–328.

Illes, J., Kirschen, M. P., Edwards, E., Stanford, L. R., Bandettini, P., Cho, M., et al. (2006). ETHICS: Incidental findings in brain imaging research. *Science, 311*(5762), 783–784.

Kamitani, Y., & Tong, F. (2005). Decoding the visual and subjective contents of the human brain. *Nature Neuroscience, 8,* 679–685.

Kay, K. N., Naselaris, T., Prenger, R. J., & Gallant, J. L. (2008). Identifying natural images from human brain activity. *Nature, 452*(7185), 352–355.

Kennedy, D. (2003, November). *Neuroethics: An uncertain future.* Program and abstracts of the 33rd Annual Meeting of the American Society for Neuroscience, New Orleans, Louisiana.

Langleben, D. (2008). Detection of deception with fMRI: Are we there yet? *Legal and Criminological Psychology, 13*(1), 1–9.

Lee, N., Brodericka, A. J., & Chamberlain, L. (2007). What is "neuromarketing"? A discussion and agenda for future research. *International Journal of Psychophysiology, 63,* 199–204.

Logothetis, N. K. (2008). What we can do and what we cannot do with fMRI. *Nature, 453,* 869–878.

Miller, G. (2008). Growing pains for fMRI. *Science, 320*(5882), 1412–1414.

Phelps, E. A., O'Connor, K. J., Cunningham, W. A., Funayama, E. S., Gatenby, J. C., Gore, J. C., et al. (2000). Performance on indirect measures of race evaluation predicts amygdala activation. *Journal of Cognitive Neuroscience, 12*(5), 729–738.

93

*Is My Mind Mine?
Neuroethics and
Brain Imaging*

Price, C. J., & Mechelli, A. (2005). Reading and reading disturbance. *Current Opinion in Neurobiology, 15,* 231–238.

Sip, K. E., Roepstorff, A., McGregor, W., & Frith, C. D. (2008). Response to Haynes: There's more to deception than brain activity. *Trends in Cognitive Sciences, 12*(4), 127–128.

Stoller, S. E., & Wolpe, P. R. (2007). Emerging neurotechnologies for lie detection and the Fifth Amendment. *American Journal of Law and Medicine 33,* 3359–3375.

Westen, D. (2007). *The political brain: The role of emotion in deciding the fate of the nation.* New York: Public Affairs.

Wolpe, P. R., Foster, K., & Langleben, D. (2005). Emerging neurotechnologies for lie-detection: Promises and perils. *American Journal of Bioethics, 5*(2), 39–49.

9

Future Minds: Transhumanism, Cognitive Enhancement, and the Nature of Persons

SUSAN SCHNEIDER

TRANSHUMANISM IS A philosophical, cultural, and political movement that holds that the human species is only now in a comparatively early phase and that its very evolution will be altered by developing technologies.[1] Future humans will, in effect, be very unlike their current incarnation in both physical and mental capacities and will be more like certain persons depicted in science fiction novels. Transhumanists share the belief that an outcome in which humans have radically advanced intelligence, near immortality,

Thanks to Vardit Ravitsky and James Hughes for their helpful comments on this chapter.

deep friendships with AI (artificial intelligence) creatures, and elective body characteristics is a very desirable end for both one's own personal development and for the development of our species as a whole. Despite its science fiction–like flavor, the issues that transhumanism presents deserve to be taken seriously because the beginning stages of this radical alteration are supposed to be the outcome of technological developments that are either here, if not generally available, or more commonly, technologies that are accepted by many in the relevant scientific fields as being on their way (Roco & Bainbridge, 2002). In the face of all these technological developments, transhumanists present a thought-provoking and highly controversial progressive bioethics agenda. Transhumanism offers intriguing perspectives on (inter alia) one's conception of the good life, the nature of persons, and the nature of mind.

This chapter will cover the basic tenets of transhumanism and will then discuss what I take to be the most important philosophical element of the transhumanist picture—its unique perspective on the nature and development of persons. Persons are traditionally regarded as being an important moral category, being the bearers of rights (if you believe in such) or at least deserving of consideration in the utilitarian calculus. And, as we shall see, considering the nature of persons through the lens of transhumanism involves pushing up against the boundaries of the very notion of personhood. Consider, for example, the enhancement debate. When one considers whether to enhance in the radical ways the transhumanists advocate, one must ask, "Will this radically enhanced creature still be me?" If not, then, on the reasonable assumption that one key factor in a decision to enhance oneself is one's own personal development, even the most progressive bioethicist will likely regard the enhancement in question as undesirable. For when you choose to enhance in these radical ways, the enhancement does not really enhance *you*. Examining the enhancement issue through the vantage point of the metaphysical problem of personal identity shall thereby present a serious challenge to transhumanism. Indeed, this is a pressing issue for any argument made for or against enhancement.

THE MAIN TENETS OF TRANSHUMANISM

TRANSHUMANISM IS BY no means a monolithic ideology, but it does have an organization and an official declaration. The World Transhumanist Association is an international nonprofit organization that was founded in 1998 by philosophers Nick Bostrom and David Pearce. Its tenets were laid out in the *Transhumanist Declaration* (World Transhumanist Association, 1998) and are reprinted here.

97

Future Minds:
Transhumanism,
Cognitive
Enhancement,
and the Nature
of Persons

The Transhumanist Declaration

1. Humanity will be radically changed by technology in the future. We foresee the feasibility of redesigning the human condition, including such parameters as the inevitability of aging, limitations on human and artificial intellects, unchosen psychology, suffering, and our confinement to the planet earth.

2. Systematic research should be put into understanding these coming developments and their long-term consequences.

3. Transhumanists think that by being generally open and embracing of new technology we have a better chance of turning it to our advantage than if we try to ban or prohibit it.

4. Transhumanists advocate the moral right for those who so wish to use technology to extend their mental and physical (including reproductive) capacities and to improve their control over their own lives. We seek personal growth beyond our current biological limitations.

5. In planning for the future, it is mandatory to take into account the prospect of dramatic progress in technological capabilities. It would be tragic if the potential benefits failed to materialize because of technophobia and unnecessary prohibitions. On the other hand, it would also be tragic if intelligent life went extinct because of some disaster or war involving advanced technologies.

6. We need to create forums where people can rationally debate what needs to be done, and a social order where responsible decisions can be implemented.

7. Transhumanism advocates the well-being of all sentience (whether in artificial intellects, humans, posthumans, or non-human animals) and encompasses many principles of modern humanism. Transhumanism does not support any particular party, politician or political platform.

This document was followed by the much longer and extremely informative *Transhumanist Frequently Asked Questions,* authored by Nick Bostrom, in consultation with dozens of leading transhumanists (Bostrom, 2003b).[2] Because the current chapter is brief and cannot touch on all elements of transhumanism, the reader is strongly encouraged to read this document for a more complete overview of transhumanism.[3]

THE NATURE OF PERSONS

I WILL NOW offer a philosophical analysis of some of the ideas expressed in this declaration. Overall, central transhumanist texts have advanced a sort of trajectory for the personal development of a contemporary human, technology permitting (Kurzweil, 1999, 2005; Bostrom, 2003b, 2005).

21st century unenhanced human → significant "upgrading" with cognitive and other physical enhancements → posthuman status → "superintelligence"

By way of illustration, suppose it is now 2025 and being a technophile, you purchase cognitive and physical enhancements as they become readily available. First, you add a mobile internet connection to your retina, then you enhance your working memory by adding neural circuitry. You are now officially a cyborg. Now skip ahead to 2040. Through nanotechnological therapies/enhancements you are able to extend your lifespan, and as the years progress, you continue to accumulate more far-reaching enhancements. By 2060, after several small but cumulatively significant alterations, you are a posthuman. Posthumans are possible future beings, "whose basic capacities so radically exceed those of present humans as to be no longer unambiguously human by our current standards" (Bostrom, 2003b). Such posthumans can be AI devices, humans who have uploaded their brains onto computers and then enhanced them, or humans who are the result of making many small but cumulatively profound enhancements (Bostrom, 2003b). At this point, your intelligence is enhanced not just in terms of speed of mental processing; you are now able to make profound connections that you were not able to make before. Unenhanced humans, or "naturals," seem to you to be intellectually disabled—you have little in common with them—but as a transhumanist, you are supportive of their right to not enhance (Bostrom, 2003b; Garreau, 2005; Kurzweil, 2005).

It is now 2600. For years, worldwide technological developments, including your own enhancements, have been facilitated by superintelligent AI. Indeed, "creating superintelligence may be the last invention that humans will ever need to make, since superintelligences could themselves take care of further scientific and technological development" (Bostrom, 2003b). And the slow addition of better and better neural circuitry has now resulted in there being no real intellectual difference in kind between you and superintelligent AI—you too are a superintelligence, a creature with "the capacity to radically outperform the best human brains in practically every field, including scientific creativity, general wisdom, and social skills" (Bostrom, 2003b).[4] The only real difference between you and an AI creature of standard design is one of origin—you were once a natural. But you are now almost entirely engineered by technology—you are perhaps more aptly characterized as a member of a rather heterogeneous class of AI life forms (Kurzweil, 2005).

This, then, is a very rough sketch of the developmental trajectory that the transhumanist generally aspires to.[5] Now, let us ask: should you

99

*Future Minds:
Transhumanism,
Cognitive
Enhancement,
and the Nature
of Persons*

embark upon this journey?[6] Here, there are deep philosophical questions that have no easy answers. For in order to understand whether *you* should enhance, you must first understand what you are to begin with. But what is a person? And given your conception of a person, after such radical changes, would you still be you or would you actually bear little relation to the person you were before? And if the latter situation is the case, why would embarking on the path to radical enhancement be something you value? For wouldn't it instead be a path that leads to your own demise, leading you away from your true self, ultimately causing you to cease to exist? In order to make such a decision one needs to understand the metaphysics of personal identity—that is, one needs to answer the question: What is it in virtue of which a self or person is supposed to continue existing over time? A good place to begin is to consider that everyday objects seem to persist over time. Consider the espresso machine in your favorite café. Suppose that five minutes have elapsed and suppose the barista has turned the machine off. Imagine asking the barista if the machine is still the same machine, despite this change. The ordinary answer is that it is of course possible for the machine to continue to be one and the same thing over time. This seems to be a reasonable case of its persistence, even though at least one of the machine's features or properties has changed. On the other hand, if the machine disintegrated or melted, then it would no longer be the same machine. It wouldn't be an espresso machine at all for that matter. So some changes do not cause a thing to cease to exist while others do. Philosophers call features or properties that are essential to a thing or person's nature "essential properties."

Now reconsider the transhumanist's trajectory for enhancement: for radical enhancement to be a worthwhile option for you, it has to represent a desirable form of personal development; at bare minimum, even if enhancement brings such goodies as superhuman intelligence and radical life extension, it must not involve the elimination of one of your essential properties. *For in this case, the sharper mind and fitter body would not be experienced by you—they would be experienced by someone else.* For even if you would like to become superintelligent, knowingly embarking on a path that trades away one or more of your essential properties would be tantamount to suicide—that is, to your intentionally causing yourself to cease to exist. So before you enhance, you had better get a handle on what your essential properties are.

Key transhumanists have grappled with this issue. For instance, Ray Kurzweil asks: "So who am I? Since I am constantly changing, am I just a pattern? What if someone copies that pattern? Am I the original and/or the copy? Perhaps I am this stuff here—that is, the both ordered and chaotic collection of molecules that make up my body and brain" (Kurzweil, 2005, p. 383).

Kurzweil is here referring to two theories at center stage in the age-old philosophical debate about what properties determine the nature of persons. The leading theories are the following:

1. The ego theory—a person's nature is her soul or nonphysical mind, and this mind or soul can survive the death of the body.[7]
2. The psychological continuity theory—you are essentially your memories and ability to reflect on yourself (Locke) and, more generally, your overall psychological configuration, what Kurzweil referred to as your "pattern."[8]
3. Materialism—you are essentially the material that you are made out of—what Kurzweil referred to as "the ordered and chaotic collection of molecules that make up my body and brain" (Kurzweil, 2005, p. 383).
4. The no self view—there is no metaphysical category of person. The "I" is a grammatical fiction (Nietzsche). There are bundles of impressions but no underlying self (Hume). There is no survival because there is no person (Buddha).

Each of these views has its own position about whether to enhance. If you hold (1) then your decision to enhance depends on whether you believe the enhanced body would retain the same soul or immaterial mind.[9] If you believe (3), then any enhancements must not alter your material substrate. In contrast, according to (2), or pattern-ism, enhancements can alter the material substrate but must preserve your memories and your overall psychological configuration. Finally, (4) contrasts sharply with (1)–(3). If you hold (4), then the survival of the person is not an issue, for there is no person to begin with. But you may strive to enhance nonetheless, to the extent that you may find intrinsic value in adding more superintelligence to the universe—you might value life forms with higher forms of consciousness and wish that your closest "continuent" should be such a creature.

Let us focus on identifying which of these conceptions conforms to the transhumanist notion of the self, at least in its most characteristic incarnation. Consider that transhumanists generally adopt a computational theory of mind. That is, the mind is essentially the program running on the hardware of the brain, where by program what is meant is the algorithm that the mind computes, something in principle discoverable by cognitive science.[10] Because, at least in principle, the brain's computational configuration can be preserved in a different medium (i.e., in silicon as opposed to carbon), with the information processing properties of the original neural circuitry preserved, the computationalist rejects the materialist view of the nature of persons.[11] Indeed, as

101

Future Minds:
Transhumanism,
Cognitive
Enhancement,
and the Nature
of Persons

Kurzweil explains, materialism seems to falter in embracing the very idea that you are what you are made up of:

> The specific set of particles that my body and brain comprise are in fact completely different from the atoms and molecules that I comprised only a short while ago. We know that most of our cells are turned over in a matter of weeks, and even our neurons, which persist as distinct cells for a relatively long time, nonetheless change all of their constituent molecules within a month.... I am rather like the pattern that water makes in a stream as it rushes past the rocks in its path. The actual molecules of water change every millisecond, but the pattern persists for hours or even years. (Kurzweil, 2005, p. 383)

Kurzweil calls his view "patternism" (2005, p. 386). Patternism is an updated version of the psychological continuity theory. Put in the language of cognitive science, as the transhumanist surely would, what is essential to you is your computational configuration—for example, what sensory systems/subsystems your brain has (e.g., early vision), the way that the basic sensory subsystems are integrated in association areas, the neural circuitry making up your domain general reasoning, your attentional system, your memories, and so on—overall, the algorithm that the brain computes. I believe that Kurzweil's appeal to patternism is highly typical of the transhumanist. Indeed, consider the appeal to patternism in the following passage of the *Transhumanist Frequently Asked Questions,* which discusses the process of uploading, a process which shall be important to our subsequent discussion.

> Uploading (sometimes called "downloading", "mind uploading" or "brain reconstruction") is the process of transferring an intellect from a biological brain to a computer. One way of doing this might be by first scanning the synaptic structure of a particular brain and then implementing the same computations in an electronic medium.... An upload could have a virtual (simulated) body giving the same sensations and the same possibilities for interaction as a non-simulated body.... And uploads wouldn't have to be confined to virtual reality: they could interact with people on the outside and even rent robot bodies in order to work in or explore physical reality.... Advantages of being an upload would include: Uploads would not be subject to biological senescence. Back-up copies of uploads could be created regularly so that you could be re-booted if something bad happened. (Thus your lifespan would potentially be as long as the universe's.).... Radical cognitive enhancements would likely be easier to implement in an upload than in an organic brain.... *A widely accepted position is that you survive so long as certain information patterns are conserved....* For the continuation of personhood, on this view, it matters little whether you are implemented on

a silicon chip inside a computer or in that gray, cheesy lump inside your skull, assuming both implementations are conscious. (Bostrom, 2003b, emphasis mine)

This is a clear appeal to patternism. And as we shall see, both patternism and the process of uploading introduce philosophical puzzles for the transhumanist case for enhancement. Indeed, they even raise problems with the transhumanist's justification for mild enhancements. As I shall now explain, such problems desperately need to be addressed.

PUZZLES

Now that we've identified the theory of personal identity that the transhumanist generally adopts, let us ask: At the point at which you enhance, being part natural and part artificial, assuming a patternist conception of the nature of persons, are you the same person you were before? Or is there some point in which you cease to exist, becoming a different person entirely? Consider first a mild enhancement—the deletion of a few memories, say, to remove bad chess playing habits and facilitate better chess strategies. Surprisingly, it is not even clear that this enhancement would be compatible with survival, according to patternism. Way back in 1785, Thomas Reid raised the following, now classic, problem for patternism:

> Suppose a brave officer to have been flogged when a boy at school, for robbing an orchard, to have taken a standard (a flag) from the enemy in his first campaign, and to have been made a general in advanced life: suppose also, which must be admitted to be possible, that, when he took the standard, he was conscious of his having been flogged at school, and that when made a general he was conscious of his taking the standard, but had absolutely lost consciousness of his flogging. (Reid, 1785/1941, p. 213)

Reid's example presents a serious challenge to the patternist theory. Identity is transitive: if A = B and B = C then A = C. Patternism holds that the boy is identical to the officer (as the officer has the boy's memory of the flogging) and the officer is identical to the general (as the general was conscious of taking the flag). But notice that patternism cannot say that the boy is identical to the general, as the general does not recall being flogged. Patternism violates the transitivity of identity. This is an abysmal result: Patternism, as it stands, is not really a theory of personal *identity*.

But perhaps the patternist could somehow modify her theory to allow that a gradual change in one's pattern preserves personhood.

103

*Future Minds:
Transhumanism,
Cognitive
Enhancement,
and the Nature
of Persons*

Here the issues grow too complex for a brief chapter, but perhaps, for instance, an understanding of the neurodynamics underlying ordinary cognitive changes could give the transhumanist a route into this problem. An appeal to dynamical systems theory would certainly be in keeping with the cognitive science orientation of transhumanism. On the assumption that people normally survive from moment to moment, we can then propose that certain therapies/enhancements should be safe by patternist standards: enhancements/therapies that modify the brain's dynamical or computational structures in a way that mimics the natural process of change in the brain. Such therapies/enhancements would preserve one's pattern because they would not be a significant departure from the brain's characteristic dynamical patterns.[12]

But notice that the new patternist theory will face the following challenge. In order for the transhumanist to justify the sort of enhancements needed to become a cyborg, a posthuman, or a superintelligent being, she will need to say that radical or unusual changes in existing structures are compatible with the survival of the person. But does patternism really allow for these enhancements? For instance, what about adding an intelligence-enhancing working memory chip so that one can perform better in law school? Would this be too sharp of a break in the existing pattern? Or what about adding a new sense (e.g., echolocation)? It appears that merely appealing to patternism is not enough to justify opting for the neural enhancements that the transhumanist envisions. Transhumanism desperately needs to develop an informative account of personhood. That is, for any theory of personal identity it defends, it needs to say which enhancements are merely changes in nonessential properties and which would be changes in essential ones. In the context of patternism, the extreme cases are clear—a memory erasure process that erased one's childhood is clearly the loss of essential property for the continuity theory because it removes much of one's memories. Mere everyday cellular maintenance by nanobots to overcome the slow effects of aging would, on this view, not affect the identity of the person. The middle-range cases are unclear. Maybe deleting a few bad chess playing habits is kosher, but what about erasing a bad relationship, as in the film *Eternal Sunshine of the Spotless Mind?* The path to superintelligence may very well be a path through middle-range enhancements. Without a firm handle on the personal identity question, the transhumanist developmental trajectory is perhaps the technophile's alluring path to suicide.

But let us press on; let us suppose that the transhumanist can offer a principled means of distinguishing suicide-inducing enhancements (so to speak) from ones compatible with survival. Nonetheless, further problems arise.

Derek Parfit's Teleportation Case

IT'S 2080 AND you are an astronaut. You attend a briefing on your next mission. You've been selected for a secret mission to a far away planet via a new means of travel. Fortunately, your trip will be quick, indeed, much of it will be at the speed of light. NASA superscientists will take a complete scan of your brain—capturing every detail of its computational configuration. Your pattern—that is, you—will be uploaded and sent to the planet, and there your brain will be reconstructed from matter that is configured precisely according to the information from the scan. In the process of scanning, your earthly brain will be destroyed, but that doesn't matter to you. For like Ray Kurzweil, you reject materialism; what is important to you is that your pattern will be safely housed in a supercomputer until, in short order, it will inhabit a new brain and body. You are being temporarily uploaded.[13]

Should you go? If you haven't studied personal identity you might be fooled into thinking you should. But we can quickly see that you wouldn't survive. There may be a person created on the planet, but it is merely your clone. We don't need to appeal to a particular theory of personal identity to see this point—the idea that it would bě you is incoherent. Consider that if the above scenario is possible, then it is also metaphysically possible (i.e., conceivable) that you were not destroyed in the process. But now, in that case, who would be on the planet? It couldn't be you. You are on Earth. And because this person is clearly not you if you weren't destroyed, it follows that it wasn't you if you were. For the life or death of another creature isn't an essential property of a person. Hence, uploading doesn't preserve personhood.

But now transhumanism is in big trouble: your duplicate on the planet has your pattern, precisely. So it must be that even an improved version of (2) is false: sameness of pattern is not sufficient for sameness of person. As a result, transhumanism cannot claim that enhancement is desirable, for its very means of deciding whether it is—its theory of personal identity—is seriously flawed. Further, we can use this result to prove that even mild enhancements are death inducing. Assume your copy on the other planet is not you, as should now be obvious. Now, consider an earlier point in your life at which time, being a good transhumanist, you had a gradual neural regeneration procedure. That is, at each doctor visit, you had 1% of your neurons replaced by silicon-based artificial neurons having the very same computational or formal properties that normally underlie your thoughts.[14] At 100% aren't you analogous to the creature on the planet, being composed of entirely new matter? Given our earlier discussion about this creature, we have reason to believe that this final product is not you. For the creature in the teleportation case was clearly not you but your replica. But, at the

105

*Future Minds:
Transhumanism,
Cognitive
Enhancement,
and the Nature
of Persons*

other end, it seems that if 1% of cells are replaced, it clearly would be you. (After all, as Kurzweil pointed out, this cell replacement process happens to us all the time.) Now, in the cases in between, the person must either be you or a replica. But crucially, which percentage is the critical percentage in which the resulting person would be you, and beyond which, the person is merely a replica? But how could there be one? A few cells couldn't make such a significant difference, could they? Since it is absurd to locate a critical percentage, it must be that there is something deeply wrong with the patternist view of the self.[15]

CONCLUSION

I HOPE ALL this has convinced you that if the transhumanist maintains patternism there are some serious issues that require working out. Indeed, as the *Transhumanist Frequently Asked Questions* indicates, the development of radical enhancements such as brain-machine interfaces, cryogenic freezing for life extension, and uploading to avoid death or simply to facilitate enhancement are key enhancements invoked by the transhumanist view of the development of the person. And, quite ironically, all of these enhancements sound strangely like the thought experiments philosophers have been appealing to for years as problem cases for various theories of the nature of persons. Given that it seems unclear whether sameness of personhood would even be preserved by any of these enhancements, it is fair to say that without further work on this topic, the transhumanist cannot support her case for enhancement. Indeed, the *Transhumanist Frequently Asked Questions* notes that transhumanists are keenly aware that this issue has been neglected:

> While the concept of a soul is not used much in a naturalistic philosophy such as transhumanism, many transhumanists do take an interest in the related problems concerning personal identity (Parfit 1984) and consciousness (Churchland 1988). These problems are being intensely studied by contemporary analytic philosophers, and although some progress has been made, e.g. in Derek Parfit's work on personal identity, they have still not been resolved to general satisfaction. (Bostrom, 2003b, section 5.4)

Our discussion also raises some general lessons for all parties involved in the enhancement debate. For when one considers the enhancement debate through the lens of the metaphysics of personhood, new dimensions of the debate are appreciated. The literature on the nature of persons is a literature that is extraordinarily rich, raising intriguing problems for commonly, and often implicitly, accepted views of the nature of persons that underlie positions on enhancement. And it seems fair to say that when a theory defends or rejects a given enhancement, it is important to determine whether its position on the enhancement in question is truly supported by, or even compatible with, the perspective of the nature of persons that the theory is sympathetic to. Further, the topic of the nature of persons is of clear relevance to the related topics of human nature and human dignity, issues that are currently key points of controversy in debates over enhancement (see, e.g., Bostrom, in press, "Dignity and Enhancement"; Fukuyama, 2002).

Perhaps, alternately, you grow weary of all this metaphysics. You may suspect that social conventions concerning what we commonly consider to be persons are all we have because metaphysical theorizing will never conclusively resolve what persons are. However, as unwieldy as metaphysical issues are, it seems that not all conventions are worthy of acceptance, so one needs a manner of determining which conventions should play an important role in the enhancement debate and which ones should not. And it is hard to accomplish this without getting clear on one's conception of persons. Further, it is difficult to avoid at least implicitly relying on a conception of persons in the context of reflecting on the case for and against enhancement. For what is it that ultimately grounds your decision to enhance or not enhance if not that it will somehow improve who you are? Are you perhaps merely planning for the well-being of your closest continuent?

NOTES

1. Julian Huxley apparently coined the term *transhumanism* in 1957, when he wrote that in the near future "the human species will be on the threshold of a new kind of existence, as different from ours as ours is from that of Peking man" (Huxley, 1957, pp. 13–17).

2. Bostrom is a philosopher at Oxford University who now directs the transhumanist-oriented Future of Humanity Institute there.

3. This document was updated in 2003 and is available at the World Transhumanist Association Web site. In addition, there are a number of excellent philosophical and sociological works that articulate key elements of the transhumanist perspective (e.g., Bostrom, 2005; Hughes, 2004a, n.d.; Kurzweil, 1999, 2005). For extensive Web resources on transhumanism see Nick Bostrom's homepage, Ray Kurzweil's newsgroup (KurzweilAI.net), the Institute for Ethics and Emerging Technologies homepage, and the World Transhumanist Association homepage.

107

Future Minds:
Transhumanism,
Cognitive
Enhancement,
and the Nature
of Persons

4. There are of course numerous nuances to this rough picture. For instance, some transhumanists believe that the move from unenhanced human intelligence to superintelligence will be extremely rapid because we are approaching a singularity, a point at which the creation of superhuman intelligence will result in massive changes in a very short period (e.g., 30 years). (Bostrom, 1998; Kurzweil, 1999, 2005; Vinge, 1993). Other transhumanists hold that technological changes will not be so sudden. These discussions often debate the reliability of Moore's law (Moore, 1965). Another key issue is whether a transition to superintelligence will really occur because the upcoming technological developments involve grave risk. The risks of biotechnology and AI concern transhumanists, progressive bioethicists more generally, as well as bioconservatives (Annis, 2000; Bostrom, 2002a, 2002b; Garreau, 2005; Joy, 2000).

5. It should be noted that transhumanism by no means endorses every sort of enhancement. For example, Nick Bostrom rejects positional enhancements (enhancements primarily employed to increase one's social position) yet argues for enhancements that could allow humans to develop ways of exploring "the larger space of possible modes of being" (2005, p. 11).

6. For mainstream anti-enhancement positions on this question see, for example, Fukuyama (2002), Kass et al. (2003), and Annas (2000).

7. For nice surveys of these four positions see Blackburn (1999) and Olson (2008).

8. See chapter 27 of John Locke's 1694 *Essay Concerning Human Understanding* (note that this chapter first appears in the second edition; it is also reprinted as "Of Identity and Diversity," in Perry, 1975). For other attempts to develop similar views see Quinton (1962) and Grice (1941), both of which are also reprinted in Perry (1975).

9. It should be noted that although a number of bioconservatives seem to uphold the soul theory, the soul theory is not, in and of itself, an anti-enhancement position. For why can't one's soul or immaterial mind inhere in the same body even after radical enhancement?

10. Computational theories of mind can appeal to various computational theories of the format of thought (e.g., connectionism, dynamic systems theory, symbolicism, or some combination thereof). See Kurzweil (2005). For philosophical background see Block (1995) and (Churchland, 1996).

11. This commonly held but controversial view in philosophy of cognitive science is called multiple realizability (Kim, 2006); Bostrom (2003a) calls it "substrate independence."

12. For a nice introduction to issues in dynamical systems theory see Scott Kelso (1997) and Walter Freeman (2000). For a more extensive discussion of the different versions of the memory theory and ways of answering Reid's objection within the metaphysics literature, as well as other objections to the theory, see the various papers in Perry (1975), especially Perry's introduction, which provides a nice overview.

13. This example is modified from a classic paper by Derek Parfit (1987).

14. This case is again inspired by Parfit (1987). Kurzweil considers similar thought experiments in his intriguing discussion of personal identity. Unfortunately, while he notes the problems with patternism, he doesn't offer a resolution (Kurzweil, 2005, pp. 382–387). The *Transhumanist FAQ* actually considers a similar case: "An alternative hypothetical uploading method would proceed more gradually: one neuron could be replaced by an implant or by a simulation in a computer outside of the body. Then another neuron, and so on, until eventually the whole cortex has been replaced and the person's thinking is implemented on entirely artificial hardware" (Bostrom, 2003b).

15. There are numerous ways that the transhumanist could respond to the preceding argument. For discussion of further patternist options see Perry (1975). Alternately, the transhumanist might instead accept a no self view, as sociologist James Hughes does in his (2004 and 2005) and in his forthcoming book, *Cyborg Buddha* (Hughes, n.d.). (Relatedly, see also the Institute for Ethics and Emerging Technology's "Cyborg Buddha" project at http://ieet.org/index.php/IEET/cyborgbuddha.)

REFERENCES

Annas, G. J. (2000). The man on the moon, immortality, and other millennial myths: The prospects and perils of human genetic engineering. *Emory Law Journal, 49*(3), 753–782.

Blackburn, S. (1999). The self. In *Think: A compelling introduction to philosophy* (pp. 129–140). Oxford: Oxford University Press.

Block, N. (1995). The mind as the software of the brain. In D. Osherson, L. Gleitman, S. Kosslyn, E. Smith, & S. Sternberg (Eds.), *An invitation to cognitive science* (pp. 377–421). New York: MIT Press.

Bostrom, N. (1998). How long before superintelligence? *International Journal of Futures Studies, 2*. Retrieved June 26, 2008, from http://jetpress.org/contents.htm

Bostrom, N. (2002a). Existential risks: Analyzing human extinction scenarios and related hazards. *Journal of Evolution and Technology, 9*.

Bostrom, N. (2002b). When machines outsmart humans. *Futures, 35*(7), 759–764.

Bostrom, N. (2003a), Are you living in a computer simulation? *Philosophical Quarterly, 53*(211), 243–255.

Bostrom, N. (2003b). *The Transhumanist Frequently Asked Questions: v 2.1*. World Transhumanist Association. Retrieved June 20, 2008, from http://transhumanism.org/index.php/WTA/faq/

Bostrom, N. (2005). History of transhmanist thought. *Journal of Evolution and Technology, 14*(1). Retrieved June 20, 2008, from http://jetpress.org/volume14/bostrom.html

Bostrom, N. (in press). *Dignity and enhancement*. Commissioned for the President's Council on Bioethics.

109

*Future Minds:
Transhumanism,
Cognitive
Enhancement,
and the Nature
of Persons*

Churchland, P. (1988). *Matter and consciousness*. Cambridge, MA: MIT Press.

Churchland, P. (1996). *Engine of reason, seat of the soul*. Cambridge, MA: MIT Press.

Clark, A. (2003). *Natural born cyborgs*. Oxford: Oxford University Press.

Freeman, W. (2000). *How brains make up their minds*. New York: Columbia University Press.

Fukuyama, F. (2002). *Our posthuman future: Consequences of the biotechnology revolution*. New York: Farrar, Straus and Giroux.

Garreau, J. (2005). *Radical evolution: The promise and peril of enhancing our minds, our bodies—and what it means to be human*. New York: Doubleday.

Grice, P. (1941). Personal identity. *Mind, 50*, 330–350.

Hughes, J. (2004a). *Citizen cyborg: Why democratic societies must respond to the redesigned human of the future*. Cambridge, MA: Westview Press.

Hughes, J. (2004b). The death of death. In C. Machado & D. A. Shewmon (Eds.), *Brain death and disorders of consciousness* (pp. 79–88). New York: Kluwer.

Hughes, J. (2005). The illusiveness of immortality. In C. Tandy (Ed.), *Death and anti-death, volume 3: Fifty years after Einstein, one hundred fifty years after Kierkegaard*. New York: Ingram.

Hughes, J. (n.d.). *Cyborg Buddha*. Manuscript in preparation. Retrieved from http://ieet.org/index.php/IEET/cyborgbuddha

Huxley, J. (1957). *New bottles for new wine*. London: Chatto & Windus.

Joy, B. (2000). Why the future doesn't need us. *Wired, 8*, 238–246.

Kass, L., Blackburn, E., Dresser, R., Foster, D., Fukiyama, F., Gazzaniga, M., et al. (2003). *Beyond therapy: Biotechnology and the pursuit of happiness: A report of the President's Council on Bioethics*. Commissioned report by the President's Council, Washington, DC.

Kelso, S. (1997). *Dynamical patterns*. New York: MIT Press.

Kim, J. (2006). *Philosophy of mind* (2nd ed.). New York: Westview Press.

Kurzweil, R. (1999). *The age of spiritual machines: When computers exceed human intelligence*. New York: Viking.

Kurzweil, R. (2005). *The singularity is near: When humans transcend biology*. New York: Viking.

Locke, J. (1694). *Essay concerning human understanding* (2nd ed.).

Moore, G. (1965). Cramming more components into integrated circuits. *Electronics, 38*(8), 11–17. Retrieved August 20, 2008, from ftp://download. intel.com/research/silicon/moorespaper.pdf

Olson, E. T. (2008). Personal identity. In E. N. Zalta (Ed.), *The Stanford encyclopedia of philosophy* (Spring 2007 Edition). Retrieved August 20, 2008, from http://plato.stanford.edu/archives/spr2007/entries/identity-personal/

Parfit, D. (1984). *Reasons and persons*. Oxford: Oxford University Press.

Parfit, D. (1987). Divided minds and the nature of persons. In C. Blakemore & S. Greenfield (Eds.), *Mindwaves* (pp. 19–28). Oxford: Blackwell Publishers.

Perry, J. (1975). *Personal identity*. Berkeley: University of California Press.

Quinton, A. (1962). The soul. *The Journal of Philosophy, 59*(15), 393–409.

Reid, T. (1785/1941). *Essays on the intellectual powers of man*. A. D. Woozley (Ed.). London: Macmillian.

Roco, M. C., & Bainbridge, W. S. (Eds.). (2002). *Converging technologies for improved human performance: Nanotechnology, biotechnology, information technology and cognitive science*. Arlington, VA: National Science Foundation/Department of Commerce.

Vinge, V. (1993, Winter). The coming technological singularity. *Whole Earth Review*.

World Transhumanist Association. (1998). *Transhumanist declaration*. Retrieved August 20, 2008, from http://www.transhumanism.org/index.php/WTA/declaration/

10

Nanotechnology and Nanomedicine: Ethical and Social Considerations

JAN JAEGER, MARISA P. MARCIN,
AND PAUL ROOT WOLPE

NANOMEDICINE IS SHAPING a new era in modern medicine that is promising to deliver extraordinary benefits. It is gradually changing medical education, medical research, and medical care to the point that our traditional beliefs and common understandings of the practice of medicine in our society might change. It is thus becoming increasingly important to understand the social and ethical implications of the rapidly emerging nanomedicine landscape, so that policies governing this field would guarantee social benefits while providing appropriate protections.

This chapter is based on research supported in part by the Nano/Bio Interface Center under a grant from the National Science Foundation NSEC DMR-0425780.

WHAT IS NANOTECHNOLOGY?

NANOTECHNOLOGY IS HARD to define. It is not an industry but rather an emerging interdisciplinary field where a mix of research, development, and production activities are united by a *common technological underpinning*. According to the National Nanotechnology Initiative (NNI) nanotechnology refers to the ability to measure, manipulate, and organize matter at the atomic scale. It is the application of the principles of engineering to create materials and structures between 1 and 100 nanometers (nm) in size. A nanometer is one billionth of a meter and invisible to the naked eye. These man-made materials are smaller than a red blood cell (~7,000 nm in length), a human hair (~80,000 nm in width) and are about the size of a virus. As a science, nanotechnology is concerned with the organization of atoms and molecules adding new functionality to current products and enabling the creation of novel products and materials (National Science and Technology Council Committee on Technology, 2000; Roco & Bainbridge, 2002, 2003; Renn & Roco, 2006).

Nanotechnology involves the creation of structures from matter in the atomic or molecular range, or at the nanoscale. Nanoscale materials are interesting to scientists because matter at this small scale changes chemical and functional properties, behaving differently than bulk materials of the same composition. For instance, materials at the nanoscale may exhibit higher conductivity and their increased surface area allows for greater reactivity with neighboring atoms and substances (Powell & Kanarek, 2006a). Managing these unique properties makes it possible for scientists to create materials and assemble molecular-sized structures with capabilities far superior to current products (Morrow, Bawa, & Wei, 2007; NNI, 2000).

Nanotechnology research and development is interdisciplinary, spanning many fields and crossing scientific disciplines. More so than other domains, it requires a wide spectrum of knowledge and involves the integration of engineering with physics, computer science, chemistry, materials, biology, and medicine (Renn & Roco, 2006). To foster collaboration between the relevant fields, a number of interdisciplinary research centers and nano-bio interface programs have been established at academic institutions and other organizations. For example, the National Cancer Institute's Nanobiology Think Tank was a collaborative outreach program designed to disseminate knowledge and promote the development of novel ideas concerning nanotechnology research and biomedical applications. Many universities involved in nanotechnology research and development have established outreach programs for high schools and summer programs for students toward the same end. Nanotechnology is therefore influencing the organization of education by gradually reversing our nation's trend of specialization of scientific disciplines and promoting interdisciplinarity (NNI, 2000; Renn & Roco, 2006).

In its current early developmental stages, nanotechnology is evoking great enthusiasm for the potential social and economic benefits it may hold. It is predicted that numerous applications will provide breakthroughs that will affect our lives on many levels. If these predictions become realities, nanotechnology may enable new technologies that would cure cancer and other debilitating and deadly physical and mental illnesses, increase agricultural yield, provide an abundant clean water supply and an efficient energy source, and enhance national security (NNI, 2000; Renn & Roco, 2006). Nanotechnologies necessary to achieve these extraordinary social benefits are in various stages of development, making some of the promises closer to reality than others.

THE SCOPE OF NANOTECHNOLOGY RESEARCH

NANOTECHNOLOGY RESEARCH IS a global endeavor with governments, industry, and private funders allocating substantial resources and implementing policies and programs to accelerate the translation of nanotechnology research into beneficial products (Sargent, 2008). Since the inception of the National Nanotechnology Initiative in 2000, the U.S. Congress has appropriated 8.4 billion dollars for nanotechnology research and development (Sargent, 2008). In 2003, the 21st Century Nanotechnology Research and Development Act was enacted (2003), allocating 3.7 billion dollars in U.S. federal funds from 2005 to 2008 to support nanotechnology research and development (Sheetz, Vidal, Pearson, & Lazano, 2005). This investment is intended to secure U.S. technological leadership, create high-wage jobs, and promote economic growth (Sargent, 2008).

Venture capital firms are heavily investing in nanotechnology research as well. In 2007, 702 million dollars of venture capital monies were invested in nanotechnology, representing a significant increase from 2004 of 497 million dollars (Sargent, 2008; Wilson, 2006).

The United States is not alone in its nanotechnology research initiatives. Strong government support exists in countries worldwide, with more than 60 nations having established their own national nanotechnology research and development programs (Renn & Roco, 2006). Estimated global annual public investments in nanotechnology reached $6.4 billion in 2006, with another $6 billion invested by the private sector (Sargent, 2008).

WHAT IS NANOMEDICINE?

ALTHOUGH THERE IS no formalized definition, nanomedicine can be considered the application of nanotechnology to the field of medicine. It concerns the use of precisely engineered nanoscale materials to develop novel medical therapies and diagnostic tools that researchers hope would overcome many of the limitations of traditional medicine (Liu, Miyoshi, & Nakamura, 2007; McNeil, 2005; Wagner, Dullaart, Bock, & Zweck, 2006; Zhang et al., 2008). Nanotechnology is expected to affect all aspects of medicine including drug development and drug delivery systems, medical devices, biotechnology products, tissue engineering products, and vaccines (Renn & Roco, 2006; Sadrieh, 2005).

Nanomedicine is not a futuristic scenario. Investments are significant and commercialization efforts are global. There are more than 38 nanomedicine products on the market, with 24 of them approved for clinical use; it is estimated that more than 200 companies are involved in nanomedicine research and development for total sales exceeding 5.4 billion dollars (Resnick & Tinkle, 2006, 2007; Wagner et al., 2006; Zhang et al., 2008). The U.S. Food and Drug Administration (FDA) reported that the number of nano-based drugs and biomedical devices increased by 67% in 2005 (Rejeski, 2006). It is estimated that by 2012, the market for nanomedical products will grow to 12 billion dollars (Resnick & Tinkle, 2007). The National Cancer Institute has launched a 144.3-million-dollar, 5-year initiative to develop new nanotechnology-based tools and approaches to the diagnosis, treatment, and prevention of cancer and metastatic disease (Alper, 2004; Kawasaki & Player, 2005).

Nanotechnology enabled medicines and diagnostic tools are expanding the fields of personalized and preventative medicine with an early focus on discovering treatments and cures for diseases associated with aging such as cancer and heart disease. The first generation of nanomedicine products and devices are in the development and production phase with many on the market satisfying varied medical and diagnostic needs. For example, there are nanomedicines designed to inhibit cancer cell growth (Morrow et al., 2007; Service, 2005) and drug delivery systems using nanosized artificially created carriers (Wagner et al., 2006), as well as dental fillers (Wagner et al., 2006) and nanoparticles used for imaging (Moghimi, Hunter, & Murray, 2005; Wagner et al., 2006). One of the most anticipated achievements of nanomedicine is more effective and safe cancer-fighting drugs that would be able to target tumors (Zhang et al., 2008).

Nanomedicine technologies that are still under development could enable the creation of sensors for in vivo monitoring, of cognitive capacity–assisting devices, and of highly advanced targeted cancer therapies (Renn & Roco, 2006). Technologies, predicted to be developed around 2010, would potentially allow for artificial organs, brain modi-fication, and tissues for scaffold engineering (Renn & Roco, 2006). Fi-nally, the most advanced category of nanotechnology, predicted to be developed around 2015–2020, would involve *nanosystems,* in which each molecule plays a different role and has its own structure (Renn & Roco, 2006). This would potentially allow the development of nanoscale ma-terials to be utilized in medicine to improve spinal nerve regeneration (Onose et al., 2007) and to detect and treat genetic deficiencies at the cellular level (Mirkin, Thaxton, & Rosi, 2004; Morrow et al., 2007; Renn & Roco, 2006). Of course, exciting claims have been made about other technologies—gene therapy comes to mind—without fulfilling their promise. So, one must weigh such claims with a certain amount of caution.

NANOMEDICINE: ETHICAL CONSIDERATIONS

HISTORY DEMONSTRATES A trend of looking through a retro-spective lens at the ethical issues raised by catastrophic events in medicine. In many cases, ethical discussion was prompted by tragedy that occurred well after a technology's inception. Thalidomide and ra-diation exposure are cases in point. We believe that it is important to educate engineers, scientists, and the general public about the ethical and social implications of nanomedicine before the science matures and a tragic event occurs (Mills & Fleddermann, 2005; NNI, 2000; Renn & Roco, 2006; Resnick & Tinkle, 2006, 2007). Early dialogue will serve to educate all stakeholders, foster public support, and ensure that appro-priate decisions are made and policies are in place to protect society (NNI, 2000; Resnick & Tinkle, 2006, 2007; Walker & Mouton, 2006).

Like all new emerging technologies, nanomedicine requires an ex-amination of safety and of the potential for unintended consequences. We believe that the scope of the ethical implications associated with nanomedicine will widen as the technology emerges and more appli-cations are tested on human subjects and make their way to market, necessitating an ongoing, evolving dialogue among all stakeholders. However, we do not believe that nanomedicine has developed to the point where it truly poses novel ethical questions. Nanomedicine can be well discussed within the well-established framework of the ethics of medical research and of emerging technologies.

SAFETY CONCERNS

WHILE THE PROMISE of nanomedicine has led the industry to rush to develop products for the medical marketplace, to date, very little is known about the potential risks to human health posed by the engineered nanomaterials that are used to make nanomedicines. Most nanomedical applications are combinations of materials, and each of these materials may have unique toxicity characteristics (Sadrieh, 2005). There is little research examining the potential toxicity of human exposure to engineered nanomaterials or nanoparticles, nor are the metrics to accurately measure toxicity in place (International Risk Governance Council, 2006; Renn & Roco, 2006; Walker & Mouton, 2006).

However what research there is into the toxic effects of nanomaterials indicates that there may be reason for concern. The occupational health community, as well as people working on safety issues in nanotechnology, are becoming concerned about the risks of exposure to engineered nanomaterials in the workplace and in products distributed for consumer consumption that may involve nanomedicines (Department of Health and Human Services, Centers for Disease Control and Prevention, National Institute of Occupational Safety and Health [NIOSH], 2006, 2007; McCauley & McCauley, 2005; Schulte & Salamanca-Buentello, 2007; Schulte et al., 2008; U.S. Environmental Protection Agency, 2007). Efforts are underway to understand more about risk to human health, but at this time only limited data is available because nanotechnology still is in the early stages of development (McCauley & McCauley, 2005; NIOSH, 2006, 2007; Schulte & Salamanca-Buentello, 2007; Schulte et al., 2008).

Currently we have to rely on the limited cellular research and animal studies on nanomaterials, along with the data developed in the study of ultrafine particulates in the workplace. Evidence suggests that some nanomaterials may cause harmful biological effects. Some of these damaging consequences can include the ability to cross the blood-brain barrier, to disperse to organs at a rapid pace, and the ability to penetrate cells (Nel, Xia, Madler, & Li, 2006; Oberdorster, 2004; Powell & Kanarek, 2006a, 2006b). While the potential harmful impact on human health from exposures to nanomaterials is not well understood, multiple studies across various scientific fields are underway focused on building upon the current body of knowledge.

Nanotechnology innovation is ahead of the policy and regulatory environment and we do not currently know the number of people working in the nanotechnology field (including nanomedicine), what materials they are exposed to, how exposures occur, and what the risks of exposures are (McCauley & McCauley, 2005; Renn & Roco, 2006; Schulte & Salamanca-Buentello, 2007; Schulte et al., 2008). Academia, industry, government, nongovernmental organizations, and international organizations need to develop measures to assess, characterize, evaluate, and manage risks of engineered nanomaterials (Renn & Roco,

2006). However slow and expensive this exercise may be, this information is crucial to policy makers and regulators charged with protecting society. A tragic event leading to public outcry may be the catalyst for overregulation of the field, similar to what happened with nuclear energy. This may be avoided by proactive thinking and discourse among stakeholders about how to manage this issue.

PUBLIC ENGAGEMENT

IN A U.S. nationwide telephone survey conducted in 2004, researchers from North Carolina State University found that over 80% of the respondents indicated they had heard "little" or "nothing" about nanotechnology (Cobb & Macoubrie, 2004, Table 1). These numbers had not improved dramatically in 2006 when another nationwide survey was conducted on behalf of the Woodrow Wilson International Center for Scholars Project on Emerging Nanotechnologies. This study found that 67% of the public had heard "little" or "nothing" about nanotechnology, with a full 42% indicating they had heard nothing at all about nanotechnology (Hart Research, 2006, p. 5). These statistics raise potential concerns, given the first generation of nanomedical advances is already here and a second generation of nanomedical applications is in the clinical trial stage.

It is not only the general public that lacks a fundamental understanding of nanomedicine and technology. A recent study (Jaeger, Marcin, & Wolpe, 2008) looked at how members of 10 institutional review boards (IRBs) (high-risk and general medical) understand clinical trials involving nanomedicines. IRBs are charged with the responsibility of reviewing clinical trial protocols to ensure that the rights and interests of the human research subjects are protected. Members of IRBs at two academic research medical institutions, both actively involved in nanotechnology research and development, were surveyed to see what they knew about nanomedicines and believed to be their responsibilities regarding an ethical and scientific review. Most of the IRB members, with the exception of community members, were associated with the home institutions and might reasonably be expected to have at least a greater exposure to, if not understanding of, nanotechnology than the public at large. Most of the IRB members were physicians, biomedical researchers, and nurses working at the institutions where the nanomedicine trials are being conducted, placing them closer to the science. In response to the question of whether they knew what nanomedicine was, 47% of the responding IRB members stated they did not. In addition, 61% of the IRB members who responded indicated that they were uncertain if the proposed study was changed by the fact that nanotechnology was used to create the drug, procedure, or therapy being studied.

Findings from these studies suggest that information about nano-medicine and nanotechnology has not been received by a good portion of the general public, including members of the medical community charged with the protection of human research subjects. The fact that the majority of IRB members themselves are unfamiliar with nanomedicine leaves little doubt that lay research participants being exposed to a nanomedicine in a clinical trial have limited comprehension of the uniqueness of the material being placed in their bodies and how little is known about how it might affect them. This means that they may not be in a position where they can reasonably understand the risks and benefits as presented to them in the informed consent process.

The issue of exposure to nanomedicine is not limited to clinical trials, as there are many nanotechnology-enhanced medical applications on the market today, many of them approved for medical use, including cancer-fighting drugs, treatment for multiple sclerosis, imaging and diagnostic applications, and pacemaker components (Service, 2005; Wagner et al., 2006; Walker & Mouton, 2006; Zhang et al., 2008). This, again, raises questions about whether the general public, as potential consumers of nanomedicines, are able to make informed and reasoned decisions in a health care setting about subjecting themselves and their families to nanomedical products.

REGULATORY CONCERNS

BECAUSE THE FDA regulates categories of products and not the technology employed in producing them, it does not regulate nanotechnology per se and purports to treat products made using nanotechnology in the same manner as all other products (Dixon, 2007). This means that there is no requirement that products, including medicines and medical devices, be labeled as containing nanoscale-engineered materials. On the surface, the FDA's position is consistent with the principle, with which we agree, that it is not the size of the matter that is important but rather its functionality. However, much remains unknown about how the functionality of materials change when they are reduced to the nanoscale, raising questions about what the public needs to know (McCauley & McCauley, 2005; Renn & Roco, 2006; Schulte & Salamanca-Buentello, 2007; Schulte et al., 2008).

Without fully understanding how the function of materials change at the nanoscale, there is no way to know for certain how they might affect the human body when used in nanomedicine. The FDA in its Task Force Report acknowledges that it is possible that certain materials produced on the nanoscale would demonstrate properties so unique and novel that they "may change the regulatory status/pathway of products" (FDA, 2007, p. 32), but to the best of our knowledge the FDA has not initiated such changes at this time.

PROTECTION OF HUMAN RESEARCH SUBJECTS

IT IS POSSIBLE that individual researchers might attempt to address safety concerns by trying to supply their potential research subjects with information about nanomedical technology at the point of informed consent. While doing so is helpful, this would not address the general lack of knowledge and may be too little and too late for the prospective subject.

Without some understanding of nanotechnology, the potential clinical research subject also may be more likely to fall prey to what is known as the "therapeutic misconception." This misconception involves the belief of a patient that as an expert his doctor knows what is best for him and would not suggest that he participate in a research study unless it offered some form of clinical benefit and might improve his condition (Appelbaum, Roth, Lidz, Benson, & Winslade, 1987; del Carmen & Joffe, 2005; Henderson et al., 2006; Lidz, Appelbaum, Grisso, & Renaud, 2004; Resnick & Tinkle, 2006). Patients generally view doctors as having a fiduciary responsibility for their well-being and not as scientists investigating disease. Adding nanotechnology to the equation only compounds the chance that therapeutic misconceptions might come into play. The average potential research subject may well believe that the "nanoness" of the product implies that it is a super product, new and cutting edge, therefore making it the best course of treatment available. Not only is the medical application being tested not a treatment, but considering it the best course of action is in startling contrast with the fact that so little is known about the potential health risks from exposure to the nanoscale materials. Physicians and clinicians must exercise a heightened level of sensitivity when enrolling subjects in trials involving nanomedicine in an effort to counterbalance the persuasive nature of what may be seen as an exciting new breakthrough.

CONCLUSION

PUBLIC ENGAGEMENT AND public education are crucial to an appropriate introduction of nanotechnology and nanomedicine into our lives over the next decades. The burden of informing the public and those working in the U.S. health care system about nanotechnology and nanomedicine cannot fall on personal physicians and clinical researchers alone. In order to ensure that our nation becomes nano-literate, we must provide fundamental education in nanotechnology across the board and not only to students of science (Mills & Fledder-mann, 2005). One of the goals of the NNI has been, from the outset, to stimulate interest about nanotechnology in children (NNI, 2000). However, some critics have stated that the necessary effort and resources to attain this goal have not been committed (Woodrow Wilson International Center for Scholars, 2006). Educational tools have been developed and are available, including those prepared by the NNI with materials suitable for even kindergartners. At the university level, many are endeavoring to help educate the public, including programs like those offered by the Nano/Bio Interface Center at the University of Pennsylvania, which is geared toward middle school students. The effort to bring nanotechnology to schools has even given rise to the peer-reviewed *Journal of Nano Education*. These efforts are laudable and are having a positive effect. However, what is truly needed is a nationwide commitment to introduce nanotechnology into the curriculum of all of America's school children. This would require considerable funding and a new perspective on how science is taught.

REFERENCES

Alper, J. (2004). US NCI launches nanotechnology plan. *Nature Biotechnology, 22*, 1335–1336.

Appelbaum, P. S., Roth, L. H., Lidz, C. W., Benson, P., & Winslade, W. (1987). False hopes and best data: Consent to research and the therapeutic misconception. *Hastings Center Report, 17*(2), 20–24.

Cobb, M. D., & Macoubrie, J. (2004). Public perceptions about nanotechnology: Risks, benefits and trust. *Journal of Nanoparticle Research, 6*, 395–405.

del Carmen, M. G., & Joffe, S. (2005). Informed consent for medical treatment and research: A review. *The Oncologist, 10*(8), 636–641.

Department of Health and Human Services, Centers for Disease Control and Prevention, National Institute of Occupational Safety and Health. (2006). *Approaches to safe nanotechnology: An information exchange with NIOSH* (draft for public comment). Retrieved September 29, 2008, from http://www.cdc.gov/niosh/topics/nanotech/safenano/pdfs/approaches_to_safe_nanotechnology_28november2006_updated.pdf

Department of Health and Human Services, Centers for Disease Control and Prevention, National Institute of Occupational Safety and Health. (2007). *Progress toward safe nanotechnology in the workplace—A report for the NIOSH Nanotechnology Research Center*. Retrieved September 29, 2008, from http://www.cdc.gov/niosh/docs/2007-123/pdfs/2007-123.pdf

Dixon, K. (2007). *FDA says no new labeling for nanotech products*. Retrieved October 31, 2007, from http://uk.reuters.com/articlePrint?articleId=UKN2514226320070725

Hart, P. D., Research Associates, Inc. (2006). *Report findings based on a national survey of adults* (conducted on behalf of The Woodrow Wilson International Center for Scholars Project on Emerging Nanotechnologies). September 19, 2006. Retrieved September 29, 2008, from http://www. nanotechproject.org/file_download/files/HartReport.pdf

Henderson, G. E., Easter, M. M., Zimmer, C., King, N.M.P., Davis, A. M., Rothschild, B. B., et al. (2006). Therapeutic misconception in early phase gene transfer trials. *Social Science & Medicine, 62,* 239–253.

International Risk Governance Council. (2006). *White paper on nanotechnology risk governance.* Retrieved September 29, 2008, from http://www.irgc. org/IMG/pdf/IRGC_white_paper_2_PDF_final_version-2.pdf

Jaeger, J., Marcin, M. P., & Wolpe, P. R. (2008). Untitled and unpublished manuscript. University of Pennsylvania.

Kawasaki, E. S., & Player, A. (2005). Nanotechnology, nanomedicine, and the development of new, effective therapies for cancer. *Nanomedicine: Nanotechnology, Biology, and Medicine, 1*(2), 101–109.

Lidz, C. W., Appelbaum, P. S., Grisso, T., & Renaud, M. (2004). Therapeutic misconception and the appreciation of risks in clinical trials. *Social Science & Medicine, 58*(9), 1689–1697.

Liu, Y., Miyoshi, H., & Nakamura, M. (2007). Nanomedicine for drug delivery and imaging: A promising avenue for cancer therapy and diagnosis using targeted functional nanoparticles. *International Journal of Cancer, 120,* 2527–2537.

McCauley, L. A., & McCauley, R. D. (2005). Nanotechnology—are occupational health nurses ready? *AAOHN Journal, 53*(12), 517–521.

McNeil, S. E. (2005). Nanotechnology for the biologist. *Journal of Leukocyte Biology, 78,* 585–594.

Mills, K., & Fleddermann, C. (2005). Getting the best from nanotechnology: Approaching social and ethical implications openly and proactively. *IEEE Technology and Society Magazine, 24*(4), 18–26.

Mirkin, C. A., Thaxton, C. S., & Rosi, N. L. (2004). Nanostructures in biodefense and molecular diagnostics. *Expert Review of Molecular Diagnosis, 4*(6), 749–751.

Moghimi, S. M., Hunter, A. C., & Murray, J. C. (2005). Nanomedicine: Current status and future prospects. *FASEB Journal, 19,* 311–330.

Morrow, K. J., Bawa, R., & Wei, C. (2007). Recent advances in basic and clinical nanomedicine. *The Medical Clinics of North America, 91,* 805–843.

National Science and Technology Council Committee on Technology, Subcommittee on Nanoscale Science, Engineering and Technology. (2000). *National Nanotechnology Initiative: The Initiative and Its Implementation Plan.* Washington, DC. Retrieved September 29, 2008, from http://www.nsf. gov/crssprgm/nano/reports/nni2.pdf

Nel, A., Xia, T., Madler, L., & Li, N. (2006). Toxic potential of materials at the nanolevel. *Science, 311,* 622–627.

Oberdorster, E. (2004). Manufactured nanomaterials (fullerenes C60) induce oxidative stress in the brain of juvenile large-mouth bass. *Environmental Health Perspectives, 112*(10), 1058–1062.

Onose, G., Ciurea, A. V., Rizea, R. E., Chendreanu, C., Anghelescu, A., Haras, M., et al. (2007). Recent advancements in biomaterials for spinal cord injury complex therapeutics. *Digest Journal of Nanomaterials and Biostructures, 2*(4), 307–314.

Powell, M. C., & Kanarek, M. S. (2006a). Nanomaterial health effects—part 1: Background and current knowledge. *Wisconsin Medical Journal, 105*(2), 16–20.

Powell, M. C., & Kanarek, M. S. (2006b). Nanomaterial health effects—part 2: Uncertainties and recommendations for the future. *Wisconsin Medical Journal, 105*(3), 18–23.

Rejeski, D. (2006). *FDA and nanotechnology: Public perceptions matter.* Woodrow Wilson International Center for Scholars Project on Emerging Nanotechnologies. Presentation. Retrieved on August 18, 2008, from http://www.nanotechproject.org/process/assets/files/2737/115_rejeskifda.pdf

Renn, O., & Roco, M. C. (2006). Nanotechnology and the need for risk governance. *Journal of Nanoparticle Research, 8*(2), 153–191.

Resnick, D. B., & Tinkle, S. S. (2006). Ethical issues in clinical trials involving nanomedicine. *Contemporary Clinical Trials, 28*(4), 433–441.

Resnick, D. B., & Tinkle, S. S. (2007). Ethics in nanomedicine. *Nanomedicine, 2*(3), 345–350.

Roco, M. C., & Bainbridge, W. S. (Eds.). (2002). *Converging technologies for improving human performance: Nanotechnology, biotechnology, information technology and cognitive science.* NSF/DOC report. Retrieved September 29, 2008, from http://www.wtec.org/ConvergingTechnologies/1/NBIC_report.pdf

Roco, M. C., & Bainbridge, W. S. (Eds.). (2003). *Nanotechnology: Societal implications—maximizing benefit to humanity.* Report of the National Nanotechnology Initiative. Retrieved September 29, 2008, from http://www.nsf.gov/crss prgm/nano/reports/nni05_si_societal_implications_2005.pdf

Sadrieh, N. (2005). *FDA considerations for regulation of nanomaterial containing products* (Power Point presentation). Retrieved August 26, 2008, from http://www.mhra.gov.uk/home/idcplg?IdcService=GET_FILE&dDoc Name=CON2022823&RevisionSelectionMethod=Latest

Sargent, J. F. (2008). *Nanotechnology: A policy primer.* Congressional Research Service (CRS) Report for Congress Order Code RL34511.

Schulte, P. A., & Salamanca-Buentello, F. (2007). Ethical and scientific issues of nanotechnology in the workplace. *Environmental Health Perspectives, 115*(1), 5–12.

Schulte, P. A., Trout, D., Zumwalde, R. D., Kuempel, E., Geraci, C. L., Castranova, V., et al. (2008). Options for occupational health surveillance of workers potentially exposed to engineered nanoparticles: State of the science. *Journal of Occupational and Environmental Medicine, 50*(5), 517–526.

Service, R. F. (2005). Nanotechnology takes aim at cancer. *Science, 310*(5751), 1132–1134.

Sheetz, T., Vidal, J., Pearson, T. D., & Lazano, K. (2005). Nanotechnology: Awareness and societal concerns. *Technology in Science, 27,* 329–345.

21st Century Nanotechnology Research and Development Act, 15 U.S.C §§ 7501 et seq (2003).

U.S. Environmental Protection Agency. (2007). *Nanotechnology white paper.* Retrieved September 29, 2008, from http://es.epa.gov/ncer/nano/publi cations/whitepaper12022005.pdf

U.S. Food and Drug Administration. (2007). *Nanotechnology task force report.* Retrieved September 29, 2008, from http://www.fda.gov/nanotechnol ogy/taskforce/report2007.pdf

Wagner, V., Dullaart, A., Bock, A., & Zweck, A. (2006). The emerging nanomedicine landscape. *Nature Nanotechnology, 24,* 1211–1217.

Walker, B., & Mouton, C. P. (2006). Nanotechnology and nanomedicine: A primer. *Journal of the National Medical Association, 98*(12), 1985–1988.

Wilson, R. F. (2006). Nanotechnology: The challenges of regulating known unknowns. *The Journal of Law Medicine and Ethics, 34*(4), 704–713.

Woodrow Wilson International Center for Scholars. (2006). *Former White House science advisor warns that nanotechnology's potential threatened by weak public education and outreach* (Press release No. 63-06, December 5, 2006). Retrieved September 29, 2008, from http://www.nanotechproject.org/ process/assets/files/6003/120506nanotechnology_neallane.pdf

Zhang, L., Gu, F. X., Chan, J. M., Wang, A. Z., Langer, R. S., & Farokhzad, O. C. (2008). Nanoparticles in medicine: Therapeutic applications and developments. *Clinical Pharmacology and Therapeutics, 83*(5), 761–769.

Part III

Bioethics at the Bedside

11

Confidentiality: An Expectation in Health Care

Anita L. Allen

H EALTH CARE PROFESSIONALS have a legal and ethical duty to keep medical information private. Physicians and nurses, along with hospitals and insurers, are required by law and professional codes to practice confidentiality. The practice of confidentiality limits "the disclosure of nonpublic information within a fiduciary, professional or contractual relationship" (Majumder, 2005, p. 33). Achieving confidentiality requires restricting information to persons belonging to a community of authorized recipients. The community authorized to receive confidential information can be smaller than a family or as large as a workforce. For example, the community of authorizer recipients of information is small where the confidence is a person's undiagnosed medical symptom secretly whispered to his spouse, but large where the confidence is the detailed medical history and insurance data needed to secure an organ for transplant. Facts, impressions, events, and data of all sorts can be deemed confidential. Confidentiality is achieved through silence, discretion, and data security.

Expectations of confidentiality surround certain relationships. Both personal and professional relationships demand confidentiality. Everyday ethics treat friendships and marriages as confidential relationships of trust in which information can be safely shared. Relationships with providers of professional services are governed by written rules of confidentiality. The doctor-patient, attorney-client, and clergy-penitent relationships are apt examples. Accountants, real estate agents, pharmacists, and tax professionals are also expected to keep certain client information quiet. So are government bureaucrats with access to the personal information recorded on tax filings, census forms, and social security disability claims. Revealing information learned in confidence may violate oaths, professional codes of conduct, business policies, or the law. Even people in illicit criminal relationships expect confidentiality for their conspiracies and abuses.

Expectations of confidentiality surround records, no less than relationships. Personal information recorded in diaries, journals, and correspondence may be confidential. Likewise, business records, medical records, academic records, and personnel files are generally described as confidential, along with banking and financial records, library records, and motor vehicle records. Video rental records and telephone transaction logs are also deemed confidential. In the United States, dozens of federal statutes and myriad state and local laws require confidential treatment of record data (Allen, 2007; Rotenberg, 2007).

Many Americans regard information about their health as appropriately private, and medical privacy as something to which they have a moral right. In fact, health information is so sensitive and personal that some people, who know that they are ill, do not share the knowledge with anyone, leaving even their closest friends and family members in the dark. Private medical knowledge precedes the creation of a confidential provider-patient professional relationship or medical record. A smoker suddenly unable to exercise without getting short of breath knows that he has a lung disorder long before he consults his primary care doctor and lets her in on the secret. When the doctor diagnoses emphysema and creates a record of her findings for specialists and insurers, she is expanding the community of authorized recipients of information about her patient's once-secret ailment. Of course, some medical conditions cannot be concealed. They are obvious to casual lay observers. If a man weighs 700 pounds, his eating disorder speaks for itself. Looking at jaundiced eyeballs the color of sunflowers leaves little doubt about liver disease.

Choosing to hide concealable symptoms of potentially serious health problems is a choice people make; but it can be a deadly choice. Quickly revealing blood in the stools, depression, or a lump in the breast is generally the better, life-saving path. Yet failure to widen the circle of confidence to include medical professionals may be prompted by a reluctance to confront death and decline; a fear of discrimination in insurance, employment, and education; and a dread of social stigma (Allen, 2003). Shame, embarrassment, and terror of surgery or other invasive medical procedures leads even educated individuals to delay seeking treatment of treatable conditions. Lack of trust in physicians and hospitals has led some individuals to suffer privately in silence.

THE VALUE OF CONFIDENTIALITY

ENCOUNTERS WITH HEALTH care professionals convert persons confronting illness into patients with charts. Everyone and every entity participating in the delivery of health care related services is ascribed the duty of patient confidentiality. Health care providers are ethically bound to keep charts and other medical information obtained in the context of care confidential. Confidentiality is a clear ethical obligation of physicians: "A physician shall respect the rights of patients...and shall safeguard patient confidences and privacy within the constraints of law" (American Medical Association, 2001). Failure to respect confidentiality can lead to legal liability. Although health care providers may lawfully share certain otherwise confidential information with insurers, researchers, public health authorities, and law enforcement, principles of confidentiality broadly pertain to health-related services and research.

American bioethicists generally agree that confidentiality is important to just and ethical health-related practices. Practicing respect for patient confidentiality benefits individuals and promotes public health. Ethicists defend confidentiality on several utilitarian grounds, each premised on the twin understandings that health is vital to human well-being and flourishing, and that a good and just society will be committed to securing public health.

First, confidentiality encourages individuals to seek essential medical care. Individuals will be more inclined to pursue medical attention if they believe they can do so privately and perhaps even secretly. Practicing confidentiality assures that, in most cases, a patient can choose when to disclose that she is unwell or declining. Others will not be told that she has abused illegal drugs, been unfaithful to her partner, or cosmetically enlarged her buttocks. As acknowledged in *North American Memorial Hospital v. Ashcroft* (2004), a dispute over Justice Department access to abortion records, medical confidentiality enables abortion patients, and indeed all patients, to exercise constitutionally protected liberties of autonomous medical decision-making (Bodger, 2006).

Second, confidentiality practices lay a foundation for frank disclosures in in-patient and out-patient settings. Individuals seeking care can be more open and honest if they believe the facts and impressions reported to health providers will not be broadcast to the world at large. People are often embarrassed and humiliated by symptoms of illness.

They may go to see a doctor and yet be reluctant to reveal bowel incontinence, loss of memory, or hallucinations.

Third, preventive medicine, early diagnosis, and treatment save money. More people sick with more chronic illnesses means higher care costs. The cost of health care and insurance might be considerably higher if people passed on routine check-ups and prompt medical attention because confidentiality was not credibly promised.

Confidentiality is arguably an ethical mandate of respect for human dignity and individual rights. Caregivers show the concern for other befitting of their status as moral persons with rational interests and feelings when they keep information about their health and health needs private. Individuals concerned about discrimination, shame, or stigma have an interest in controlling the flow of information about their health. Some patients believe they own personal information about themselves, especially genetic information, and should control its release. Confidentiality is required by fair relations with government and businesses. Ideals of fairness embodied in so-called fair information practice standards embraced in the United States and Europe provide that personal data collected about individuals should be accurate, secure, and disclosed to third-parties only with consent (Rothstein, 2005).

OPENNESS IS A TREND

POLLING DATA STRONGLY and consistently suggests that most Americans believe the confidentiality of medical records is important (Patientprivacyrights.org, 2008). However, speaking openly and publicly about health-related matters has emerged as a cultural trend, suggesting a decrease in the felt importance of medical privacy and confidentiality. Disclosures that would have been considered indelicate, embarrassing, or stigmatizing 30 years ago are freely offered today. Celebrities and public officials have taken the lead, turning, for example, AIDS, erectile dysfunction, dementia, Parkinson's disease, prostate enlargement, and breast cancer into topics of ordinary conversation (Barron, 1998; Stevenson, 1991).

But the polling data and the openness trend are not inconsistent. People who speak openly about their health generally prefer to do so on their own terms. They want some control over health information, a say in who is told what. It is not unusual for patients to want health professionals to respect their medical privacy by limiting disclosures to those with a need to know. But patients can have idiosyncratic preferences. Some patients may be open with their family members but not with their friends. Or they may be open with nonjudgmental friends and coworkers but not with critical, scolding parents. A person who shares health-related information on the Web with millions of strangers may be too shy to share information over coffee with siblings they know well.

CONFIDENTIALITY REMAINS RELEVANT

THE UNITED STATES may have entered an era of greater openness about medical matters, including cancer, HIV/AIDS and other serious illnesses. But medical and behavioral health professionals ought to respect the privacy preferences of their patients. The ethical tradition of medical confidentiality has not outlived its relevance. Many people are still particular about when and whether they share health information. With justification, many people are still concerned that they will suffer emotional and economic harm if others learn their health status. Mental and other behavioral health care consumers continue to face stigma and discrimination in a world in which getting what they need requires a virtual surrender of confidentiality to family members, doctors, psychiatrists, psychotherapists, neuropsychologists, social workers, teachers, school administrators, hospitals, insurers, and law enforcement.

Public concern about medical confidentiality is reflected in privacy rules promulgated under the Health Insurance Portability and Accountability Act (HIPAA).

The U.S. Congress enacted HIPAA in 1996. HIPAA patient privacy and data security rules developed by the Department of Health and Human Services went into effect starting in 2003 (Annas, 2003; Rothstein, 2005). HIPAA requires that new patients receive a privacy notice and consent in advance to some disclosures of health information. Under HIPAA, patients do not have a private right of action to sue health care providers who do not conform to the rules. Moreover, numerous exceptions for research, law enforcement, and reporting mean that patient's medical information is widely disclosed without their consent. In court challenges, including *Acara v. Banks* (2006), federal judges have held that HIPAA grants neither an explicit nor an implied right for individuals to sue health care providers. But complaints by individuals may be reported to regulatory bodies empowered to enforce HIPAA's rules (Goldfein, n.d.).

The concern for medical confidentiality is also reflected in the special protection genetic data receives under state laws. A recent federal statute, the Genetic Information Nondiscrimination Act (GINA), prohibits basing employment or insurance decisions on information about a person's DNA or genetic predispositions (Allen, 2007, p. 587; Rao, 2006).

BREACH OF CONFIDENTIALITY

AMERICAN CASE LAW offers a unique window into current confidentiality practices and expectations. In *Whalen v. Roe* (1977) the Supreme Court stated that the Fourteenth Amendment protects the individual's interest in informational privacy. However, the court upheld the validity of a New York state statute that required pharmacists to report the names of persons purchasing certain prescription medications prone to abuse, on the ground that the state had implemented measures to protect confidentiality. In the face of recent data breaches in retailing and health care, such promises of confidentiality carry uncertain weight with the general public. On August 22, 2007, someone broke into the offices of the Pennsylvania Department of Public Welfare in Harrisburg and stole two computers housing data concerning mental health patients receiving state services. Patients were encouraged not to unduly worry about the breach because most of the information on the computers was protected by multiple security passwords, did not identify consumers by name, and contained only coded information relating to treatment.

Unauthorized disclosures of personal information are the essence of so-called breach of confidentiality lawsuits. In these personal injury cases, plaintiffs seek monetary damages because they believe they have been injured by defendants' nonconsensual disclosure of confidential information. Interesting variants on medical breaches of confidentiality are cases in which a health care provider reveals a patient's confidences to a member of the patient's family and intends no harm by it.

In *Humphers v. First Interstate Bank* (1985), for example, a physician was sued after he disclosed his patient's identity to the adult daughter she had placed for adoption in infancy. In *Bagent v. Blessing Care Corporation* (2007), an Illinois hospital and hospital phlebotomist were sued by a patient whose sister was told of the patient's positive pregnancy test. The phlebotomist falsely assumed the patient had discussed the pregnancy with her sister. Even a spouse cannot be presumed a confidant. In *Gracey v. Eaker* (2002) a married couple sued their marriage counselor for breach of confidentiality. The therapist sometimes met with the spouses separately. The couple alleged that the therapist revealed sensitive and personal information that neither spouse had disclosed to the other.

Some people expect confidentiality even when they are doing wrong. In *Morris v. Consolidation Coal Co.* (1994) an employer videotaped an employee engaging in physical labor at his home despite claiming a serious disability for which he was receiving workers' compensation benefits. The employer showed the videotape to the employee's doctor. The physician then wrote a report stating that he could no longer certify a back injury. The employee sued the physician alleging breach of physician-patient confidentiality relationship. He also sued his employer for interference with his confidential relationship with his physician.

The foregoing cases attest to the prudence of seeking consent before making informational disclosures of any sort, even disclosures to persons deemed entitled to the information or likely to already have it. In some instances, a health care provider may be required to breach patient confidentiality. Psychotherapists are required by state law to report child abuse and neglect about which they learn in the course of therapy. State law may also require that therapists warn potential victims of patients' violent intentions. *Tarasoff v. Regents of the University of California* (1976) imposed a duty to warn on California mental health providers. Generally speaking, however, psychotherapists are expected to keep their patients' secrets. They are not permitted to reveal infidelity, closeted sexual orientation, or ruined finances. The American Psychological Association's (APA) ethical code requires that "Psychologists respect…the rights of individuals to privacy, confidentiality, and self determination" (APA, 2002).

Invasion of privacy tort cases alleging intrusion upon seclusion or publication of private fact sometimes involve wrongful disclosure of confidential medical information. In *Doe v. High-Tech Inst.* (1998), a professor had one of her students secretly tested for HIV/AIDS. A medical assistant trainee, the student had informed the instructor (on the basis of an anonymous blood test) that he was HIV positive and asked that she keep the information confidential. Instead the instructor asked a lab that tested all of her students for rubella to also test the plaintiff for HIV. The lab reported the positive test results to the Colorado Department of Health and informed the school. The student sued for invasion of privacy.

Medical information can also be acquired by witnessing medical events or procedures. A patient may wish to exclude both strangers and physicians from intimacies occurring in the hospital. In *Knight v. Penobscot Bay Medical Center* (1980) a physician gave the husband of a nurse permission to observe the delivery of the plaintiff's child while he was waiting for his wife to complete her shift. The plaintiff sued the hospital for invasion of privacy. In *Estate of Berthiaume v. Pratt* (1976), a dying man objected to being disturbed and photographed by a physician who wanted images of the man's surgical wound for scientific purposes. A posthumous suit by the man's estate alleged invasion of privacy—the man had wanted to spend his final hours alone with his wife.

Finally, individuals' medical confidentiality expectations are protected by the rules of evidence, though not perfectly (Denike, 2003). Courts may order disclosure of medical confidences. In *Ex parte Father*

Paul G. Zoghby (2006), a married woman accused her parish priest of sexual assault and indecencies. The woman sued only after being disappointed with the church's failure to discipline the priest. In the course of litigation, the plaintiff requested that the archdiocese produce Zoghby's psychiatric records. The church defendants objected, alleging confidentiality and the physician-patient privilege. Unfortunately for the priest, he had voluntarily signed an affidavit authorizing disclosure of his psychiatric records to a church superior charged with investigating the sexual impropriety allegations. The trial court granted the plaintiff's motion to compel production of the medical evidence, on the ground that the priest had effectively waived the physician-patient privilege by signing the affidavit.

CONCLUSION

Confidentiality has value. It confers autonomy and control over information; prevents shame and violations of modesty; and, perhaps most importantly, frees individuals from the burdens of stigma, inequality, and discrimination. The practice of confidentiality has continued in an era of increased, voluntary openness about medical information in everyday life. Indeed, the number and variety of state and federal laws mandating confidentiality by medical professionals has increased in the last dozen years. Moreover, personal injury suits alleging breach of confidentiality or invasion of privacy, along with suits asserting evidentiary privileges, reflect the reality that expectations of confidentiality of medical records and relationships remain strong.

REFERENCES

Acara v. Banks, 470 F.3d 569 (5th Cir. 2006).

Allen, A. L. (2003). *Why privacy isn't everything*. Lanham, MD: Rowman and Littlefield.

Allen, A. L. (2007). *Privacy law and society*. Minneapolis, MN: West Publishing Co.

American Medical Association. (2001). *Principles of medical ethics*. Retrieved on August 13, 2007, from http://www.ama-assn.org/ama/pub/category/2512.html

American Psychological Association. (2002). *Ethical principles of psychologists and code of conduct*. Retrieved August 13, 2007, from http://www.apa.org/ethics/code2002.html#principle_e

Annas, G. (2003). HIPAA regulations—A new era of medical-record privacy? *New England Journal of Medicine, 348*(15), 1486–1490.

Bagent v. Blessing Care Corporation, 2007 WL 121319 (Ill. 2007).

Barron, J. (1998, November 26). Actor Michael J Fox reveals that he is suffering from Parkinson's disease. *New York Times*, p. B2.

Bodger, J. A. (2006). Taking the sting out of reporting requirements: Reproductive health clinics and the constitutional right to informational privacy. *Duke Law Journal, 56*, 583–609.

Denike, M. (2003). Sexual inequality and the crisis of confidentiality: The myth and the law on personal records. In C. M. Koggel, C. Levin, & A. Furlong (Eds.), *Confidential relationships: Psychoanalytic, ethical, and legal contexts* (pp. 133–150). New York: Rodopi.

Doe v. High-Tech Inst., Inc., 972 P.2d 1060 (Colo. Ct. App. 1998).

Estate of Berthiaume v. Pratt, 365 A.2d 792 (Me. 1976).

Ex parte Father Paul G. Zoghby, 2006 WL 3239971 (Ala. 2006).

Goldfein, R. (n.d.). *Comparison of Pennsylvania Confidentiality of HIV-Related Information Act (Act 148) and federal Health Insurance Portability and Accountability Act*. Retrieved August 13, 2007, from http://www.aidslawpa.org/comparativechart.pdf

Gracey v. Eaker, 837 So. 2d 348 (Fla. 2002).

Humphers v. First Interstate Bank, 298 Ore. 706 (Or. 1985).

Knight v. Penobscot Bay Medical Center, 420 A.2d 915 (Me. 1980).

Majumder, M. (2005). Cyberbanks and other virtual research repositories. *Journal of Law, Medicine and Ethics, 33*, 31–43.

Morris v. Consolidation Coal Co., 191 W.Va. 426, 446 S.E.2d 648 (W.Va. 1994).

North American Memorial Hospital v. Ashcroft, 362 F.3rd 923 (7th Cir. 2004).

Patientprivacyrights.org. (2008). *Health privacy polls*. Retrieved August 13, 2008, from http://www.patientprivacyrights.org/site/PageServer?pagename=Polls#July2004Harris

Rao, R. (2006). A veil of genetic ignorance? Protecting genetic privacy to ensure equality. *Villanova Law Review, 51*, 827–840.

Rotenberg, M. (2007). *Sourcebook on privacy law*. Washington. DC: Electronic Privacy Information Center.

Rothstein, M. A. (2005). Currents in contemporary ethics: Research privacy under HIPAA and the common rule. *Journal of Law, Medicine and Ethics, 33*, 154–158.

Stevenson, R. (1991, November 8). Magic Johnson ends his career, saying he has AIDS infection. *New York Times*. Retrieved July 17, 2007, p. A1.

Tarasoff v. Regents of the University of California, 17 Cal.3d 425 (1976).

Whalen v. Roe, 429 U.S. 589 (1977).

12

Hospital Ethics Committees and Ethics Consultants

JAMES J. McCARTNEY

HOSPITAL ETHICS COMMITTEES (HECs) began to make their presence felt in hospitals and other health care services in the 1970s and 1980s, and the role of bioethics consultants developed shortly thereafter, first in nonprofit health care organizations and then in for-profit pharmaceutical and biomedical companies and in for-profit health care systems. Many questions have been raised about the utility, suitability, and competence of both HECs and bioethics consultants, and some of them will be discussed in this chapter.

THE DEVELOPMENT OF HOSPITAL ETHICS COMMITTEES

LIKE A RIVER formed by several tributaries, many events and issues in health care led to the creation of HECs. The first of these emanated from the medical-moral committees established by Catholic hospitals in the 1960s and 1970s and occasionally even before that. These committees were somewhat narrow in scope, focusing almost exclusively on the issues of abortion and sterilization. Eventually they tried to ensure the implementation of the *Ethical and Religious Directives for Catholic Health Facilities,* published in 1971 (National Conference of Catholic Bishops, 1971). After the publication of the *Directives,* committees also began to focus on end-of-life issues such as brain death, termination of treatment, ventilator support, and do not resuscitate orders, by this time developing into full-fledged HECs. Many continue to use the revised *Directives* for guidance and focus (Bernt, Clark, Starrs, & Talone, 2006; United States Conference of Catholic Bishops, 2001).

In 1976, the case *In re Quinlan* was decided by the Supreme Court of New Jersey. This case involved a young woman, Karen Ann Quinlan, who had ingested drugs and other harmful substances that had put her into a coma and eventually left her in a persistent vegetative state. Her father petitioned to become her legal guardian so that he could have the ventilator that was supporting her respiration removed, convinced that if Karen Ann could speak for herself, she would have wanted this burdensome medical intervention discontinued. Interestingly, the Quinlans were Catholic and they made this decision with the full support of their parish priests and the local bishop. After decisions in the lower courts rejected Mr. Quinlan's petition, the New Jersey Supreme Court reversed on appeal, affirmed Mr. Quinlan's request and appointed him Karen Ann's legal guardian. In the *Quinlan* decision, the Supreme Court also said that the attending physician's prognosis that a patient is in a coma or a persistent vegetative state should be reviewed by a hospital ethics committee or some comparable body and that an assessment of the physician's prognosis should be made. The court held that this process would enable a more broad-based decision to be legally binding without the possibility of criminal or civil proceedings. The court compared this process to a panel of judges reviewing cases at the appellate level, arguing that this type of review is usually more fair and thorough than review by one judge alone (*In re Quinlan,* 1976). A more recent application of this approach is found in the Texas Advance Directives Act of 1999. This statute is unique because it provides a process by which conflicts between a patient, or surrogate decision-maker, and the caregivers about the perceived futility of a particular therapeutic approach can be resolved by an HEC. If after following a defined protocol, the committee concurs with the caregivers that a particular level of care is inappropriate, the caregivers may override a patient's or family's wishes for continued aggressive therapy and withhold or withdraw potentially life-saving treatments with legal protection (Texas Advance Directives Act, 1999).

But HECs cannot always assume they are acting according to the law or have legal protection. In the case of Ashley X, a hysterectomy was performed on a child at the parents' request and with the concurrence of the HEC at Seattle Children's Hospital. However, the Washington Protection and Advocacy System, a private group with federal investigative authority, ruled that Seattle Children's Hospital violated Ashley's rights by performing a hysterectomy without a court order.

A third factor that influenced the development of HECs were the great advances in medical science and technology, especially those related to end-of-life care. This fact was averred to by the Quinlan Court at about the same time that hospitals realized that they needed new policies developed to deal with the ever increasing complexity of health care. Thus, many HECs were created to develop clinical care policies that took into consideration the rapid development of applied medical science.

A final element in the development of HECs was the availability of so-called professional ethicists made possible by the growth and development of bioethics think tanks such as the Hastings Center in New York, and degree-granting programs with concentrations in bioethics such as the one at the Kennedy Institute of Ethics at Georgetown University in Washington, DC. Professionally trained bioethicists were looking for jobs and convinced many hospitals of the need to use their services to either create or enhance an HEC to deal with emerging ethical problems in the care and treatment of patients.

THE FUNCTION OF HOSPITAL ETHICS COMMITTEES

THE ACTIVITIES OF early HECs can be summarized as having five primary functions:

1. Education of physicians and staff concerning clinical ethics.
2. Education of the public in issues of clinical ethics.
3. Retrospective and concurrent case review.
4. Policy development.
5. Consultation and counseling (McCartney, 1989).

Membership and participation in a HEC was a learning experience in itself as physicians and staff began to examine cases and issues in clinical ethics from a multidisciplinary perspective. Many times HECs presented ethics grand rounds to the whole clinical staff of the institution, and occasionally some HECs took their show on the road, sending a team of three or four ethics committee members to other health care institutions to present a program in clinical ethics for physicians and staff there. Many ethics committees also sponsored annual programs for the public, to educate people on the use of advance directives, explain current understandings of brain death, and to present other issues of clinical ethics believed to be of general interest.

Early HECs often used cases, both as instruments of education and as a way of providing consultation and review. Generally, historical cases were discussed for educational purposes, not in order to assign praise or blame, but to see which ethical issues had been considered and which ignored in the context of clinical decision-making. Some of these cases were drawn from the bioethics literature available at the time, but some were actual cases submitted by physicians and nurses to help everyone on the committee gain deeper insights into the ethical dilemmas health care professionals often faced.

One of the main activities of early HECs was the development of institutional policies dealing with refusal of treatment, cardiopulmonary resuscitation, ability to make health care decisions, and brain death, among others. These policies were generally submitted to the medical staff and to the hospital administration for review and approval. Policy development also provided a good way to educate committee members about the developing ethical dilemmas that new biotechnologies spawned.

Finally, individuals or small groups of ethics committee members were called on to provide consultation on specific cases, or in some cases to provide counseling and support to patients and families who had to make difficult health care choices. Generally, families received a great deal of support from committee members who realized the anguished decisions people often had to make.

The most significant change in function for HECs came about in the early 1990s when hospitals themselves began to be seen as ethical (or unethical) agents in their own right. This led to the development of organizational ethics, which considered ethics in the financial, marketing, access, and overall patient care policies of hospitals. Many HECs were asked to include these organizational ethics issues into their purview, but some HECs had a clinical ethics subcommittee as well as an organizational ethics subcommittee, each of which acted somewhat independently from the other. Eventually, many HECs developed or reviewed mission and values statements and created values-based decision-making processes (Ells, 2006; Iltis, 2005b; McCartney, 2005; Rorty, 2000).

A final impetus for the expanded development of HECs was provided by the Joint Commission on Accreditation of Healthcare Organizations (JCAHO), which mandated in 1992 that hospitals who wished to be accredited must establish some procedure for assuring that patient rights and organizational ethics standards are met (JCAHO, 1992). The JCAHO did not specifically mandate the creation of HECs, but most health care organizations that did not have them created them at this time. Many health care organizations also hired a professional bioethics consultant if there was not one on staff already, either to work with the HEC or as a substitute for a HEC. The role and functions of bioethics consultants will now be considered in greater detail (Nilson & Fins, 2006).

BIOETHICS CONSULTANTS

As ENGELHARDT (2003) points out, it is very difficult to describe or define the nature and scope of the activities of bioethics consultants because they take on many roles, such as legal advisor, group facilitator, medical consultant, family counselor, philosopher, or theologian. They also have various levels of training, ranging from taking a 1-week intensive course in bioethics at the Kennedy Institute of Ethics to earning a PhD in philosophy with a concentration in bioethics at such institutions as Rice University or Georgetown University. Bioethics consultants may have a great deal of clinical experience or very little, depending on their previous training and courses of study. And finally, not surprisingly in a secular pluralistic culture, bioethicists subscribe to many different ethical theories and hold bioethical convictions that often conflict with each other and with the individuals and institutions they are hired to serve. All these elements militate against attempting to establish a set of core competencies that bioethics consultants should possess.

Bioethics consultants are often hired by health care organizations to bring ethical expertise to the HEC, but occasionally they are hired as a substitute for a HEC. As Engelhardt points out, secular organizations hire bioethicists not because of their ethical commitments, but often because of their philosophical acumen in sorting out ethical arguments and helping to assure that ethical discourse includes many different points of view. That is, secular health care organizations are more interested in process (in accord with the law), not in the personal convictions of the bioethics consultants. Religious health care organizations, on the other hand, usually hire bioethics consultants who are at least conversant with and respectful of the mission and values of the organization; their preference is to hire those who are enthusiastic supporters of this mission and these values (Dubois, 2003). In the last few years, bioethics consultants have been hired by for-profit organizations such as pharmaceutical companies and bioengineering firms. This has raised a number of controversial issues such as possible conflicts of interest and the question of intellectual freedom, issues that have yet to be resolved in a satisfactory way (DeVries & Bosk, 2004; Iltis, 2005a; Jansen & Sulmasy, 2003; Post, 2003; Spielman, 2005).

EDUCATION AND CREDENTIALING

MOST MEMBERS OF HECs have little formal training in ethics generally, and less in biomedical or business ethics. Members are usually chosen because they are available, interested, and are perceived by administrators and/or physicians to be people of integrity.

However, most take their membership seriously and are usually very open to programs of self-education but are generally opposed to any attempts to establish criteria for membership (credentialing). As mentioned previously, many HECs use bioethics or organizational ethics cases presented by an ethics consultant as an educational methodology. Other committees take time each month to discuss a section of a classical textbook on bioethics, usually one focused on mid-level bioethical principles, such as *Principles of Biomedical Ethics* by Tom Beauchamp and James Childress (2001) or a comparable text.

HECs that present programs of public education do so to educate their own membership as well as the public at large. Some committees include the medical librarian of the institution as a member of the HEC who is responsible for ordering bioethics and business ethics journals and is requested to supply articles relating to issues the HEC is currently discussing. Religious organizations often invite theologians and mission and values directors to the HEC to present insights of theological ethics and values-based decision-making relevant to that religious tradition (Iltis, 2005b; McCartney, 2005).

More recently, educational modules (and the possibility of earning degrees in bioethics) have been developed for use over the Internet. Members of HECs are encouraged to access these modules during their free time so that not much committee time is taken up with ethics education. While using these modules as a supplement is a good idea, it should not take the place of ongoing education at the committee level because shared learning is an important element of developing trust in and creating mutual respect for committee members, which is essential if HEC members are to collaborate as a team.

As indicated above, most of those who serve on HECs are opposed to the idea of credentialing, believing that it is important to get as many health care professionals as possible involved in the work of the ethics committee by allowing rotation of members on a decided-upon schedule. However, HECs generally agree that continuing education of members is necessary or at least very important. Thus, most HECs have established procedures to assure that continuing education happens on a regular basis. Some authors have proposed that a set of core competencies for HEC members be established as goals (not as requirements), so that member education in ethics would be more structured and take into consideration the many demands made on the time of those serving on HECs (Pape & Manning, 2006).

Bioethics consultants who work in a clinical setting are generally required to possess a higher level of competency than that required for nonethicist members of HECs. Clinical ethicists must know how to communicate with patients and health care professionals and ask questions ethically relevant to patients' care and treatment. They are also expected to provide insights relating to the ethical values and dilemmas at issue in each particular case. They must be able, if possible, to communicate patients' values to their surrogates so that they might be better able to make decisions based on patients' implied wishes when there is no written advance directive. Effective performance of these tasks takes a great deal of training and knowledge, and clinical ethicists should have some kind of credential that shows they have been taught the skills necessary for their work. The problem is that in this area one size does not fit all: ethics consultants are variously (and not exclusively) lawyers, physicians, philosophers, theologians, social workers, priests, ministers, rabbis, and imams. Is there any credential that would cover individuals coming from any and all of these groups? This is the dilemma that professional societies like the American Society for Bioethics and the Humanities have been grappling with for several years, with no resolution of this problem presently in sight.

It seems that a sensible bare minimum requirement for aspiring ethics consultants would be that they possess a master's degree in a field in which ethics is at least part of the curriculum, and that they continue their education by taking at least one course in ethics (or its equivalent) every year they are employed. To require anything further or more uniform would be unwieldy and would sacrifice the multidisciplinary nature of much clinical ethics work. Engelhardt (2003) raises several important questions about the desirability and possibility of credentialing ethics consultants; however, it should be possible to establish at least a bare minimum of necessary training and education, without which a person should not be able to present himself or herself as an ethics consultant in the clinical context.

BIOETHICS CONSULTANTS IN THE FOR-PROFIT WORLD

MOST BIOETHICS CONSULTING is performed within the context of not-for-profit health care organizations. However, in recent years bioethicists have been hired as ethics consultants for pharmaceutical companies, biotechnology developers, and for-profit health care systems. This situation has raised many questions about the responsibilities of these bioethics consultants to the companies who hired them, to their own ethical values and commitments, to the bioethics community, and to the public at large. Most of these concerns focus around the issue of conflicts of interest, but other problems have been raised as well (DeVries & Bosk, 2004; Iltis, 2005a; Jansen & Sulmasy, 2003; Rasmussen, 2005).

Conflicts of interest can easily arise because the bioethicist is being paid by the company whose protocols and products he or she is evaluating. In this situation, can the ethicist objectively evaluate a protocol or project if a negative evaluation might cost the company millions of dollars in lost revenue? Could the ethicist be fired for providing negative evaluations? Are companies hiring ethicists merely as a marketing ploy, to provide an ethical veneer for their protocols and products? One solution that has been used by biomedical ethics consultants to minimize the possibility of conflicts of interest is to disclose the fact that they are employed by the company whose activities are being discussed in any reports or articles written by them. While this is better than nothing, it does not really resolve the fundamental issues that arise when bioethics consultants are paid by the same companies whose protocols and products they are assigned to evaluate.

A solution to this dilemma might be found by looking at Data Safety Monitoring Boards (DSMBs). DSMBs are required by law in research protocols involving human subjects. DSMBs are not the institutional review boards that evaluate the protection of human subjects in research protocols in the first place and monitor them on an ongoing basis. Rather, DSMBs are created to review the data being generated from the research to make sure that none of the arms of the study are producing statistically significant adverse effects. Unless absolutely necessary, DSMBs do not know which arm of the study is the control and which arm is the experiment. What is important in the context of for-profit ethics consultants is the way in which DSMBs are established (National Institutes of Health, 1998).

Companies or industries needing to establish a DSMB must generally contract for a specified amount of time with another organization that in no way stands to benefit from the success or failure of the research. This company then hires the members of the DSMB (usually two or three physicians, an ethicist, and a biostatistician). The DSMB is hired for the duration of the research protocol and examines the data at specified intervals based on the size and duration of the study. The DSMB may stop the investigation at any time if it discovers any statistically significant pattern of adverse events in any arm of the study. A majority of the DSMB (including the ethicist and the biostatistician, who are usually required to be present) decide at every meeting whether to allow the investigation to continue or demand that it be stopped. This arrangement insulates the members of the DSMB from any conflict of interest, because the organization that hires them as well as they, themselves, must be disinterested in the results of the study itself.

Perhaps a similar type of arrangement could be used for the hiring of bioethics consultants. This approach might not provide long-term job security for the consultants because the organization that hired them would be hired by the for-profit company for a specific amount of time (though there is no reason that this contract would have to be of short duration); nevertheless, it would insulate ethicists from conflicts of interest and would allow them a measure of personal integrity and the ability to serve the public and common good more freely and effectively. Admittedly, this is a somewhat bureaucratic solution to the conflicts of interest problem, but for-profit companies who are really concerned about disinterested ethical evaluation of their protocols and products should see this as a structural solution that has worked very effectively in the case of the unbiased operation of DSMBs.

CONCLUSION

THIS CHAPTER HAS focused on the origin and development, as well as the education and credentialing, of HECs and bioethics consultants, and the activity and regulation of bioethics consultants in the for-profit sphere. As technological tools continue to promote information exchange (e.g., podcasts, chat rooms, blogs), more demands may be made on members of HECs to enhance their education in ethics and the clinical setting. It might also be necessary to set up criteria for service on a HEC besides the willingness to be present and participate, such as demanding a certain number of continuing education credits each year that could be obtained by listening to specific podcasts, attending lectures, or participating in Web-based instructional programs.

With regard to conflicts of interest generated by the hiring of ethicists by for-profit corporations, the DSMB model serves only as an example of one way that has been used to minimize conflicts of interest in the public sphere. This model could hopefully serve as a template for structures that would assure that ethicists are able to serve the common good by helping for-profit companies become more ethically responsible—a goal to which ethicists must commit themselves if they are to be faithful to their profession.

REFERENCES

Beauchamp, T., & Childress, J. (2001). *Principles of biomedical ethics* (5th ed.). New York: Oxford University Press.

Bernt, F., Clark, P., Starrs, J., & Talone, P. (2006). Ethics committees in Catholic hospitals. *Health Progress, 87*(2), 18–26.

DeVries, R. G., & Bosk, C. L. (2004). The bioethics of business: Rethinking the relationship between bioethics consultants and corporate clients. *Hastings Center Report, 34*(5), 28–32.

Dubois, J. (2003). Editor's introduction: The varieties of clinical consulting experience. *HEC Forum, 15*(4), 303–309.

Ells, C. (2006). Healthcare ethics committees' contribution to review of institutional policy. *HEC Forum, 18*, 265–275.

Engelhardt, H. T. (2003). The bioethics consultant: Giving moral advice in the midst of moral controversy. *HEC Forum, 15*(4), 362–382.

Iltis, A. S. (2005a). Bioethics consultation in the private sector. *HEC Forum, 17(2)*, 87–93.

Iltis, A. S. (2005b). Values based decision making: Organizational mission and integrity. *HEC Forum, 17*(1), 6–17.

In re Quinlan, 70 N.J. 10 (1976).

Jansen, L. A., & Sulmasy, D. P. (2003). Bioethics, conflicts of interest and the limits of transparency. *Hastings Center Report, 33*(4), 40–43.

Joint Commission on Accreditation of Healthcare Organizations. (1992). *Hospital accreditation manual* (Sections R11 and R12). Chicago: Author.

McCartney, J. J. (1989). Health care ethics committees in south Florida: A comparison and contrast. *HEC Forum, 1*(6), 351–358.

McCartney, J. J. (2005). Values based decision making in healthcare: Introduction. *HEC Forum, 17*(1), 1–5.

National Conference of Catholic Bishops. (1971). *Ethical and religious directives for Catholic health facilities*. Washington, DC: United States Catholic Conference.

National Institutes of Health. (1998). *NIH policy for data and safety monitoring*. Retrieved November 25, 2007, from http://grants.nih.gov/grants/guide/notice-files/not98-084.html

Nilson, E. G., & Fins, J. J. (2006). Reinvigorating ethics consultations: An impetus from the "quality" debate. *HEC Forum, 18*(4), 298–304.

Pape, D., & Manning, S. (2006). The educational ladder model for ethics committees: Confidence and change flourishing through core competency development. *HEC Forum, 18*(4), 305–318.

Post, L. F. (2003). Clinical consulting: The search for resolution at the intersection of medicine, law, and ethics. *HEC Forum, 15*(4), 338–351.

Rasmussen, L. M. (2005). The ethics and aesthetics of for-profit bioethics consultation. *HEC Forum, 17*(2), 94–121.

Rorty, M. V. (2000). Ethics and economics in healthcare: The role of organizational ethics. *HEC Forum, 12*(1), 57–68.

Spielman, B. (2005). Professional independence and corporate employment in bioethics. *HEC Forum, 17*(2), 146–156.

Texas Advance Directives Act, Texas Health and Safety Code, ch 166 (1999).

United States Conference of Catholic Bishops. (2001). *Ethical and religious directives for Catholic health care services* (4th ed.). Retrieved November 25, 2007, from http://www.usccb.org/bishops/directives.shtml

13

Ethical Issues in Nursing Practice

Connie M. Ulrich and Mindy B. Zeitzer

NURSING IS A discipline that is critical to the health and welfare of all nations and the backbone of any health care system. Without a sufficient supply of nurses to care for the public's needs, the public's health is at risk. Unfortunately, the United States is currently experiencing a nationwide nursing shortage and it is estimated that 500,000 additional nurses will be needed by the year 2025 (United Press International, 2008). This represents a potential public health crisis; at a time when we are facing an unprecedented nursing shortage and a need for qualified nurse providers, recruitment and retention efforts should focus on long-term solutions, not simply quick fixes. Regrettably, ethics dialogue is not generally part of this solution, as nurses leave the profession, in part, because of unresolved ethical issues. In the past, nurses were more subordinate than they are today, and changes in the profession continue to address the legitimate role of nursing in society.

In light of these changes, nurses still face ethical challenges that stem from their unique position in the health care system. Historical issues of subordination, limited autonomy, lack of respect, and perception of powerlessness continue to haunt the profession and create sources of frustration, distress, and dissatisfaction. Ultimately, many nurses leave their positions. Therefore, it is important to define and discuss the ethical issues that the nursing profession faces in order to improve not only recruitment and retention of nurses but also address patient-centered care, the overall public good, and the future of health care.

Defining the field of nursing ethics is germane to this process. What is nursing ethics and how is this field addressing ethical issues specific to nursing practice? Is it a separate and distinct field of scholarly inquiry, an amalgam of medical ethics and/or something subsumed under medicine's umbrella? Importantly, how has this message been conveyed to relevant stakeholders to assist nurses within the health care system, if at all? The purpose of this chapter is to provide an overview of the ethical problems in nursing practice and to discuss some of the shared ethical issues that cut across various specialties. We will also discuss the term *nursing ethics,* its historical beginnings, and the importance of this field to the nursing profession, and we will suggest long-term solutions for key constituents, including administrators, policy makers, and the public at large.

HISTORICAL BACKGROUND

NURSES HAVE ENCOUNTERED ethical problems in their clinical and professional practice since the early 19th century. In her *Notes on Nursing,* Florence Nightingale (1859) discusses the importance of ethical actions such as listening to patients, upholding confidentiality, and putting patients' needs first. These acts of beneficent caring reflect early indicators of a nursing ethic or what might be considered essential ethical duties of the profession. In fact, Nightingale (1859) noted that nursing was a specialty and that the knowledge of nursing was essentially separate and distinct from that of medicine. And since 1900, not a single decade has passed without at least one publication on nursing ethics, with the earliest nursing text being published in 1886 (Jameton, 1984; Luckes, 1886). Additionally, although we believe that nursing ethics is a legitimate field of scientific inquiry, there continues to be no general consensus on whether it is distinct from other subdisciplines of applied ethics, such as medical ethics (Fry & Veatch, 2000; Volker, 2003).

Ethics courses were commonly included in nursing curriculum until World War II (Jameton, 1984). In the early 1900s, nursing ethics focused on nursing character and virtues, such as discipline, because professional behavior was perceived as part of moral character (Perry, 1906; Volbrecht, 2002). Loyalty, obedience, and nursing duties were major foci of nursing ethics during this time. The Nightingale pledge, first used in 1893, emphasized loyalty as a key virtue of the nurse and of nursing ethics (Winslow, 1984). This was further enforced in Aikens's text (1916) on nursing ethics, a standard book for over 20 years (Winslow, 1984). Indeed, this sense of loyalty to physicians and others in authoritative positions precluded nurses from questioning the judgment or patient treatment prescriptions of other members of the health care team. To question a physician was to create doubts about his or her character, ultimately diminishing the confidence of the patient that was considered essential to illness management (Winslow, 1984). Of course, this behavior created difficult moral dilemmas for many nurses, which to some degree still exists today. Where the nursing profession's loyalty lies is an ethical question that even now creates conflict in the provision of patient care and has only intensified with increased autonomy within nursing, technological and genetic advancements, cost concerns, and an aging society.

As the mid-1900s approached and World War II started, nursing curriculum adopted courses in science and health care technology and omitted nursing ethics from the curriculum. At this time, the American Nurses Association (ANA) and the International Council of Nurses (ICN) adopted their codes of ethics (ANA, 1950; ICN, 1953). These codes of ethics outlined essential principles and duties of the profession and served as a guiding force for ethical conduct. Hospitals and other health care institutions also began adopting codes and regulations for nurses to follow rather than providing ethics training as part of their core educational requirements.

By the late 1900s, nurses rediscovered and refined their own ethics. In 1973, the ICN revised the beginning of their code of ethics from "The nurse is under an obligation to carry out the physician's orders intelligently and loyally" (*Code for Nurses*, 1965) to "The nurse sustains a cooperative relationship with co-workers in nursing and other fields" (*Code for Nurses*, 1973). The *ICN Code of Ethics for Nurses* (*ICN Code of Ethics for Nurses*, 2006) now includes the statement, "The nurse's primary professional responsibility is to people requiring nursing care," emphasizing the nurse's responsibility to the patient and human rights rather than duties and loyalty to physicians and others. These codes are not stagnant; they are frequently revisited and updated as issues arise within the profession and societal needs change.

Sara Fry, Anne Davis, Patricia Benner, and other early nursing ethics leaders set the stage for a fuller discussion of the ethical problems nurses encounter in their daily practice, and they are credited for their honest and candid portrayal of and dialogue on many sensitive ethical issues. With societal changes, nurses have gained greater independence and can fully participate in ethical decision-making related to patient care. As nurses have become more autonomous, however, the need for ethics education in nursing curriculums has resurfaced, and we believe that nursing ethics needs to be defined as a legitimate field of inquiry within academia.

Fry and Veatch (2000) agree that while nursing ethics falls under the umbrella of bioethics, it is not the same as medical ethics. While nursing and medicine face similar ethical issues, there are also distinct issues because the physician-patient relationship is inherently different from the nurse-patient relationship. Nevertheless, we need to identify what it is that makes nursing ethics unique. Is it the holistic and healing relationship that nurses have with patients? Is it the nature of the ethical issues that arise or that are inherently imbedded within the practice? Is it the in-between role of nurses who must function between physicians, patients, and differing hierarchal positions within institutions (Bishop & Scudder, 2001; Engelhardt, 1985; Hamric, 2001; Volker, 2003)? Or maybe it is a combination of these and other criteria?

ETHICAL ISSUES IN NURSING PRACTICE

NURSES ARE CONFRONTED with complex ethical challenges on a daily basis. These present themselves in various manners in a myriad of nursing specialties. In his text on nursing ethics, Jameton (1984) first described three different types of moral problems in nursing: moral uncertainty, moral dilemma, and moral distress. Today, nurses experience all three types of moral problems with serious consequences for the profession and the health care needs of society. First, moral uncertainty exists when nurses do not know the ethically correct action in a given situation, and this may lead to silence "out of deference to the judgment of others, out of fear that their comments will be ignored, or out of uncertainty that what they might have to say is really not that important" (Bird, 1996, p. 1). Second, moral dilemmas occur in nursing when (two or more) competing morally correct courses of action can be equally justified (Beauchamp & Childress, 2001; Purtilo, 2005). In choosing one course of action over the other, the nurse is between a rock and a hard place that potentially threatens her integrity. The nurse chooses a morally correct action, but in doing so, a sense of wrongdoing by not choosing "the other thing that is also right" may arise (Purtilo, 2005, p. 39). Third, moral distress occurs when the agent knows the morally correct action but is precluded from taking it because of external constraints on his/her practice—organizational, legal, authoritative power, or simply time pressures. Here, a nurse might ask him/herself, Why am I continuing to participate in providing care that I believe is morally wrong and only creates more suffering? Moral distress, then, often leads to feelings of anger, frustration, and guilt, contributing to nurse burnout, turnover, and nurses leaving the profession (Corley, 1995; Corley, Elswick, Gorman, & Clor, 2001; Elpern, Covert, & Kleinpell, 2005; Kelly, 1998; Sundin-Huard & Fahy, 1999; Wilkinson, 1987/1988).

Each nursing specialty presents its own unique set of ethical issues for nurses, most likely because of the nature of the patients' illnesses, social commitment to treatment, the technology, the organization, and the relationship of professionals delivering care (e.g., the relationship between nurses and their coworkers, physicians, other professionals; Redman & Fry, 2000). Research has highlighted these particular ethical problems in specialties such as community health, acute care and hospital-based care, mental health, critical care, home care, oncology, diabetes care, nephrology, rehabilitation, pediatric care, administration, and managed care. For example, critical care nurses are often confronted with conflicts related to prolonging a patient's life without benefit while mental health nurses struggle with delivery of care to a patient against his/her will. Although these issues differ, basic ethical principles of "doing good," "avoiding harm," "respecting patient rights," and "providing just care" are universal (see Table 13.1).

It is not unusual for nurses to struggle with balancing the benefits and burdens of patient care, including discontinuing or initiating treatments, particularly in terminally ill patients. Other particular concerns include respecting patient autonomy by respecting the right to refuse care, following or not following patients' advance directives, issues of informed consent, administering life-prolonging aggressive therapies, and compromising professional and personal integrity.

While studies have shown that nurses experience unique issues within specialties, a few ethical issues cut across nursing practice in general. These include: quality of care, adequacy of staffing and resource allocation, and autonomy. Frequently identified issues include informed consent, advance directives, restraint use, patient-provider relationship, use of aggressive therapies to prolong life, patient advocacy/protecting patient rights, providing high-risk care (risk to providers), and nurse-physician relationships (Butz, Redman, Fry, & Kolodner, 1998; Ferrell & Rivera, 1995; Killen, Fry, & Damrosch, 1996; Redman & Fry, 1996, 1998a, 1998b, 2000, 2003; Redman, Hill, & Fry, 1997; Severinsson & Hummelvoll, 2001; Ulrich, Soeken, & Miller, 2003). These day-to-day ethical challenges that nurses must grapple with receive little attention (Hamric, 2000). However, the individual and collective research results beg serious pragmatic and normative questions about what can and ought to be done that will make a difference for nurses.

WHY IS ADDRESSING ETHICAL PROBLEMS IN NURSING IMPORTANT?

As trained professionals, nurses are moral agents caring for the intimate needs of the ill and infirmed, acting on their professional knowledge for the betterment of the patient. Moral agency has been conceptualized as an "action based upon self-embodied

TABLE 13.1   Ethical Issues in Nursing Practice Categorized by Guiding Ethical
Principles and Values

Beneficence	—Administering life-prolonging aggressive therapies.
	—Balancing the risks and benefits to patients.
	—Discontinuing or initiating treatments such as dialysis, particularly with regard to terminally ill patients.
	—Undertreating pain.
	—Over- or undertreating patients.
	—Using or not using physical or chemical restraints.
	—Overriding patient care needs by business decisions.
	—Staffing patterns that limit patient access to nursing care.
	—Patient advocacy.
	—Quality of medical care patients receive.
Respect for persons	—Balancing the risks and benefits to patients.
	—Approaching a mentally ill patient.
	—Creating a good relationship with the patient.
	—Respecting patients' autonomy.
	⋄ Right to refuse treatment.
	⋄ Do not resuscitate orders.
	⋄ Following or not following advance directives.
	⋄ Informed consent.
	⋄ Respecting or not respecting informed consent for treatment.
	⋄ Deciding the ethically correct action for a patient.
	—Respecting patients' rights.
	⋄ Providing care against the patient's will.
	⋄ Patients' rights.
	⋄ Protecting the child's rights.
	⋄ Protecting patient rights and human dignity.
	⋄ Use or nonuse of physical or chemical restraints.
Justice	—Administering life-prolonging aggressive therapies.
	—Discontinuing or initiating treatments such as dialysis, particularly with regard to terminally ill patients.
	—Over- or undertreating patients.
	—Deciding what is right and what should be done.
	—Overriding patient care needs by business decisions.
	—Having to follow various medical or institutional practices.
	—Dealing with payment issues.
Professional/ personal integrity	—Communication.
	—Recognizing own values and norms that influence actions.
	—Compromising personal values and ethics.
	—Concern over becoming agents for the health plan rather than patient advocates.
	—Providing care with possible risks to nurses' health.
	—Providing care with risk to self.
	—Nurse-physician relationships.
	—Child/parent/practitioner relationship.

Note. Table is not exhaustive (Butz et al., 1998; Ferrell & Rivera, 1995; Killen et al., 1996; Redman & Fry, 1996, 1998a, 1998b, 2000, 2003; Redman et al., 1997; Severinsson & Hummelvoll, 2001; Ulrich et al., 2003).

principles and knowledge to facilitate a perceived positive outcome for the patient, family, or society" (Raines, 1994, p. 7). But technological innovations, along with an aging society, changing cultural demography, and fragility within the health care system, have created complex ethical challenges for nurses and threaten their agency. Questions continually arise regarding the appropriate and ethical use of technology, the fair and judicial use of limited resources, and equality of health care. Today, "it is not enough to recognize that something is morally wrong; to truly be good moral agents, we also must know how to confront wrongful behavior" (Cooper, 2004, p. 82).

It seems plausible to question if nurses are considered good moral agents if they perceive there are some ethical problems they can do nothing about, report powerlessness, fail to confront ethical conflicts in patient care for fear of reprisal, are morally distressed (i.e., the agent knows the morally right course of action but is inhibited from carrying out the action because of institutional or other identified constraints), and if 25% or more want to leave their positions (Danis et al., 2008; Hamric & Blackhall, 2007; Hamric, Davis, & Childress, 2006; Jameton, 1984; Ulrich et al., 2007). If nurses are so unsatisfied and distressed, how can they act to facilitate positive outcomes for patients—particularly when they face a history of subordination? Despite these problems, one of nurses' primary roles is patient advocacy. But if they perceive such powerlessness, how do they advocate for appropriate patient care? There seems to be a disconnect between the manner in which nurses accept responsibility in their professional roles and the manner in which they perceive their effectiveness, particularly when it comes to difficult ethical decisions.

Among these other problems that nurses perceive, about one out of four nurses report physical symptoms associated with ethical problems (e.g., headaches, stomach aches, tension in neck or shoulders) and/or report burnout and emotional exhaustion, and many simply feel disrespected within health care settings (Laschinger, 2004; Ulrich et al., 2007). Limited perceived organizational support for ethical issues in nursing practice raises concerns about the ability to openly voice dissent and challenge assumptions/practices related to ethical decision-making in patient care. Indeed, several authors posit a relationship between health outcomes of hospital employees including nurses (i.e., absences due to sickness) and perceived levels of organizational justice (Elovainio, Kivimaki, & Vahtera, 2002).

Addressing ethical challenges in nursing practice is imperative if we want to retain qualified professionals, maintain the quality and personal nature of the nurse-patient relationship, and improve the health and well-being of patients, families, and the providers who care for them. Unfortunately, merely 23% of nurses have received ethics education, and Grady et al. (2008) report a significant relationship between ethics education and nurses' ability to take moral action. Ethics education is necessary but not sufficient to resolve all of the ethical problems that nurses experience; it can, however, assist providers to articulate and advocate for their moral positions, potentially increasing their negotiating power within health care institutions. As Lützén, Cronqvist, Magnusson, and Anderson (2003) commented: "Leaving nursing may be the last resort for some and one way of avoiding the negative consequences of moral stress, and subsequent ill health, but this does not solve any problems for the common good of health care" (p. 320). In a similar way, for those who choose to stay in their positions, ethical numbing or adaptability may occur where a go along to get along mentality is perceived as necessary when personal values conflict with institutional constraints (Mohr & Mahon, 1996; Ulrich, 2001; Wynia, Cummings, VanGeest, & Wilson, 2000). But this too has consequences. What harm do we do ourselves and others if we remain in our positions but are morally mute (Bird, 1996)?

CONCLUSION

As NURSES CONTINUE to struggle with a multitude of ethical problems in the workplace, it has become imperative that we concentrate our efforts on finding solutions to overcome these challenges. More empirical bioethics research and ethical discourse among key stakeholders will allow us to identify the best strategies that help nurses address the ethical challenges in their practice. In doing so, they can meet their most fundamental role of patient care and patient advocacy in a manner that upholds their moral integrity. It is no longer acceptable to avoid, dismiss, or diminish the ethical problems that nurses encounter. Throughout the history of nursing, ethics has served as a cornerstone of professional conduct, beneficent care, and societal good. The ethical problems then and now are real and are dramatically affecting nurses and patient care. If nursing is to continue in its healing, caring, and advocacy traditions, we must take nursing ethics seriously as a discipline in order to create necessary change.

REFERENCES

Aikens, C. A. (1916). *Studies in ethics for nurses*. Philadelphia: W. B. Saunders Company.

American Nurses Association. (1950). A code for nurses. *American Journal of Nursing, 50,* 196.

Beauchamp, T. L., & Childress, J. F. (2001). *Principles of biomedical ethics* (5th ed.). Oxford: Oxford University Press.

Bird, F. B. (1996). *The muted conscience: Moral silence and the practice of ethics in business.* Westport, CT: Greenwood Publishing Group.

Bishop, A., & Scudder, J. (2001). *Nursing ethics: Therapeutic caring presence* (2nd ed.). Boston: Jones and Bartlett Publishers.

Butz, A., Redman, B. K., Fry, S. T., & Kolodner, K. (1998). Ethical conflicts experienced by certified pediatric nurse practitioners in ambulatory settings. *Journal of Pediatric Health Care, 12*(4), 183–190.

Code for nurses. (1965). Geneva: International Council of Nurses.

Code for nurses. (1973). Geneva: International Council of Nurses.

Cooper, D. E. (2004). *Ethics for professionals in a multicultural world.* Upper Saddle River, NJ: Pearson/Prentice Hall.

Corley, M. C. (1995). Moral distress of critical care nurses. *American Journal of Critical Care, 4*(4), 280–285.

Corley, M. C., Elswick, R. K., Gorman, M., & Clor, T. (2001). Development and evaluation of the moral distress scale. *Journal of Advanced Nursing, 33*(2), 250–256.

Danis, M., Farrar, A., Grady, C., Taylor, C., O'Donnell, P., Soeken, K., et al. (2008). Does fear of retaliation deter requests for ethics consultation? *Medicine, Health Care and Philosophy, 11*(1), 27–34.

Elovainio, M., Kivimaki, M., & Vahtera, J. (2002). Organizational justice: Evidence of a new psychosocial predictor of health. *American Journal of Public Health, 92,* 105–108.

Elpern, E. H., Covert, B., & Kleinpell, R. (2005). Moral distress of staff nurses in a medical intensive care unit. *American Journal of Critical Care, 14*(6), 523–530.

Engelhardt, H. T. (1985). Physicians, patients, health care institutions—and the people in between: Nurses. In A. H. Bishop & J. R. Scudder (Eds.), *Caring, curing, coping: Nurse, physician, patient relationships* (pp. 62–79). Birmingham: University of Alabama Press.

Ferrell, B. R., & Rivera, L. M. (1995). Ethical decision making in oncology: A case study approach. *Cancer Practice, 3*(2), 94–99.

Fry, S. T., & Veatch, R. M. (2000). *Case studies in nursing ethics* (2nd ed.). Boston: Jones and Bartlett Publishers.

Grady, C., Soeken, K., Danis, M., O'Donnell, P., Taylor, C., Farrar, A., et al. (2008). Does ethics education influence the moral action of practicing nurses and social workers? *American Journal of Bioethics, 8*(4), 4–11.

Hamric, A. B. (2000). Moral distress in everyday ethics. *Nursing Outlook, 48,* 199–201.

Hamric, A. B. (2001). Reflections on being in the middle. *Nursing Outlook, 49,* 254–257.

Hamric, A. B., & Blackhall, L. J. (2007). Nurse-physician perspective on the care of dying patients in intensive care units: Collaboration, moral distress, and ethical climate. *Critical Care Medicine, 35*(2), 422–429.

Hamric, A. B., Davis, W. S., & Childress, M. D. (2006). Moral distress in health care professionals: What is it and what can we do about it? *The Pharos of Alpha Omega Alpha-Honor Medical Society, 69*(1), 16–23.

ICN code of ethics for nurses. (2006). Geneva: International Council of Nurses.

International Council of Nurses. (1953). International code of nursing ethics. *American Journal of Nursing, 53,* 1070.

Jameton, A. (1984). *Nursing practice: The ethical issues.* Englewood Cliffs, NJ: Prentice-Hall.

Kelly, B. (1998). Preserving moral integrity: A follow-up study with new graduate nurses. *Journal of Advanced Nursing, 28*(5), 1134–1145.

Killen, A. R., Fry, S. T., & Damrosch, S. (1996). Ethics and human rights issues in perioperative nurses: A subsample of Maryland nurses. *Seminars in Perioperative Nursing, 5*(2), 77–83.

Laschinger, H. S. (2004). Hospital nurses' perceptions of respect and organizational justice. *Journal of Nursing Administration, 34,* 354–364.

Luckes, E. C. E. (1886). *Hospital sisters and their duties.* London: J. and A. Churchill.

Lützén, K., Cronqvist, A., Magnusson, A., & Anderson, L. (2003). Moral stress: Synthesis of a concept. *Nursing Ethics, 10*(3), 312–322.

Mohr, W. K., & Mahon, M. M. (1996). Dirty hands: The underside of marketplace health care. *Advances in Nursing Science, 19*(1), 29–37.

Nightingale, F. (1859). *Notes on nursing: What it is and what it is not.* London: Harrison & Sons.

Perry, C. M. (1906). Nursing ethics and etiquette. *American Journal of Nursing, 6,* 450–451.

Purtilo, R. (2005). *Ethical dimensions in the health professions* (4th ed.). Philadelphia: Elsevier Saunders.

Raines, D. A. (1994). Moral agency in nursing. *Nursing Forum, 29,* 5–11.

Redman, B. K., & Fry, S. T. (1996). Ethical conflicts reported by registered nurse/certified diabetes educators. *Diabetes Educator, 22*(3), 219–224.

Redman, B. K., & Fry, S. T. (1998a). Ethical conflicts reported by certified registered rehabilitation nurses. *Rehabilitation Nurse, 23*(4), 179–184.

Redman, B. K., & Fry, S. T. (1998b). Ethical conflicts reported by registered nurse/certified diabetes educators: A replication. *Journal of Advanced Nursing, 28*(6), 1320–1325.

Redman, B. K., & Fry, S. T. (2000). Nurses' ethical conflicts: What is really known about them? *Nursing Ethics: An International Journal for Health Care Professionals, 7*(4), 360–366.

Redman, B. K., & Fry, S. T. (2003). Ethics and human rights issues experienced by nurses in leadership roles. *Nursing Leadership Forum, 7*(4), 150–156.

Redman, B. K., Hill, M. N., & Fry, S. T. (1997). Ethical conflicts reported by certified nephrology nurses (CNNs) practicing in dialysis settings. *American Nephrology Nurses Association Journal, 24*(1), 23–31.

Severinsson, E., & Hummelvoll, J. K. (2001). Factors influencing job satisfaction and ethical dilemmas in acute psychiatric care. *Nursing and Health Sciences, 3*(2), 81–90.

Sundin-Huard, D., & Fahy, K. (1999). Moral distress, advocacy and burnout: Theorizing the relationships. *International Journal of Nursing Practice, 5,* 8–13.

Ulrich, C. M. (2001). Practitioners' perceptions on ethical aspects of managed care. *Dissertation Abstracts International, 62,* B1326.

Ulrich, C. M., O'Donnell, P., Taylor, C., Farrar, A., Danis, M., & Grady, C. (2007). Ethical climate, ethics stress, and the job satisfaction of nurses and social workers in the United States. *Social Science and Medicine, 65*(8), 1708–1719.

Ulrich, C. M., Soeken, K. L., & Miller, N. (2003). Ethical conflict associated with managed care. *Nursing Research, 52*(3), 168–175.

United Press International. (2008). *Nurses should prepare for fewer nurses.* Retrieved May 12, 2008, from http://www.upi.com/NewsTrack/Health/2008/03/28/patients_should_prepare_for_fewer_nurses/1560/

Volbrecht, R. M. (2002). *Nursing ethics: Communities in dialogue.* Upper Saddle River, NJ: Prentice Hall.

Volker, D. L. (2003). Is there a unique nursing ethic? *Nursing Science Quarterly, 16*(3), 207–211.

Wilkinson, J. M. (1987/1988). Moral distress in nursing practice: Experience and effect. *Nursing Forum, 23*(1), 16–29.

Winslow, G. (1984). From loyalty to advocacy: A new metaphor for nursing. *The Hastings Center Report, 14*(3), 32–40.

Wynia, M. K., Cummings, D. S., VanGeest, J. B., & Wilson, I. B. (2000). Physician manipulation of reimbursement rules for patients: Between a rock and a hard place. *Journal of the American Medical Association, 283*(14), 1858–1865.

14

Conscientious Refusals by Physicians

HOLLY FERNANDEZ LYNCH

PHYSICIANS OFTEN ENTER the profession of medicine because they wish to help others, serve patients in need, and generally do good. However, what should happen when patients request services that are legally permissible but that their physicians find morally objectionable, such as abortion, the withdrawal of life-sustaining treatment, or the purposeful creation of deaf children? Do these physicians have a responsibility to do whatever their patients ask, or should they be allowed to refuse on grounds of personal conscience?

Many state legislatures and professional organizations answer these questions in favor of the physician, often without regard to the burden this approach may impose on patients vulnerable to the collective professional monopoly. Such one-sidedness has led to considerable criticism, and the gravity of conflicts of conscience between doctors and patients has only been compounded as technology pushes forward into morally controversial territory. Although patient access concerns are clearly a fundamental issue in need of resolution, it is essential to recognize that forcing physicians to provide services they deem to be ethically impermissible may not be the best way to achieve this goal, especially given the desirability of maintaining a role for morally serious physicians with a wide variety of perspectives. Developing a compromise capable of balancing the interests of patients and their physicians is imperative, but unfortunately this has proven to be quite difficult.

HISTORICAL BACKGROUND

LEGISLATION FORMALLY PROTECTIVE of physician conscience, often referred to as "conscience clauses," first began to appear around the time that the Supreme Court handed down its revolutionary decision in *Roe v. Wade*. Concerned that newly established negative rights against state interference in reproductive decision-making would soon turn into positive entitlements that could be demanded from individual doctors, Congress passed the first federal conscience clause, known as the Church Amendment, in 1973. Prompted by similar fears, as well as reactions against the patient autonomy movement and increasing secularization of the public sphere, the vast majority of states followed suit, passing a flurry of refusal legislation initially focused on abortion, contraceptive services, and sterilization (Charo, 2005; Minow, 2001).

Today, 46 states, the District of Columbia, and the federal government have statutes shielding physicians who refuse to participate in abortion procedures from an incredibly broad array of consequences, such as liability to patients, negative employment actions, and professional discipline. Several states extend this protection to doctors who will not engage in the provision of contraceptive and sterilization services, assisted reproduction, human cloning, fetal experimentation, euthanasia, physician-assisted suicide, and, most frequently, to doctors who refuse to participate in withholding or withdrawing life-sustaining treatment. Laws in Illinois, Mississippi, and Washington prevent physicians from having to provide *any* medical service to which they are morally opposed. Increasingly, conscience clauses reach beyond physicians to cover other health care providers, such as nurses and pharmacists, as well as health care institutions, such as hospitals and insurers (Smearman, 2006; Swartz, 2006, Wardle, 1993).

LEGAL ANALYSIS

ONE OF THE most interesting—and least discussed—aspects of conscience clauses is whether the protection they offer is really necessary against the backdrop of what physicians could expect without them. First, it may be the case that physicians can, and often do, protect themselves by simply avoiding fields where they are likely to be asked to provide services they find morally objectionable. However, such self-selection may become more difficult as controversial technologies and procedures infiltrate nearly every medical specialty; as stem cell research advances, for example, it will no longer be sufficient for physicians committed to the moral inviolability of the unborn to steer clear of the specialties traditionally responsible for abortions. If these doctors were to refuse, what would happen to them in the absence of legislative protection?

With regard to liability to patients, probably not much. Existing case law and statements of professional ethics convey the well-established rule that initiation of the physician-patient relationship is entirely voluntary for both parties. Physicians are free to refuse to accept a prospective patient for any reason not prohibited by law or contract, such as discriminatory bases for refusal (Dietz, Jacobs, Leming, & Kennel, 2006a; American Medical Association, 2001, 2003). Because physicians have no duty of care to non-patients, prospective patients who are refused services based on a physician's moral beliefs have no basis on which to bring a lawsuit, offering physicians another level of protection completely outside the realm of conscience clause legislation. Even current patients seem out of luck, given that in the absence of an emergency, a physician can terminate an existing relationship so long as he provides the patient with sufficient notice of his intention to do so (Dietz et al., 2006b). Thus, in many ways, statutory elimination of any duty that could be used to form a malpractice case against a refusing physician may be redundant, since it already appears that in many cases, no such duty exists.

Nonetheless, conscience clauses are doing some work (Lynch, 2008). On the employment front, they often supplement Title VII's protection against discrimination on the basis of an employee's religious beliefs by offering protection of secular moral refusals and requiring accommodation of an employee's conscience without regard to the hardship such accommodation may impose on the employer (see, e.g., *Swanson v. St. John's Lutheran Hosp.*, 1979). More importantly, they prevent state medical boards from demanding that physicians provide certain services regardless of their moral objections as a condition for obtaining or retaining their license to practice medicine, which these boards might otherwise be able to do under existing Free Exercise jurisprudence (see, *Employment Division v. Smith*, 1990). Thus, conscience clauses do protect physicians, but they often go too far. When *should* physicians have a duty to satisfy patient requests and when *should* they be able to refuse?

OPPOSING PERSPECTIVES

MUCH OF THE existing debate surrounding conflicts of conscience in health care contrasts the rights of patients with the rights of physicians, but this trumping approach is not very helpful.

First, as a legal matter, patients have very few positive rights to health care services in this country, which is one of the most frequent and stinging critiques of the American system. Even those services to which they can claim an entitlement do not generally involve a claim on any particular physician (Lynch, 2008). Thus, a woman may be free to obtain an abortion, for example, but no one has any concrete legal obligation to actually provide her with one.

On the other hand, conscience clauses themselves do impart on physicians a legal right to refuse, but the existence of these statutes lies within the discretion of policy makers—conscience clause protection appears to be neither constitutionally mandated nor constitutionally prohibited. Religious individuals are not entitled under the First Amendment's Free Exercise Clause to exemptions from valid and neutral state laws of general applicability governing conduct but not beliefs, such as duties of care or licensing requirements covering all health care professionals, although the Establishment Clause will tolerate broad religious exemptions to such laws (American Civil Liberties Union, 2002; Lynch, 2008). For these reasons, reliance on legal rights to resolve the conscience clause debate will prove fruitless. Instead, a normative analysis of moral rights and duties is in order, though commentators have resorted to trumping in this realm as well.

At one extreme, some commentators on medical professionalism argue that physicians, simply by virtue of becoming physicians, have an absolute obligation to provide all medical services within their professional specialty, regardless of any moral objections they may harbor toward a particular service and regardless of the existence of more compromising alternatives. These opponents of conscientious refusal suggest that if the moral stakes are so high for refusing physicians, they should simply not enter the profession in the first place; a person who is afraid of flying cannot complain when he is denied a job as a pilot, and a physician who will not perform abortions cannot object to being excluded from the fields of obstetrics and gynecology.

Physicians, these opponents argue, must advance the patient's self-defined interests, imposing only those limits already set by law, and perhaps by widely accepted tenets of medical ethics. They should act as nothing more than technical accomplices whose sole function is to resolve problems of information and skill asymmetry, providing all of the facts truthfully and without judgment, which the patient can then apply in accord with his or her own values to select the desired medical service. When they act otherwise, physicians are accused of unacceptably encumbering their patients and behaving selfishly. The bottom line for these critics is that physicians have voluntarily taken on their responsibilities, while patients are in a vulnerable position of relying on doctors for care. From this perspective, patients win (Blustein & Fleischman, 1995; Rhodes, 2006; Savulescu, 2006).

At the opposite end of the spectrum are those commentators who claim that professionals have no obligation of moral neutrality. In response to arguments that conscientious objectors should find another profession, they point out that nearly all clinical decisions involve value judgments. Thus, to exclude only those physicians whose value judgments are based on religion or other personal moral beliefs is an unacceptable preferential imposition of one set of values as the only acceptable values in a pluralistic society. This side of the debate also stresses the fact that simple legality or public consensus surrounding a particular medical service does not automatically confer moral acceptability. Since no one has an obligation to perform morally wrong acts, whether a professional or not, refusing physicians should actually be praised for their unwillingness to ignore their conscientious beliefs, for they may in fact be right.

Supporters of conscience clause protection reject the notion that physicians are nothing more than instruments for the advancement of the patient's will, noting instead that physicians are morally responsible for the actions they take as professionals, regardless of whether they were requested by another. Finally, they claim that autonomy is a right applicable to all persons regardless of role, such that respect for autonomy cannot be a solely patient-driven concept but must also be applicable to physicians, who should not be expected to ignore their personal beliefs simply because they are acting in their professional capacity. From this angle, doctors win (Collett, 1999; May, 2001; Pellegrino, 1989, 1993, 2000, 2002).

Unfortunately, neither of these perspectives adequately contends with access issues. Too many of those who suggest that refusing physicians should leave the profession, or at the very least the specialty responsible for providing the objectionable service, ignore that such a drastic solution is unnecessary in the vast majority of situations where patient access can be preserved even if the patient is unable to obtain the desired service from a given physician. More troublesome is that these opponents fail to recognize the serious problems associated with eliminating refusing physicians entirely, particularly the lack of diversity of opinion that this would breed within the profession, the important moral debate and counsel of restraint that could be lost, and the fact that refusers can often provide a plethora of other desired services to their patients (Lynch, 2008). Why not treat them as subspecialists who choose to restrict their practice for personal reasons, just as other physicians may restrict the hours during which they are willing to see patients or choose to focus on a particular disease or procedure that they find most interesting, even if patients may have a stronger need

for some other specialty? On the other side of the spectrum, proponents of conscience clause protection stress that patients should not
be allowed to impose their views on their doctors, while ignoring the
reality that when a patient cannot find another physician willing to
provide the requested service, the refusing physician has unacceptably
imposed his view on the patient.

THE VALUE OF INSTITUTIONAL SOLUTIONS

CLEARLY, ACCESS CONCERNS are at the heart of this debate,
but attempts to resolve them by focusing on the responsibilities
of individual physicians seem destined for stalemate. Instead, a more
broadly acceptable solution may be possible by abstracting to an institutional level. The profession of medicine holds a collective monopoly
over the provision of a variety of legal medical services resulting from
a social contract crafted to protect patients and the community from
dangerous and immoral practices and providers. This monopoly, combined with understandings of professional altruism and the needs of
society, creates an obligation on the profession to secure the availability of services only it can provide. Notably, individual physicians do
not always bear this monopoly power themselves, particularly when
other physicians are reasonably available to the patient. For this reason, it is often—though not always—possible to bifurcate the responsibilities of individual doctors and the responsibilities of the collective
group in order to mitigate the access concerns raised by conscientious
refusal (Charo, 2005, 2007; Dresser, 2004).

In fact, this sort of compromise solution has proven capable of balancing the interests of professionals and patients in both the pharmacy
and end-of-life contexts (Lynch, 2008). For example, several states have
responded to recent refusals by pharmacists to fill prescriptions for
contraceptives by imposing an obligation on pharmacies to ensure
that patients can access their medications, rather than forcing individual pharmacists to perform. Similarly, courts have required hospitals to comply with a patient's wishes to forego artificial nutrition and
hydration without demanding that any particular doctor be involved.
In these cases, it is not up to any individual professional to satisfy the
patient's demand, but rather the burden is placed on some higher-level
institution. This way, individual professionals can remain true to their
personal beliefs and patients can readily access the medical services
they desire. In other words, both parties win.

Executing this division of responsibility in other contexts will be a
challenge, since medical care is quite frequently rendered outside of the
hospitals and pharmacies that can bear the burden of accommodating
both patients and doctors. Which institution can implement the

concrete measures that are needed to ensure that patients have reasonable access on a broader scale to physicians who will not lodge conscientious objections against their requests? Voluntary professional organizations might take steps in the right direction, but state licensing boards are the preferable institutions capable of preventing and resolving denials of patient access (Lynch, 2008). By monitoring supply and providing incentives for willing physicians to practice in areas where conscientious refusals threaten patient access, these boards are in the position to guarantee that the monopoly power of the profession never (or at least rarely) trickles down to individual physicians.

However, boards taking on this new role will have their work cut out for them. What counts as reasonable access? Is it too much to ask patients to seek services from an alternate physician who is 20 miles away, and does the answer to that question depend on what type of services the patient seeks? Are there any legal medical services that the profession has no obligation to provide, perhaps things like sex-selective abortions or breast augmentation for adolescent girls? Are there any types of physician refusals that are unacceptable even if the patient can obtain the desired service elsewhere with no problem at all? And what steps should the profession take to calibrate the supply of willing physicians and the demand for their services?

Many of these questions are quite difficult, though they are not intractable (Lynch, 2008). Reasonable access could be measured in comparison to the level of access patients could expect if they resided in a similar geographic area whose physicians felt no need for conscientious refusal, and patients can often be expected to sacrifice some level of convenience in order to respect the beliefs of physicians. Broad social discussion could conclude that the profession can limit its services only on the basis of its scientific expertise and what is legal, or perhaps broader moral limits are appropriate. Easiest of all, refusals based on objections to the patient who is requesting the service, rather than to the service itself, should be deemed unacceptable. When invidious discrimination is at issue, access is not the only concern; the avoidance of dignitary harm is essential as well. Unfortunately, however, even when these issues are resolved, there are likely to remain some cases in which the institutional solution will fail to ensure patient access, leaving individual refusing physicians once again at odds with patients.

HARD CASES AND BASELINE OBLIGATIONS

WHEN THESE FAILURES occur, the individual physician finds himself in the position of the sole gatekeeper of the medical monopoly such that bifurcation of responsibilities is no longer possible. The patient is uniquely vulnerable to *this* physician—if she refuses to provide the desired service, the patient will not be able to obtain it from any other source. Concern for the equality of citizens, in the sense that they should be able to access medical services regardless of where they live, the threat of informal rule by an oligarchy of physicians, and the value of diversity in terms of the medical services that are available are all factors suggesting that physicians finding themselves in the position of the last doctor in town have a professional obligation to provide the requested service regardless of their personal moral objections. Physicians can appropriately object, but they cannot appropriately obstruct (Cantor & Baum, 2004).

Importantly, however, while this conclusion seems technically correct, the practical consequences of actually enforcing such professional responsibilities would likely do more harm than good. Physicians can only have an obligation to perform the services that fall within their technical competence, so if they avoid competence, they can avoid the obligation. Because this approach simply moves the refusal to an earlier point in the physician's career, leaving access problems intact, would it be appropriate to force physicians to learn and maintain the competence to perform even objectionable services? Physicians who truly find the service morally wrong would sooner leave the profession than provide it, or at least relocate to a geographic area with access to other willing providers so as to avoid bearing the profession's responsibility.

Unfortunately, these disincentive effects would only exacerbate access problems, leaving some patients in precisely the same position they would have been in had the last doctor in town been permitted to refuse, and potentially harming an even broader scope of patients who desire unobjectionable services but who now have no physician to provide them. Therefore, while physicians should be strongly encouraged to respond to patient demands when the patient has no practicable alternative, and in fact may have a professional duty as the last doctor in town, for consequential reasons, they should not be punished for failing to do so in any way beyond social reprehension and loss of patients (Lynch, 2008).

Then again, some professional responsibilities are so essential that they should be enforced under all circumstances, whether the physician is the last doctor in town or not. As described above, bigoted physicians ought to be denied protection for prejudiced and inequitable refusals. Additionally, due to the importance and value of doctor-patient matching on the basis of shared moral beliefs, as well as the fact that advanced knowledge of a physician's grounds for refusal will help minimize conflicts, physicians must disclose the sorts of refusals patients can expect as early in the relationship as possible. Because of the unacceptable consequences that would stem from allowing physicians to refuse services when a patient is facing a true medical emergency, protection of a physician's conscience cannot be extended to such contexts. Physicians also have an obligation to inform patients about all reasonable treatment options, even if the physician himself is unwilling to provide them, so that the patient is at least made aware of the need to seek an alternate provider. Finally, despite valid concerns of complicity, the refusing physician likely has a responsibility to help patients connect with those alternate providers through direct referrals, or potentially through indirect referrals to some higher-level source of information, such as the state licensing board or professional associations.

Conscientious refusers must engage in deep self-reflection and should be open to reconsidering their views in light of patients' unique situations. However, so long as physicians engage in respectful dialogue with their patients rather than condemnation or proselytizing, patients need not be shielded from the physician's moral reasons for refusal. In most circumstances, it goes too far to exclude refusing physicians entirely from the profession of medicine, but if a physician cannot satisfy even these highly constrained responsibilities, then he truly should find a different specialty or leave the profession altogether (Lynch, 2008).

CONCLUSION

I N MANY CASES, the profession as a whole can resolve conflicts of conscience and access problems by working to ensure that individual physicians unwilling to provide certain services on grounds of conscience do not find themselves in the monopolist's position. When it cannot, physicians standing as the last available option for the patient do have a professional obligation to provide access regardless of their personal beliefs, although legally enforcing this duty would likely have undesirable consequences. Society stands to benefit if it chooses to respect the moral integrity of physicians by allowing them to subspecialize based on their conscientious beliefs, because physicians "who refuse, withdraw, or disassociate themselves from certain practices or procedures on grounds of conscience may well be among the more thoughtful and effective members of a healthcare team" (Benjamin, 2004, p. 515). On the other hand, the public has a clear interest in being assured access to a variety of desired medical services. Therefore, the most ideal solution to the conscience clause debate will be a nuanced, context-dependent compromise—not the sort of winner-take-all approach that so thoroughly pervades current discussion.

REFERENCES

American Civil Liberties Union Reproductive Freedom Project. (2002). *Religious refusals and reproductive rights: The report.* Retrieved June 6, 2007, from www.aclu.org/FilesPDFs/ACF911.pdf

American Medical Association. (2001). *Principles of medical ethics* § VI. Retrieved August 13, 2008, from www.ama-assn.org/ama/pub/category/2512.html

American Medical Association. (2003). Potential patients. *Current opinions of the Council on Ethical and Judicial Affairs* § 10.05 (2)(b). Retrieved August 13, 2008, from www.ama-assn.org/ama/noindex/category/11760.html

Basic Health Plan-Health Care Access Act, Wash. Rev. Code § 70.47.160 (West 2006).

Benjamin, M. (2004). Conscience. In Stephen G. Post (Ed.), *The encyclopedia of bioethics* (pp. 513–517). New York: Macmillan Reference USA.

Blustein, J., & Fleischman, A. R. (1995). The pro-life maternal-fetal medicine physician: A problem of integrity. *The Hastings Center Report, 25,* 22–26.

Cantor, J., & Baum, K. (2004). The limits of conscientious objection—May pharmacists refuse to fill prescriptions for emergency contraception? *The New England Journal of Medicine, 351,* 2008–2012.

Charo, R. A. (2005). The celestial fire of conscience—Refusing to deliver medical care. *The New England Journal of Medicine, 352,* 2471–2473.

Charo, R. A. (2007). *Health care provider refusals to treat, prescribe, refer, or inform: Professionalism and conscience.* Retrieved June 6, 2007, from http://www.acslaw.org/node/4214.

Church Amendment, 42 U.S.C. § 300a-7 (1973).

Collett, T. S. (1999). The common good and the duty to represent: Must the last lawyer in town take any case? *South Texas Law Review, 40,* 137–179.

Dietz, L. H., Jacobs, A., Leming, T. L., & Kennel, J. R. (2006a). Creation and nature of relationship. *American jurisprudence, 2nd, physicians, surgeons, and other healers, 61,* § 130.

Dietz, L. H., Jacobs, A., Leming, T. L., & Kennel, J. R. (2006b). Duty to give proper notice before withdrawal. *American jurisprudence, 2nd, physicians, surgeons, and other healers, 61,* § 117.

Dresser, R. S. (2004). Freedom of conscience, professional responsibility, and access to abortion. *Journal of Law, Medicine, and Ethics, 22,* 280–285.

Employment Division v. Smith, 494 U.S. 872 (1990).

Health Care Right of Conscience Act, 745 Ill. Comp. Stat. Ann. 70/3 (West 2006).

Lynch, H. F. (2008). *Conflicts of conscience in health care: An institutional compromise.* Cambridge, MA: MIT Press.

May, T. (2001). Rights of conscience in health care. *Social Theory and Practice, 27,* 111–128.

Minow, M. (2001). On being a religious professional: The religious turn in professional ethics. *University of Pennsylvania Law Review, 150,* 661–688.

Mississippi Health Care Rights of Conscience Act, Miss. Code Ann. § 41-107-3 (2005).

Pellegrino, E. D. (1989). Character, virtue, and self-interest in the ethics of the professions. *Journal of Contemporary Health Law and Policy, 5,* 53–73.

Pellegrino, E. D. (1993). Patient and physician autonomy: Conflicting rights and obligations in the physician-patient relationship. *Journal of Contemporary Health Law and Policy, 10,* 47–68.

Pellegrino, E. D. (2000). Commentary. Value neutrality, moral integrity, and the physician. *Journal of Law, Medicine, and Ethics, 28,* 78–80.

Pellegrino, E. D. (2002). The physician's conscience, conscience clauses, and religious belief: A Catholic perspective. *Fordham Urban Law Journal, 30,* 221–244.

Rhodes, R. (2006). The ethical standard of care. *American Journal of Bioethics, 6,* 76–78.

Roe v. Wade, 410 U.S. 113 (1973).

Savulescu, J. (2006). Conscientious objection in medicine. *British Medical Journal, 332,* 294–297.

Smearman, C. A. (2006). Drawing the line: The legal, ethical, and public policy implications of refusal clauses for pharmacists. *Arizona Law Review, 48,* 469–540.

Swanson v. St. John's Lutheran Hosp., 597 P.2d 702 (Mont. 1979).

Swartz, M. (2006). Conscience clauses or unconscionable clauses: Personal beliefs versus professional responsibilities. *Yale Journal of Health Policy, Law, and Ethics, 6,* 269–350.

Wardle, L. D. (1993). Protecting the rights of conscience of health care providers. *Journal of Legal Medicine, 14,* 177–230.

15

Mediation and Health Care

Edward J. Bergman and Autumn Fiester

MEDIATION HAS EXISTED for as long as people have had differences (Moore, 1996, chap. 1). Today, mediation has become a process of choice for many, particularly those skeptical of the costs of litigation in both human and economic terms. Mediation, as a party-driven process rather than a formal system to which disputants outsource problems for resolution by third parties, is often compelling for those who value assumption of personal responsibility and principles of self-determination. As a dispute resolution process, mediation has gained tremendous momentum over the last few decades and flourishes in both private and court-connected settings as the dominant form of alternative/complementary dispute-resolution process (Bergman & Bickerman, 1998). Health care mediation represents a comparatively recent application of the process to previously unaddressed categories of cases. Notwithstanding its relative infancy, notable and successful examples of health care mediation exist, in particular, the groundbreaking efforts of Nancy Dubler and her colleagues at Montefiore Hospital in New York (Dubler & Liebman, 2004).

Mediation is a form of assisted negotiation by which parties can resolve or prevent a dispute by achievement of consensus. The mediator is a neutral third party who assists by acting as communication facilitator, resource expander, educator, process manager, translator, generator of creative options, reality tester, and searcher for compatible interests (Moore, 1996, chap. 1; Riskin & Westbrook, 1987). To perform these roles effectively, mediators must possess a mastery of negotiation principles. The parties' perception of a mediator's neutrality is critical for success because the parties' willingness to divulge information is often dependent on trust that the mediator will not use information revealed by a party against the provider of that information. A mediator inspires trust, in part, by her perceived neutrality but also as a function of her professional stature, inclusive of age and relevant experience, practical intellect, listening skills, level of empathy, warmth, respectfulness, dignity, nonjudgmental nature, and an infinite range of personal characteristics viewed as positive in one privy to sensitive information (Moore, 1996, chap. 7). We will see that health care mediation presents unique challenges with respect to the neutrality aspect of mediation.

Beyond mediator neutrality, the mediation process in legal and/or commercial contexts is typically characterized by strict confidentiality. Just as trust in the mediator leads to candor and an open exchange of information, confidentiality enhances trust in the process, increasing the likelihood that failed attempts at mediation will leave the parties in no worse position than they previously occupied. Special problems associated with confidentiality in health care mediation will be addressed later in this chapter.

Mediation's most salient characteristic is its consensual, noncoercive nature. When a successfully mediated outcome is achieved, the parties themselves generate that outcome, contrary to what occurs in the arbitration or adjudication of a dispute where judges, juries, or arbitrators impose verdicts, judgments, or awards. Ownership of outcomes is widely believed to result in high levels of satisfaction with the mediation process and is similarly associated with a greater likelihood of voluntary compliance with resolutions reached (Moore, 1996, chap. 14).

Because a mediator does not determine outcomes, the process allows for mediator caucuses with parties, separately, without fear of bias. Mediation is a flexible process which, in its ideal form, provides a safe forum for the expression of intense feelings, allowing for catharsis rarely experienced in more formal and authoritarian modes of dispute resolution governed by rules of evidence and procedure. This has been referred to as the moral space in which meaningful dialogue occurs (Walker, 1993). Parties are given a voice, encouraged to tell their own stories, and, in consequence, often feel empowered as never before. Sometimes catharsis and empowerment result in healing that renders the stated reason for mediation secondary or even moot.

Mediation ideally includes all parties possessing an interest in the subject matter of a dispute (Marcus, Dorn, Kritek, Miller, & Wyatt, 1995, chap. 12). When all stakeholders participate, the likelihood of an outcome that would seriously injure or offend nonparticipating, interested parties is diminished (Gray, 1989).

As in any negotiation, a third party with sufficient power and leverage may ultimately mandate the outcome of its choice (Shell, 1999, chap. 6). In health care mediation, the party empowered to make a decision in the absence of agreement, whether physician or patient, must be persuaded that alternative viewpoints are deserving of respect and consideration in order to forego exercise of that power. Unintended consequences such as the loss of valued relationships or damage to reputation may otherwise ensue. A skilled mediator can diminish the likelihood of such interests being overlooked in favor of more apparent and immediate gains (Shell, 1999, chap. 4).

CLASSES OF HEALTH CARE DISPUTES

CREATION OF INSTITUTIONAL POLICIES AND RELATED DISPUTES

INNUMERABLE POLICY ISSUES arise in the course of the operation and governance of health care institutions. Managed care issues, credentialing, departmental and hospital-wide administrative procedures, legal compliance, development and enforcement of safety regulations, disciplinary matters, budgetary allocations, staff size, expansion decisions, and exclusive provider arrangements are a few of an infinite number of policy concerns (Marcus et al., 1995, chap. 7). Mediation can be an effective tool in the realm of policy to facilitate the creation of shared visions (Gray, 1989) or to resolve disputes between individuals or factions within the institution. Although we acknowledge the utility and potential of institutional policy mediation, this chapter deals primarily with health care mediation in the context of caregiver, patient, surrogate, and family disputes.

DISPUTES THAT ALLEGE MEDICAL ERROR (MEDICAL MALPRACTICE)

ALSO BEYOND THE scope of this chapter are disputes over alleged medical error, which can be resolved through mediation either before or after suit has been filed, and which do not turn on ethical concerns. These malpractice disputes focus on whether negligence has been committed by virtue of a caregiver's deviation from the standard of care expected within the relevant medical community, whether the injury sustained was legally caused by such negligence, and the extent of damages suffered in consequence of the negligence.

Once litigation has commenced, these cases may be referred to mediation in conjunction with court-connected programs, or by the parties themselves, in common with any other class of civil disputes (Bergman & Bickerman, 1998). Indeed, some medical institutions and insurance carriers have begun to experiment with mediation as a mandatory precursor to litigation (Drexel University College of Medicine, 2004).

COMMUNICATION, PERSONALITY, AND INFORMATION-BASED DISPUTES

MEDIATION IN THE health care setting and outside the court system involving disputes between caregivers, patients, surrogates, and families is often referred to as bioethics mediation (Dubler & Liebman, 2004). Because many commentators have concluded that the great majority of these disputes are caused by communication problems, personality differences, or inadequate information (Dubler & Liebman, 2004), we favor the term *health care mediation* as inclusive of those disputes that do not involve ethical conflicts in the sense that term is commonly understood yet involve disputes between caregivers, patients, surrogates, and families. For example, if a patient takes issue with her physician's prescribed treatment, which is presented as mandatory and not subject to question, but discovers, in mediation, that the physician considered and ruled out alternatives for reasons which the patient ultimately accepts, the dispute may be resolved.

Similarly, if a patient declines to accept a treatment recommendation based on the perception that a physician is patronizing her, a candid dialogue in which resentment is expressed and reconciliation achieved may resolve the dispute without reference to traditional ethical principles. If, as has been posited, a majority of disputes in the clinical setting take the preceding form, it may be misleading to say that mediation in the health care context is necessarily bioethics mediation.

CLASSICAL BIOETHICAL DISPUTES

HEALTH CARE MEDIATION also encompasses disputes that *can* be characterized as bioethical in the traditional sense. These include disputes as to the medical futility of prospective treatment, the right of a patient to refuse treatment, and the painful class of disputes that involve end-of-life decisions (Dubler & Liebman, 2004; Hoffmann, 1994). Each of these types of dispute can occur even where communication is exemplary, personality conflicts are not in evidence, and each party possesses all relevant information.

SPECIAL CHARACTERISTICS AND PROBLEMS IN HEALTH CARE MEDIATION

NEUTRALITY

AS NOTED PREVIOUSLY, mediation in legal and commercial settings relies on the presumption of mediator neutrality. Neutrality is predicated, in part, on the fact that mediation does not ordinarily require an outcome in conformity with external norms, notably legal principles, though it may be influenced by those norms because of the likelihood of their application in the event that mediation is unsuccessful (Bergman & Bickerman, 1998). In consequence, the mediator is freed from the role of enforcer of external norms, and the parties are free to resolve their dispute creatively, without reference to the limitations of available legal remedies, the likely outcome of a court-proceeding or the atypical nature of their settlement.

Critics have asserted that, because health care mediation requires that any outcome reached conform to both legal and ethical requirements, a health care mediator cannot maintain the level of neutrality necessary for an effective process (American Society for Bioethics and Humanities, 1998; Gibson, 1999a; Marcus et al., 1995).

While this premise is initially compelling, it will not survive in-depth analysis. First, we have seen that most health care disputes are not ultimately ethical disputes in the sense contemplated by the aforementioned critics. Second, some commentators believe that the use of so-called principlism in clinical bioethics is misplaced because disputes in this realm cannot be resolved by the application of abstract principles such as beneficence, nonmaleficence, and patient autonomy, which, while important considerations, often compete with one another for primacy and are not amenable to balancing by experts but only by those whose lives and values are implicated in the medical situation at hand (Charon & Montello, 2002; Clouser & Gert, 1999). Third, it is widely believed that most true bioethics disputes are not susceptible of resolution by a single definitive answer but by a range of outcomes, all of which may satisfy legal and ethical requirements (American Society for Bioethics and Humanities, 1998; Caplan & Bergman, 2007; Fiester, 2007a; Hoffmann, 1994). Few outcomes embraced by patients, surrogates, families, and health care providers, after a process in which facts and emotions are elicited, alternatives considered, and consensus reached, are likely to violate legal or ethical norms. Where decisions contemplated by the parties appear flagrantly contrary to widely accepted ethical norms or manifestly illegal, a skilled mediator can carefully examine a proposed outcome, seek advice and, where appropriate, disassociate himself from what he believes to be unlawful or unethical, thus terminating the mediation. This situation, though relatively rare, also occurs in contexts other than health care mediation (Gibson, 1999b; Golann, 1996, chap. 1). Fourth, the articulated neutrality problem is not unique to health care mediation but arises in other realms, notably environmental mediation, where the literature posits the unacceptability of outcomes that violate public policy or that affect future generations negatively (Susskind & Weinstein, 1980). These concerns have engendered lively debate but have not halted environmental mediation or brought it into disfavor. Fifth, it has been suggested that neutrality be redefined for health care mediation as impartiality toward the parties, as distinct from neutrality as to outcomes (Perlman, 2001). Finally, it has been proposed that the neutrality dilemma be resolved by the presence of a bioethicist, not as mediator but as a party to the mediation or through review of mediated outcomes by ethics boards (Hoffmann, 1994). These cumbersome alternatives are intended to relieve the health care mediator of her role as the repository of ethical correctness. All proposed options demand further study before conclusions can be drawn.

A simpler neutrality issue has yet to be adequately addressed. Of the health care mediation initiatives to date, many involve the use of mediators employed by the medical institution whose providers are party to the mediation process. An associated problem is the appearance or fact of bias in favor of the institutionally sponsored point of view (Marcus et al., 1995). Independent mediation services represent an alternative, subject to further analysis of economic and logistical issues relevant to the feasibility of that model (Caplan & Bergman, 2007). Penn's Center for Bioethics is actively engaged in examining the viability of independent health care mediation services.

POWER IMBALANCES

HEALTH CARE MEDIATION is notable for the extreme nature of its power imbalances. Patients and their families are typically hampered by anxiety and alienation caused by unfamiliarity with the institutional setting, debilitation caused by injury or illness, the strange jargon and complexity of medical discourse, distrust of the system, and consequent feelings of powerlessness (Caplan & Bergman, 2007; Dubler & Liebman, 2004).

While mediation cannot perfectly redress power imbalances, the very existence of a forum in which to air grievances—assisted by a professional who actively listens and hears parties' concerns, who translates new and seemingly incomprehensible information into manageable components, who questions health care provider and patient alike, and conveys empathy and respect—favorably alters the odds of achieving patient empowerment.

ABSENCE OF THE PATIENT

HEALTH CARE MEDIATION often takes place in the absence of the primary interested party—the patient. When end-of-life decisions or futility issues are at stake, the patient is typically incapacitated and represented by surrogates. Some have opined that the surrogate's imperfect knowledge of a patient's history and wishes makes mediation inappropriate (Hoffmann, 1994). This perspective is difficult to embrace unless formal legal proceedings with a panoply of witnesses are viewed as feasible in every such case or alternative processes are deemed superior to mediation for the ascertainment of patient preferences. The time required for decision-making in a formal context could result in a patient's demise prior to resolution. While the aforementioned concerns merit attention, the issues presented are complex and ultimately beyond the scope of this chapter. There is a countervailing fact unique to health care mediation—that is, all of the parties, unless otherwise reflected in the course of mediation, presumptively have the best interests of the patient in common (Dubler & Liebman, 2004). In non–health care settings, agents frequently appear in mediation on behalf of principals. The difference is that in most (but not all) instances, designated agents can confirm the principal's agreement with prospective outcomes or with strategies for achieving prospective outcomes. In health care mediation, the agent for an incapacitated patient derives her authority from an advance directive, from appointment by a court as legal guardian, or by statutory designations that can differ by jurisdiction (Jonsen, Siegler, & Winslade, 2002; Mcnikoff, 2001). In all of the foregoing circumstances, the right of the agent to make decisions on behalf of the principal is clear. Conflicts occur primarily where there is no advance directive, no guardianship appointment, and no relevant statute, or where the statute in question sets forth criteria for the exercise of power by a surrogate that an interested party alleges have not been followed.

TRAINING, CREDENTIALING, AND FUNDING

AS REMAINS TRUE in the many types of disputes in which mediation has an established track record, training, credentialing, and funding of mediation and mediation initiatives (including resources for pilot programs and related research on methodology, criteria for effectiveness, and specialized education) are certain to remain foreground concerns for years to come. Only commitment, experience, and a substantial investment of resources will yield information prerequisite to the establishment of a vital health care mediation culture possessed of a proven cadre of skilled professionals focused on attainment of excellence in the field.

MEDIATION AND MORAL UNCERTAINTY

HEALTH CARE MEDIATION is often criticized for taking the ethics out of ethics consultation, on the premise that a neutrally negotiated outcome will allow any and all options to be put on the table, regardless of their moral defensibility or justifiability. Conversely, we argue that mediation actually provides a built-in moral safety net because mediation demands that all interested voices be heard; it resists the tendency in ethics consultation to privilege some positions or values (perhaps the morally flawed ones) over others. Mediation can grapple with moral uncertainty because it strives to obtain moral consensus about what the contextually right answer actually is (Fiester, 2007b).

Many clinical ethics conflicts involve genuine ethical ambivalence: there is more than one applicable moral principle, those relevant moral principles often conflict, and there is more than one ethically justified option as a legitimate outcome of the conflict (Caplan & Bergman, 2007). In these cases, different parties will appeal to principles that support their own preferred outcomes. The avoidance of bias requires a process that does not take sides and does not render definitive judgments. Conventional ethics consultations frequently violate these norms (Fiester, 2007b).

Conventional approaches to ethics consultation that provide authoritative recommendations in conflicts fraught with uncertainty should be viewed as ethically suspect because the committee or its designee has no greater access to the moral truth of the matter than the patient, the family, or the clinical staff. If all parties apply valid moral principles in support of treatment preferences, there is no prima facie reason to adopt the view of the ethics consultant or ethics committee merely because they carry the imprimatur of their institution. Self-proclaimed authority, as it happens, is not a persuasive moral credential (Fiester, 2007b).

If there are legitimate moral claims on various sides of a clinical ethics dispute, mediation provides an appropriate mechanism for conflict resolution in cases of moral uncertainty because it works toward consensus about *outcome,* even where consensus about principles or values is not possible. Mediation facilitates the creation of a shared solution between parties without taking a stand as to which moral principles or claims trump others.

CONCLUSION

CRITICISM AND SKEPTICISM of health care mediation have undoubtedly slowed its universal adoption to date. The nature of these protests is, however, analogous to those voiced long ago by critics of classical mediation in the legal or commercial setting. Yet mediation as a dispute-resolution mechanism has thrived and been widely embraced as effective on both humanistic and efficiency-based grounds.

While critical perspectives present challenges to the mediation community that are healthy and deserving of attention, they ultimately remind us that mediation, in common with other democratic processes, including adjudication and legislation, is inherently delicate and relies on the strengths of individual practitioners for effectiveness.

Beyond the critiques already examined, some distinguished legal scholars have opined that mediation, and settlement in general, are suspect because of the element of compromise (common but not universal in the fashioning of mediated outcomes), which replaces a grand notion of justice with a watered-down result that all can accept but none can cheer (Fiss, 1984). Fortunately, this perspective has become marginalized in the face of competing realities. People have the right to resolve disputes in the manner they see fit, both with respect to outcomes and preferences as to process. In every U.S. state and federal jurisdiction, the vast majority of civil cases settle prior to adjudication. The question should thus be framed not as settlement versus adjudication but as how to maximize the quality and timing of the settlement process. This old saw has been resurrected by critics of health care mediation who opine that a consensual dispute-resolution process is inherently incapable of yielding the correct ethical result just as mediation in the legal setting does not render justice (Fiester, 2007b; McThenia & Shaffer, 1985). These are interesting philosophical debates, but they are inapposite to the critical needs of real people in crisis whose right to self-determination is at stake. The notion of a correct ethical result is predicated on the questionable premise that clinical ethics is the province of experts rather than the examined decisions of patients, families, and caregivers possessed of the relevant facts, which are then weighed and balanced in the context of a calculus that incorporates life experience, value systems, religious beliefs, cultural influences, and relationships.

REFERENCES

American Society for Bioethics and Humanities. (1998). *Core competencies for healthcare ethics consultation.* Glenview, IL: Author.

Bergman, E. J., & Bickerman, J. G. (1998). *Court-annexed mediation: Critical perspectives on selected state and federal programs.* Bethesda, MD: Pike & Fischer.

Caplan, A. L., & Bergman, E. J. (2007). Beyond Schiavo. *Journal of Clinical Ethics, 18,* (4), 340–345.

Charon, R., & Montello, M. (2002). *Stories matter: The role of narrative in medical ethics.* New York: Routledge.

Clouser, K. D., & Gert, B. (1999). A critique of principlism. In Nancy S. Jecker, Albert R. Jonsen, & Robert A. Pearlman (Eds.), *Bioethics: An introduction to the history, methods, and practice* (pp. 147–157). Sudbury, MA: Jones and Barlett Publishers.

Drexel University College of Medicine. (2004). *Mediation program brochure.* Philadelphia: Philadelphia Health & Education Corporation.

Dubler, N., & Liebman, C. J. (2004). *Bioethics mediation.* New York: United Hospital Fund of New York.

Fiester, A. (2007a). The failure of the consult model: Why "mediation" should replace "consultation." *American Journal of Bioethics, 7*(2), 31–32.

Fiester, A. (2007b). Mediation and moral aporia. *Journal of Clinical Ethics, 18*(4), 355–356.

Fiss, O. (1984). Against settlement. *Yale Law Journal, 93,* 1073, 1075, 1076–1078, 1082–1090.

Gibson, K. (1999a). Mediation in the medical field: Is neutral intervention possible? *Hastings Center Report, 29*(5), 6–13.

Gibson, K. (1999b). Mediator attitudes toward outcomes: A philosophical view. *Mediation Quarterly, 17*(2), 197–211.

Golann, D. (1996). *Effective strategies for lawyers and mediators.* Boston: Little Brown and Company.

Gray, B. (1989). *Collaborating: Finding common ground for multiparty problems.* San Francisco: Jossey-Bass.

Hoffmann, D. E. (1994). Mediating life and death decision. *Arizona Law Review, 36,* 821–877.

Jonsen, A. R., Siegler, M., & Winslade, W. J. (2002). *Clinical ethics: A practical approach to ethical decisions in clinical medicine* (5th ed.). New York: McGraw-Hill.

Marcus, L. J., Dorn, B. C., Kritek, P. B., Miller, V. G., & Wyatt J. B. (1995). *Renegotiating healthcare.* San Francisco: Jossey-Bass.

McThenia, A., & Shaffer, T. (1985). For reconciliation. *Yale Law Journal, 94,* 1660.

Menikoff, J. (2001). *Law and bioethics: An introduction.* Washington, DC: Georgetown University Press.

Moore, C. W. (1996). *The mediation process: Practical strategies for resolving conflict* (2nd ed.). San Francisco: Jossey-Bass.

Perlman, D. (2001). *Mediation and ethics consultation: Towards a new understanding of impartiality.* Retrieved April 1, 2007, from http://www.mediate.com/articles/perlman.cfm

Riskin, L. L., & Westbrook, J. E. (1987). *Dispute resolution and lawyers.* St. Paul, MN: West Publishing.

Shell, G. R. (1999). *Bargaining for advantage.* New York: Viking.

Susskind, L., & Weinstein, A. (1980). Towards a theory of environmental dispute resolution. *Environmental Affairs, 9,* 311–357.

Walker, M. U. (1993). Keeping moral space open: New images of ethics consulting. *Hastings Center Report, 23*(2), 33–40.

16

The Moral Education of Medical Students

Judah L. Goldberg

A T FIRST GLANCE, it might not be obvious that the moral education of medical students should be a topic of general interest. Though bioethicists have certainly championed for the inclusion of ethics in medical school curricula, actual goals and methods of instruction would seem to be a question of pedagogy more than of genuine moral inquiry. Just as ethicists in general have traditionally left the task of imbuing moral skills to school educators and psychologists, so too has the moral development of future physicians been seen as a practical, nonmoral issue that belongs primarily to the medical profession and its academic arm.

This chapter argues, however, that the moral education of medical students deserves a place on the bioethics agenda for several reasons. First, the subject of moral education is not so easily separated from that of moral theory. For instance, when a review of the medical literature describes a fundamental split in the medical community about whether ethics instruction "is a means of creating virtuous physicians" or "a means of providing physicians with a skill set for analyzing and resolving ethical dilemmas" (Eckles, Meslin, Gaffney, & Helft, 2005, p. 1145), it is hard not to notice the parallel to the centuries-old rivalry between Aristotelian, virtue ethics, on the one hand, and Kantian, rule-based ethics, on the other. If bioethicists would encourage educators to frame their own debates within this larger context, then bioethicists themselves should perhaps more actively flesh out the pedagogic consequences of the moral theories they promote.

Second, while methods of education might not have moral implications, setting priorities in education certainly does. For instance, whether a medical school emphasizes good service more or less than ensuring equity in health care is a moral choice, not just an educational one, and certainly one that bioethicists can weigh in on.

Third, and perhaps most importantly, if the field of bioethics is not purely theoretical but takes moral outcomes seriously, future physicians constitute one of the most important targets for influence and intervention. At the practical end of virtually all health care law, policy, and regulation stands a health care worker who will decide how, when, and at what cost to pursue a given moral goal. It would be foolish to invest energies in moral deliberation and policy formation while taking a backseat in planning the training of those who will effectively control the clinical environment and serve as the flesh-and-blood moral agents at the center of so many conflicts.

This chapter outlines two major areas of current discussion with regard to moral education for medical students: content and method. The earliest experiments in bioethics instruction for medical students took traditional, didactic lessons in moral theory and applied them to the kinds of clinical dilemmas that have become prototypical for modern bioethics. More recently, increased recognition of the broader range of challenges to ethical behavior that physicians contend with, on the one hand, and the limitations of didactic teaching, on the other, have proliferated further thinking along each of these axes. At the moment, the field remains ripe for innovation, which will hopefully further enrich the medical school experience.

CONTENT

UNQUESTIONABLY, THE INCLUSION of bioethics in medical school curricula is a welcome development in the history of medical education. Whereas generations of medical students were expected to absorb a vague set of guiding values by osmosis, today's students enjoy explicit instruction in well-anchored, widely accepted moral principles and their application to clinical medicine. The history of ethics courses has generally followed that of the field of bioethics in general. Clinical bioethics has by and large abandoned fundamental discussions of moral philosophy over time and instead works with the more pragmatic principlism theory developed by Beauchamp and Childress (2001). Principlism maintains that independent of any specific moral theory, the four cardinal principles of autonomy, nonmalefi-cence, beneficence, and justice can guide almost any dilemma that arises in the clinical context. Following this approach, ethics courses instruct their students to use these principles to identify the morally salient features of a case, clarify what moral principles are at stake, and understand what response the principles would dictate.

Furthermore, bioethics instruction has moved further and further away from the teaching of theory to case-based instruction, which fo-cuses discussions of ethics around actual clinical scenarios. Whether through small-group discussions, written essays, or some other me-dium, students are called upon to apply the principles of autonomy, nonmaleficence, beneficence, and justice to specific moral dilemmas culled from the clinical experience.

What emerges from these two trends together is a fairly standard mode of teaching bioethics that might look like this: The students are posed with a particular case description (e.g., an elderly man whose children request that his diagnosis be withheld from him). The stu-dents must correctly describe the ethical problem (deception might be a violation of the patient's autonomy), identify the relevant principles (autonomy of the patient; nonmaleficence in not wanting to deliver potentially damaging news), and provide a sound argument for priori-tizing one principle over another in this case or suggest a resolution that respects both of them. Of course, this last part has a subjective component, in that different individuals may come to vastly differ-ent conclusions. It is important to note, however, that this subjective component is inherent to the principlism framework itself, rather than to any particular teaching method, and must be tolerated in any educa-tional framework that is rooted in principlism.

At the same time, commentators have noted that this form of bio-ethics does not sufficiently address the full range of concerns that the public and the medical profession have about exemplary medical prac-tice. Critiques have come from a variety of directions. In the mid-1990s, a landmark essay by two medical students at the University of Pennsyl-vania, Christakis and Feudtner (1993), called for a recentering of ethi-cal training for medical students. Ethics curricula focused on complex questions that medical students, as the junior members of the team, are not usually called upon to negotiate, Christakis and Feudtner noted, whereas the very real and vexing challenges to courage, honesty, and empathic care that constitute the unspoken side of medical school were being ignored. When a student is ordered to forge a resident's signa-ture, for instance, the four principles are at best strained to respond and more realistically are plainly unhelpful. Subsequent studies by them (Feudtner, Christakis, & Christakis, 1994) and others (Caldicott & Faber-Langendoen, 2005; Satterwhite, Satterwhite, & Enarson, 2000) documented the tumultuous ethical life of the medical student and helped turn attention toward other possible components for medical education. Fiester (2007), on the other hand, believes that the "principlist paradigm" (p. 684), as she terms it, is too narrow even for the limited domain of classic bioethical dilemmas. The list of possible problems identified by the principlist paradigm is too short, the conflicts too clichéd, and the possible solutions generated too constricted. Broad and sensitive moral intuitions are blunted as students are taught to squeeze their conception of ethical care into just these four principles.

Fox's critique runs deeper. Wondering "Is Medical Education Asking Too Much of Bioethics?" (1999) Fox suggests that the field of bioethics has been co-opted by medical educators for a larger, and ultimately inappropriate, agenda. Not only is bioethics providing guidance for ethical practice, but it has also become the latest substitute for a broad and probing engagement with the social and cultural dimensions of medical practice. What is lacking for Fox is not more relevant material or a wider range of ethical values, but attention to the full scope of medical practice in the current health care environment. Yes, today's fledgling doctors will have to make both medical and ethical decisions, but they will also be pivotal figures in our ongoing public discussions about access to care, about the intersection between poverty and disease, and about the evolving meanings of health and illness. Woe to the society whose physicians believe that four solitary principles can navigate all value-laden aspects of health care.

These concerns, and others, have led the medical community to consider other value systems that can supplement principlism as a basis for professional development. Two trends in particular, humanism and professionalism, have gained prominence. While humanistic medicine is not a novel concept, it has been reinvigorated by the Arnold P. Gold Foundation, "a public foundation fostering humanism in medicine" founded in 1988, whose programs and initiatives now involve 93% of American medical and osteopathic schools (Arnold P. Gold Foundation, n.d.). Furthermore, several medical schools now incorporate the humanities into their curricula, including such diverse activities as literature, creative writing, art, film, and theater (DasGupta & Charon, 2004; Montgomery, Chambers, & Reifler, 2003; Rucker & Shapiro, 2003). As opposed to bioethics, which focuses on policy formation and conflict resolution, humanism addresses the nuances of everyday interactions between provider and patient. Sensitivity, empathy, and compassion are its hallmarks, rather than the stoic pillars of principlism.

Professionalism, too, emphasizes some of these same elements, but it emerges from a different source. Whereas humanism appeals to a broader value system that transcends medicine or health care per se, professionalism encourages practitioners to embody the ideals of the medical tradition. One position statement on medical professionalism has summarized these values as (a) "competence," (b) "honesty," (c) "patient confidentiality," (d) "appropriate relations with patients," (e) "improving quality of care," (f) "improving access to care," (g) "just distribution of finite resources," (h) "commitment to scientific knowledge," (i) "maintaining trust by managing conflicts of interest," and (j) "commitment to professional responsibilities" (American Board of Internal Medicine Foundation, American College of Physicians, & European Foundation of Internal Medicine [ABIM Foundation], 2002). Professionalism as an educational goal, in fact, did not start with medical schools, but with professional organizations and residency (postmedical school) training programs that were concerned about "medicine's contract with society" (ABIM Foundation, 2002). In 1999, the Accredited Council for Graduate Medical Education (ACGME), which is charged with regulating residency education, named professionalism as one of the six core competencies that should frame residency education (ACGME Outcome Project, 1999). Over time, the language of professionalism has trickled down to medical schools as well.

Both humanism and professionalism highlight some of the aspects of medical education and practice that principlism does not capture. At the same time, concern exists about the ways in which they are manifest in medical education and their ultimate implications for the practice of medicine. Professionalism, for instance, while calling for "compassion, integrity, and respect for others" (ACGME Outcome Project, 2007) ultimately looks to the traditions of medicine themselves as its measuring stick rather than to universal, lay values (Goldberg, 2008). Its definition is set by physicians alone, and certain issues, such as physician entanglement with pharmaceutical companies, have been conspicuously missing from its agenda (Hafferty, 2006). Thus a student steeped in professionalism may indeed grow into a good doctor, but only insofar as the medical profession itself defines one. This should hardly be reassuring to the lay public and totally misses the depth that Fox is looking for.

Humanism seems to be more promising, but here, too, questions remain. First and foremost is whether medical education is adopting a model of medicine in humanism or humanism in medicine. In other words, are educators actually framing health care within larger aspirations for general human welfare and flourishing, or are they just sticking the label of humanism onto already clichéd virtues of medical practice, such as compassion? The former bespeaks the kind of thoughtful examination of medicine and its social role that Fox envisions; the latter smacks of veiled professionalism. Though the jury is still out on this question, a tendency among both educators and professional organizations to conflate humanism with professionalism is threatening to drain humanism of its moral potency for medicine (Goldberg, 2008). To be sure, a renewed emphasis on compassion, sensitivity, and integrity in medical education is welcome, whether in the guise of humanism, professionalism, or any other -ism. However, the deeper the educational process encourages medical students to probe, and the more critically they reflect, on medicine and on themselves, the richer they will emerge.

METHOD

THE TRADITIONAL MODEL of bioethics instruction, consisting of didactic teaching followed by some forum for students to practice and apply ethical principles, developed out of both pragmatic and theoretical considerations. Practically, Fox, Arnold, and Brody (1995) observe that "many of the pioneers of formal medical ethics education began their careers as teachers of moral philosophy or theology" (p. 762). As such, "these early ethics educators brought the objectives and methods of liberal arts courses into medical schools" (Fox et al., 1995, p. 762). Medical ethics instruction was an offshoot of the undergraduate classroom. Chronologically, it took place during the first 2 years of medical school, when the bulk of formal instruction happens, rather than in the last 2, when students spend most of their time involved in patient care. Its goal was analysis and reflection, rather than character refinement or behavioral change, and its pedagogic method was correspondingly cognitive.

This framework, though, was also based on theoretical assumptions. Specifically, it embraced what Feudtner and Christakis (1994) later termed the "ethical homunculus" (p. 7) myth: the belief that ethical doctors are born (or more accurately, accepted), not made. The seemingly mature college graduates who enter medical school, argued medical educators, are fully formed human beings, physically, cognitively, emotionally, and ethically. While their minds are open to fill with information, their essential character has been cast long before the first day of medical school and will be immutable to the best, or worst, influences of the medical profession. The guardians of physician integrity, went this argument, are to be found on the admissions committees, who should be filtering out less than scrupulous candidates, whereas ethics instructors can do nothing more than lecture about ethical theory and sharpen the instruments of the analytical toolbox.

As appealing as this neat picture may have been for medical educators, it was never quite consistent with the observations of social scientists. In any case, the myth was eventually shattered by Hafferty and Franks (1994), who meticulously described the "hidden curriculum" of medical education (p. 865). In addition to the formal curriculum of medical schools, explained Hafferty and Franks, there exists a hidden curriculum, an entire culture of behaviors, practices, attitudes, and values that students imbibe over the course of medical education. Whereas the formal curriculum dominates the classroom, the hidden curriculum owns the unregulated environment of the hospital ward, where the would-be doctors of tomorrow are initiated into the unspoken traditions of medicine—the good, the bad, and the ugly. Where others saw a benign training ground for clinical skills, Hafferty and Franks saw a mind-bending process that touched students to their core and altered their very conceptions of self. Of greatest irony, they observed, was that the ethical homunculus myth had actually worked its way into the received tradition. Medical students were learning that they would not really change through the training experience, even though they already were.

Two other sources of critique of traditional ethics instruction are worth noting. First is the repeated observation that when medical students do lapse, the gap is not in reasoning but in action. Christakis and Feudtner (1993) write that "one of the central riddles of unethical behavior is that, much of the time, the perpetrators sense what they ought to do but instead do something that they believe is wrong" (p. 251). Consider, for example, the following account they cite:

> Following morning "lightening" rounds (during which we had seen 20 patients in half an hour), my resident asked me to write progress notes in five charts. I felt uneasy because I had not actually examined these patients and wasn't sure anybody had done a routine morning physical exam. But at the time, I complied. (Christakis & Feudtner, 1993, p. 251)

The ethics of false documentation were apparent to this student, and yet he or she faltered. At issue were not beneficence or nonmaleficence, but power, hierarchy, and a lack of courage. This is something that classic bioethics did not anticipate and has little to offer in response. As Christakis and Feudtner add, "It is not clear that learning about ethical principles or legal standards, an objective of many existing curricula, will alter this phenomenon" (Christakis & Feudtner, 1993, p. 251).

Coupled to this is a critique from the field of psychology, which observes that medical ethics curricula have been formulated and implemented without reference to the actual psychological processes by which ethics is learned and practiced. The weak correlation between moral reasoning and action, for instance, has long been known to moral psychologists (Blasi, 1980). As far back as 1982, James Rest, a moral psychologist at the University of Minnesota, tried to alert ethicists to this and other concerns about ethics teaching in an article titled "A Psychologist Looks at the Teaching of Ethics" (Rest, 1982). History suggests that his message went unheeded then and, with few exceptions, has still not been absorbed by the mainstream medical community.

If educators want to take the moral education of medical students seriously, they could benefit greatly from the vast, rich field of moral psychology. In particular, they should take note of the prominent role that current psychological research gives to intuitive, reflexive responses rather than to deliberative, laborious ethical analysis. Conditioning toward desired behavior is not seen as petty or juvenile but has been incorporated into innovative, integrated models for ethics education that relate to both reasoning and action (Narvaez, 2005, 2006). While teachers of ethics have in the past sidelined talk of moral character, contemporary moral psychology has returned it to center stage.

The implications of this collection of sociological, clinical, and psychological data for medical education are enormous. All lines of reasoning converge on the ward experience as the place where ethics is learned and negotiated. Educators will succeed in actually influencing their students' moral development to the extent that they can control and modulate the clinical experience. All the classroom time in the world—whether in the first year or fourth year of medical school, whether through discussion groups or role-playing, whether taking on complex ethics cases or the mundane conflicts of medical students— will do little to alter the crushing power of the hidden curriculum. Students need to learn, practice, and refine their moral responses in real-time and with effective feedback if their teachers want to nurture true "ethical expertise" (Narvaez, 2005, p. 139). And of course, this is only possible and meaningful if the clinical teaching environment itself is structured in a way that reflects strong ethical intuitions and supports their growth.

CONCLUSION

O N   T H E   O N E hand, the pioneers of ethics teaching in medical schools have much to show for their work over the last 30 years. Ethics now occupies a prominent spot on the medical education agenda and has managed to pry away precious time and energy for itself from competing segments of the curriculum. Early models of instruction have evolved over time, increasingly focusing on issues immediately relevant to medical students and incorporating opportunities for student discussion and reflection. Moreover, the field of medical education now recognizes that the moral upbringing of virtuous physicians is a multidimensional process of which bioethics is only one piece. Recent attention to humanism and professionalism has considerably rounded out the picture.

But for all of the accomplishments to date, the field of moral education for medical students is arguably still very much in a formative stage. This is a time for deep exploration and inquiry, not consolidation. Educational undertakings in medical schools remain largely uninformed of the insights of moral psychologists, let alone their advice for how to plan effective programming and measure its impact. And while true humanism could offer a way of nurturing the human soul as it trudges its way through the boot camp of medical school, right now the initiative risks being hijacked by the catechisms of professionalism.

In sum, the medical community needs to take moral education seriously. Like the parents of young schoolchildren, it needs to first recognize that education is happening during these years, for better or worse. Identities are coming into formation; habits of thought and action are digging in. The potential for either positive or negative growth is enormous, and no lecture series or ethical formulae can counter the immersive experience of school, locker room included. This is not a time to rest easy. It is a time for the parents of medicine to think long and hard about what they want their children to become.

REFERENCES

Accredited Council for Graduate Medical Education Outcome Project. (1999). *Minimal program requirements language*. Retrieved April 30, 2008, from http://www.acgme.org/outcome/comp/compMin.asp

Accredited Council for Graduate Medical Education Outcome Project. (2007). *Common program requirements: General competencies*. Retrieved April 30, 2008, from http://www.acgme.org/outcome/comp/GeneralCompetencies Standards21307.pdf

American Board of Internal Medicine Foundation, American College of Physicians, & European Foundation of Internal Medicine. (2002). *Medical professionalism in the new millennium: A physician charter*. Retrieved April 30, 2008, from http://www.abimfoundation.org/professionalism/pdf_ charter/ABIM_Charter_Ins.pdf

Arnold P. Gold Foundation (n.d.). *Main page*. Retrieved April 30, 2008, from http://www.humanism-in-medicine.org

Beauchamp, T. L., & Childress, J. F. (2001). *Principles of biomedical ethics* (5th ed.). New York: Oxford University Press.

Blasi, A. (1980). Bridging moral cognition and moral action: A critical review of the literature. *Psychological Bulletin, 88*(1), 1–45.

Caldicott, C. V., & Faber-Langendoen, K. (2005). Deception, discrimination, and fear of reprisal: Lessons in ethics from third-year medical students. *Academic Medicine, 80*, 866–873.

Christakis, D. A., & Feudtner, C. (1993). Ethics in a short white coat: The ethical dilemmas that medical students confront. *Academic Medicine, 68*, 249–254.

DasGupta, S., & Charon, R. (2004). Personal illness narratives: Using reflective writing to teach empathy. *Academic Medicine, 79*, 351–356.

Eckles, R. E., Meslin, E. M., Gaffney, M., & Helft, P. R. (2005). Medical ethics education: Where are we? Where should we be going? A review. *Academic Medicine, 80*, 1143–1152.

Feudtner, C., & Christakis, D. A. (1994). Making the rounds: The ethical development of medical students in the context of clinical rotations. *Hastings Center Report, 24*(1), 6–12.

Feudtner, C., Christakis, D. A., & Christakis, N. A. (1994). Do clinical clerks suffer ethical erosion? Students' perceptions of their ethical environment and personal development. *Academic Medicine, 69*, 670–679.

Fiester, A. (2007). Why the clinical ethics we teach fails patients. *Academic Medicine, 82*, 684–689.

Fox, E., Arnold, R. M., & Brody, B. (1995). Medical ethic education: Past, present, and future. *Academic Medicine, 70*, 761–769.

Fox, R. C. (1999). Is medical education asking too much of bioethics? *Daedalus, 128*(4), 1–25.

Goldberg, J. L. (2008). Humanism or professionalism? The White Coat Ceremony and medical education. *Academic Medicine, 83*, 715–722.

Hafferty, F. (2006). The elephant in medical professionalism's kitchen. *Academic Medicine, 81*, 906–914.

Hafferty, F. W., & Franks, R. (1994). The hidden curriculum, ethics teaching, and the structure of medical education. *Academic Medicine, 69*, 861–871.

Montgomery, K., Chambers. T., & Reifler, D. R. (2003). Humanities education at Northwestern University's Feinberg School of Medicine. *Academic Medicine, 78*, 958–962.

Narvaez, D. (2005). The neo-Kohlbergian tradition and beyond: Schemas, expertise and character. *Nebraska Symposium on Motivation, 51*, 119–163.

Narvaez, D. (2006). Integrative ethical education. In M. Killen & J. Smetana (Eds.), *Handbook of moral development* (pp. 703–733). Mahwah, NJ: Lawrence Erlbaum Associates.

Rest, J. R. (1982). A psychologist looks at the teaching of ethics. *Hastings Center Report, 12*(1), 29–36.

Rucker, L., & Shapiro, J. (2003). Becoming a physician: Students' creative projects in a third-year IM clerkship. *Academic Medicine, 78*, 391–397.

Satterwhite, R. C., Satterwhite, W. M., & Enarson, C. (2000). An ethical paradox: The effect of unethical conduct on medical students' values. *Journal of Medical Ethics, 26*, 462–465.

17

Disability Perspectives on Bioethics

Carol Schilling

BOTH *BIOETHICS* AND *disability* resist stable definitions, making a discussion of their relevance to each other a challenge to both intellectual coherence and practical decision-making. This instability might partially explain the limited scope of scholarship on the intersections of bioethics and disability studies (Kuczewski, 2001; Tremain, 2008). Bioethics, a relatively new discipline, remains open to debates about its methods, its intellectual and institutional allegiances, its construction of authority, and its spheres of academic and social responsibility (Chambers, 2000; Rosenberg, 1999), all of which have complicated relationships to disability. Disability is a protean concept including both physical and cultural contents that, separately or combined, can designate individual and collective identities that profoundly affect ways of living fully in the world (Davis, 2006a; Lane, 2002; Silvers, 2001; Wendell, 1996). The Americans With Disabilities Act (1990) referred definitions to the courts, where meanings are determined as cases are argued. While disability is a category that a person can be born into, it is also one that, in the course of a lifetime, any human can instantly slip—or crash—into.

Since neither term can be fully analyzed in a short chapter, I will take their fluidity as a given and explore actions taken up in the name of bioethics and disability. For the sake of brevity, I'll rely on the phrase *disability perspective* to represent the perspectives of academic and advocacy projects regarding persons living as disabled in a culture. I do so while acknowledging that this shorthand phrase sets aside controversies within and between those projects and obscures important differences among groups of persons with disabilities. The field of disability studies is itself dynamic. Its founding project of identifying and solidifying a marginalized group and countering negative descriptions of it has transitioned to both recognizing diversity within the group and unsettling the category itself by challenging the construction of normalcy (Davis, 2006b).

MEDICAL AND SOCIAL MODELS OF DISABILITY

FROM A BIOMEDICAL perspective, disability primarily denotes a functional, measurable, biological impairment that affects a particular bodily or cognitive activity. Bioethics, with origins in the clinic and sites of medical research, has readily absorbed such a medical model of disability. With philosophical foundations aligned with medical imperatives to do no harm, to do good (to correct impairments or to alleviate the suffering impairments are presumed to cause), to respect persons (typically by granting autonomy over decision-making), and to treat persons equally (Beauchamp & Childress, 1994), bioethics has customarily intersected with disability in the clinic and its allied research sites over matters of protection from harm, correction of impairments, and interventions for alleviating pain and suffering. Where disability is concerned, bioethics has typically entered disputes concerning cures (such as cochlear implants), genetic testing, prenatal interventions, abortion, and ending a life. Bioethics' participation in these interventions is often premised on the assumption that living with a disabling impairment inevitably causes suffering that can be alleviated by a cure or, failing that, by ending a life (Singer, 1993, pp. 169–174, 181–191).

Those taking a disability perspective have, of course, endorsed bioethics projects that exposed and condemned practices that harm disabled, nonconsenting, or other persons who become vulnerable in clinical sites: the subjects of Nazi medical experiments, of the Willowbrook study of hepatitis, and of the Tuskegee study of syphilis. However, the disability perspective challenges the medical model of disability as primarily an impairment, an intrinsic or inevitable source of suffering, or a condition awaiting clinical interventions. Many persons regarded as disabled claim that whether one experiences the world as a disabled person is determined less by bodily conditions or functions than by social attitudes and environmental designs that restrict participation in the life of a culture: a social model of disability.

From a disability perspective, the category *disability* has been constructed in opposition to the category *normal,* resulting in the social exclusion of the former and the social advantage of the latter (Coleman, 2006; Davis, 2006c). A disability perspective reminds us that the normal design of the built environment accommodates a restricted range of human capabilities. The fact that cultures across time and place have considered a widely varying range of conditions (mobility impairment, deafness, stature, extreme facial scarring, imbecility, homelessness) as signs of disability, and pretexts for stigma and exclusion, offers credibility to the social model. So does the fact that expectations for individual human productivity differ across cultures allowing the same impairment to register as a disability in one culture, but not another (Wendell, 1996, pp. 37–39). The distinction between disability as an impairment and as the experience of living with an impairment resembles the familiar distinctions made between disease as a biomedical event and illness as the experience of living with a disease (Kleinman 1988; Toombs, 1993; Wendell, 1996). Each model suggests different responses to disability that give rise to ethical complexities and negotiations.

DEBATING CURES, REPAIRS, AND CARE

THE DISABILITY PERSPECTIVE has an uneasy relationship with contemporary medicine's unprecedented ability to cure and its ethic to do so, challenging two of medicine's fundamental assumptions. The first links the principle of beneficence to the project of correcting flaws, which is premised on the narrow construction of a standardized, acceptable body. The second presumes that living with a significant chronic impairment ineluctably leads to suffering, which medicine has a duty to relieve by performing corrections or allowing death. While people who acquire a disabling condition later in life often accept those assumptions, people living with a congenital disability or a long-standing acquired disability often challenge the same assumptions. Members of the latter group, such as the congenitally disabled attorney Harriet McBryde Johnson (2003), who counters Peter Singer's (1993) utilitarian position, explain that living their lives in and through bodies regarded as nonstandard, while complicated, can be pleasurable and rewarding. Quality of life research, as rehabilitation medicine has cast the phrase and the project, often restrains medical and popular assumptions that living with a disability inevitably leads to feelings of inadequacy, frustration, or a wish to die (Gill & Feinstein, 1994; Tulsky & Rosenthal, 2003; Whiteneck, 1994). Compelling narrative accounts of persons living with disabilities describe the ordinary pleasures and sorrows, as well as specific challenges, of their lives (Cole, 2004; Dubus, 1991; Hammell, 2000; Knighton, 2006; Mairs, 1986, 1996).

Emphasizing the need for social interventions, many persons with disabilities advocate (in rehabilitation clinics, journals, the arts, and on Web sites) accommodation and care that enable education, employment, and participation in the life of a family and a community. Such accommodations include barrier-free environments, personal care assistants, flexible and accessible medical systems, assistive technologies, affordable medical insurance, management of cognitive disabilities and, more generally, an ethic of inclusion. Attending to systems of care for persons with disabilities would extend the typical domain of bioethics from its microlevel focus on the individual and expressions of autonomy to broader social concerns. Paramount among these concerns is the fair distribution of adequate, dependable resources. The familiar example in bioethics literature of Larry McAfee, a quadriplegic who prevailed in his legal pursuit to end his life but did not do so after securing both funding for care and social recognition, calls attention to how what is framed as a right-to-die question can more accurately be described as the case of an inadequate system of chronic care (Pence, 2000). Some argue that the search for cures, which make arresting news bulletins, diverts too many resources from such systems of care. For a spinal cord injured person, for example, dependable, compassionate aides and a customized, controllable wheelchair with a cushion that prevents life-threatening pressure sores immediately enhance daily living and repair some effects of the injury.

While a cure is unavailable to many, it is undesirable to others. Some have invested considerable psychological, social, and economic resources in learning to live a decent life with a disability. At some points, a cure would require making energy-exhausting practical and existential alterations once again. Sometimes a cure reduces anatomical function and the pleasures of life. Such was the case of the blind man Oliver Sacks calls Virgil in "To See and Not See." After a successful surgery, he found that becoming sighted was so disorienting and physically painful that he experienced suffering and social isolation he never knew with blindness (Sacks, 1995). In addition, many who accept their disabilities fear that their acceptance might be confused with what some regard as a morally questionable act of giving up or malingering. Some encounter physicians who hold such beliefs or feel demoralized in the presence of a patient who cannot be cured or whose condition worsens (Mairs, 1986). Some fear the extent to which physicians and insurance providers refuse maintenance care or life-saving interventions because certain impairments are irreversible and the lives of those so impaired seem not worth living. Presently, Anita Silvers reminds us, medicine and bioethics "burden disabled individuals with having to persuade the nondisabled world of the comparative harmlessness of many impairments" (Silvers, 2001, p. 57). Medical and bioethics education can take steps to ease that burden.

Perhaps the most compelling challenge to both medical and social models of disability, as well as microlevel constructions of bioethics, is posed by those speakers of American Sign Language (ASL) who identify themselves not as persons with impairments *or* disabilities, but as members of a particular minority culture, the Deaf-World. They base their cultural claim primarily on the act of communicating in a common language, which has a unique grammar and distinctive art forms, that between half a million and a million people share (Lane & Grodin, 1997, p. 233; Mitchell, Young, Bachleda, & Karchmer, 2006). This community, which relies on vision to communicate and to navigate the world, shares customs and values as well. In these ways, the Deaf community distinguishes itself not only from the larger population, but also from the almost 29 million U.S. citizens with hearing loss who communicate primarily in English or another spoken language (Agrawal, Platz, & Niparko, 2008). The Deaf culture also defines health and well-being in ways that value deafness, interpreting cures for deafness as harm: "harm to bodily integrity" or "psychological harm" in one view (Burke, 2008, pp. 73, 74) and harm to a minority culture in another (Lane & Grodin, 1997). From the perspective of the Deaf-World, what others might regard as a beneficent medical act by physicians—implanting cochlear devices to enable hearing—instead registers as harm. In fact, opinions about the efficacy as well as the ethics of cochlear implants vary, especially regarding children born with profound deafness (Lane & Grodin, 1997, pp. 235–236; Nichols & Geers, 2006). Furthermore, there are Deaf-World adults who wish to increase the possibility of having deaf children through their choice of partners or genetic screening (Lane & Grodin, 1997, pp. 242–244; Tucker, 1998).

Arguments challenging the perspective of the Deaf-World move between micro and macro concerns. One focuses on the individual who is unable to communicate with the larger world and might in the future (in the case of a child) prefer doing so in uncomplicated ways, or might like to control his voice or to hear the voices of her children (Tucker, 1998). The other considers the cost to the larger community of providing services and technologies to moderate the effects of deafness that one has, in Tucker's word, "elected" (Tucker, 1998). The justice concern questions the moral ground of hearing persons to compel the Deaf to implant cochlear devices or be denied resources. It also questions members of the Deaf-World who insist, as some do, that parents refrain from providing cochlear implants to ensure the continuity of Deaf culture.

TREATING NEWBORNS

THE RESPONSES TO deafness and other disabilities expose the ways surrogacy and best-interest decisions are centrally about how disability is understood. (See also a father's account of such decision-making in Galli, 2000.) This understanding also enters decisions about withholding life-preserving, ordinary medical treatments from newborns (often those born prematurely) with significant physical or cognitive impairments, or both. These circumstances entail questions about who—parents, physicians, ethics committees—should decide and what counts as justification. Depending on the severity of an infant's condition, primary justifications not to treat include the status of these infants as persons, the perceived quality of their psychosocial lives, the expectation of physical pain and ongoing medical treatments that could constitute burden to themselves, and the perceived burdens of their care to others (Harrison, 2006; Kuhse & Singer, 1985; Robertson, 1998).

On the one hand, low estimates of the experience of living with a disability and expectations of its burdens are rallied in arguments not to treat. On the other hand, arguments premised on the construction of personhood or sanctity of life have led to measures such as the Baby Doe rulings that require treating all infants (Morrow, 2000). The arguments based on personhood point to instances in which nonpersonhood has been invoked throughout history to deprive those labeled nonpersons (women, slaves, and ethnic minorities) of liberty and to justify policies of genocide. The disability perspective typically points to these instances. While respecting the lessons of history, other perspectives question both the ethics of treating newborns who will spend their lives in medical systems and the framing of these treatments as miracles (Guyer, 2006).

Further complications arise in the case of disabled newborns. One concerns agency and the process by which decisions are made. Parents depend almost entirely on physicians' medical accounts of particular congenital conditions, the prospects of a child's quality of life, and the value of treatments offered. It has been suggested that the way physicians describe these matters is directed by their own preferences about treating newborns, and these descriptions, in turn, direct parents' decisions (Kuhse & Singer, 1985, pp. 62–63). Other complications appear in omissions made by those arguing against and those advocating maximal treatments. Generally, the arguments against treatments assume poor quality of life and significant burdens to the parental caregivers. Yet these arguments do not consider the difference that improved social conditions for those living with a disability or policies providing financial and other support for the caregivers can make. Similarly, arguments advocating the maximal treatment of newborns remain unaccompanied by efforts to support the disabled infants, the children or adults they become, or the families that care for them. These issues regarding how disability is understood and responded to pertain as well to conditions that medical technology now detects prior to birth.

DISABILITY IN THE LIFE CYCLE

WHEREAS THE MEDICAL model of disability distinguishes bodies that have deficits from those that do not, the social model distinguishes persons with disabilities as an oppressed group, ironically reinforcing notions of normalcy. However, disability theorists as well as the World Health Organization (WHO) are offering a more inclusive conceptualization, one that understands disability as a condition of the human life cycle that calls for a combination of functional enhancements and gracious physical and social accommodations (Davis, 2006b; Shakespeare, 2006; WHO, 2002). Humans begin and often end a full life with incapacitating conditions that include lack of independent mobility, levels of cognition that prevent independent living, and, often at the end, lost or diminished vision and hearing. We can sustain this capacious understanding of disability while acknowledging that some conditions at birth and some diseases and impairments in the course of a life, where most disabling conditions occur, are more devastating than others. Once disability is regarded as "a universal human experience" (WHO, 2002, p. 3) rather than an unanticipated, alienating, individual experience, disabling conditions can be prepared for when constructing social, medical, educational, employment, and family systems. Doing so would acknowledge human fragility and the limits of medicine to sustain bodies considered to be perfect. Such acknowledgment would parallel the way contemporary medicine is reconsidering vigorous use of technologies that prolong dying and is attempting, instead, to respect death's inevitability.

CONCLUSION

MAINSTREAMING DISABILITY WITHIN the life cycle, as well as within culture, opens or reconfigures areas of interest for bioethics. Attention to disability extends the principle of respect for persons beyond autonomous decision-making to include respect for ways of living with a range of conditions and capacities. This respect would compel consideration of ethical responsibility to those with cognitive disabilities (Kittay, 2005). Disability concerns would emphasize everyday ethical principles and values that enhance dignity and capacities to participate in social life and in the world in general, which are obscured by headline-making instances of what is framed as the right to die (Kane & Caplan, 1990). The ethics of care and the conditions of family or other intimate caregivers, whom medical and social systems unquestioningly call into service, would need further research and consideration, including the construction of a vocabulary of justice that acknowledges dependency and reciprocity as features of the life cycle (Kittay, 1999; Kittay & Feder, 2002; National Alliance for Caregiving and AARP, 2004; Silvers, Wasserman, & Mahowald, 1998). Ethics committees would need to be scrutinized for the relationship of their members to disability. Clearly, a token person with a disability or token family caregiver cannot represent the range of experiences disabling conditions issue or the range of responses to them. But committees can include enough members with varying relationships to disability in its diverse manifestations to ensure rich and rigorous conversations. Finally, mainstreaming disability would untangle the question of whether bioethics should enter or endorse disability activism from the assumption that to do so entails acting on behalf of a special interest group (Kirschner, 2001; Silvers, 2001; Singer, 2001; Sisti & Caplan, 2001).

REFERENCES

Agrawal, Y., Platz, E. A., & Niparko, J. K. (2008). Prevalence of hearing loss and differences by demographic characteristics among U.S. adults: Data from the National Health and Nutrition Examination Survey, 1999–2004. *Archives of Internal Medicine, 168*(14), 1522–1530.

The Americans With Disabilities Act. Retrieved August 14, 2008, from http://www.gov/ada/adatext.html

Beauchamp, T. L., & Childress, J. F. (1994). *Principles of biomedical ethics* (4th ed.). New York: Oxford University Press.

Burke, T. B. (2008). Bioethics and the deaf community. In K. A. Lindgren, D. DeLuca, & D. J. Napoli (Eds.), *Signs and voices: Deaf culture, identity, language, and arts* (pp. 63–74). Washington, DC: Gallaudet University Press.

Chambers, T. (2000). Centering bioethics. *Hastings Center Report, 30*(1), 22–29.

Cole, J. (2004). *Still lives: Narratives of spinal cord injury*. Cambridge, MA: MIT Press.

Coleman, L. M. (2006). Stigma: An enigma demystified. In L. J. Davis (Ed.), *The disability studies reader* (2nd ed., pp. 145–155). New York: Routledge.

Davis, L. J. (Ed.). (2006a). *The disability studies reader* (2nd ed.). New York: Routledge.

Davis, L. J. (2006b). The end of identity politics and the beginning of dis-modernism: On disability as an unstable category. In L. J. Davis (Ed.), *The disability studies reader* (2nd ed., pp. 231–242). New York: Routledge.

Davis, L. J. (2006c). Constructing normalcy: The bell curve, the novel, and the invention of the disabled body in the nineteenth century. In L. J. Davis (Ed.), *The disability studies reader* (2nd ed., pp. 3–16). New York: Routledge.

Dubus, A. (1991). *Broken vessels: Essays*. Boston: David R. Grodin.

Galli, R. (2000). *Rescuing Jeffrey*. Chapel Hill, NC: Algonquin.

Gill, T. M , & Feinstein, A. R. (1994). A critical appraisal of the quality of quality-of-life measurements. *Journal of the American Medical Association, 272*(8), 619–626.

Guyer, R. L. (2006). *Baby at risk: The uncertain legacies of medical miracles for babies, families, and society*. Sterling, VA: Capital Books.

Hammell, K. (2000, April). Living from the neck up: Society and high quadriplegia. *New Mobility*, 53–56.

Harrison, H. (2001). Making lemonade: A parent's view of "quality of life" studies. *The Journal of Clinical Ethics, 12*(3), 239–250.

Johnson, H. M. (2003, February 16). Unspeakable conversations. *The New York Times Magazine*, 50–55, 74, 78–79.

Kane, R. A., & Caplan, A. L. (Eds.). (1990). *Everyday ethics: Resolving dilemmas in nursing home life*. New York: Springer Publishing.

Kirschner, K. L. (2001). Rethinking anger and advocacy in bioethics. *The American Journal of Bioethics, 1*(3), 60–62.

Kittay, E. F. (1999). *Love's labor: Essays on women, equality, and dependency*. New York: Routledge.

Kittay, E. F. (2005). At the margins of moral personhood. *Ethics, 116*, 100–131.

Kittay, E. F., & Feder, E. K. (Eds.). (2002). *The subject of care: Feminist perspectives on dependency*. Lanham, MD: Rowan & Littlefield.

Kleinman, A. (1988). *The illness narratives: Suffering, healing, and the human condition*. New York: Basic Books.

Knighton, R. (2006). *Cockeyed: A memoir*. New York: Public Affairs of Perseus Books.

Kuczewski, M. G. (2001). Disability: An agenda for bioethics. *The American Journal for Bioethics, 1*(3), 36–44.

Kuhse, H., & Singer, P. (1985). *Should the baby live? The problems of handicapped infants*. New York: Oxford University Press.

Lane, H. (2002). Do deaf people have a disability? *Sign Language Studies, 2*(4), 356–379.

Lane, H., & Grodin, M. (1997). Ethical issues in cochlear implant surgery: An exploration into disease, disability, and the best interests of the child. *Kennedy Institute of Ethics Journal, 7*(3), 231–251.

Mairs, N. (1986). On being a cripple. In *Plaintext* (pp. 9–20). Tucson: University of Arizona Press.

Mairs, N. (1996). *Waist-high in the world: A life among the nondisabled*. Boston: Beacon Press.

Mitchell, R. E., Young, T. A., Bachleda, B., & Karchmer, M. A. (2006). How many people use ASL in the United States? Why Estimates Need Updating. *Sign Language Studies, 6*(3), 306–335.

Morrow, J. (2000). Making mortal decisions at the beginning of life: The case of impaired and imperiled infants. *Journal of the American Medical Association, 284*, 1146–1147.

National Alliance for Caregiving and AARP. (2004, April). *Caregiving in the U.S.* Retrieved September 21, 2006, from http://www.caregiving.org/data/04finalreport.pdf

Nichols, J. G., & Geers, A. E. (2006). Effects of early auditory experience on the spoken language of deaf children at 3 years of age. *Ear and Hearing, 27*(3), 286–298.

Pence, G. E. (2000). Requests to die: Elizabeth Bouvia and Larry McAfee. In *Classic cases in medical ethics: Accounts of cases that have shaped medical ethics, with philosophical, legal, and historical backgrounds* (3rd ed., pp. 56–84). New York: McGraw Hill.

Robertson, J. A. (1998). Involuntary euthanasia in defective newborns. In G. E. Pence (Ed.), *Classic works in medical ethics: Core philosophical readings* (pp. 218–228). New York: McGraw Hill.

Rosenberg, C. E. (1999). Meanings, policies, and medicine: On the bioethical enterprise and history. *Daedalus, 128*(4), 27–46.

Sacks, O. (1995). To see and not see. In *An anthropologist on Mars: Seven paradoxical tales* (pp. 108–152). New York: Random House.

Shakespeare, T. (2006). The social model of disability. In L. J. Davis (Ed.), *The disability studies reader* (2nd ed., pp. 197–204). New York: Routledge.

Silvers, A. (2001). A neutral ethical framework for understanding the role of disability in the life cycle. *The American Journal of Bioethics, 1*(3), 57–58.

Silvers, A., Wasserman, D., & Mahowald, M. B. (Eds.). (1998). *Disability, difference, discrimination: Perspectives on justice in bioethics and public policy.* New York: Rowman & Littlefield.

Singer, P. (1993). *Practical ethics* (2nd ed.). Cambridge, UK: Cambridge University Press.

Singer, P. (2001). Response to Mark Kuczewski. *The American Journal of Bioethics, 1*(3), 55–56.

Sisti, D. A., & Caplan, A. L. (2001). Help wanted: Entrepreneurs needed to serve bioethics' outsiders. *The American Journal of Bioethics, 1*(3), 48–49.

Toombs, S. K. (1993). *The meaning of illness: A phenomenological account of the different perspectives of physician and patient.* Dordrecht: Kluwer.

Tremain, S. (Guest Ed.). (2008). Reconfiguring disability: From bioethics to biopolitics [Special issue]. *Journal of Bioethical Inquiry, 5*(2-3).

Tucker, B. P. (1998). Deaf culture, cochlear implants, and elective disability. *Hastings Center Report, 28*(4), 6–14.

Tulsky, D. S., & Rosenthal, M. (2003). Measurement of quality of life in rehabilitation medicine: Emerging issues. *Archives of Physical Medicine Rehabilitation, 84*(Suppl. 2), S1–S2.

Wendell, S. (1996). *The rejected body: Feminist philosophical reflections of disability*. New York: Routledge.

Whiteneck, G. G. (1994). Measuring what matters: Key rehabilitation outcomes. *Archives of Physical Medicine Rehabilitation, 75*, 1073–1076.

World Health Organization. (2002). *Towards a common language for functioning, disability, and health*. Geneva: Author.

18

Ethical Issues in Caregiving

Rabbi Gerald I. Wolpe

Informal Caregiver–A nonpaid caregiver who is not a health care professional. Usually a member of the patient's family, it also includes a friend or associate who assumes health care responsibilities.

THE CARE AND support of the ill by informal caregivers have a long recorded history. Ancient documents, including the Bible, underscore the expected familial response to the needs of the afflicted. Often couched as religious law, the obligation is clear. "Thou shalt not stand idly by the blood of your brother" (Leviticus 19:16).[1] Hands-on-care within the home was considered a moral responsibility and a vital part of the response to illness and disease. The extent of institutional care in that period and the ritual of communication with healers by the ill and family are still a subject of study. Archeology and anthropological studies have revealed ancient forms of surgery and professional healing. Religious law defined disease and religious authorities crafted the response. However, it is also clear that the closeness of familial and tribal relationships resulted in mandatory informal caregiving.

The rise of an extended network of formal health care in the first half of the 20th century created a new interaction of family with the

Disclosure. The author has been a spousal caregiver for 22 years.

professional health care provider. The placing of the informal care-giver outside of the care protocol by the professional health care de-liverers during that period was a historical change. It came as a result of the expansion of hospitals, nursing homes, and other care facilities. It also created an authoritative stance of physicians and put medical protocols entirely in the hands of the health care professional. The pa-tient and family caregiver had little consultant role.[2] Institutional care demanded its own rules. Family contact with the patient, information about treatment or lack of treatment and accountability became en-tirely under the direction of the health care professional. The length of hospital stays, nature of clinical care, impact of third-party insurance payment, and end of treatment were put entirely in the hands of the professional health care community.

Unexpectedly, beginning in the 1970s, a reversal began. Unforeseen societal shifts reintroduced the vital role of the informal caregiver. The dramatic rise in the importance of the informal caregiver in the health care delivery system presented both wider health care possibili-ties and a complex series of new definitions and ethical conflicts. Legal overview and new economic realities chipped away at the health care institution, and community and home health care became a major set-ting. Rosalynn Carter, the former First Lady, indicated that there are only four kinds of people in the world: those who have been caregivers, those who are currently caregivers, those who will be caregivers, and those who will need caregivers. The informal caregiver had returned to a traditional role and importance.

BIOETHICS AND CAREGIVING

A COMBINATION OF historical events including participation of German doctors in the Nazi atrocities, revelation of American medical experiments on humans, impact of new medical technology, and so forth resulted in the rise of bioethics as an influential discipline (Walter & Klein, 2003). The keynote theme of ethical issues in health care included the recognition of the informal caregiver as a major par-ticipant in acute and, especially, chronic illness. The disruptive impact of illness on family life and resultant ethical dilemmas slowly brought the status of the caregiver into the health care delivery system (Levine, 2004). Statistical studies of home care, a new discipline, are sobering and startling.

More than 25 million Americans provide ongoing care to ill and dis-abled family members and friends. "Despite their numbers and their provision of what would cost more than $250 billion in services each year—nearly twice our combined expenditures for home health and nursing home care—family caregivers have been largely invisible to health care providers and policy makers" (Tallon, 2002, p. x). Eighty percent of the informal caregivers are women, with a rapidly growing category of male caregivers above the age of 80. Sixty percent of the caregivers are married. More than one-third have been engaged in caregiver activities for more than 10 years. Nearly 75% reported that they provided all or most of the care for their family member. The lengthening of life spans has resulted in longer periods of chronic aging needs. Home care is not only more common but exists for a longer period of time.

New economic realities affected the availability of hospitals for all medical needs. Ventilator therapy and artificial nutrition channeled through infusion pumps are applicable in homes as much as in medical institutions. The growth of high-tech home medicine has been explosive. The instruction of caregivers to become technologically adept is an arduous process with the understandable stress of fear of inadequacies and failure. The time and effort needed for the application of high-tech home care has resulted in the creation of agencies of home assistance. They have been helpful but also have added to the caregiver's administrative task of the care dossier. Managing home care schedules and appropriate treatment is ongoing and time consuming.

Informal caregivers are not a monolithic group. Parents, spouses, children, extended family members, and friend caregivers face varying challenges but also share common dilemmas.

CARE OF THE ELDERLY

"BARRING MAJOR UNFORESEEN developments, we are entering an unprecedented phase of our history—indeed, of human history—featuring (1) a new age structure of society, (2) longer and more vigorous old age for millions, (3) new modes of dwindling and dying, and (4) a likely shortage of available caregivers" ("Taking Care," 2005).

The projected aging of the U.S. population has forced revised attention to the impact of the demographic shift. "Between 2000 and 2050, the population of Americans age 45 to 64 is expected to grow modestly from 61 to 85 million while the population 65 and over is expected to grow from 34 to 79 million, with the cohort 85 and above more than quadrupling, from 4 million to 18 million" ("Taking Care," 2005).

The dramatic extension of life is attributable to the remarkable strides in medical care and preventive medicine. This growth in personal longevity is an unprecedented achievement but also engenders major social challenges. Traditional role-playing among the generations has been revised. Four existing generations in one family can create two so-called sandwich generations with obligations and demands from two directions. For example, a couple arriving at the traditional retirement age of 65 may find long-awaited plans to be thwarted by needs of older parents, children, or grandchildren. The extension of life may provide more years of health and vigor but it also creates a longer period of chronic illness and care demands (Johnson, 2008).

Extended periods of disability, total dependence, and dementia create scenarios of stress and inner conflict. The financial drain, in itself, can destroy retirement funds of elderly patients as well as the caregiver. Family disputes as to the priority of existing means can strain marital, sibling, and parental relationships. This stress can extend to decisions about institutionalization in nursing homes, site of home care, and sharing of caretaking duties. Health care decisions based on economic needs are a constant challenge.

Even the creation of innovative programs can cause ethical conflict. The growth of hospice care for the terminally ill has been a vital aid to caregivers (see chapter 66). The difficult period of watching a loved one in the final time of life can be eased by the management of pain, compassionate support of the caregiver, and guidance at the time of death. Yet major religious traditions and philosophies resist the abandonment of continued hope and oppose the acceptance of death. Families still resist the honest discussion of death with the patient. Hospice sends a clear signal to all, including the patient, that it is terminal care (Groopman, 2004).

SPOUSAL CAREGIVING

SPOUSAL PARTICIPANTS WHO were providing care and experiencing caregiver strain had mortality risks 63% higher over the four years of the study than those participants whose spouses did not require care (Shulz & Beach, 1999). Parallel studies indicate a high rate of divorce among parental caregivers and divisive strain among family members. More than 50% of caregivers turned first to other family members for assistance, and nearly 66% reported receiving little or no help from them. Family responsibility does not fit into the firm categories of more legalistic, contractual notions of responsibility. Health care professionals tend to be impatient with the demands of the families during health protocols. This has particular impact in spousal caregiving. There is usually strong interplay among members of the family, and that relationship can cause confusion in negotiations with paid professionals.

The age of the spousal caregiver is a vital factor. When illness or accident occurs at a younger age, the long-term adjustment can be brutal.

There are the death of expectations and the strain on loyalty and commitment. In many cases institutionalization takes place to allow the caregiver more independence for a meaningful life. The conflict with children, in-laws and extended family is constant. This is especially true when major life and death decisions are in question.

Familial differences regarding major decisions can explode into legal confrontation at any point and even receive national attention. The Terri Schiavo tragedy is a case in point (Quill, 2005). The dispute between her husband and parents was a media spectacle and national political and religious leaders joined in the fray. Bioethicists and legal scholars contributed their insights toward some understanding of the categories involved. The importance of advanced directives was reflected in the conflicting claims about cessation of care and the basic authority of her husband and parents (Power of Attorney and Health Care Directives, 2007). The discouraging low number of people with advanced directives and health care directives have exacerbated the difficulty in ascertaining the desire of the patient and the desired surrogate for substitute decisions (see chapter 64). The identity of the caregiver who is primus inter pares (first among equals) in making life decisions for the patient is essential and is a major decision to be encouraged in all cases of informal caregiving.

PARENTAL CAREGIVING

MANY OF THE previously mentioned issues pertain to parental caregiving. However, an added issue is the rights of the child. Parents must make decisions, and it is assumed that those decisions are motivated by what is best for the child (see chapter 39). In most cases, the child has no part in what is decided for the future. For varying reasons, courts and medical authorities may be forced to make vital decisions in loco parentis. The inherent conflict with that process has disturbing ethical undertones. Setting aside the natural authority of parents can be traumatic at the least.

In all cases of parental caregiving, the level of inner parental conflict is intense. The sickness and death of grandparents and parents, as painful as it can be, is still part of a natural course of life. Marriage vows affirm love for better or for worse, indicating a recognition that the course of married life may include disease or accident. However, the illness or challenged condition of a child is an anomaly. Disappointment and sense of guilt are constant as well as a major disruption in family life. Attention to a sick child may diminish parental time for other children as well as for the spouse, and resentment becomes operant. The financial burden may become overwhelming, and parental love for the child could become conditioned. Marriages falter, and the constant concern about the future of the child becomes the focus of family life.

Understandably, the nature of the illness also is varied. The specificities of dementia, head injury, terminal illnesses, genetic diseases, physical disabilities, and so forth call for varying forms of needed care, both in time investment and physical-emotional effort. Health advocates may be helpful in financing research and clinical response for particular illnesses and treatments but they also can be adamant in their opposition to certain medical procedures, which may create conflict if the parents hold a different position.

CONCLUSION

WHAT IS COMMON to different types of caregiving is the constant conflict between personal needs and wants and the sense of obligation to the patient. Often the caregiver's life is defined by the needs of the ill. The relationship with health care professionals is mostly patient-oriented and the needs of the caregiver tend to be ignored or minimized. Many factors create an unrelenting fatigue that is both emotional and physical: other family obligations, work demands, absence of a nuclear family or extended family support, intimidating issues related to health care plans, insurance, constant financial strain, the agony of watching loved ones in distress, and change of identification—child becomes parent and vice versa. A sense of guilt is constant as different demands and needs test the caregiver. Shorter stays in the hospital also require long negotiations with the health care delivery system. No one is ever prepared for the transition from acute to chronic care and the change in care responsibilities. The stress of this adjustment is ongoing and debilitating. As indicated above, major areas of attention have arisen regarding advance directives and the appointment of surrogates for health decisions of the patient (Caring Connections, n.d.). This is a vital component of the new need for decision-making during care and when ending care.

The motto of the spousal caregiver organization Wellspouse is "When one person is ill, two need help." The recognition of the informal caregiver as a vital participant in the health care delivery system is a result of many factors.

That recognition has awakened its own demands. Because of the endless demands of caregiving, illness of the caregiver has become a serious issue, and so-called caregiving syndrome is a growing area of attention. The strain placed upon family members is common and destructive. In addition, the trend toward greater participation of the informal caregiver is exacerbated by faster discharge from hospitals and newer home care techniques. The demographic reality of a new age structure in our society also awakens awareness of the growing shortage of caregivers. Our mobile society results in the scattering of family and the inability of children, parents, siblings, and so forth to be available. The alternative to nuclear families also causes ambiguity as to the identification of family and appropriate caregivers (e.g., divorce and mixed families). This issue calls for expanding social attention and planning.

The awareness of these trends and the importance of the caregiver in the healing process have resulted in a separate category of study. Ethical issues in informal caregiving require bioethical insights with specific attention to the inherent endemic conflicts. Home care support is a growing trend, and statistical studies are vital. The rising use of hospice care, community social and health support and greater attempts of the health delivery system to respond to the worth of caregiving are encouraging signs of integrating medical and social concerns and assistance. It also demands a greater exposure in the training of the health professional so that the new partnership with the informal caregiver will be effective. The ancient mandate has its new character, and with the growing dependence on the informal caregiver, it will become an important factor in health care and healing.

NOTES

1. Rabbinic interpretation uses this verse to legitimize medical response to illness.

2. Reaction to this process in cases of dying and death became highly publicized legal issues with major contention between the medical and legal communities and informal caregiver advocacy groups.

REFERENCES

Caring Connections, a program of the National Hospice and Palliative Care Organization (NHPCO). (n.d.). *Advance directives*. Retrieved September 3, 2008, from http://www.caringinfo.org/PlanningAhead/AdvanceDirectives.htm

Groopman, J. (2004). *The anatomy of hope: How people prevail in the face of illness*. New York: Random House.

Johnson, M. (2008). Strains and drains, long-term care. *Virtual Mentor, 10* (6), 397–400.

Levine, C. (Ed.). (2004). *Always on call, when illness turns families into caregivers* (expanded ed.). Nashville, TN: Vanderbilt University Press.

Power of Attorney and Health Care Directives. (2007). *Final law*. Mayo Clinic. com—Living Will and Advanced Directives. Retrieved September 1, 2008, from http://www.mayoclinic.com/health/living-wills/HA00014

Quill, T. (2005). Terri Schiavo—A tragedy compounded. *New England Journal of Medicine, 352*(16), 1630–1633.

Shulz, R., & Beach, S. R. (1999). Caregiver as a risk factor for mortality. *Journal of the American Medical Association, 282*(23), 2215–2219.

"Taking care": Ethical caregiving in our aging society. (2005). Washington, DC. The President's Council on Bioethics.

Tallon, J., Jr. (2002). Foreword. *Making room for family caregivers*. New York: United Hospital Fund Report.

Walter, J. K., & Klein, E. P. (Eds.) (2003). *The story of bioethics*. Washington, DC: Georgetown University Press.

Part IV

Research Ethics

19

Research Misconduct and Fraud

Barbara K. Redman

URING THE 1990S, professor Eric T. Poehlman studied aging, menopause and obesity and submitted 17 grant applications that were based on fabricated data. In October 2000, a junior member of Poehlman's laboratory became convinced that he had altered data. A 6-year investigation found that Poehlman had committed scientific fraud for more than 12 years and expended $2.9 million in research funding based on grant applications with false and fabricated data. He was debarred for life from receiving Public Health Service (PHS) research funds, agreed to retract or correct 10 scientific articles (Office of Research Integrity [ORI], 2005), and as a result of criminal prosecution was sentenced to 366 days in prison followed by 2 years of supervised release (Gravois, 2006).

Although one of the most egregious, the Poehlman case raises questions of how the misconduct could have gone on for so long without discovery, how much of the rest of his work was also affected, and why he did it. In a letter to the judge, Poehlman said he had convinced himself that it was acceptable to falsify data because: the research questions were worthy of study, it was okay to misrepresent supposedly minor pieces of data to increase the odds the grant would be funded, he felt pressure from his institution to produce and to fund his lab, and he was ambitious (ORI, 2005). Had Poehlman's work been part of a multisite trial, statistical programs that detect data discrepant from other centers might have triggered an audit. As it was, although members of his lab had suspicions, the fabrication was undetected for more than a decade.

The definition of research misconduct consistent across many federal agencies including the U.S. Department of Health and Human Services (USDHHS) Office of Research Integrity (ORI) is "fabrication, falsification or plagiarism in proposing, performing or reviewing research, or in reporting research results. Fabrication is making up data or results and recording or reporting them. Falsification is manipulating research materials, equipment, or processes, or changing or omitting data or results such that the research is not accurately represented in the research record. Plagiarism is the appropriation of another person's ideas, processes, results, or words without giving appropriate credit. Research misconduct does not include honest error or differences of opinion" (ORI, 2005, p. 1).

"A finding of research misconduct requires that there be a significant departure from accepted practices of the relevant research community, and the misconduct be committed intentionally, knowingly, or recklessly, and the allegation be proven by a preponderance of the evidence" (USDHHS, 2005, p. 28386). ORI regulations govern funds applied or received from the PHS, which includes the National Institutes of Health, although many institutions receiving such grants adopt the policy for all research activities. A summary of ORI findings of scientific misconduct in clinical trials from 1992 to 2002 found the most frequent offence to be fabrication or falsification of data (88%); falsification of credentials was found in 8% of cases, and plagiarism in 10% (Reynolds, 2004).

Recent policy governing research misconduct dates from the Health Research Extension Act of 1985. Investigative processes have developed from informal ones traditional to the scientific community to those that ensure due process at the ORI level (Mello & Brennan, 2003). ORI's role has evolved from direct investigation and judgment of cases of alleged misconduct to oversight and facilitation of institutional investigations. The agency also plays an educational role for the responsible conduct of research.

Allegations of research misconduct are usually reported by individuals to the institution or to ORI; less than 10% result in a finding of research misconduct. Retaliation against the complainant is common (Pascal, 2006). Many cases in which there is a finding of research misconduct are concluded by an agreement in which respondents voluntarily exclude themselves from U.S. government grants and contracts and often from advising the PHS for a period of time. They may be subject to supervision or required to have the accuracy of their work certified. They may be debarred, which means they may not receive or benefit from federal funds. A settlement may also require affected publications to be retracted or corrected (Reynolds, 2004). It is important to note that these policies do not cover privately funded research, although studies to support action by the Food and Drug Administration for approval of products and many other federal agencies are covered by similar policies.

Other countries, most recently Australia, are faced with a need to construct a system for handling allegations of research misconduct, precipitated from lessons learned in handling contentious cases. While most countries have taken an ad hoc approach to the problem, others are taking the next step of formalizing a structure, with the ORI serving as a model (Finkel, 2007). After years of discussion, in March of 2006, the United Kingdom created a national Research Integrity Office that intends to establish guidelines and give advice (Marshall, 2006).

Research misconduct is a very basic form of dishonesty, usually involving public funds. It hinders scientific progress, violates norms of trust and transparency of methods and data to other scientists, and raises questions about whether the historical policy of allowing the scientific community to self-govern should continue. Federal regulatory policy, evolving over a long series of scandals involving investigators whose misconduct has been undetected for prolonged periods of time, has been resisted at every step by the scientific community.

A persistent but still unanswered question of the extent of research misconduct has yielded estimates ranging from 1 in 10,000 active researchers to 100 times this level (Steneck, 2000). A large survey of early and mid-career scientists based in the United States and funded by the National Institutes of Health (NIH) asked respondents to report their own behaviors. They reportedly engaged in a range of behaviors extending far beyond fabrication, falsification, and plagiarism (FFP) that can damage the integrity of science, including changing the design, methodology, or results of a study in response to pressure from a funding source, or dropping observations or data points from analyses based on a gut feeling they were inadequate (Martinson, Anderson, & De Vries, 2005).

Fraud in scientific research has been defined as "the knowing breach of the standard of good faith and fair dealing as understood in the community, involving deception or breach of trust, for money" (Sheehan, 2007, p. S63). It can involve falsifying data or documents, or knowingly failing to comply with regulations protecting research participants. Fraud can be committed by individuals, institutions, or corporations in the context of research (Sheehan, 2007).

It is important to note that allegations of research misconduct can be used by parties with financial interests in a product to discredit an investigator or a line of research. The case of Dr. Herbert Needleman is illustrative. In 1979, Dr. Needleman published a study concluding that very low exposures of children to lead caused mental impairment. A lead industry consultant filed a complaint of research misconduct for bias. Though eventually cleared, Needleman spent years and thousands of dollars defending himself and his work. There is no penalty for attacking a scientist's integrity with exaggerated or even wholly specious charges (McGarity, 2006).

This chapter takes the position that current policy represents a narrow slice of possible and desirable policy. It addresses basic questions including outcomes that should be expected from research misconduct policy, and notes that the current regulatory approach touches little of the process of constructing and using scientific knowledge and focuses on a limited number of causes for misconduct. It then considers alternative policy instruments and makes the case for evidence-based policy.

GOAL AND PRESSURE POINTS

CURRENT POLICY APPEARS to have been enacted for the political purpose of punishing and ridding the scientific community of so-called bad apples, thus sustaining the view that aberrant individuals are the cause of this problem. The reporting of an accelerating number of cases across the world raises the question of whether current methods of identification are adequate.

The applicable federal regulation identifies its purpose as protecting the health and safety of the public, promoting the integrity of PHS-supported research and the research process, and conserving public funds (USDHHS, 2005). I propose that the goals of regulation should be conceived more broadly. For example, they might include the following.

1. Protection of scientific capital (knowledge, scientists, institutions, resources, norms of science)
2. Support of fair competition in science
3. Containment of harms to end users

The social system for production and use of scientific knowledge provides a series of pressure points at which research misconduct can be thwarted; however, few of the involved actors/institutions even acknowledge their role in doing so. Funders of scientific knowledge do not require that it be certified as free of fabrication, falsification or plagiarism, as they could by further oversight and development of data verification analysis. Second, publication in the best possible journals is necessary to sustain a scientific career. Yet a recent study of high-impact biomedical journals showed that few had publicly stated policies on research misconduct (Redman & Merz, 2006). Third, while PubMed notes retraction of studies for a variety of reasons, including research misconduct, subsequent citations of these studies frequently do not recognize the retraction, and retraction notices due to research misconduct are obfuscated by language suggesting simple scientific error or inability to reproduce (Redman, Yarandi, & Merz, in press).

Fourth, because they employ the scientists, institutions are in a strong position to thwart and punish research misconduct. Those receiving PHS funds must have an active assurance on file with ORI stating that they have developed and will comply with a process for responding to allegations of research misconduct. In addition to ORI sanctions, institutions can impose their own, which may include letters of reprimand being issued and retained in the respondent's personnel file, requiring supervision by a senior faculty member, subjecting grants and publications to special monitoring and review, and requiring a course or counseling in the responsible conduct of research.

And finally, authoritative bodies such as the United Nations Educational, Scientific and Cultural Organization (UNESCO) found among its member nations lack of societal will to set clear normative (ethical) standards to hold the scientific community responsible and accountable, including for research misconduct. This is still the situation after 10 years of debate and discussion (Scholze, 2006). Thus, none of these pressure points is fully used to thwart scientific misconduct

There is some evidence of tightening standards. A committee called to advise the journal *Science,* after some high-profile retractions, concluded that new and more rigorous policies are necessary. It acknowledges that current procedures are based on an assumption of trust; however, a small number of papers submitted are either intentionally misleading or substantially distorted by self-interest. The committee recommended audits for high-impact papers and for occasional randomly chosen papers, availability of primary data, and rethinking of penalties for authors who knowingly submit distorted or faulty work (Bauman, 2006).

It is important to note that current sanctions occur largely against scientists or staff and rarely against institutions because the actionable behaviors are falsification or fabrication of data or records, which by definition must be committed by an individual. Yet one of the most plausible explanations for ethical misconduct in organizations is the effect of climate. The Organizational Climate Measure, developed with young scientists, captures important elements of organizational environment. These include perceptions of organizational justice, adequate financial support, and clear role definitions, all of which are correlated with ethical scientific behavior (Gaddis et al., 2003). Active institutional monitoring of the conditions in which scientists work and their perspectives on organizational justice may point to needed areas of reform.

Although education in the responsible conduct of research (RCR) is clearly necessary and required for NIH research training grants, its effect on research misconduct has not been established. While core standards and knowledge of RCR have never been defined, content analysis of current materials showed scientific misconduct as a core instructional area that should be expanded beyond rules to include values in science, moral reasoning skills, the scientific method and objectivity, and self-deception (Heitman & Bulger, 2005). A study testing new graduate students in the sciences confirmed the implicit claim that standard graduate science education does not provide adequate grounding in the core concepts and standards of RCR and that a single course early in a student's graduate career is probably insufficient to impart even core concepts and standards in a lasting way (Heitman, Olsen, Anestidou, & Bulger, 2007).

Wider adoption of standards by all stakeholders, universal requirement of effective RCR training, as well as effective regulation of research misconduct could strengthen science's moral commitments. Scientific morality could change dramatically in a generation—witness the effect 40 years later of Henry K. Beecher's classic paper on the ethics of using human subjects (Beecher, 1966). This paper and others ended the era of researcher paternalism and precipitated the move to a period of regulatory protection. It is still cited today as evidence of how practice at a particular time, even in the best scientific institutions, can be revealed as unethical and raises the question, what current practices will be so judged in the future?

ALTERNATIVE POLICY APPROACHES

CURRENTLY, SEVERAL POLICY tools are used to attain compliance with research misconduct regulations: education in RCR; punishment that denies respondents access to grant money and advisory service and may require publication retraction or correction; grants for research in research misconduct and for development of standards and educational materials; annual reports from institutions; and advice. Occasionally, the institution must repay grant money. Other potential policy instruments including institutional fines would move beyond the bad apple theory and acknowledge that toxic institutional environments can lead to research misconduct.

The common approach to ethical concerns in research has been to establish regulations, which has set up an adversarial relationship with scientists. Some believe that, devoid of deeper ethical analysis, a purely regulatory approach is destined to fail because it assumes that the ethically correct course involves only compliance with rules. In recognition of the complexity of determining ethically appropriate behavior, a few institutions are establishing research ethics consultation services, which bridge concerns about subjects as well as about the responsible conduct of research, a core service much like biostatistics (de Melo-Martin, Palmer, Fins, & Joseph, 2007). The service at Stanford University yields confidential advice but has an obligation to report misconduct if consultants discover it (Pilcher, 2006).

Institutions, including government, can develop punishment strategies that optimize deterrence. Those lacking substantial enforcement resources might impose high penalties, while a government with sufficient resources might impose a lower penalty but enforce the law against all or almost all violators (Sunstein, 2005). Current evidence suggests minimal investment by institutions, government, or the profession in enforcement and modest penalties. Increasing one or the other should improve deterrence.

Although policies are political, a body of empirical work on consequences of a policy will help to create agreement and make it harder for narrow political interests to prevail. A very limited body of evidence on research misconduct leaves basic questions unanswered: Have research misconduct cases yielded poorer quality data than science with other kinds of errors? How much harm is done to subjects, to end users of the fabricated or falsified research, to other scientists who depend on prior research, to those found guilty, and how much money is wasted? Is punishment of offenders more effective than is an active effort to rehabilitate them? As countries around the world face scandalous cases of research misconduct and global collaborations are common, what is the best balance between cultural adaptation of policies or their harmonization?

Because misconduct has been found to be more prevalent in resource-poor environments with perceptions of injustice (Martinson, Anderson, Crain, & De Vries, 2006), would coordination of federal investment in scientific workforce development with appropriate levels of research support for the pool of scientists reduce misconduct? Martinson (2007) notes that all attention is on the size or distribution of the pool of NIH dollars; far less attention has been paid to whether too many biomedical scientists are being produced. The current mismatch between number of scientists and research resources may be adversely affecting the integrity of research (Martinson, 2007).

Implicit in current policy is the assumption that scientists are completely rational and ought to be able to withstand any amount of environmental pressure such as the current plateau of NIH research funding, which may result in dismantling productive research teams

built up over years and possibly loss of a generation of new investigators (Heinig, Krakower, Dickler, & Korn, 2007). As it currently stands,
research misconduct policy aims at the individual scientist or staff
member. It does not contain any expectations of policy makers for creating conditions supportive not only of economic payoff from science
but also for its ethical practice.

Evidence from the policy sciences provides perspective. The conflicting values inherent in policy may be dealt with by balancing them,
by cycling between values, or by use of firewalls between policy areas
(Thacher & Rein, 2004). Current policy of excluding bad apples seems
unlikely to change since the science community continues in this protective belief. It should be noted that to my knowledge, no one found
guilty of research misconduct has reoffended, supporting effectiveness of current policy. What have not been examined are side effects of
this policy such as ruined careers, scientific productivity lost because
of lack of rehabilitation, and the notion that investment in improved
surveillance systems is not necessary because research misconduct is
rare and bad apples are hard to detect.

The firewall between protection of research subjects (Office of
Human Research Protection) and research misconduct (ORI) likely allows each of these areas of research ethics to develop. But with the
recognition that the institutional review board (IRB) system may be
in need of reform, why not consider merging the two? Such a merger
would encourage follow up of scientific projects after IRB approval,
would provide a needed focus on harm from research misconduct,
and would likely increase researchers' understanding of misconduct.

CONCLUSION

WHILE FABRICATION OR falsification of data and plagiarism
are carried out by individual actors, current research misconduct policy avoids assigning responsibility for proper oversight to institutions that receive federal grants, to purchasers/funders, and to the
publishers of scientific knowledge. It also neglects to acknowledge the
responsibility of policy makers for establishing conditions that would
reasonably be understood to support the responsible conduct of science, for articulating clear goals for the regulation of research misconduct, and for determining whether they are met.

The field's attention to training in RCR is laudable but insufficient.
Driven by scandal, current policy supports the common supposition of
the bad apple that must be excised, leaving the field once again pure.
What is more likely needed is a system-wide change of incentives and
oversight for a higher standard of research integrity.

REFERENCES

Bauman, I. (2006). *Report from committee examining* Science's *peer review process.* Retrieved December 7, 2006, from http://www.sciencemag.org/cgi/data/314/5804/1353/DC1/1

Beecher, H. K. (1966). Ethics and clinical research. *New England Journal of Medicine, 2/4,* 1354–1360.

de Melo-Martin, I., Palmer, L. I., Fins, J. J., & Joseph, J. (2007). Developing a research ethics consultation service to foster responsive and responsible clinical research. *Academic Medicine, 82,* 900–904.

Finkel, E. (2007). New misconduct rules aim to minister to an ailing system. *Science, 317,* 1159.

Gaddis, B. H., Helton-Fauth, W., Scott, G., Schaffer, A., Connelly, S., Mumford, M., et al. (2003). Development of two measures of climate for scientific organizations. *Accountability in Research, 10,* 253–288.

Gravois, J. (2006). Former professor gets one year in jail for faking data on grant application. *The Chronicle of Higher Education, 52*(45), A10.

Heinig, S. J., Krakower, J. Y., Dickler, H. B., & Korn, D. (2007). Sustaining the engine of U.S. biomedical discovery. *New England Journal of Medicine, 357,* 1042–1047.

Heitman, E., & Bulger, R. E. (2005). Assessing the educational literature in the responsible conduct of research for core content. *Accountability in Research, 12,* 207–224.

Heitman, E., Olsen, C. H., Anestidou, L., & Bulger, R. E. (2007). New graduate students' baseline knowledge of the responsible conduct of research. *Academic Medicine, 82,* 838–845.

Marshall, E. (2006). Crime scene investigation: How to handle misconduct. *Science, 312,* 1465.

Martinson, B. C. (2007). Universities and the money fix. *Nature, 449,* 141–142.

Martinson, B. C., Anderson, M. S., Crain, A. L., & De Vries, R. (2006). Scientists' perceptions of organizational justice and self-reported misbehaviors. *Journal of Empirical Research on Human Research Ethics, 1,* 51–66.

Martinson, B. C., Anderson, M. S., & De Vries, R. (2005). Scientists behaving badly. *Nature, 435,* 737–738.

McGarity, T. O. (2006). Defending clean science from dirty attacks by special interests. In W. Wagner & R. Steinzor (Eds.), *Rescuing science from politics* (pp. 24–45). New York: Cambridge University Press.

Mello, M., & Brennan, T. A. (2003). Due process in investigations of research misconduct. *New England Journal of Medicine, 349,* 1280–1286.

Office of Research Integrity. (2005, March 17). *Press release—Dr. Eric T. Poehlman.* Retrieved September 9, 2008, from http://ori.hhs.gov/misconduct/cases/poehlman.shtml

Pascal, C. B. (2006). Complainant issues in research misconduct: The Office of Research Integrity Experience. *Experimental Biology and Medicine, 231,* 1264–1270.

Pilcher, H. (2006). Dial "E" for ethics. *Nature, 440,* 1104–1105.

Redman, B. K., & Merz, J. F. (2006). Research misconduct policies of high impact biomedical journals. *Accountability in Research, 13,* 247–258.

Redman, B. K., Yarandi H. N., & Merz, J. F. (in press). *Empirical developments in retraction.* Manuscript submitted for publication.

Reynolds, S. M. (2004). ORI findings of scientific misconduct in clinical trials and publicly funded research, 1992–2002. *Clinical Trials, 1,* 509–516.

Scholze, S. (2006). Setting standards for scientists. *EMBO Reports, 7,* S65–S67.

Sheehan, J. G. (2007). Fraud, conflict of interest, and other enforcement issues in clinical research. *Cleveland Clinic Journal of Medicine, 74*(Suppl. 2), S63–S67.

Steneck, N. H. (2000). *Assessing the integrity of publicly funded research.* ORI Research Conference on Research Integrity. Retrieved September 9, 2008, from http://ori.hhs.gov/research/extra/conference_2000.shtml

Sunstein, C. R. (2005). On psychology of punishment. In F. Parisi & V. L. Smith (Eds.), *The law and economics of irrational behavior* (pp. 339–357). Stanford, CA: Stanford University Press.

Thacher, D., & Rein, M. (2004). Managing value conflict in public policy. *Governance, 17,* 457–486.

United States Department of Health and Human Services. (2005). *Public Health Service policies on research misconduct; final rule.* 42 CFR (Code of Federal Regulations) parts 50 and 93. Fed Reg; 70, 28370–28400.

20

Ethical Issues in Innovative Surgery

Angelique M. Reitsma

During the last decades, major improvement has been made in the area of human subject research protections. Nowadays, it would be unthinkable to enroll a patient or a healthy volunteer into a clinical trial without his informed consent, a requirement that was not obvious to early investigators. Regardless of these significant advancements, informed consent for all *surgical* research is still not taken for granted. A form of surgical research, innovative surgery, is an elusive entity within clinical research. It somehow evades the currently accepted standards for human subject research such as obtaining informed consent for research participation and prior institutional review board (IRB) review. As this chapter argues, current federal regulations and governmental bodies do not have a firm grasp on surgical innovation, and therefore patients are sometimes at risk of becoming unknowing participants of (informal) research studies.

First, let us consider the existing regulations that guide research with human subjects. In the United States, the development of new drugs and medical devices is closely monitored by the federal government. The Food and Drug Administration (FDA) regulates biologics, devices, and drugs by reviewing their safety and efficacy for a given indication before granting approval for marketing and distribution. The labeling (package insert) summarizes what the FDA has deemed the safe and effective use of the product, and so-called off-label use of a product, although allowed, may be subject to regulatory scrutiny.

When a surgery does not include a device, biologic, or drug, the FDA has no jurisdiction over it.

The Department of Health and Human Services (DHHS) has set forth regulations pertaining to all human subject research in the federal rule 45 CFR 46, also dubbed "The Common Rule" (Code of Federal Regulations, 2005) because it has been adopted by almost all federal agencies. The Common Rule sets out definitions for research (systematic investigations designed to develop or contribute to generalizable knowledge) and for human subject (a living person from whom data is obtained either through direct interaction or via the use of personal identifiable information or bodily samples). Every person participating in a research study should do so willingly and voluntarily, with prior informed consent and protected by the safeguards that the Common Rule provides (such as prior IRB review of studies to assess the risk-benefit ratio of the proposed trial and the provision that a participant can voluntarily withdraw from the study at any given time). All research involving human participants that is performed with federal support (such as NIH grants) or within facilities that receive federal money (for example through Medicare and Medicaid), falls under this regulation. This implies that surgical research conducted *without* direct or indirect federal funding is beyond the jurisdiction of the DHHS' Office of Human Research Protection (OHRP).

HISTORY

THE SLIPPERY CONCEPT of innovation could be applied to all areas of medicine, but surgery has especially used the term. The somewhat exceptional position of innovative surgery within the realm of research and apparent lack of ethical regulations specifically governing surgical innovation has been long recognized. Internist Henry Beecher wrote as early as 1961:

> Ideally, all surgical interventions should be controlled. When real hazard is involved in a new and unproven procedure, it may be urgent to determine the value of such intervention. This is only possible with a proper plan. One may question the moral or ethical right to continue with casual or unplanned new surgical procedures—procedures which may encompass no more than a placebo effect—when these procedures are costly of time and money, and dangerous to health or life. (Beecher, 1961, p. 1103)

A group of surgeons wrote 25 years later:

> When large numbers of innovative treatments are being continuously introduced into clinical practice, rigorous testing is mandatory for the

protection of individual patients and the just use of limited resources. This holds true with even greater force in light of the evidence that many innovations show no advantage over existing treatments when they are subjected to properly controlled study. They may even be less effective, or harmful. (Roy, Black, & McPeek, 1986, p. 119)

Pediatricians (Frader & Caniano, 1998) suggested that

The era of limitations on health care expenditures and renewed concern about the human burden of unproven medical interventions may herald a sea change in attitudes toward surgery. (p. 239)

Frader and Flanagan-Klygis (2001) repeated the call for formal assessment of surgical interventions. Increasingly, from the surgical community proper, there is a call for vigilance toward cavalier innovators and reckless acceptance of procedures and techniques that have not been scientifically tested (Bunker, Hinkley, & McDermott, 1978; Casler, 2003; Cronin, Millis, & Siegler, 2001; Jones, 2000; Josefson, 2000; Love, 1975; Margo, 2001; McKneally, 1999; Moore, 2000; "Qualms About Innovative Surgery," 1985; Strasberg & Ludbrook, 2003; Ward, 1994; Waring, 1999).

The momentum for policy change seems to be building. The professional discourse on this issue is intensifying, and publications and presentations are on the rise (Kornetsky, 2001; McKneally & Kornetsky, 2003). At the same time, the call for evidence-based surgery is growing stronger (Jarvik & Deyo, 2000; Petrelli, 2002). The American College of Surgeons, the most authoritative professional fellowship representing U.S. surgeons, has made it one of its important goals (Jones & Richards, 2003). In 2004, the director of the Association of American Medical Colleges' (AAMC) Council of Academic Societies Affairs contacted the presidents of five major surgical societies, suggesting that leaders of the surgical community should provide guidance on this issue. The objectives of this project were to: (a) clarify the distinction between variations (minor modifications not requiring specific disclosure), innovations (modifications of potential significance to the patient, requiring disclosure), and research (systematic investigations designed to develop or contribute to generalizable knowledge); and (b) suggest guidelines to surgeons and hospitals for appropriate implementation and oversight of surgical innovations. The Society of University Surgeons (SUS) chose to pursue this initiative, and a statement, composed by a working group that included surgeons and a bioethicist, recently appeared in a surgical journal (Biffl et al., 2008).

A few years before this initiative was taken, bioethicists from the University of Virginia conducted a 2-year study into the ethics of surgical innovation. The results and conclusions of this project were published in the surgical literature (Reitsma & Moreno, 2002, 2005), and recommendations for policy change appeared in a book published in the summer of 2006 (Reitsma & Moreno, 2006). The rising demand for more ethically sound innovation in surgery from both the surgical, the bioethical, and the lay arena appears to be an open invitation for increased and better applicable regulation of clinical surgical research.

THE MORAL PROBLEM

THE ETHICAL ISSUES that surgical innovation may bring about are multifaceted. Surgical innovation is not an unequivocally negative entity but rather an intrinsic part of surgery that is necessary for progress and future improvement of the practice of surgery. As such, it has decidedly positive moral elements. However, other elements and some forms of surgical innovation *do* give rise to moral concern.

The first and perhaps most obvious concern is the threatened respect for a patient's *autonomy*. Respect for autonomy is not a mere ideal in health care; it is a professional obligation (Beauchamp & Childress, 2001). Autonomy, or self-determination, is expressed in the doctrine of informed consent. A patient's right to self-determination is in jeopardy when he or she is not presented with the complete information about the nature of the procedure (experimental versus accepted) and given the opportunity to elect or reject an offered treatment. Good clinical practice in surgery and the standard of professional practice dictates that every surgeon should present a patient with all the pertinent information about and alternatives to a suggested procedure, including the nonoperative treatment modalities. This becomes particularly stringent if the suggested procedure is experimental. Pertinent information needed to come to an informed decision is knowledge about the expected outcome and the risks and benefits of a certain procedure. If such information is unavailable, because the procedure has not yet been adequately evaluated, true informed consent and subsequent autonomous decision-making is hampered.

A *paternalistic* act occurs when decisions that are necessarily within the scope of patient preference and a duty to disclose are overridden by the physician. It seems apparent that the consideration of risks and benefits involved in a surgical procedure is necessarily a part of a patient's preference and should be readily disclosed by the treating surgeon. This is unfortunately not always a given in the case of surgical innovation. When risks and benefits are partly or largely unknown, as in innovative surgeries, they cannot be fully disclosed nor adequately considered. The authorization process would still be ethically acceptable as long as all factors are laid out and a patient is willing to voluntarily undergo a procedure with a (partly) unknown risk-benefit ratio. A possible scenario would be a desperate situation, where no other therapies are available and the surgeon and his patient agree on using an experimental procedure in a last effort to treat the patient, who would otherwise be facing certain worsening of symptoms or perhaps even demise. In a less dramatic situation, however, a surgeon may not feel as compelled to share every bit of information about an innovative procedure with a patient. In general, risk assessment should involve the patient as a decision-maker and, when the procedure is highly experimental, the insight of an IRB as well.

The principle of *nonmaleficence* dictates that a physician should refrain from causing harm to the patient and also includes obligations not to impose *risks* of harm. In cases of risk imposition, law and morality recognize a standard of due care that determines whether the agent that is causally responsible for the harm is legally or morally responsible as well. What constitutes harm in the case of surgical innovation can vary. When performing an experimental procedure of unproven utility, a surgeon exposes a patient to unknown risks. These risks can be of great magnitude (the ultimate being death) or of relatively small impact. Jones termed this practice "reckless experimentation," adding that it should always be condemned, regardless of estimated risks (Jones, 2006).

The principle of *beneficence* consists of three moral norms: (a) one ought to prevent evil or harm, (b) one ought to remove evil or harm, and (c) one ought to promote or do good. Applying these norms to surgical innovation leads to a multifold analysis. When no other therapy is available for a particular patient or diagnosis, performing an experimental procedure can be an act of beneficence when opposed to doing nothing. Also, striving to improve surgical care is an act of beneficence and is a trait of the virtuous surgeon. The good surgeon, as determined by most U.S. professional surgical societies, should always aim to better his or her practice and the profession as a whole. Promoting the well-being of future patients is a beneficent act. Failing to improve means becoming eventually outdated, leading to a situation where a surgeon can only offer obsolete and old-fashioned operations to patients. In essence, innovation is an intrinsic and vital part of surgery. Without it, there would be no progress. But progress is never linear; sometimes a few side steps are taken. Such side steps might be clinical trials, where a surgical technique is put to the test to establish its efficacy and safety. Or they might include monitoring the outcomes of a newly developed procedure clinically, perhaps not in a formal study but nonetheless via a model that is experimental in nature. Patients involved in these very side steps deserve adequate protection because the procedures are not of proven utility.

The principle of *justice* mandates that health care and (scarce) resources should be distributed evenly and fairly. In the context of research, it demands that research subjects be selected fairly and without putting undue pressure on one particular gender or social or racial group. If a medical experiment is formulated into a research protocol, which is subsequently submitted to an IRB for review, attention will be given to fair subject selection. IRBs have guidelines and formulas for even distribution among the various population denominators, to ensure a just selection system. When experimental surgeries are not submitted to IRBs and performed without protocol and without prior patient population determination, it is highly unlikely that patients will be selected randomly, fairly, or evenly across the general population. This may not only confound the scientific results of the informal study, but it also represents an unjust method of patient selection. Certain patient groups may be more heavily burdened, depending on the expected outcomes of the procedure.

When a surgeon presents an innovative procedure as an accepted therapy, the information she is giving is arguably *deceptive*. Unintentionally, the patient is given a false sense of security that the procedure he is undergoing is of proven utility, when in fact it is not. The surgeon in turn may subconsciously mislead herself into thinking she is doing the right thing for the patient by submitting him to an experimental procedure. The underlying assumption leading to this is, again, that new equals better, when in fact this has not yet been scientifically proven. This is usually done as a framing error, where a procedure is termed a *new treatment*. This situation is not unique to surgery; it occurs often in medicine as well. For example, the off-label use of FDA-approved drugs by physicians is in fact a clinical experiment presented as a validated treatment.

Another way of thinking about the self-deception a surgeon experiences is the existence of bias toward the innovative therapy. This is illustrated by a lack of equipoise.

Equipoise is the existence of true uncertainty about the effectiveness of therapeutic modalities, and it is the basis and prerequisite of any (randomized) clinical trial. If equipoise exists, it is considered ethical to randomize patients or healthy volunteers to test the hypothesis that the new therapy is better than the old one. If in the heart and mind of a surgeon bias exists toward an innovative procedure, true equipoise is absent. This is an added impediment for innovative procedures to find their way into a formal research protocol and through IRB review. Even if the effectiveness, safety, and long-term outcomes of the innovation are unknown, when the performing surgeon is biased toward its (supposed) merits, it will not be put to the test.

SAFETY AND EFFICACY ISSUES

MANY OF THE operations that are currently in use have never been formally tested in a rigorous scientific trial. They were originally introduced into clinical care as so many other procedures before and after them: as innovative therapies. As such, they were simply implemented in surgical practice without additional safeguards to protect the patients who underwent these experimental procedures. This has been and largely still is accepted and constitutes everyday surgical practice. Only when the implications of the procedure are enormous, and the risks and stakes are high (life and death issues, e.g., in the case of fetal surgery, heart surgery, and live liver graft transplantations), the surgical profession and the public alike are alerted about their introduction and rightfully demand that first studies be done to establish efficacy and safety (Lyerly, Cefalo, Socol, Fogarty, & Sugarman, 2001; Lyerly, Gates, Cefalo, & Sugarman, 2001; Lyerly & Mahowald 2001). Live donor liver graft transplantations, for example, have received a lot of attention from professionals and sometimes caused outrage (Cronin et al., 2001; Moreno, 2002). This was especially the case when two healthy donors died after donating a portion of their livers. Transplant surgeons such as Cronin complain that the true morbidity and mortality rate, let alone the overall efficacy of this innovation, are still largely unknown, while the procedure gains widespread use and popularity regardless.

The less high-profile innovative surgeries, however, escape this added scrutiny and eventually find their way into standard clinical care. After a while, the novelty wears off these innovations and they become established techniques, with or without scientific testing. While the *safety* of these procedures will eventually be established through the regular surgical mechanisms (i.e., morbidity and mortality conferences, case reports, etc.) and by way of malpractice suits if necessary, their true *effectiveness* may never be known if a randomized controlled clinical trial is never done. When put to the test, some of these much-hyped procedures may prove partially or completely ineffective, at times no better than a placebo (Starling et al., 2000). This has been shown in the case of internal mammary artery ligation for angina pectoris in the 1950s and, more recently, in an arthroscopic knee surgery trial (Moseley et al., 2002; Kolata, 2002). This latter trial is a perfect example of how a new procedure gains wide acceptance and is reimbursed by third-party payers even in the absence of strong scientific evidence. When the evidence was finally sought, it turned out that the procedure was no better than the sham surgery, the placebo.

THE POWER OF MONEY

THERE ARE SEVERAL reasons *why* surgical innovations are continually introduced into practice without prior formal scrutiny, and reimbursement is one of them. The cost of an experimental technique may not be covered by insurance companies, while the standard of care is. Modifying a procedure up to the point of making it highly experimental but still booking it as standard technique will (hopefully) ensure needed reimbursement. The financial incentives to study new drugs (heavily sponsored by pharmaceutical companies) are absent in surgery; this significantly reduces the external entrepreneurial push to innovate within the clinical trial model. Unless a drug or medical device is involved, there is no financial gain for companies to be made; hence the surgical community has a hard time finding the money to conduct clinical trials involving an experimental procedure alone. These financial disincentives to innovate within the scientific model are considerable and a formidable obstacle to change.

WHAT'S IN A NAME: IDENTIFYING EXPERIMENTAL INNOVATIONS

HOW IS IT possible that surgical innovation evades the scrutiny of existing safeguards for human subject research? One reason is that surgeons themselves do not regard their modifications and innovations as clinical research (Reitsma & Moreno, 2003). Innovations are therefore not assessed within a formal research protocol, and are not being submitted for IRB review before implementation of the procedure. Invisible to IRBs, innovations go forward without external oversight. Innovations are not readily defined as research especially if they constitute incremental modifications. Also, standard of care is more difficult to define in the surgical domain because every surgeon may have a preferred style of performing the same procedure.

The first and foremost problem for the effective oversight of surgical innovations is therefore their vague definition. To aid in the identification and definition of research-like innovations, using certain criteria may be helpful. Sometimes the nature of the innovations is such that they become quite experimental and necessarily enter the realm of research activities. Criteria that would make an innovation a research activity have been discussed by several experts on the matter and have been narrowed down to a few common denominators. Important criteria distinguishing incremental improvements from experimental innovations are:

1. intent (if the surgeon plans to perform an innovation with the intent of testing a hunch, informal hypothesis, or theory about it),

2. extent of departure from standard of care (if significantly different from currently accepted procedure),

3. outcomes (risks and benefits are largely unknown or not adequately described in international professional literature), and

4. extent of risks involved (greater perceived risk indicates greater need for scientific scrutiny). (Criteria adapted with permission from Reitsma & Moreno, 2006.)

CONCLUSION

APPLYING STANDARDS TO assess surgical innovations may aide surgeons in identifying an innovative technique needing to follow the research track. The exact structure of this research track and whether it should take the formal IRB route or follow some internal oversight model are issues about which surgeons should reach consensus. Some surgeons feel that the surgical community should be allowed to maintain some degree of professional autonomy in overseeing innovation, thereby bypassing the IRB model in certain cases. If and when this is ethically and scientifically acceptable is still open for debate. It will be fascinating to follow the discourse in the professional literature. The end of an era of unfettered innovating may very well be in sight, although the implementation of new, more applicable, and perhaps more stringent guidelines for introducing surgical innovations will take time, effort and buy-in from all relevant parties—surgeons, patients, policy makers, journal editors, and others—to become a reality.

REFERENCES

Beauchamp T. L., & Childress, J. F. (2001). *Principles of biomedical ethics* (5th ed.). New York: Oxford University Press.

Beecher, H. K. (1961). Surgery as placebo. A quantitative study of bias. *Journal of the American Medical Association, 176,* 1102–1107.

Biffl, W. L., Spain, D. A., Reitsma, A. M., Minter, R. M., Upperman, J., Wilson, M., et al. (2008). Responsible development and application of surgical innovations: A position statement of the Society of University Surgeons. *Journal of the American College of Surgeons, 206*(3), 1204–1209.

Bunker, J. P., Hinkley, D., & McDermott, W. V. (1978). Surgical innovation and its evaluation. *Science, 200*(4344), 937–941.

Casler, J. D. (2003). Clinical use of new technologies without scientific studies. *Archives of Otolaryngoly and Head and Neck Surgery, 129*(6), 674–677.

Code of Federal Regulations. (2005). Title 45, Public Welfare, Department of Health and Human Services. Part 46: Protection of Human Subjects.

45 CFR 46. Retrieved October 30, 2008, from http://www.hhs.gov/ohrp/ humansubjects/guidance/45cfr46.htm

Cronin, D. C., Millis, J. M., & Siegler, M. (2001). Transplantation of liver grafts from living donors into adults—too much, too soon. *New England Journal of Medicine, 344*(21), 1633–1637.

Frader, J. E., & Caniano, D. A. (1998). Research and innovation in surgery. In L. B. McCullough, J. W. Jones, & B. A. Brody (Eds.), *Surgical ethics* (pp. 216–241). New York: Oxford University Press.

Frader, J. E., & Flanagan-Klygis, E. (2001). Innovation and research in pediatric surgery. *Seminars in Pediatric Surgery, 10*(4), 198–203.

Jarvik, J. G., & Deyo, R. A. (2000). Cementing the evidence: Time for a randomized trial of vertebroplasty. *American Journal of Neuroradiology, 21*(8), 1373–1374.

Jones, J. W. (2000). Ethics of rapid surgical technological advancement. *Annals of Thoracic Surgery, 69*(3), 676–677.

Jones, J. W. (2006). The surgeon's autonomy: Defining limits in therapeutic decision making. In A. M. Reitsma & J. D. Moreno (Eds.), *Ethical guidelines for innovative surgery* (pp. 75–92). Hagerstown, MD: University Publishing Group.

Jones, R. S., & Richards, K. (2003). Office of evidence-based surgery. Charts course for improved system of care. *Bulletin of the American College of Surgeons, 88*(4), 11–21.

Josefson, D. (2000, December 16) University must tell patients that they were research "guinea pigs." *British Medical Journal, 321*(7275), 1487A.

Kolata, G. (2002, July 11). Arthritis surgery in ailing knees is cited as sham. *New York Times, Health.* Retrieved October 30, 2008, from http://query. nytimes.com/gst/fullpage.html?res=9E02E0D71230F932A25754C0A9649 C8B63&sec=&spon=&pagewanted=2

Kornetsky, S. (2001). *Guidelines, concepts and procedures for differentiating between research and innovative therapy* [Internal memo]. Boston, MA: Children's Hospital Boston.

Love, J. W. (1975). Drugs and operations. Some important differences. *Journal of the American Medical Association, 232*(1), 37–38.

Lyerly, A. D., Cefalo, R. C., Socol, M., Fogarty, L., & Sugarman, J. (2001). Attitudes of maternal-fetal specialists concerning maternal-fetal surgery. *American Journal of Obstetrics and Gynecology, 185*(5), 1052–1058.

Lyerly, A. D., Gates, E. A., Cefalo, R. C., & Sugarman, J. (2001). Toward the ethical evaluation and use of maternal-fetal surgery. *Obstetrics and Gynecology, 98*(4), 689–697.

Lyerly, A. D., & Mahowald, M. B. (2001). Maternal-fetal surgery: The fallacy of abstraction and the problem of equipoise. *Health Care Analysis, 9*, 151–165.

Margo, C. E. (2001). When is surgery research? Towards an operational definition of human research. *Journal of Medical Ethics, 27*(1), 40–43.

McKneally, M. F. (1999). Ethical problems in surgery: Innovation leading to unforeseen complications. *World Journal of Surgery, 23*(8), 786–788.

McKneally, M. F., & Kornetsky, S. (2003, October). *Protecting participants in surgical innovation: Ideas and experiments from Canada and the US.* Presented at the American Society for Bioethics and Humanities/Canadian Bioethics Society in Montreal, Canada, October 23–26.

Moore, F. D. (2000). Ethical problems special to surgery: Surgical teaching, surgical innovation, and the surgeon in managed care. *Archives of Surgery, 135*(1), 14–16.

Moreno, J. D. (2002). *Donation disaster: A high price for the gift of life.* abcNews.com. Retrieved January 25, 2002, from http://abcnews.go.com/Health/story?id=116999&page=1

Moseley, J. B., O'Malley, K., Petersen, N. J., Menke, T. J., Brody, B. A., Kuykendall, D. H., et al. (2002). A controlled trial of arthroscopic surgery for osteoarthritis of the knee. *New England Journal of Medicine, 347*(2), 81–88.

Petrelli, N. J. (2002). Clinical trials are mandatory for improving surgical cancer care. *Journal of the American Medical Association, 287*(3), 377–378.

Qualms about innovative surgery. (1985). *Lancet, 1*(8421), 149.

Reitsma, A. M., & Moreno, J. D. (2002). Ethical regulations for innovative surgery: The last frontier? *Journal of the American College of Surgeons, 194*(6), 792–801.

Reitsma, A. M., & Moreno, J. D. (2003). Surgical research, an elusive entity. *American Journal of Bioethics, 3*(4), 52–53.

Reitsma, A. M., & Moreno, J. D. (2005). The ethics of innovative surgery: US surgeons' definitions, knowledge and attitudes. *Journal of the American College of Surgeons, 200*(1), 103–110.

Reitsma A. M., & Moreno, J. D. (Eds.). (2006). *Ethical guidelines for innovative surgery.* Hagerstown: MD: University Publishing Group.

Roy, D. J., Black P., & McPeek, B. (1986). Ethical principles in surgical research. In H. Troidl, W. O. Spitzer, B. McPeek, & D. S. Mulder (Eds.), *Principles and practice of research: Strategies for surgical investigators.* New York: Springer-Verlag.

Starling, R. C., McCarthy, P. M., Buda, T., Wong, J., Goormastic, M., Smedira, N. G., et al. (2000). Results of partial left ventriculectomy for dilated cardiomyopathy: Hemodynamic, clinical and echocardiographic observations. *Journal of the American College of Cardiology, 36*(7), 2098–2103.

Strasberg, S. M., & Ludbrook, P. A. (2003). Who oversees innovative practice? Is there a structure that meets the monitoring needs of new techniques? *Journal of the American College of Surgeons, 196*(6), 938–948.

Ward, C. M. (1994). Surgical research, experimentation and innovation. *British Journal of Plastic Surgery, 47*(2), 90–94.

Waring, G. O., III. (1999). A cautionary tale of innovation in refractive surgery. *Archives of Ophthalmology, 117*(8), 1069–1073.

21

Unique Aspects of Informed Consent in Emergency Research

Jill M. Baren

RESEARCH ON CRITICALLY ill or injured patients is logistically difficult but must proceed in order to demonstrate the safety and effectiveness of therapies that have the potential to decrease morbidity and mortality (Bircher, 2003). Obtaining prospective informed consent is the standard by which all human research should be conducted; however, when patients are incapacitated secondary to critical illness or injury, there must be a mechanism for such patients to potentially benefit from experimental therapies while maintaining the same if not greater protection of their rights as research subjects.

In 1996, federal guidelines, harmonized between the Food and Drug Administration (FDA) and the Department of Health and Human Services (DHHS), were instituted to permit such research to take place under emergency circumstances (Department of Health and Human Services [DHHS], 1996; "Protection of Human Subjects," 1996). Known as the Final Rule, these regulations permit selected research to proceed with a waiver of informed consent (WIC) or emergency exception from informed consent (EFIC). For the purpose of this chapter, the terms WIC and EFIC will be used interchangeably and represent the same concept of foregoing prospective informed consent. The regulations are explicit in outlining the conditions under which emergency research may proceed and in requiring special protections for patients who are incapacitated with a life-threatening condition.

HISTORICAL CONTEXT

THE *BELMONT REPORT* issued in 1979 delineated ethical standards by which research involving human subjects should abide (Belmont Report, 1979). Among the principles of beneficence, justice, and respect for persons, the latter specifies that individuals ought to be treated as autonomous agents, and that those with diminished autonomy should be additionally protected (Morris, 2005). These so-called vulnerable individuals are traditionally represented by the following populations: prisoners, children, and pregnant women/fetuses/neonates (Baren & Fish, 2005). The interpretation of vulnerable populations, however, historically excluded patients stricken with sudden, acute, emergent illness or injury—such as trauma, stroke, or cardiac arrest—and who therefore were similarly unable to exercise their autonomy.

To address this particular vulnerability, the FDA in 1981 established rules (FDA, 1981) providing guidance by which clinical research involving these patients should be ethically conducted (FDA, 1981). The FDA outlined that (a) the subject population must be in a life-threatening situation, (b) informed consent cannot be obtained from the patient, (c) time is not sufficient to obtain consent from a surrogate, and (d) no alternative therapy is available to provide an equal or greater likelihood of saving the subject's life (Bateman, Meyers, Schumacher, Mangla, & Pile-Spellman, 2003; Bircher, 2003). Researchers investigating emergent conditions, however, found many problems with the FDA guidelines. Specifically, the FDA rules were written so as to favor the one-time, so-called compassionate use of an emergent therapy rather than requiring a placebo-controlled clinical trial (Bateman et al., 2003). Furthermore, condition (d) at face value made investigational trials nearly impossible, as an experimental therapy would not need to be tested if it were already known to be of equal or better value when compared to standard therapy.

To complicate matters, DHHS through the National Institutes of Health (NIH) issued their own set of guidelines addressing this particular issue in 1981, invoking the term *Waiver of Informed Consent* (DHHS, 1981). Though similar in many ways to the FDA rules, the DHHS/NIH guidelines required a distinct set of criteria for research to proceed with a waiver. DHHS/NIH rules proposed that (a) the research entail minimal risk (with minimal risk defined as the risk associated with daily life or a routine physical), (b) the waiver does not adversely affect patient rights and welfare, (c) the research could not be done without a waiver, and

(d) subjects will be informed after their participation (Bateman et al., 2003; Bircher, 2003). As was clear to investigators involved with emergent and critical research, the major problem posed by DHHS/NIH rules was the definition of minimal risk, which essentially precluded all emergency-related research because death was always considered a potential risk.

In an attempt to sidestep these conflicting rules and often impracticable conditions, throughout 1979–1991 the concept of deferred consent, rather than waiver or exception from consent, was successfully used by investigators to attain institutional review board (IRB) approval (Abramson & Safar, 1990). Ultimately, however, the concept of deferred consent was determined by the Office for Protection from Research Risks (OPRR) in 1993 to be the same as a waiver of consent and therefore subject to DHHS/NIH rules (Bateman et al., 2003; Bircher, 2003). The OPRR also concurrently imposed a stricter interpretation of the standard for minimal incremental risk in human subjects research, such that all research unable to attain patient informed consent was essentially shut down (Bircher, 2003). The release of this ruling in a report by OPRR thus began a 3-year moratorium on all acute and critical care research foregoing prospective informed consent in the United States (Biros, Fish, & Lewis, 1999).

IMPETUS FOR THE CREATION OF THE FINAL RULE

PRIOR TO THE creation of the current research regulations governing emergency research (known as the Final Rule) in 1996, the FDA and DHHS/NIH guidelines failed to explicitly address how emergency-related research would be allowed to take place. Investigators as well as IRBs were left without a guide as to how any emergency research foregoing prospective informed consent could be sanctioned. With the moratorium as a great cause for concern, activism on the part of a broad community of researchers resulted in the formation of the Coalition of Acute Resuscitation and Critical Care Researchers. The Coalition held a Consensus Conference in 1995, and provided the impetus for the FDA and DHHS to amend their guidelines (Bircher, 2003; Biros, Runge, Lewis, & Doherty, 1998). Following a period of public comment upon the release of consensus recommendations, additional professional association meetings dedicated to this issue were held, and the Final Rule was released in 1996 (Biros et al., 1998; DHHS, 1996; "Protection of Human Subjects," 1996).

PROVISIONS OF THE FINAL RULE

AMONG THE MANY important changes codified in the Final Rule, it is important to note first that the Final Rule decisively unified the formerly disparate DHHS and FDA guidelines. As ethical justification for foregoing prospective informed consent, the Final Rule implies that because patients in acute and critical condition are incapable of exercising their autonomy, a best interest standard is undertaken on the part of the investigator such that the patient is assumed to desire the preservation of his or her life (Biros et al., 1999). Nonetheless, the Final Rule stipulates that the investigator must make every effort to attain proxy consent during the therapeutic window. In these terms, the Final Rule claims not to violate the right of research subjects' autonomy as articulated in the *Belmont Report* (Belmont Report, 1979). Additionally, the broad language in the Final Rule permits the use of placebo in addition to standard therapy in emergency medical conditions (DHHS, 1996; "Protection of Human Subjects," 1996).

Another important change required by the Final Rule is that the research team must perform so-called community consultation, whereby members of the community from which subjects in the study will likely arise are allowed to voice input prior to beginning the trial. Although community opposition does not automatically preclude a study from taking place, it is within the IRB's discretion to suggest that investigators redesign a protocol. Furthermore, the Final Rule also requires investigators to perform public notification of a planned trial in the forms of prestudy, ongoing, and poststudy public disclosures. In keeping with respect for local community norms, the Final Rule notes that its regulations are preempted by state law that may prohibit any research that seeks EFIC. The Final Rule also states that there must be ongoing review by an independent investigational data monitoring committee (DMC) to assure that investigators abide by the aforementioned stipulations (DHHS, 1996; "Protection of Human Subjects," 1996).

CURRENT USE OF THE FINAL RULE

DESPITE THE IMPROVEMENTS and revisions introduced into the conduct of emergency research by the Final Rule, emergency research studies that attempt to use EFIC continue to be very difficult to perform. In the 12 years since the passage of the Final Rule, research using EFIC has been sparse (Schmidt, Lewis, & Richardson, 2005). Both investigators and IRBs note confusion about and lack of specific guidance within the regulations, specifically with regard to satisfactorily demonstrating that one has met the requirements of community consultation and public disclosure. Other concerns include the continued lack of a meaningful threshold for permissible risk as well as a failure to articulate a moral basis for community consultation (McRae & Weijer, 2003).

Specifically with regard to the requirement for community consultation, both investigators and the regulatory community have found it difficult to define the target community of interest and the community at large (Biros et al., 1999). In studies using EFIC, the most common form of community consultation has been community meetings, although a myriad of other approaches have also been utilized (Baren & Biros, 2007). The most common form of public disclosure has been newspaper advertisements about a planned trial. Press releases, newspaper articles, and community meetings have similarly been utilized. The requirements of community consultation and public disclosure have proven to be prohibitively expensive for some investigators; one study was prematurely terminated secondary to the slow enrollment of subjects and the expensive costs of community consultation (Baren & Biros, 2007).

There exists strong skepticism over the effectiveness of community consultation techniques and whether they can truly define a community's values (Baren & Biros, 2007). Additionally, there exists no consensus on how information gathered from community consultations and public disclosure should be used by the IRB (Biros et al., 1998; Ernst & Fish, 2005; Mosesso & Cone, 2005). And, finally, there is little to no substantive evaluation of the community consultation and public disclosure efforts associated with a trial; thus there is no foundation on which future investigators may learn effectively from prior efforts (Baren & Biros, 2007).

KEY ISSUES

ETHICAL ACCEPTABILITY OF THE FINAL RULE

THREE GENERAL CRITICISMS of the conduct of research without informed consent have been well articulated by ethicists and scientists alike (Fost, 1998): (a) Consent is an absolute principle, (b) the standard for consent in research should be higher than that required for standard clinical care, and (c) patients would not want to be enrolled into a clinical trial without their consent, thus leaving no justification for giving a placebo without consent. These are compelling arguments that deserve careful consideration.

Informed consent is a major mechanism for protecting human subjects but is neither necessary nor sufficient for ethically responsible research. The use of EFIC is akin to the concept of presumed consent invoked frequently in clinical emergency situations. There is large public support for providing emergency treatment without consent using the presumption that patients would consent if they could. It is understood that this presumption is not absolute assurance that the patient would consent; rather it is based on the likelihood that a so-called reasonable person would be highly likely to consent. Unavoidably in such a setting, some patients would be treated against their wishes, but the decision to err on the side of treatment is the lesser of two evils. Presumed consent authorizes a physician to use his/her best judgment and in such situations makes an educated guess as to what the patient's autonomous wishes might be.

Many believe that the regulatory infrastructure of a clinical trial provides more protection to a patient than that received in the course of routine clinical care during which a given physician might exercise considerable liberty in choosing therapies for patients, in some cases, perhaps experimental therapies. This practice may be more common in emergency and critical care settings where physicians frequently make judgments involving unconscious patients in need of urgent, life-saving interventions. The process of conducting research on critically ill or injured patients, with its attendant need for IRB approval, justification of sample size and study design, minimization of subject risk, continuing IRB review, and dissemination of results through the peer review process reduces the potential for harm compared to unregulated use of innovative or experimental therapies outside the research process. EFIC requires even greater protections for subjects compared to those offered in a usual clinical trial in the form of community consultation, public notification and disclosure, FDA review, and independent data safety monitoring requirements.

Although not extensive, the literature contains some empirical data indicating that the use of EFIC can be consistent with the preferences of many potential research subjects (Biros, 2005; McClure et al., 2003). Several investigators with experience conducting emergency research using EFIC have published convincing evidence that the majority of families and patients are in agreement with what was done and would have provided prospective informed consent had it been feasible to have such a discussion prior to enrolling the patient (Abramson & Safar, 1990; Sloan et al., 1999). Giving people the opportunity to receive an experimental therapy that holds the prospect of direct benefit seems to be consistent with what patients and families prefer, and foregoing prospective informed consent does not seem to be morally problematic in these circumstances.

Use of Placebo

USE OF PLACEBO in emergency research using EFIC has been labeled *nontreatment*, which has a negative connotation. Given that no satisfactory or proven treatments are known to exist for a large number of critical illnesses, injuries, and emergent conditions, the use of placebo should be considered to be no more harmful (or helpful) than an experimental treatment, provided a trial is designed properly and there is true clinical equipoise (Fost, 1998).

CONCLUSION

EMERGENCY RESEARCH MUST take place so that potentially effective therapies can be proven for use in clinical settings where only the most realistic estimates of human subject risk and benefit can be demonstrated; otherwise there is a societal risk that advances in care will be based on consensus as opposed to the best information. The effect of EFIC on the advancement of science within the emergency research community remains to be seen. There is mounting evidence that additional revisions to the Final Rule are needed to address barriers identified during implementation of the rule and from research on the rule itself (Baren & Biros, 2007; Biros, 2005; Mosesso & Cone, 2005; Schmidt et al., 2005). If applied conscientiously, the use of EFIC in emergency research trials is ethically justifiable and likely to be ethically acceptable to those who conduct, regulate, or participate in such research.

REFERENCES

Abramson, N. S., & Safar, P. (1990). Deferred consent: Use in clinical resuscitation research. Brain Resuscitation Clinical Trial II Study Group. *Annals of Emergency Medicine, 19*(7), 781–784.

Baren, J. M., & Biros, M. H. (2007). The research on community consultation: An annotated bibliography. *Academic Emergency Medicine, 14*(4), 346–352.

Baren, J. M., & Fish, S. (2005). Resuscitation research involving vulnerable populations: Are additional protections needed for emergency exception from informed consent? *Academic Emergency Medicine, 12*(11), 1071–1077.

Bateman, B. T., Meyers, P. M., Schumacher, H. C., Mangla, S., & Pile-Spellman, J. (2003). Conducting stroke research with an exception from the requirement for informed consent. *Stroke, 34*, 1317–1323.

Belmont report. (1979). Retrieved December 5, 2005, from http://www.hhs.gov/ohrp/humansubjects/guidance/45cfr46.htm

Bircher, N. G. (2003). Resuscitation research and consent: Ethical and practical issues. *Critical Care Medicine, 31*(Suppl. 5), S379–S384.

Biros, M. H. (2005). The ethical conduct of resuscitation research: Setting the stage for change. *Academic Emergency Medicine, 12*(11), 1015–1016.

Biros, M. H., Fish, S. S., & Lewis, R. J. (1999). Implementing the Food and Drug Administration's Final Rule for waiver of informed consent in certain emergency research circumstances. *Academic Emergency Medicine, 6*(12), 1272–1282.

Biros, M. H., Runge, J. W., Lewis, R. J., & Doherty, C. (1998). Emergency medicine and the development of the Food and Drug Administration's Final Rule on informed consent and waiver of informed consent in emergency research circumstances. *Academic Emergency Medicine, 5*(4), 359–368.

Department of Health and Human Services (DHHS), 45 CFR § 46.116 (1981).

Department of Health and Human Services (DHHS). (1996). Protection of human subjects; informed consent and waiver of consent requirements in certain emergency research; final rules. (Codified at 21 CFR.50, et al, 45 CFR.46). *Federal Register, 61*(192), 51500–51533.

Ernst, A. A., & Fish, S. S. (2005). Exception from informed consent: Viewpoint of institutional review boards—balancing risks to subjects, community consultation, and future directions. *Academic Emergency Medicine, 12*(11), 1050–1055.

Food and Drug Administration (FDA), 21 CFR § 50.23 (1981).

Fost, N. (1998). Waived consent for emergency research. *American Journal of Law and Medicine, 24*(2–3), 163–183.

McClure, K. B., DeIorio, N. M., Gunnels, M. D., Ochsner, M. J., Biros, M. H., & Schmidt, T. A. (2003). Attitudes of emergency department patients and visitors regarding emergency exception from informed consent in resuscitation research, community consultation, and public notification. *Academic Emergency Medicine, 10*(4), 352–359.

McRae, A. D., & Weijer, C. (2002). Lessons from everyday lives: A moral justification for acute care research. *Critical Care Medicine, 30*(5), 1146–1151.

McRae, A. D., & Weijer, C. (2003). Waiver of consent for emergency research. *Annals of Emergency Medicine, 42*(4), 550–564.

Morris, M. C. (2005). An ethical analysis of exception from informed consent regulations. *Academic Emergency Medicine, 12*(11), 1113–1119.

Mosesso, V. N., & Cone, D. C. (2005). Using the exception from informed consent regulations in research. *Academic Emergency Medicine, 12*(11), 1031–1039.

Protection of human subjects; informed consent—FDA. Final Rule. (1996). *Federal Register, 61*(192), 51498–51533.

Schmidt, T. A., Lewis, R. J., & Richardson, L. D. (2005). Current status of research on the federal guidelines for performing research using an exception from informed consent. *Academic Emergency Medicine, 12*(11), 1022–1026.

Sloan, E. P., Koenigsberg, M., Houghton, J., Gens, D., Cipolle, M., Runge, J., et al. (1999). The informed consent process and the use of the exception to informed consent in the clinical trial of diaspirin cross-linked hemoglobin (DCLHb) in severe traumatic hemorrhagic shock. *Academic Emergency Medicine, 6*(12), 1203–1209.

22

The Ethics of Inclusion and Exclusion in Clinical Trials: Race, Sex, and Age

DIANA ZUCKERMAN

FOR WHITES ONLY is an offensive phrase from another era. Whether applied to schools, water fountains, restaurants, or rest rooms, it is completely unacceptable in the United States today. But more than 40 years after the civil rights demonstrations that shook America, a different kind of racial exclusion is pervasive, unreported, and unnoticed: medical products that are sold to everyone but are tested on Whites only.

When you see prescription medication advertised on television, it does not tell you whether that medicine is for Whites only. When a physician prescribes the medication, he or she does not say that the medication was studied primarily on White patients and therefore is not proven safe or effective for any other racial or ethnic group. Each medication has a label that describes the risks and benefits—in mind-numbing and often microscopic detail—but these labels fail to mention if the product was studied on diverse populations and whether either the risks or benefits are more likely for some racial and ethnic groups compared to others.

Federal law requires the U.S. Department of Health and Human Services to include people representing diverse racial and ethnic backgrounds in research studies (Department of Health and Human Services [DHHS], 1993; DHHS, 1997a). There are many agencies within the department that abide by this law: for example, studies conducted by or funded by the Centers for Disease Control and Prevention (CDC), the Administration on Children, Youth and Families, the Substance Abuse and Mental Health Administration, or any of the institutes comprising the National Institutes of Health (NIH) are required to include diverse populations when the research is relevant to those populations. The one health agency exempted from these requirements is the Food and Drug Administration (FDA), which is the federal agency responsible for ensuring the safety of packaged food and the safety and effectiveness of prescription drugs, medical devices, vaccines, and other biologics.

Since the FDA regulates products responsible for 25% of the U.S. economy, and has the responsibility of protecting all Americans, excluding the FDA from diversity requirements is not logical. There is an explanation, however: unlike other federal health agencies, the FDA relies on studies conducted by and paid for by the private sector, rather than by taxpayers (DHHS, 2007). Therefore, the justification is that since private companies are paying for and conducting the studies, the federal government should not tell them what to do.

This explanation is somewhat disingenuous. Although the FDA generally offers written guidance to industry about the studies they believe should be conducted, rather than requirements, companies that make medical products understand that their products are more likely to be approved by the FDA if they conduct the studies as the FDA suggests. If the FDA only approved products when the studies provided the information that the FDA asked for in their guidance documents, companies would take the guidance more seriously. Unfortunately, the FDA's official guidance regarding diversity in clinical trials does not even urge or suggest that companies include substantial numbers of people representing specific racial or ethnic backgrounds in their studies. Instead, the guidance merely suggests how the companies should categorize racial and ethnic groups and urges them to evaluate racial and ethnic groups separately (DHHS, 2005). That means that a company could abide by the FDA guidance by excluding people of specific racial or ethnic backgrounds or by including just a few such people as long as they are correctly categorized and separately analyzed—even if the number is too small to provide meaningful information.

245

*The Ethics of
Inclusion and
Exclusion in
Clinical Trials:
Race, Sex, and Age*

The lack of people from diverse racial or ethnic backgrounds in clinical trials reviewed by the FDA is part of a larger problem that faces the FDA: making sure that medical products are safe and effective for the vast majority of people who are likely to use them. Generally, medical products are approved after being tested on relatively small numbers of mostly young, healthy, White men but then are used by men and women of a wide range of ages and races, some of whom are in fair or poor medical condition and many of whom are taking numerous other medications at the same time. These medical products may also be taken by children, even if no studies have proven their safety or effectiveness for children. Prior to 1989, most clinical trials excluded children or the elderly, and prior to 1993, most clinical trials excluded women (DHHS, 1995).

RACIAL DISPARITIES

I T I S W E L L - E S T A B L I S H E D that there are health disparities between Whites and other minority groups in the United States, for a wide range of diseases and causes of death, including infant mortality, heart disease, and certain cancers. Much of those disparities are due to health care inequities; Whites tend to have better health insurance coverage and more money to spend on health care, and that means better access to better doctors. Discrimination within the health care system has been found to also favor Whites (Council on Ethical and Judicial Affairs, 1990), stress may increase health risks for Blacks (Baum, Garofalo, & Yali, 1999), and there are eating habits and cultural influences that could help explain these disparities (Kieffer et al., 2004; Shankar et al., 2007). So it is perhaps not surprising that the lack of diversity in clinical trials has rarely been blamed. But there is growing evidence that it is likely to be at least one of the causes of health disparities.

The human genome project tells us that what we think of as racial groups are culturally rather than biologically defined. The genetic differences between various racial or ethnic groups are very minor, and skin color, hair, and other superficial features that are associated with what is called race are very unlikely to affect physiological responses to a medical treatment. However, there are health differences between racial and ethnic groups that can't be explained by access to medical care or types of medical care, and there are documented racial and ethnic differences in how people respond to some medical products. Research indicates that there are genetic differences that tend to vary across race that are responsible for variations in the safety and effectiveness of certain classes of drugs, such as beta blockers and angiotensin-converting enzyme (ACE) inhibitors (Burroughs, Maxey, & Levy, 2002). What we do not know is how often this happens, exactly which medical products are involved, and what impact this has on the health of people representing different racial or ethnic groups.

SCIENTIFIC SUPPORT FOR DIVERSITY IN CLINICAL TRIALS

POLYMORPHISMS ARE NATURALLY occurring variants in genes and the products they encode, such as enzymes. These variants occur in all human genes, and some vary significantly according to race and affect how drugs are metabolized, absorbed, or excreted (Burroughs et al., 2002). As a result of these variations, some classes of drugs will be safer or more effective for some individuals than others, resulting in different doses or even the need to avoid certain drugs. For example, genetic traits that result in the poor metabolism of a drug can result in an overdose for a susceptible individual. Racial and ethnic categories are imprecise substitute measures that can help predict which individuals are likely to benefit more from a specific drug and which are likely to benefit less (Burroughs et al., 2002). Age and sex also affect drug response, and so can health habits and environmental factors such as smoking, alcohol, drug use, and climate. However, genetic factors are of particular importance (Burroughs et al., 2002).

Recent studies on breast cancer illustrate the practical implications of genetic variations for African American women. It has long been known that African American women are less likely to be diagnosed with breast cancer but more likely to die from the disease. Experts assumed that the higher death rate was due to later diagnosis or inadequate health care, but more recent research indicated that these racial disparities were maintained even for women diagnosed at the same time and receiving similar treatment (Field et al., 2005). In 2007, research indicated that African American women are more likely to have estrogen-receptor negative breast cancer, a type of breast cancer that is not responsive to tamoxifen or other hormones that are frequently used for breast cancer treatment (Li, Malone, & Daling, 2002). If African American women had been studied separately in clinical trials for hormone treatment when these products were first reviewed by the FDA, it would have been obvious years earlier that there was a racial difference in response to treatment. However, the lack of diversity in clinical trials delayed that finding.

African Americans have higher rates of heart disease and are more likely to die from heart disease than Whites, and this situation might also be related to lack of diversity in clinical trials. ACE inhibitors, often the first choice of drug therapy for heart failure, are more effective

247

*The Ethics of
Inclusion in
Exclusion in
Clinical Trials:
Race, Sex, and Age*

for Whites, for example, according to large-scale clinical trials suggesting ACE inhibitors alone "may not represent ideal therapy" for African Americans (Durand, 2004, p. 42).

In response to the findings regarding ACE inhibitors, the FDA approved a prescription drug for heart failure patients, BiDil, for African Americans, based on its greater success for that specific group compared to White patients (Sankar & Kahn, 2005). This is the first time that a drug was approved specifically for African American patients, and although this may be progress, it does not provide the essential information needed regarding the safety and effectiveness of thousands of other medical products that were approved for all patients despite lack of evidence regarding safety and effectiveness for African Americans or other people of color or specific ethnic groups. In fact, it could be argued that it is inadequate to specify that a specific treatment is more effective for African Americans without also specifying which other treatments are not or might not be effective for that minority group or other people of specific racial or ethnic backgrounds.

Genetic variations may affect disease pathways that may have a major impact on a drug's effectiveness on individuals. For example, only 5%–7% of Chinese people have the e4 polymorphism, which is a major risk factor for Alzheimer's disease, compared to 10% in other Asian and American Indian groups, and 20%–30% in African Americans and Africans (Burroughs et al., 2002). This polymorphism makes tacrine, a drug for Alzheimer's disease, less effective, and also makes the patient more likely to suffer from memory loss as an adverse reaction to lorazepam (Burroughs et al., 2002).

Polymorphism also creates variations in acetylation, resulting in people who acetylate slowly or those who acetylate quickly. Burroughs et al. (2002) found that 52%–62% of Whites are slow acetylators compared to 7%–34% of Chinese and Japanese populations. This may affect specific drug therapies, such as desipramine, an antidepressant, and perphenazine, an antipsychotic. Indeed, many Asians may have a weaker response to antidepressants because they may be slow metabolizers of the enzyme cytochrome P4502D6 (CYP4502D6). Similarly, The Cancer Institute in Singapore noted differences in Whites and Asians in response to particular cancer drugs (Wang, 2002). Beta-adrenergic receptors make a person less sensitive to beta blockers for asthmatics (Burroughs et al., 2002). In addition, Puerto Ricans and Mexicans with asthma were shown to differ from each other in responsiveness to another asthma drug, albuterol (Choudhry et al., 2005). However, that information is not listed on the medication's label.

As previously noted, the human genome project has made it clear that the popular definition of race is not supported by genetic differences. That makes race difficult to precisely define. Multiracial backgrounds and the existence of people who are unsure of their racial or ethnic background make this issue even more complex. For example, if a medication is less safe or effective for someone with East Asian descent, what is the likely outcome for someone who is a mixture of East Asian and other ethnicities?

Several years ago, the FDA reviewed the extent to which racial and ethnic differences were specified in clinical trials for new molecular entities (Evelyn et al., 2001a). A retrospective review of 185 approved new molecular entities was completed in 2001, based on approvals between 1995 and 1999 that involved data on 493,347 people enrolled in 2,581 clinical trials. Race could only be ascertained in 53% of the study participants; no race was specified in the other 47%. Of those that specified race, 83% were White; 8% were Black; 1% were Asian, Pacific Islander or Native Hawaiian; 3% were Hispanic/Latino; and less than 1% were American Indian or Alaskan Native. Studies conducted outside the United States contributed to the underrepresentation of people of diverse racial or ethnic backgrounds. However, rates for Hispanic/Latino participation were substantially below their representation levels in the United States even in the studies conducted in the United States.

The researchers also evaluated whether information about race was included in the product label, which is the main source of information to physicians and patients about a product's safety and effectiveness. Labeling for 84 of the 185 products tested (45%) included some type of statement about race, and only 15 products (8%) noted differences due to race, primarily in pharmacokinetics, followed by efficacy and safety. Only one label recommended a change in dosage based on racial differences; that was to increase the dosage of a hypertensive drug for Blacks. Overall, 10 products were noted to differ for Blacks, 1 for Hispanics/Latinos, and 5 for Asians.

INCLUDING WOMEN IN CLINICAL TRIALS

FOR MUCH OF the 20th century, women were typically excluded from clinical trials. One reason was that researchers assumed that a woman's hormonal cycle could influence the outcome of studies. In addition, women of child-bearing age could become pregnant, and would therefore need to be excluded from an ongoing study. Liability concerns also were raised because medical products tested in clinical trials could potentially harm offspring. These exclusionary policies were meant to protect women and children but resulted in the lack of information about the safety and effectiveness of medications for half of the population (Mastroianni, Faden, & Federman, 1994).

249

*The Ethics of
Inclusion and
Exclusion in
Clinical Trials:
Race, Sex, and Age*

It was only 15 years ago that the federal government required women to be included in clinical trials. The NIH Revitalization Act of 1993 ensures the inclusion of both women and minorities as NIH research subjects. However, pregnant women are still excluded. While it makes sense to protect against prenatal risks, many pregnant women take medication, and some of those medications may be necessary to save their lives while pregnant. Therefore, the lack of research data on pregnant women can be harmful.

The most infamous example of lack of data on medication used by pregnant women is thalidomide, which was marketed to pregnant women in 1958, primarily overseas, but also as part of research studies in the United States. The drug was described as effective at combating prenatal nausea and helping pregnant women to sleep. By 1962, 8,000 children born to women taking thalidomide had been born with limb deformities, with many lacking functional arms or legs (Mastroianni et al., 1994).

Similarly, the drug diethylstilbestrol (DES) was prescribed to millions of pregnant women from 1938 until 1971 to help prevent miscarriage. By 1971, it was determined that those pregnant women had given birth to girls who were significantly more likely to develop cancers of the cervix or vagina. Referred to as DES daughters, many of them became infertile or experienced ectopic pregnancies or preterm deliveries (CDC, *Facts About DES and Reproductive Complications*). DES sons were found to be at an increased risk of epididymal cysts, and women who had taken the drug were found to have a moderately increased risk for breast cancer (CDC, *About DES*).

Protections of human subjects in the 1970s were geared more toward warning patients about risks rather than ensuring that medical treatments were adequately studied on women and diverse populations. For example, in 1974, the U.S. Department of Health, Education, and Welfare established a system of institutional review boards (IRBs), a more formal version of the research review committee, as one mechanism for the protection of human research subjects. The responsibilities given to IRBs included the reviewing of risk-benefit ratios, confidentiality protections, informed consent processes and documents, and procedures for selection of subjects to ensure that selection is equitable (Mastroianni et al., 1994). However, with the threat of AIDS in the 1980s, inclusion of women and minorities in clinical trials was pushed to the forefront of discussions.

By the 1990s, the participation rate of women in clinical trials was approaching that of their male counterparts. A retrospective review of clinical trials of new drugs and labeling conducted from 1995–1999 (Evelyn et al., 2001b) revealed that women were participating in FDA-reviewed research at rates from 42%–55% during this 5-year time frame.

The study found that two-thirds of the products tested contained statements about sex, although only 22% described actual effects, primarily regarding pharmacokinetics but also in relation to safety and efficacy. Differences were noted more in cardio-renal and metabolic/endocrine products, followed by neuropharmacological, antiviral, oncologic products, and special pathogens. Thirty-two of the 185 products reviewed listed sex differences in the effects of the drugs. Most (81%) of these had labeling statements to note the differences found, but six (19%) did not have a labeling statement. None of the labels recommended a different dosage for women.

AGE DIVERSITY IN CLINICAL TRIALS

AGE DIFFERENCES IN reactions to medical treatment have also posed challenges to researchers and the FDA. Prior to the 1990s, most drugs and biological products were not tested on children, because of financial and ethical concerns.

When adults participate in clinical trials they are required to provide informed consent. If children are to participate, the parents or guardian must provide informed consent. Many adults barely look at informed consent documents before they sign them for themselves, instead trusting the physician to protect them from harmful research. However, when providing informed consent for their children, parents might be more cautious, especially for studies involving children whose lives do not depend on an experimental treatment. Medical products approved only for adults can almost always legally be used for children as an off-label use, which is the term for uses that were not approved by the FDA as shown on the product's label. Therefore, companies had little financial incentive to go to the expense and risk of conducting studies of children. There would have been more incentive if there were competition—if at least one company was getting their medical products approved for children—but in most cases companies were competing against other companies that also had not tested their products on children. The main exception was vaccines that are intended primarily for children and therefore needed to be tested on them.

Before laws were changed to ensure more studies of children, only about 20% of drugs approved by the FDA were labeled for pediatric use. Many of the other 80% of drugs sold in the United States were given to children off-label, with doctors prescribing the medicine based on data from clinical trials in adult populations (DHHS, 2006). For most of these 80% of medical products, dosages were extrapolated from adult

251

*The Ethics of
Inclusion and
Exclusion in
Clinical Trials:
Race, Sex, and Age*

populations, reduced proportionately to the child's lower weight. This approach failed to consider other physiological differences between children and adults, particularly in regard to metabolism rates. Sometimes the recommended dosage of medicine was not enough, sometimes it was too much. Doctors simply used their best judgment or avoided the decision altogether.

Not surprisingly, ineffective treatment and adverse reactions were some of the noted consequences. Sometimes, the results were very serious. For example, chloramphenicol, an antibiotic, causes so-called gray baby syndrome, a condition where the baby turns blue. After 23 infant deaths were reported, it was determined that the immature livers of these infants were unable to clear chloramphenicol from the body, "allowing toxic doses of the drug to accumulate" (DHHS, 1997b, p. 8).

Voluntary measures to persuade pharmaceutical companies to conduct pediatric clinical trials were largely unsuccessful at first. Barriers included the need for specialized equipment and personnel, the concerns about issues of consent, and the lack of financial incentives to test products in children (DHHS, 2006). Progress was very slow until regulations were put in place to improve those incentives.

- In 1977, the American Academy of Pediatrics called for clinical trials on children.
- In 1979, the FDA added a section to the labels of medical products specifically for information on indications and dosage for children, if they were available.
- In the 1980s, concerns about HIV and AIDS among children brought attention to the need to conduct HIV/AIDS trials on newborns and children.
- In 1994, in response to Congressional pressure, the FDA finally issued a regulation requiring manufacturers of marketed drugs to survey existing data and to determine whether the data were sufficient to support additional pediatric use information in the drug's labeling. If the data existed, manufacturers were encouraged to submit a supplemental application to request a labeling change. If the information was insufficient, the rule required the labeling of the drug to state that "safety and effectiveness in pediatric patients have not been established" (Biotechnology Industry Organization, n.d.).

In 1997, the FDA Modernization Act required the FDA to list which drugs most needed pediatric labeling. Section 111 of the law offered an extension of patent exclusivity as an incentive to pharmaceutical companies to test their drugs on children. Companies that were willing to conduct research on children could apply to the FDA for a 6-month extension on their patent in exchange for the research. If the FDA determined that the research would be worthwhile, the company could make many millions or even billions of dollars in exchange for a study that might cost a few million dollars to conduct and analyze.

In the same way that manufacturers did not conduct studies of children until there was a financial incentive to do so, most manufacturers have avoided studying their medical products on elderly patients, many of whom take other medications at the same time and are at higher risk of serious complications, compared to younger patients. Pharmaceutical companies and other companies making medical products have found it was easier to conduct studies on younger, healthier patients, and there was less concern about risks making their products look unsafe. However, the reality is that elderly patients often take many medications at the same time and may be especially vulnerable to certain side effects. By excluding those higher risk patients from clinical trials, manufacturers are not able to provide useful information about safety and effectiveness for older patients, who in some cases are the majority of patients who would be taking the medications that are being studied.

INCLUSION AND EXCLUSION
IN CLINICAL TRIALS

M ORE RESEARCH IS needed to evaluate the safety and effectiveness of medical products for children and the elderly. However, the lack of research on adults or children from a wide range of racial and ethnic backgrounds may be even more urgent, and those studies should include sufficient numbers so that each group can provide meaningful information for specific racial and ethnic groups. Including a small number of people representing one group is not enough to provide meaningful data that can be generalized to the entire population. On the other hand, including a small number of individuals representing each of several different groups in a much larger population of Whites will tell us nothing about the safety or effectiveness for people of these specific racial or ethnic backgrounds but could possibly provide results that would be misleading for Whites or others. For example, if a medication is more effective for Whites, combining the groups would make the product seem less effective than it is for Whites, and possibly make it seem more effective than it is for people of various other racial or ethnic backgrounds. Similarly, if a product is dangerous for one ethnic group, combining all groups into one sample would most likely make the risks seem negligible rather than statistically significant.

CONCLUSION

A GROWING BODY OF research indicates that racial and ethnic differences can influence the safety and effectiveness of medical products. While the need for diversity in clinical populations is sometimes obvious, such as studies of skin cancer or vitamin D deficiency, where skin color would have a clear physical effect, most potential disparities in the safety or effectiveness of medical products are not obvious. Moreover, even if we do not know *why* certain disparities in treatment outcome exist, it is still useful to know *that* they exist, in order to improve medical treatment and reduce health disparities. Companies that make medical products are currently urged to include diverse populations in studies submitted to the FDA, but they are not required to do so. This voluntary policy has not been effective.

Efforts to improve racial and ethnic diversity in clinical trials should be the next frontier for civil rights and human rights, because it could help ensure that medications are as effective for people of various racial or ethnic backgrounds as they are for Whites. Studying potential differences for men and women of varying ages is also important. Requirements for diversity and separate data analysis for different racial, ethnic, and age groups are long overdue. Like other rights movements, these are battles that have already been fought and won for other groups. Whereas the women's rights movement followed the civil rights movement, in clinical trials the struggle for racial and ethnic diversity follows successful efforts to include women and children.

APPENDIX: INCLUSION IN UNETHICAL EXPERIMENTS

E GREGIOUS ETHICAL BREACHES from the past most often affected marginalized people, including people of certain racial or ethnic backgrounds. The best known example was the Tuskegee syphilis study, which targeted African American males. Unfortunately, this was not an exception. There were other questionable or clearly unethical studies, although none as horrific as the unfounded claim that the U.S. government intentionally created the AIDS epidemic as a form of genocide.

The lack of people of diverse racial or ethnic backgrounds in legitimate clinical trials is all the more outrageous in light of the unethical use of people of specific racial or ethnic backgrounds as unwitting guinea pigs in clinical trials. Here are some examples of that terrible history:

1845–1849

J. Marion Sims uses three Alabama slave women to develop new techniques to repair vesicovaginal fistulas, without the use of anesthesia. Only after success does he attempt to do the same with White women (Gamble, 2004).

1931

Dr. Cornelius Rhoads, a pathologist, conducts a cancer experiment in Puerto Rico for The Rockefeller Institute for Medical Investigations. Dr. Rhoads intentionally infects his Puerto Rican subjects with cancer. Thirteen of the subjects die. Despite Rhoads's written statements that "what the island needs is not public health works…but something to totally exterminate the population," Rhoads is exonerated and goes on to establish U.S. Army Biological Warfare facilities in Maryland, Utah, and Panama, and is later named to the U.S. Atomic Energy Commission (Duster, 2006, p. 491). Rhoads is also responsible for radiation experiments on prisoners, hospital patients, and soldiers. Years later, the American Association for Cancer Research honors him by naming its exemplary scientist award the Cornelius Rhoads Award (Duster, 2006).

1955–1957

In order to learn how cold weather affects human physiology, researchers give a total of 200 doses of iodine-131, a radioactive tracer that concentrates almost immediately in the thyroid gland, to 85 healthy Eskimos and 17 Athapascan Indians living in Alaska. They study the tracer within the body by blood, thyroid tissue, urine and saliva samples from the test subjects. Due to the language barrier, no one tells the test subjects what is being done to them, making informed consent impossible (Committee on Evaluation of 1950s Air Force Human Health Testing in Alaska Using Radioactive Iodine-131, Commission on Geosciences, Environment, and Resources, Commission on Life Sciences, National Research Council, 1996).

1963

Chester M. Southam, who injected Ohio State Prison inmates with live cancer cells in 1952, performs the same procedure on 22 senile, African American female patients at the Brooklyn Jewish Chronic Disease Hospital in order to watch their immunological response. Southam tells the patients that they are receiving "some cells," but leaves out the fact that they are cancer cells. He claims he does not obtain informed consent from the patients because he does not want to frighten them by telling them what he is doing. He temporarily loses his medical

255

The Ethics of
Inclusion and
Exclusion in
Clinical Trials:
Race, Sex, and Age

license for fraud, deceit, and unprofessional conduct (Faden & Beauchamp, 1986).

1988–2001

The New York City Administration for Children's Services begins allowing foster care children living in about two dozen children's homes to be used in NIH-sponsored experimental AIDS drug trials. These children—totaling 465 by the program's end—experience serious side effects, including inability to walk, diarrhea, vomiting, swollen joints, and cramps. Children's home employees are unaware that they are giving the HIV-infected children experimental drugs rather than standard AIDS treatments. Approximately 99% were Hispanic or African American (Doran, 2004).

1990

The CDC and Kaiser Permanente of Southern California inject 1,500 6-month-old Black and Hispanic babies in Los Angeles with an experimental measles vaccine that had never been licensed for use in the United States. Adding to the risk, children less than 1 year old may not have an adequate amount of myelin around their nerves, possibly resulting in impaired neural development because of the vaccine. The CDC later admits that parents were never informed that the vaccine being injected into their children was experimental (Ladson-Billings & Donner, 2005).

1992

Columbia University's New York State Psychiatric Institute and the Mount Sinai School of Medicine give 100 boys, between the ages of 6 and 10, 10 milligrams of fenfluramine (Fen-phen) per kilogram of body weight in order to test the theory that low serotonin levels are linked to violent or aggressive behavior. Most are African American or Hispanic, and all were the younger brothers of juvenile delinquents. Parents of the participants received $125 each, including a $25 Toys'R'Us gift certificate (Pine et al., 1997).

REFERENCES

Baum, A., Garofalo, J. P., & Yali, A. M. (1999). Socioeconomic status and chronic stress: Does stress account for SES effects on health? *Annals of the New York Academy of Sciences, 896,* 131–144.

Biotechnology Industry Organization. (n.d.). *History of pediatric studies, rule, legislation and litigation.* Retrieved December 24, 2007, from http://www.bio.org/reg/action/pedhist.asp

Burroughs, V. J., Maxey, R. W., & Levy, R. A. (2002). Racial and ethnic differences in response to medicines: Towards individualized pharmaceutical treatment. *Journal of the National Medical Association, 94*(10 Suppl.), 1–26.

Centers for Disease Control and Prevention. (n.d.) *About DES*. Retrieved December 24, 2007, from http://www.cdc.gov/des/consumers/about/index.html

Centers for Disease Control and Prevention. (n.d.). *Facts about DES and reproductive complications*. Retrieved December 24, 2007, from http://www.cdc.gov/des/partners/download/DES&ReproductiveRisksFS.pdf

Choudhry, S., Ung, N., Avila, P. C., Ziv, E., Nazario, S., Casal, J., et al. (2005). Pharmacogenetic differences in response to albuterol between Puerto Ricans and Mexicans with asthma. *American Journal of Respiratory and Critical Care Medicine, 171,* 563–570.

Committee on Evaluation of 1950s Air Force Human Health Testing in Alaska Using Radioactive Iodine-131, Commission on Geosciences, Environment, and Resources, Commission on Life Sciences, National Research Council. (1996). *The Arctic Aeromedical Laboratory's thyroid function study: A radiological risk and ethical analysis*. Washington, DC: National Academy Press.

Council on Ethical and Judicial Affairs. (1990). Black-White disparities in health care. *Journal of the American Medical Association, 263,* 2344–2346.

Department of Health and Human Services. (1993). *National Institutes of Health Revitalization Act of 1993 subtitle B—clinical research equity regarding women and minorities*. Retrieved December 24, 2007, from http://orwh.od.nih.gov/inclusion/revitalization.pdf

Department of Health and Human Services. (1995). Investigational new drug applications and new drug applications. *Federal Register, 60*(174), docket no. 95N-0010. Retrieved December 24, 2007, from http://www.fda.gov/OHRMS/DOCKETS/98fr/95n-0010-npr0001.htm

Department of Health and Human Services. (1997a). *Policy statement on inclusion of race and ethnicity in DHHS data collection activities*. Retrieved December 24, 2007, from http://aspe.hhs.gov/datacncl/inclusn.htm

Department of Health and Human Services. (1997b). *Regulations requiring manufacturers to assess the safety and effectiveness of new drugs and biological products in pediatric populations*. 21 CFR Parts 201, 312, 314, and 601 (Docket No. 97N-0165) RIN 0910-AB20. Retrieved December 24, 2007, from http://www.fda.gov/cder/guidance/pedrule.pdf

Department of Health and Human Services. (2005). *Guidance for industry: The collection of race and ethnicity data in human trials*. Retrieved December 24, 2007, from http://www.fda.gov/cder/guidance/5656fnl.pdf

Department of Health and Human Services. (2006). Drug research and children. *Special Report from FDA Consumer Magazine, 4*. Retrieved December 24, 2007, from http://www.fda.gov/fdac/special/testtubetopatient/children.html

Department of Health and Human Services. (2007). *The Food and Drug Administration's oversight of clinical trials*. Retrieved December 24, 2007, from http://oig.hhs.gov/oei/reports/oei-01-06-00160.pdf

Doran, J. (2004, November 30). New York's HIV experiment. *BBC News*. Retrieved March 13, 2008, from http://news.bbc.co.uk/2/hi/programmes/this_world/4038375.stm

Durand, J. B. (2004). Heart failure management in African Americans: Meeting the challenge. *The Journal of Clinical Hypertension, 6*, 42–47.

Duster, T. (2006). Lessons from history: Why race and ethnicity have played a major role in biomedical research. *Journal of Law, Medicine and Ethics, 34*(3), 487–496.

Evelyn, B., Toigo, T., Banks, D., Pohl, D., Gray, K., Robins, B., et al. (2001a). Participation of racial/ethnic groups in clinical trials and race-related labeling: A review of new molecular entities approved 1995–1999. Reprinted from the *Journal of the National Medicine Association, 93*(Suppl.). Retrieved January 15, 2008, from http://www.fda.gov/cder/reports/race_ethnicity/race_ethnicity_report.htm

Evelyn, B., Toigo, T., Banks, D., Pohl, D., Gray, K., Robins, B., et al. (2001b). *Women's participation in clinical trials and gender-related labeling: A review of new molecular entities approved 1995–1999*. Retrieved January 15, 2008, from http://www.fda.gov/cder/reports/womens_health/women_clin_trials.htm

Faden, R. R., & Beauchamp, T. L. (1986). *A history and theory of informed consent*. Oxford: Oxford University Press.

FDA Modernization Act of 1997 (FDAMA). (1997). Retrieved August 11, 2008, from http://www.fda.gov/cdrh/modact/modern.html

Field, T. S., Buist, D. S., Doubeni, C., Enger, S., Fouayzi, H., Hart, G., et al. (2005). Disparities and survival among breast cancer patients. *Journal of the National Cancer Institute Monographs, 35*, 88–95.

Gamble, V. N. (2004). Under the shadow of Tuskegee: African Americans and health care. In N. Worcester & M. H. Whatley (Eds.), *Women's health: Readings on social, economic, and political issues* (4th ed., pp. 108–115). Dubuque, IA: Kendall/Hunt Publishing Company.

Kieffer, E. C., Willis, S. K., Odoms-Young, A. M., Guzman, J. R., Allen, A. J., Two Feather, J., et al. (2004). Reducing disparities in diabetes among African-American and Latino residents of Detroit: The essential role of community planning focus groups. *Ethnicity and Disease, 14*(2 Suppl. 1), S27–S37.

Ladson-Billings, G., & Donner, J. (2005). The moral activist role of critical race theory scholarship. In N. K. Denzin & Y. S. Lincoln (Eds.), *The SAGE handbook of qualitative research* (3rd ed.). Sage Publications.

Li, C. I., Malone, K. E., & Daling, J. R. (2002). Differences in breast cancer hormone receptor status and histology by race and ethnicity among women 50 years of age and older. *Cancer Epidemiology Biomarkers, 11*(7), 601–607.

Mastroianni, R., Faden, R., & Federman, D. (Eds.) (1994). *Women and health research: Ethical and legal issues of including women in clinical studies*. Washington, DC: National Academy Press.

Pine, D. S., Coplan, J. D., Wasserman, G. A., Miller, L. S., Fried, J. E., Davies, M., et al. (1997). Neuroendocrine response to fenfluramine challenge in boys. *Archives of General Psychiatry, 54,* 839–846.

Sankar, P., & Kahn, J. (2005). BiDil: Race medicine or race marketing? *Health Affairs Web Exclusive,* W5, 455–463.

Shankar, S., Klassen, A. C., Garrett-Mayer, E., Houts, P. S., Wang, T., McCarthy, M., et al. (2007). Evaluation of a nutrition education intervention for women residents of Washington, DC, public housing communities. *Health Education Research, 22*(3), 425–437.

Wang, L. (2002). Oncology group spans Southeast Asia, Australia. *Journal of the National Cancer Institute, 94,* 1426–1429.

23

The Use of Placebo-Control Groups in Clinical Trials

SUSAN S. ELLENBERG

THE USE OF placebos in clinical research has long been controversial. In the days before informed consent requirements became rigorously enforced, the primary concern about use of placebos was the possibility of deception—research participants who agreed to participate in a study on the assumption that they would receive therapy might instead receive an inactive substance (Bok, 1974).

Another concern that regularly arises relates to the use of placebo controls in a study of a promising experimental treatment for a serious disease for which no satisfactory treatments are yet available. Despite the fact that in such situations the standard of care (no treatment or noncurative treatment) may be well defined, there may be pressure from patients, physicians, or advocacy groups to make the promising new treatment available to all. Such concerns have been (and continue to be) the subject of published debates, particularly in the context of cancer trials (Gehan & Freireich, 1974; Hellman & Hellman, 1991), but also in regard to studies of treatments for AIDS (Byar et al., 1990), amyotropic lateral sclerosis (Munsat, 1996), and other similarly serious diseases or conditions.

More recently, concerns about use of placebos have focused on the appropriateness of offering placebo treatment to some participants in a clinical trial when treatments known to be effective for the condition under study are available (Freedman, Weijer, & Glass, 1996a, 1996b; Rothman & Michels, 1994). Unfortunately, the scientific considerations for using placebos in trials are complex and often poorly understood, thereby complicating the dialogue around the ethical issues.

Placebo control groups play an important role in drug development. When investigators, and ultimately regulatory authorities, want to know whether a treatment has a beneficial effect on the condition being treated and is acceptably safe, the simplest and most reliable way to answer this question is to perform a study in which some participants are randomly assigned to receive the treatment and others to receive a placebo. Control groups generally are important to control for the sorts of changes that can be observed for reasons other than the administration of treatment, such as natural fluctuations in the condition under study and the "regression to the mean" phenomenon (Barnett, van der Pols, & Dobson, 2005) whereby people who are entered onto a study because they exceed a threshold on some clinical or laboratory measure will tend to be somewhat closer to the threshold when next measured, regardless of treatment. A placebo control provides the additional protection afforded by blinding—which means that trial participants do not know whether they are receiving drug or an inert substance, the observed drug effect cannot be influenced by their expectations, and the comparison of effects in those receiving and not receiving the active drug can be considered to be unbiased (Friedman, Furberg, & DeMets, 1998).

There is little debate about the appropriateness of placebo controls in certain situations: for example, in evaluating a treatment for which there is no current proven therapy (except in cases such as those cited previously). Another uncontroversial example is use of placebos purely to achieve blinding—as, for example, in a study comparing a lower dose and a higher dose of the same therapy in which all participants would take the number of doses consistent with high dose therapy but for those assigned to the low dose, some of those doses might be placebo rather than active drug. Finally, there is general agreement that it is *not* appropriate to use placebo controls when studying a new treatment for a serious disease for which alternative proven effective therapies are available and considered standard of care. In such cases, where a participant not receiving active treatment might be subject to irreversible harm, the control treatment must be an active agent known to benefit people with the condition under study, even if this adds scientific complexity.

Controversies have arisen, however, regarding the ethics of assigning a participant to a placebo instead of an active treatment when there are active treatments that have been shown effective, regardless of the circumstances. These controversies are of two primary types, each of which raises distinct issues:

- Is it ethical to assign participants to a placebo when effective agents are available, as long as no irreversible harm will result from remaining untreated for the duration of the study?
- Is it ethical to assign participants to a placebo when effective agents have been identified and are available in some regions but not where the study is taking place, even if the known effective agents have been shown to prevent irreversible harm in the regions where they have been evaluated?

PLACEBO CONTROLS IN DRUG DEVELOPMENT

THE FIRST OF these issues was brought to wide public attention in 1994 by Rothman and Michels, who attacked the common use of placebos in drug development. For example, it is common to evaluate new agents for symptomatic conditions such as allergies, aches and pains, depression, and anxiety in placebo-controlled trials. Rothman and Michels criticized the practice in such circumstances of leaving an individual untreated with any active agent for the duration of the study, thus subjecting that individual to the risk of discomfort and/or worsening of the disease, when effective treatment alternatives are known. Others agreed, often elaborating on the philosophical and ethical principles underlying the scientific considerations (Freedman et al., 1996a, 1996b; Weijer, 1999).

Rothman and Michels and their supporters were countered by others who argued that there is no reason to avoid placebo controls when it cannot harm the patient to go without active treatment for a short period of time, patients are fully informed about treatments available outside the trial, and there is no other reliable way to evaluate new treatments for many types of conditions (Ellenberg & Temple, 2000; Emanuel & Miller, 2001; Levine, 2002; Miller & Brody, 2002; Temple & Ellenberg, 2000).

If known effective treatments were always suitable as control treatments for evaluating new drugs, there would be no need to use placebo controls in settings where treatments have already been shown effective. Interpreting a study in which one treatment is shown to be more effective than another is straightforward. But many new drugs are developed, not with the expectation that they will be more effective than existing drugs but that they will have some other advantage—for example, fewer or less severe side effects, greater convenience of use, or lack of interaction with other medications likely to be taken concomitantly. To evaluate such drugs, one must show that they are effective without showing superiority to an existing drug. There are two ways to accomplish this. First, and by far the simplest and most efficient way, is to show that the new drug is better than a placebo. The second way would be to show that the new drug's efficacy is similar enough to that of the existing drug to support the conclusion that the new drug is indeed effective.

The second approach often proves complicated. In many situations, the size of the effect of an available drug is not well defined, as the effect size seen in the clinical trials of this agent when compared to a placebo may have varied widely. This is often the case in many medical areas, especially for drugs intended to alleviate symptoms rather than to cure or prevent disease (Jones, Jarvis, Lewis, & Ebbutt, 1996; Lasagna, 1979; Tramer, Reynolds, Moore, & McQuay, 1998). Clearly, if a drug that is accepted as effective showed little or no effect when compared to a placebo in some studies, it becomes difficult to interpret a study in which a new drug appears to show about the same effect as the active control. One would have to know whether in *this* study the active control would have appeared better than placebo, and by how much. To avoid this difficulty, and to ensure that drugs made available to the public are indeed effective, placebo controls have been routinely employed in circumstances where interpreting studies with active controls would be difficult and where there is no risk to study participants of any permanent harm. Proponents of the use of placebo controls in such situations point out that the alternative is either increasing the risk of approving new drugs that are ineffective or not approving any new drugs that cannot be shown more effective than available drugs, regardless of any advantage in safety, convenience, or cost.

One way to couch the debate is in terms of the trial participants—are they study subjects only (as, for example, in a phase 1 study in normal volunteers) or are they also patients? One might argue that someone suffering from depression, for example, who enters a short-term (typically 8–12 weeks) study to evaluate a new antidepressant is not really seeking medical treatment. A course of 8–12 weeks of an antidepressant is long enough to see whether the drug appears to be working, but is far shorter than an expected course of treatment. At the end of the period of observation, study participants will have to seek treatment with available drugs if they wish to be treated for their depression. Those who argue that assigning such individuals to a placebo is unethical clearly view these individuals as patients, and the physicians who enter them onto studies as caregivers who, by randomizing to active treatment or placebo, are violating their obligation to offer the best possible treatment to those under their care. Those who argue that placebo controls are perfectly appropriate in such trials view these individuals as people who are volunteering to participate in a medical experiment, and that the risks they face by doing so (possible delay in obtaining relief of symptoms, side effects of drug) are acceptable in a context of full informed consent and the ability to withdraw from the study at any time.

PLACEBO CONTROLS WHEN ACTIVE TREATMENTS ARE UNAVAILABLE IN TRIAL SETTING

THE SECOND CONTROVERSY presents different and perhaps more difficult challenges. It arose following the dramatic finding in 1994 that a regimen of AZT given to an HIV-infected pregnant woman during pregnancy and labor cut the risk of transmitting the infection to the infant by more than half (Connor et al., 1994). This study, usually referred to as the "076" trial (per the numbering system used by the AIDS Clinical Trials Group, which conducted the trial) was and remains one of the historic milestones in treatment and prevention of HIV/AIDS. The 076 trial was conducted in the United States; following the release of results, placebo-controlled trials of simplified treatment regimens were initiated in Africa and Asia. The regimens were substantially simplified in order to address feasibility issues; investigators felt that a regimen requiring a series of prenatal visits was not workable in developing countries where health care facilities were limited and prenatal care was not available. There was also concern about whether environmental factors, such as coinfections with other pathogens, diet, and other similar factors, might affect the efficacy (and perhaps the safety) of AZT. Thus, there was uncertainty about the effects of this modified regimen in developing countries, and hence the trials included a placebo control.

Shortly after the initiation of these trials there was an outcry, led by Lurie and Wolfe of Public Citizen's Health Research Group (Lurie & Wolfe, 1997). Lurie and Wolfe argued that the 076 regimen that had been shown to be highly effective in the United States should be the control arm in any further studies of approaches to prevent perinatal transmission of HIV. Responses by Varmus and Satcher (1997), and others (Abdool Karim, 1998; Halsey, Sommer, Henderson, & Black, 1997; Levine, 1998; Resnik, 1998; Susser, 1998) pointed out that a study designed as Lurie and Wolfe advocated might well yield no information useful to the population in which it was studied; for example, if the simplified regimen was demonstrated to be inferior to the 076 regimen (a not implausible outcome), the critical question of whether the simplified regimen was effective at all would remain unanswered. Thus, such a study would be of no value to the population in which it was conducted, because the full 076 regimen was considered not implementable in developing countries, and even the full 076 regimen might not have the same effect in these countries as it had in the United States. Finally, there were concerns that the safety of this regimen might not be comparable in the two settings, given the vast differences in prenatal and fundamental health care.

This particular controversy was quickly resolved; faced with a growing global perception that these trials would doom infants in the developing world to unnecessarily elevated risk of HIV infection and early death, the trials were modified and the placebo arms were eliminated. But other similar cases arose. Was it generally ethical to conduct placebo-controlled trials of new drugs for serious diseases and conditions in countries with populations having limited access to treatments considered to be standard of care in the developed world? Controversies arose, for example, about a proposed placebo-controlled trial of a new drug to treat respiratory distress syndrome in infants in countries where the standard treatment available in the United States was not routinely given (Charatan, 2001). The argument that it was wrong to conduct a trial in a poor country that would be considered unethical in the United States was countered by the argument that the proposed trial would offer better care to all trial participants, including those on the placebo, than they would otherwise receive, that a trial with an active control would not be interpretable because of the issue noted earlier—prior trials of active agents had shown widely varying effect sizes—and finally that the most relevant trial for that country would be a trial testing the new agent against that country's current standard of care. These counterarguments have not been found persuasive by those who fear the exploitation of populations in poorer countries to more efficiently develop medications intended for marketing and use in wealthier countries.

While the case against conducting trials in developing countries that would be considered unethical in the United States or other developed countries is emotionally compelling, especially when children are involved, there are some logical gaps. First, the notion that such trials are by definition exploitative seems to assume that scientists and policy makers in developing countries are unable to determine what research is most appropriate in their own countries. There are certainly examples of studies conducted in developed countries that would not have been considered ethical in the United States for reasons relating to standards of care. For example, placebo-controlled trials of acellular pertussis vaccines were carried out in Sweden and Italy (Greco et al., 1996; Gustafsson, Hallander, Olin, Reizenstein, & Storsaeter, 1996). The whole-cell pertussis vaccine given routinely to children in the United States at that time was considered overly reactogenic in many countries, who welcomed the opportunity to conduct a study that might identify an alternative pertussis vaccine that would prove more acceptable. If a developed country has the right to reject a control treatment or vaccine used as standard treatment in the United States because it was not relevant to the question of interest to their population, one might wonder why a developing country should not have the same privilege.

Second, it would be virtually impossible to conduct clinical trials in developing countries if the standard of care in developed countries had to be made available to trial participants, either as a control treatment or as background treatment for all participants. Malaria prevention provides an apt example. There are no proven malaria preventives, so a placebo-controlled trial of a vaccine or other treatment to prevent malaria would be ethical anywhere. But such trials could not be conducted in a developed country because the incidence of malaria is far too low. The Centers for Disease Control and Prevention (CDC) wanted to study the use of insecticide-treated bed nets in a malaria-endemic area to see whether such nets could reduce the risk of malaria. The control group would be untreated bed nets. We know, however, that the best way to prevent malaria is to keep all the doors and windows of the house tightly shut, so mosquitoes cannot get in. In the tropical climates where malaria is a problem, one cannot keep doors and windows closed without some mechanical system of ventilation and cooling. It could be concluded, then, that testing treated bed nets would be unethical, because we already know the best way to prevent exposure to malaria-infected mosquitoes—construct air-conditioned homes!

THE DECLARATION OF HELSINKI

THE DEBATES ABOUT the appropriate use of placebo controls involved the World Medical Association's (WMA) Declaration of Helsinki (DH; WMA, 2004) from the start. In the 1994 paper of Rothman and Michels, the DH was cited as the basis for considering unethical the use of placebo controls when known effective treatments were available. The version of the DH extant at the time included the following wording:

> In any medical study, every patient—including those of a control group, if any—should be assured of the best proven diagnostic and therapeutic method. (WMA, 1989)

Rothman and Michels interpreted this wording as precluding the use of placebo controls when proven therapy had been identified. Others, however, pointed out that this wording, taken literally, seemed to preclude any further comparative studies once any therapy had been "proven," since those receiving an experimental treatment would not be treated with the "best proven" method—surely this had not been the intent of the framers—and thus the wording could not be so clearly interpreted as Rothman and Michels argued. Debate regarding the meaning of the DH wording (which had been in place since 1975 without leading to earlier speculation about its implication for the use of placebo controls) led the WMA to initiate consideration of a revision. The result of these deliberations, put forth in 1996, simply added the clarification that placebo controls were appropriate when there was no known effective therapy, a position that had never been controversial. Recognizing that this 1996 revision had not resolved the debate, and energized by the issues raised by the 076 trial described previously, the WMA commissioned further deliberations, and a new revision was issued in 2000. This revision included a statement that unambiguously supported the views of Rothman/Michels and Wolfe/Lurie—if there was a treatment known to be effective for a disease or condition, then any further study of new treatments could not ethically use a placebo control. The new wording was as follows:

> The benefits, risks, burdens and effectiveness of a new method should be tested against those of the best current prophylactic, diagnostic, and therapeutic methods. This does not exclude the use of placebo, or no treatment, in studies where no proven prophylactic, diagnostic or therapeutic method exists. (WMA, 2000)

The 2000 revision of the DH clarified the WMA position but did nothing to settle the debate. Further deliberations were undertaken and in 2003 a clarification to the DH was added that in effect reversed the changes in the 2000 revision:

> The WMA hereby reaffirms its position that extreme care must be taken in making use of a placebo-controlled trial and that in general this methodology should only be used in the absence of existing proven therapy. However, a placebo-controlled trial may be ethically acceptable, even if proven therapy is available, under the following circumstances:
>
> ‹ Where for compelling and scientifically sound methodological reasons its use is necessary to determine the efficacy or safety of a prophylactic, diagnostic or therapeutic method; or
> ‹ Where a prophylactic, diagnostic or therapeutic method is being investigated for a minor condition and the patients who receive placebo will not be subject to any additional risk of serious or irreversible harm.
>
> All other provisions of the Declaration of Helsinki must be adhered to, especially the need for appropriate ethical and scientific review. (WMA, 2003)

The current wording, including the clarification, now allows for the conduct of placebo-controlled trials in the context of evaluation of drugs for symptomatic conditions when no serious consequences of remaining untreated for the duration of the trial are expected. With regard to the evaluation of treatments for serious diseases in developing countries where treatments that would be used as an active control in a developed country are not available, the current wording is negative but perhaps somewhat ambiguous. An advocate of placebo controls in such circumstances might argue, at least for some kinds of treatments, that placebo controls are "necessary to determine the efficacy or safety" of the treatment under study, on the grounds that the issues of concomitant care, diet, and other factors that could influence outcome are so different in developing countries that one cannot assume that the benefits and risks shown in regions such as the United States and western Europe would apply universally. But this argument is less than compelling as medical advances established in the developed world are routinely applied in less developed settings to the extent feasible, without such concerns being raised.

In 2007, a call for comment on the 2004 version of the DH was issued by the WMA, and in October 2008 a new version was released. With regard to the issue of placebo controls, the sense of the 2008 version has not changed from the "clarified" 2004 version.

OTHER STATEMENTS OF ETHICAL PRINCIPLES

THE WORLD HEALTH Organization's Council for International Organizations of Medical Sciences (CIOMS) first issued its International Guidelines for Ethical Conduct of Biomedical Research in 1982. A revised document was published in 1993 and, in the wake of the controversy about use of placebos (and other issues pertaining to research in developing countries), CIOMS developed further revisions that were published in 2002 (CIOMS, 2002). The 2002 guidelines are consistent with the clarification of the DH with regard to placebo controls:

> As a general rule, research subjects in the control group of a trial of a diagnostic, therapeutic, or preventive intervention should receive an established effective intervention. In some circumstances it may be ethically acceptable to use an alternative comparator, such as placebo or "no treatment".
>
> Placebo may be used:
>
> - when there is no established effective intervention;
> - when withholding an established effective intervention would expose subjects to, at most, temporary discomfort or delay in relief of symptoms;

when use of an established effective intervention as comparator would not yield scientifically reliable results and use of placebo would not add any risk of serious or irreversible harm to the subjects. (CIOMS, 2002)

In contrast to the DH, the CIOMS guideline goes on to directly address the issue of placebo-controlled trials to evaluate treatments for serious diseases in developing countries when effective treatments have been identified and are in use in the developed world. It includes a lengthy discussion of the differing perspectives and, while not endorsing any particular perspective, does not completely close the door to use of placebo-controlled trials in such circumstances. Careful consultation with experts is recommended when considering whether a scientifically valid result could be obtained from a trial without a placebo control group.

The CIOMS guidelines add commentary that includes emphasis on the importance of adhering to scientific principles in the design and interpretation of studies and on the increased reliability of conclusions when placebo controls are included.

The International Conference on Harmonization (ICH), a collaboration among industry and regulatory scientists in Europe, Japan, and the United States, issued a document titled *Choice of Control Group in Clinical Trials* (ICH, 2001). Although this document is not fundamentally a statement of ethical principles, it does address ethical issues relating to the conduct of clinical research involving investigational therapies from the perspective of regulatory authorities and drug development scientists. This document is also permissive with regard to the use of placebo controls in the circumstances described in the previous documents.

CONCLUSION

THE USE OF placebo controls, a mainstay of drug development and virtually universally accepted in many circumstances, remains controversial in others. Perhaps the most contentious issue beginning in the late 1990s is the ethical acceptability of placebo-controlled trials in developing countries when effective treatments have been identified and are in use in developed countries. Debate continues as to whether the most appropriate control for trials of treatments for serious diseases is the standard of care in the region where the study is being conducted, or the highest level of standard of care anywhere in the world.

REFERENCES

Abdool Karim, S. S. (1998). Placebo controls in HIV perinatal transmission trials: a South African's viewpoint. *American Journal of Public Health, 88*, 564–566.

Barnett, A. G., van der Pols, J. C., & Dobson, A. J. (2005). Regression to the mean: What it is and how to deal with it. *International Journal of Epidemiology, 34*, 215–220.

Bok, S. (1974). The ethics of giving placebos. *Scientific American, 231*, 17–23.

Byar, D. P., Schoenfeld, D. A., Green, S. B., Amato, D. A., Davis, R., De Gruttola, V., et al. (1990). Design considerations for AIDS trials. *New England Journal of Medicine, 323*, 1343–1348.

Charatan, F. (2001). Surfactant trial in Latin American infants criticized. *BMJ, 322*, 575.

Connor, E. M., Sperling, R. S., Gelber, R., Kiselev, P., Scott, G., O'Sullivan, M. J., et al. (1994). Reduction of maternal-infant transmission of human immunodeficiency virus type 1 with zidovudine treatment. *New England Journal of Medicine, 331*, 1173–1180.

Council for International Organizations of Medical Sciences (CIOMS). (2002). *International ethical guidelines for biomedical research involving human subjects*. Geneva: Author.

Ellenberg, S. S., & Temple, R. (2000). Placebo-controlled trials and active-control trials in the evaluation of new treatments. Part 2: Practical issues and specific cases. *Annals of Internal Medicine, 133*, 464–470.

Emanuel, E. J., & Miller, F. G. (2001). The ethics of placebo-controlled trials—a middle ground. *New England Journal of Medicine, 345*, 915–919.

Freedman, B., Weijer, C., & Glass, K. C. (1996a). Placebo orthodoxy in clinical research. I: Empirical and methodological myths. *Journal of Law, Medicine and Ethics, 24*, 243–251.

Freedman, B., Weijer, C., & Glass, K. C. (1996b). Placebo orthodoxy in clinical research. II: Ethical, legal and regulatory myths. *Journal of Law, Medicine and Ethics, 24*, 252–259.

Friedman, L. M., Furberg, C. D., & DeMets, D. L. (1998). *Fundamentals of clinical trials* (3rd ed.). New York: Springer-Verlag.

Gehan, E. A., & Freireich, E. J. (1974). Non-randomized controls in cancer clinical trials. *New England Journal of Medicine, 290*, 198–203.

Greco, D., Salmaso, S., Mastrantonio, P., Guiliano, M., Tozzi, A. E., Anemona A., et al. (1996). A controlled trial of two acellular vaccines and one whole-cell vaccine against pertussis. Progetto Pertusse Working Group. *New England Journal of Medicine, 334*, 341–348.

Gustafsson, L., Hallander, H. O., Olin, P., Reizenstein, E., & Storsaeter, J. (1996). A controlled trial of a two-component acellular, a five-component acellular, and a whole-cell pertussis vaccine. *New England Journal of Medicine, 334*, 349–355.

Halsey, N. A., Sommer, A., Henderson, D. A., & Black, R. E. (1997). Ethics and international research. *British Medical Journal, 315*, 965–966.

Hellman, S., & Hellman, D. (1991). Of mice but not men: Problems of the randomized clinical trial. *New England Journal of Medicine, 324*, 1585–1589.

International Conference on Harmonization. (2001). *Choice of control group in clinical trials, guideline E10.* Retrieved November 13, 2008, from http://www.fda.gov/cder/guidance/4155fnl.htm

Jones, B., Jarvis, P., Lewis, J. A., & Ebbutt, A. F. (1996). Trials to assess equivalence: The importance of rigorous methods. *British Medical Journal, 313*, 36–39.

Lasagna, L. (1979). Placebos and controlled trials under attack. *European Journal of Clinical Pharmacology, 15*, 373–374.

Levine, R. J. (1998). The "best proven therapeutic method" standard in clinical trials in technologically developing countries. *IRB: A Review of Human Subjects Research, 20*, 5–9.

Levine, R. J. (2002). Placebo controls in clinical trials of new therapies for conditions for which there are known effective treatments. In H. A. Guess, A. Kleinman, J. W. Kusek, & L. W. Engel (Eds.), *The science of the placebo* (pp. 264–280). London: BMJ Books.

Lurie, P., & Wolfe, S. M. (1997). Unethical trials of interventions to reduce perinatal transmissions of the human immunodeficiency virus in developing countries. *New England Journal of Medicine, 337*, 853–856.

Miller, F. G., & Brody, H. (2002). What makes placebo-controlled trials unethical? *American Journal of Bioethics, 2*, 3–9.

Munsat, T. L. (1996). Issues in clinical trial design I: Use of natural history controls. A protagonist view. *Neurology, 47*(Suppl. 2), S96–S97.

Resnik, D. B. (1998). The ethics of HIV research in developing nations. *Bioethics, 12*, 286–306.

Rothman, K. J., & Michels, K. B. (1994). The continued unethical use of placebo controls. *New England Journal of Medicine, 331*, 394–398.

Susser, M. (1998). The prevention of perinatal HIV transmission in the less-developed world. *American Journal of Public Health, 88*, 547–548.

Temple, R., & Ellenberg, S. S. (2000). Placebo-controlled trials and active-control trials in the evaluation of new treatments. Part 1: Ethical and scientific issues. *Annals of Internal Medicine, 133*, 455–463.

Tramer, M. R., Reynolds, D. J., Moore, R. A., & McQuay, H. J. (1998). When placebo controlled trials are essential and equivalence trials are inadequate. *British Medical Journal, 317*, 875–880.

Varmus, H., & Satcher, D. (1997). Ethical complexities of conducting research in developing countries. *New England Journal of Medicine, 337*, 1003–1005.

Weijer, C. (1999). Placebo-controlled trials in schizophrenia: Are they ethical? Are they necessary? *Schizophrenia Research, 35*, 211–218.

World Medical Association. (2008). *Declaration of Helsinki.* Retrieved November 13, 2008, from http://www.wma.net/e/policy/b3.htm

24

Forbidden Knowledge

William R. LaFleur

D URING RECENT YEARS the topic of forbidden knowledge has gained increased attention from the general public and bioethicists in particular. This is because new technologies have opened an area where it is pressingly relevant—an individual patient's right to keep information about his or her own genetic history private and, most especially, out of the hands of insurers who might use it to deny or limit coverage. To some extent this problem results from the peculiarities of the current system of providing—but also limiting—medical care in the United States. In the present situation, which is forced by what has been described as a growing deluge of genetic information, it appears to be ethically mandated to forbid designated others from having access to knowledge that is already possessed by some, especially if the norms of privacy and of nondiscrimination in coverage are prioritized. The legal enforcement of this notion is the objective of proposed federal legislation, the Genetic Information Nondiscrimination Act (GINA). A strong case not only for this act's passage but also for other safeguards—such as the creation of a genetic test registry and the regulation of genetic testing labs—has been set forth (Rugnetta, Russell, & Moreno, 2008).

Our debates about gate-keeping in this domain are, however, only the most current and society-engaging twist in what have, in fact, been millennia-long contestations over the possession of knowledge. And things other than principles have usually been at stake. Even in the aforementioned contemporary case, in which some might argue that any forbidding of access to information puts in jeopardy the values of an open society, there is good reason to assume that the interest in this matter on the part of insurers is largely economic.

It seems clear, therefore, that consideration of the topic of forbidden knowledge may not be divorced from an awareness of why some individuals or groups will have an interest in forbidding others' access to knowledge and, on the other side, why others will insist on gaining such access. This is so because the recognition that knowledge is power surely did not commence with the person, Francis Bacon (1561–1626), who expressed that truth so pithily. In fact, knowledge's inherent power was implicitly acknowledged by early physicians' interest in forbidding the sharing of what they knew with persons outside their own profession; part of the "oath" attributed to Hippocrates (c. 430 BCE states: "Whatever I see or hear professionally or privately, which ought not to be divulged, I will keep secret and tell no one" (quoted in Lloyd, 1978, p. 67). Some kind of *interestedness* on the part of each type of knowledge forbidder appears to have been fairly constant within history.

RELIGION AND FORBIDDEN KNOWLEDGE

THIS CHAPTER'S FOCUS, however, will be on the history of forbidding or allowing inquiry into still unknown or vaguely known domains—and on the present state of questions related to the ethics of such research. It is clear that in much of the history of the West, arguments based on religion had a powerful role in the construction of rationales for forbidding certain kinds of inquiry. Theologians claiming to *know* what domains of inquiry to disallow long ago appealed to biblical authority, citing a supposedly historical fall from Edenic bliss due in part to a curiosity-based transgression of boundaries. Biblical cautions about human pride in the Tower of Babel legend and in Greek myths about Prometheus and Pandora added to concerns in the West about transgressive curiosity, a theme that had a large role in medieval Christian writing.

Tertullian (c. 160–225 CE), often called the "Father" of the Latin Church, had a large role in defining truth as God's property and human curiosity (*curiositas*) as disallowed. In Tertullian's view "freely chosen *ignorantia* [ignorance] can thus become an act of acknowledgement of the exclusive divine right of possession of the truth and disposition over it" (Blumenberg, 1983, p. 302). Likewise for Lactantius (c. 250–c. 325 CE) God's majesty required that He intend to keep things secret from humans—and have a plan for implementing this. "God had protected

Himself by making man the last of His creations so that he should not acquire any insight into the process of creation" (Blumenberg, 1983, p. 304). Such religion-based proscriptions on inquiry had a deep impact in the West's history and were bound to make the revalorization of curiosity in Europe's Renaissance appear to be an antireligious movement.

The writings of Francis Bacon changed things dramatically. His *Novum Organum* of 1620 saw a precedent for science in Adam's naming of animals and charged as "evil" any assumption that "the inquisition of nature is in any part interdicted or forbidden" (Bacon, 1620/1978, pp. 288–289). And John Milton (1608–1674) surely was absorbing his epoch's increased interest in science when he revised the interpretation of Genesis by pointing to what has been called "the paradox of the fortunate Fall" (quoted in Shattuck, 1996, p. 49). With this turnabout what had been assumed boundaries around domains of inquiry were, at least theologically, poised for erasure.

In East Asia the fact that there was only one known human dissection before the 11th century suggests that the Chinese had a "taboo against opening the body" (Lloyd & Sivin, 2002, p. 220). If so, this likely arose out of respect for ancestors who had literally given a person his or her body. This was less a religious proscription on inquiry than a deeply enculturated inhibition, one working in sync with an alternative channeling of interest in the body's functioning and in alternative ways to maintain health. Expertise in acupuncture and in how to deploy a vast herbal and mineral pharmacological knowledge base would, we may assume, have given their possessors a vested professional interest in retaining a cultural taboo on dissection. In 18th-century Japan, curiosity about the body's internal organs and functions, stimulated by known books imported from Europe, intensified so much that physicians such as Genpaku Sugita (1733–1817) sought to augment indigenous East Asian methods with knowledge gained by dissecting the body (Sugita, 1815/1969). One result has been that differing domains of knowledge about the body, regarded by many as complementary, inform medical practices in much of contemporary East Asia (Lock, 1980).

In the West the view that certain domains of inquiry are proscribed by religion has over recent centuries lost ground, due largely to the sequential falsification of predictions that what had been ecclesiastically disallowed would also prove to be inaccessible in fact. Research has routinely penetrated such postulated barriers—for instance, by showing linkages between *homo sapiens* and other species, in making extraterrestrial travel a reality, and in ongoing projects to replicate and create life. Although language about the risks of "playing God" and of violating so-called natural law continue to play a role in some debates about scientific inquiry and biotechnological engineering (Peters, 1997), the notion that some things fall within areas that are, by divine intent, *inherently* forbidden to humans was effectively challenged already by Renaissance practices and by the priority that the Enlightenment gave to rationality. Funkenstein (1986), however, sees another kind of continuity with earlier Christianity in the Enlightenment figures' educational, even "missionary," zeal. "In many countries the *illuminati, Aufklärer, philosophes* set out to reform humanity and society through knowledge and reasoning" (Funkenstein, 1986, p. 357).

The early modern era was much fascinated by ethnographic and anatomical "curiosities" and what might be learned from them; some, such as the French mathematician Maupertuis (1698–1759), at one time a president of the Berlin Akademie, advocated doing experiments that would actively produce what were termed "curiosa." He proposed isolating groups of preliterate children to learn through them about the formation of languages and ideas. Doing experiments on condemned prisoners also, he wrote, ought to go forward undeterred by "the appearance of cruelty." Quoting this, Blumenberg comments: "Experiments on living people here appear as the logical consequence of a *curiosité* that posits itself as absolute" (Blumenberg, 1983, p. 411). Rescher views Maupertuis as an instance of a laissez faire approach that evolved only in the 18th century, the extreme opposite of wholesale regulation, and equally unacceptable (Rescher, 1987, p. 3).

CRUELTY TO THE FOREFRONT

IT IS INSTRUCTIVE to note that Maupertuis felt compelled to claim that experiments on living prisoners gave only the appearance, not the reality, of *cruelty*. His argument, unconvincing as it is, shows that a fundamental change was taking place in Western thinking about what might constitute a reason to forbid certain kinds of knowledge acquisition. Theological strictures were yielding to the claims of reason, but, on the other hand—as seen for instance in Voltaire (1694–1778)—a sensitivity to what is morally objectionable in cruelty was rising. This would be a change that would have continuing resonance and import even centuries later when the discipline of bioethics would be formed. Reasons for forbidding certain kinds of research inquiry might, after the Enlightenment, now be shaped by *humanistic* concerns. "The age of reform that began in the eighteenth century was fueled by an increasing revulsion against cruelty" (Shklar, 1984, p. 35).

Montaigne (1533–1592) already had explicitly listed cruelty "as the extreme of all vices" (Montaigne, 1588/1958, p. 313). Although he was a Catholic, it can be assumed that he had the Inquisition's methods in mind when holding that "Christianity had done nothing to inhibit cruelty" (Shklar, 1984, p. 11). Nevertheless, the Enlightenment's elevation of rationality often was in tension with the no-cruelty criterion. Montaigne would countenance no cruelty to animals but, in contrast, Descartes (1596–1650) so stressed rationality as a prerequisite for sensing pain that he famously—or infamously—justified research that would involve the public vivisection of animals.

This tension has, in fact, never been resolved and continues to influence a wide range of debates today about what should or should not be allowed not only in research agendas but in therapeutic options. Even a wide consensus holding that permissible research will necessarily avoid cruelty does not itself provide a clear guideline when what is involved comes under the category of risk—risk to the researcher, risk to the subjects of an experiment, or risk to a whole community (Rescher, 1987, p. 14). Since putatively all new knowledge would again become forbidden if experiments were required to be totally risk-free, the solution to this dilemma, as shaped during the second half of the 20th century, was the mechanism of informed consent.

The obtaining of informed consent from risk-bearing *individuals* has become the default method in our time for a social distinction between research deemed licit and that which is to be forbidden. Questions remain about its just applicability in the case of individuals who, because they deeply need or desire the financial benefits given to research subjects, will tend to screen-out information about risks to themselves, especially if they are subjects in multiple studies. Even more problematic are the risks that research might pose to whole communities—especially because neither being informed nor consenting will likely be possible when those most adversely affected comprise a multitude, are scattered, are victims of so-called collateral damage, or even would be members of future generations. Although it merits ever closer scrutiny, the long and pervasive influence of utilitarianism and consequentialism in Anglo-American contexts leads to a ready-to-hand assumption that these ethical dilemmas of research might be solved by a *calculation* of likely suffering and benefits (Pernick, 1985).

THE 20TH CENTURY

DISCUSSIONS OF THE ethics of experimenting with human subjects intensified in post–World War II America—partially in response to the realization of how horrendously cruel some midwar experimentation had been. During the Nazi era, Germany had carried out at least two dozen projects using coerced human subjects, many of whom were killed in the process. But it needs to be recognized that even morally tainted data can expand the realm of what is known and prove useful. The usefulness, especially in military contexts, of some of the information gained in such despicable ways was indicated by the eagerness of the victorious Allies to confiscate and retain it (Caplan, 1992). Likewise, midwar experiments in Manchuria carried out clandestinely by Japan's Unit 731, an army medical unit, involved not only coerced subjects but vivisections and the killing of research subjects. In the postwar context the U.S. military refrained from prosecuting those most responsible in exchange for privileged acquisition of the data that had been collected by this Japanese unit (Harris, 1994; Tsuneishi, 2007).

Should access to such bodies of knowledge be forbidden? One perspective holds that to deprive present and future generations of the benefits of its potential use would be "misguided puritanism" (Rescher, 1987, p. 4). While holding that editors of journals should not publish new data if it had been obtained by immoral means, Caplan recognizes the power of the scientific community's desire to know and that, in reality, it is "often too late to talk of ignoring or excising [immorally obtained data] from biomedicine" (Caplan, 1997, p. 26). He deplores the fact that data such as that obtained from the infamous Tuskegee experiment, for instance, will be frequently cited but without mention of the egregious ethical violations involved in the conduct of that experiment and the human suffering it unquestionably caused.

In fact, the accumulated evidence of unethical and horrendous rationalized research having been carried out during the 20th century has given new urgency to the question of forbidden knowledge. So-called normal science has even to this day not yet been able to absorb the implications of Robert Oppenheimer's jolting 1947 statement that, in creating the atomic bomb, "physicists have known sin, and this is a knowledge they cannot lose" (quoted in Shattuck, 1996, p. 177). Although we may assume that his use of the term *sin* does not in itself throw the question of forbidden knowledge back into the arena of religion and theology, there can be no doubt that deep questions about legitimizing what might be inherently unethical research persist.

This is to say that in our own time the question of forbidding certain kinds of knowledge is given urgency not by religion or divine mandates but what we know of *history*, especially our relatively recent history and what it tells of man's inhumanity to man as evidenced in certain programs for knowledge acquisition. One concern about depending on the informed consent rule as adequate for filtering out unethical modes of research is that, although this rule's application envisions societies at peace, the de facto situation of our world is one in which war and anticipated wars are the ongoing contexts in which the most morally egregious research is conducted (LaFleur, 2007). Is normal science not, then, an illusion? Böhme, insisting that we scrutinize the interestedness of its early advocates, locates "socially institutionalized science within the framework of nation-state egotism" and calls attention to the fact that "for Bacon one of the most important dimensions of scientific-technological development in terms of use was war" (Böhme, 1992, pp. 4–5).

This may help explain why a recent study involving 51 interviews of American researchers found among them no "coherent ethos regarding the production of forbidden knowledge." Inconsistently, researchers "decried external regulations" but "recognized the right of society to place limits on what and how science is done" (Kempner, Perlis, & Merz, 2005, p. 854).

It is not only the rights of society but also the *risks to* society that are most mooted in these matters. In the postwar discussions of experimenting on human subjects, Henry Beecher articulated what has become the common optimism about the capacity of the informed consent rule to curb violations—although he admitted the difficulties and saw as erroneous the "bland assumption that meaningful or informed consent is readily available for the asking" (Beecher, 1966/1999, p. 422).

Hans Jonas (1903–1993), having barely evaded death in the Holocaust and subsequently writing on biology and philosophy, was much less sanguine. Today seen, especially in Germany and Japan, as an early advocate of ecological responsibility, Jonas was wary of what is deceptive in an unfounded rhetoric about progress. "Unless the present state is intolerable, the melioristic goal is in a sense gratuitous.... Our descendents have a right to be left an unplundered planet; they do not have a right to new miracle cures" (Jonas, 1980, p. 117). And Jonas was a critic of what he detected as a hidden religiosity in much of the rhetoric about scientific progress.

CONCLUSION

A⊤ **THE** **CONCLUSION** of his magisterial study, *Theology and the Scientific Imagination From the Middle Ages to the Seventeenth Century*, the late Amos Funkenstein did not exclude awareness of the current state of affairs when commenting: "The dialectics of open and closed knowledge characterizes the history of science from its outset" (Funkenstein, 1986, p. 358). Perhaps we are, as suggested by Amy Gutmann, especially today poised between the force of Jonas's arguments for an "ethics of caution" and what has continuing relevance in what in Benjamin Franklin (as a scientist) could be called a "heuristics of hope" (Gutmann, 2006). Whether, at least in matters having to do with knowledge that should or should not be disallowed, the tension of whether these two will remain positive or take a negative and ultimately destructive turn cannot at this time be known.

REFERENCES

Bacon, F. (1620/1978). *Novum organum*. In F. Baumer (Ed.), *Main currents of Western thought* (pp. 280–289). New Haven, CT: Yale University Press.

Beecher, H. K. (1966/1999) Ethics and clinical research. In H. Kuhse & P. Singer (Eds.), *Bioethics: An anthology* (pp. 421–428). Oxford: Blackwell Publishers.

Blumenberg, H. (1983). *The legitimacy of the modern age* (R. M. Wallace, Trans.). Cambridge, MA: MIT Press.

Böhme, G. (1992). *Coping with science*. Boulder, CO: Westview Press.

Caplan, A. L. (Ed.). (1992). *When medicine went mad: Bioethics and the holocaust*. Totowa, NJ: Humana.

Caplan, A. L. (1997). *Am I my brother's keeper? The ethical frontiers of biomedicine*. Bloomington: Indiana University Press.

Funkenstein, A. (1986). *Theology and the scientific imagination from the Middle Ages to the seventeenth century*. Princeton, NJ: Princeton University Press.

Gutmann, A. (2006). *Welcome remarks: Penn's Center for Bioethics 10th anniversary*. Speech delivered May 1. Philadelphia, PA (unpublished). Retrieved September 4, 2008, from http://www.bioethics.upenn.edu/symposium/

Harris, S. H. (1994). *Factories of death: Japanese biological warfare, 1932–45, and the American cover-up*. New York: Routledge.

Jonas, H. (1980). Philosophical reflection on experimenting with human subjects. In *Philosophical essays: From ancient creed to technological man* (pp. 105–131). Chicago: University of Chicago Press.

Kempner, J., Perlis, C. S., & Merz, J. F. (2005). Forbidden knowledge. *Science, 307*, 854.

LaFleur, W. R. (2007). Introduction: The knowledge tree and its double fruit. In W. R. LaFleur, G. Böhme, & S. Shimazono (Eds.), *Dark medicine: Rationalizing unethical medical research* (pp. 1–12). Bloomington: Indiana University Press.

Lloyd, G. E. R. (Ed.). (1978). *Hippocratic writings*. New York: Penguin Books.

Lloyd, G., & Sivin, N. (2002). *The way and the word: Science and medicine in early China and Greece*. New Haven, CT: Yale University Press.

Lock, M. M. (1980). *East Asian medicine in urban Japan: Varieties of medical experience*. Berkeley: University of California Press.

Montaigne, M. (1588/1958). Of cruelty. In D. Frame (Ed.), *The complete essays of Montaigne* (pp. 306–318). Palo Alto, CA: Stanford University Press.

Pernick, M. S. (1985). The calculus of suffering in 19th century surgery. In J. W. Leavitt & R. L. Numbers (Eds.), *Sickness and health in America: Readings in the history of medicine and public health* (pp. 98–112). Madison: University of Wisconsin Press.

Peters, T. (1997). *Playing God? Genetic determinism and human freedom*. New York: Routledge.

Rescher, N. (1987). *Forbidden knowledge and other essays on the philosophy of cognition*. Dordrecht, Netherlands: D. Reidel Publishing Company.

Rugnetta, M., Russell, J., & Moreno, J. (2008). *Genetic nondiscrimination: Policy considerations in the age of genetic medicine*. Washington, DC: Center for American Progress.

Shattuck, R. (1996). *Forbidden knowledge: From Prometheus to pornography*. New York: St. Martin's Press.

Shklar, J. N. (1984) *Ordinary vices*. Cambridge, MA: Harvard University Press.

Sugita, G. (1815/1969). *Dawn of Western science in Japan* (R. Matsumoto et al., Trans.). Tokyo: The Hokuseido Press.

Tsuneishi, K. (2007). Unit 731 and the human skulls discovered in 1989: Physicians carrying out organized crimes. In W. R. LaFleur, G. Böhme, & S. Shimazono (Eds.), *Dark medicine: Rationalizing unethical medical research* (pp. 73–84). Bloomington: Indiana University Press.

Conflict of Interest in American Universities

Perry B. Molinoff

CONFLICT OF INTEREST exists when a primary interest or goal is compromised or influenced by a secondary goal. At a university or academic medical center, the primary goal typically involves scholarship or the welfare of patients. Although we often think of conflict of interest as being primarily financial, there are many other conflicts or potential conflicts that are accepted as being part of the natural order in an academic environment. For example, obtaining convincing data on an important question has enormous potential benefits for an investigator. Benefits can include publications in prestigious journals, invitations to meetings, receipt of grants or prizes, as well as academic success, including, for example, the award of tenure. All of these potential rewards could cloud professional judgment. It is hard to measure or even to explicitly identify secondary influences like these, and we generally accept the fact that these pressures exist. In part because it is easier to identify financial conflicts of interest, most emphasis has been on the identification, disclosure, and management of financial conflicts of interest. It is worth pointing out that the existence of a conflict of interest doesn't necessarily mean that an offense has been committed. It may, however, raise questions in the mind of an observer as to whether certain results should be taken at face value.

In some cases the conflict is sufficiently blatant that most observers would conclude that inappropriate behavior has indeed taken place. For example, if the maker of a medical device offers a consultancy to the physician who chooses which of a variety of competing devices is to be used exclusively at his or her institution, then the presumption is that the maker of the device is trying to *buy* acceptance. Similarly, when administrators responsible for financial aid are consultants to companies that provide aid to students at their institution, then most observers would believe that the integrity of the situation has been undermined. A grey area is the amount of money required for a potential conflict to be seen as significant. What would be a small sum to one person could be very significant to another. The Department of Health and Human Services has taken the position that a significant financial interest does not exist if the interest for the investigator (and his or her spouse and children) does not exceed $10,000 and does not represent more than a 5% ownership interest in a single entity (Code of Federal Regulations, 2000). Most universities have accepted this guidance, although some have set lower limits and others have accepted equity interests up to $25,000. A further complication arises from the fact that it may be difficult or impossible to value an equity interest, as in the case of a start-up that is not publicly traded. Some institutions have taken the position that an equity interest that cannot be valued is by definition a significant financial interest.

HISTORICAL BACKGROUND

UNTIL RECENTLY THERE was little public oversight of biomedical science. Occasional examples of scientific fraud were thought of as aberrations, and improper behavior of any kind, let alone conflict of interest, was not even on the radar screen. The integrity of individual scientists was assumed, and universities were self-policing. Most potential conflicts were handled by disclosure of the nature of the conflict. Things changed in 1980 with the passage of the Bayh-Dole Act (Bayh-Dole Act, 1980). Under this act, ownership of intellectual property generated at universities and supported by federal funds resided at the university. The goal was to increase technology transfer by incentivizing universities to commercialize the scientific discoveries made by their faculties. Bayh-Dole had its intended effect but, by virtue of an increase in the possibility of financial reward, it may also have contributed to an erosion of trust in the academic enterprise. There is no doubt that Bayh-Dole has increased technology transfer for universities. The number of patents submitted on behalf of academic investigators has increased from approximately 250 per year before Bayh-Dole to thousands per year at the present time. This has led to an increase in revenue to both universities and to individual investigators. It has also increased the incentives for both investigators and institutions to encourage the patenting and licensing of new technology. Accompanying these increased incentives has come increased scrutiny. Several well-publicized instances involving potential or actual conflict of interest have taken place, and the ability of academia to police itself has been called into question. In some instances, patient deaths occurred in clinical trials in which the investigators had a financial interest. This is not to suggest that the investigators were necessarily driven or even influenced by the potential for financial gain. However, the possibility of such gain raises suspicion and leads to the asking of questions that should never have to be asked. One consequence of the media scrutiny that is initiated following the unexpected death of a patient in a clinical trial is the call for stricter and more burdensome scrutiny. For example, the recent death of a patient involved in a clinical trial at the National Institutes of Health (NIH) led to a significant strengthening of the rules relating to conflict of interest as applied to employees of the NIH. In this case, one of the clinical investigators running the trial in which the subject died was also receiving significant compensation from the company sponsoring the trial. The response of the NIH to this event was to require that senior employees divest interest in what were called "substantially affected organizations" in excess of $15,000 (Health and Human Services, 2005). Restrictions of outside activities included prohibitions of teaching, speaking, and writing for these types of organizations. Other prominent instances of conflict of interest included direct involvement of academic investigators with hedge funds and with extensive marketing efforts of pharmaceutical companies. The recent controversy in which the inventor of the Jarvik artificial heart became involved in direct-to-consumer advertising as a spokesman for Pfizer and the marketing of Lipitor is a case in point.

The federal government has regulated conflict of interest in federally sponsored research since 1995. The AAMC (Association of American Medical Colleges, Task Force on Financial Conflicts of Interest in Clinical Research, 2001) and the AAU (Association of American Universities, Task Force on Research Accountability, 2001) have been active in working with their constituencies to recommend approaches and to increase the visibility of the importance of being aware of and managing conflicts of interest both on the part of individuals and institutions. A survey carried out by the AAMC and reported in 2004 documented the progress made in bringing institutional practices related to at least individual conflicts of interest into a consistent framework (Ehringhaus & Korn, 2004).

The prevalence and extent of the financial relationships between investigators, academic institutions, and industry have been described and reported on by a number of investigators (see Bekelman, Li, & Gross, 2003). There is no question that support of academic investigators by the for-profit sector has been increasing. The growth of the private sector and its realization that it benefits from the capture of intellectual output from academia have taken place in parallel with a flattening of the budget of the NIH. This scenario has increased the willingness of academic investigators to look for and embrace nonfederal sources of support that are increasingly available from the private sector. In 2003 Bekelman et al. published a systematic review titled "Scope and Impact of Financial Conflicts of Interest in Biomedical Research, a Systematic Review" (Bekelman et al., 2003). They reported that between 23% and 28% of biomedical investigators received funding from industry, that 43% reported receiving research-related gifts, and approximately one-third of investigators had financial ties with companies. A great deal of concern has recently been expressed with regard to conflicts of interest of advisors to the FDA. The importance of the outcome of advisory committee meetings to the pharmaceutical industry cannot be overstated. Complicating this issue is the fact that in many instances a significant percentage of the physicians who have experience with and knowledge of the drug being considered have done research on or otherwise consulted for the company that is developing the particular agent. It is interesting that a bill was introduced in Congress in 2007 calling for elimination of waivers granted to allow an investigator with an acknowledged conflict of interest to participate in FDA deliberations. If this bill had become law, it would likely have had a significant impact on the ability of the FDA to recruit panels, and it might well have resulted in less knowledgeable panels. On the other hand, the presence of individuals on these panels with significant ties to industry and to the company whose product is being reviewed undermines public confidence in the fairness of the process and raises questions about whether the health and well being of the public is being adequately protected.

In an attempt to respond to concerns about the effects of conflicts of interest, the federal government implemented a set of regulations in 1995 that mandated disclosure of potential conflicts of interest by individuals applying for grants from the NIH or the National Science Foundation (NSF). This regulation is limited in scope in a number of ways. In the first place, it requires disclosure only to institutional officials who, in turn, identify the existence of conflict of interest to NIH and certify that it has been managed. Secondly, it requires disclosure only if the potential conflict relates to a project for which federal funding is being sought. Thus, the federal guidelines do not require disclosure by a conflicted investigator who is supported by private sources of funding. It should be noted that most institutions have established systems by which disclosure is required, regardless of the potential source of the funds. In many cases, a part of the routing sheet for a grant or for a protocol being submitted for institutional review board (IRB) approval involves identifying potential sources of conflict of interest. The regulations require each institution to have procedures in place to review, evaluate, and manage conflicts that are identified. The regulations further require grantee institutions to certify that existing conflicts of interest (but not the nature of the conflict or other details) will be reported to the Public Health Service awarding component prior to the expenditure of any funds under that award; that these conflicts have been managed, reduced, or eliminated; and that any subsequently identified conflicts will be reported" (Department of Health and Human Services, Office of the Inspector General, National Institutes of Health, 2008, p. 1–23). Although the regulations mandate that institutions develop policies related to identifying and managing conflicts of interest, they do not specify how conflicts should be managed, leaving that to the discretion of each individual institution. In addition, although certification is required, specific reporting is not. Thus, the NIH was unable to provide an accurate count of even the number of conflict of interest reports that had been received let alone the types of conflict that had been reported (Department of Health and Human Services, Office of the Inspector General, National Institutes of Health, 2008). This subject is further discussed later in this chapter.

FINANCIAL DISCLOSURE POLICY FOR RESEARCH AND SPONSORED PROJECTS AT THE UNIVERSITY OF PENNSYLVANIA AND AT OTHER UNIVERSITIES

IN RESPONSE TO the aforementioned federal mandate, the University of Pennsylvania and most other institutions have developed procedures to obtain financial disclosure by investigators and others responsible for the design, implementation, and reporting of a research project ("Financial Disclosures and Presumptively Prohibited Conflicts for Faculty," 2001). Prior to submission of a grant proposal or a project involving human subjects, investigators are asked to certify that neither they "[n]or their spouses and dependant children have any Significant Financial Interests that would reasonably appear to be affected by the activities proposed to be funded, thus creating a potential conflict of interest." A "Significant Equity Interest means any ownership interest, stock options, or other financial interest whose value cannot be readily determined through reference to public prices." A "Significant Financial Interest includes a Significant Equity Interest... but does not include an equity interest that when aggregated for the Investigator and the Investigator's spouse and dependent children, meets both of the following tests: does not exceed $10,000 in value as determined through reference to public prices or other reasonable measure of fair market value; and does not represent more than five percent (5%) ownership interest in any single entity" ("Financial Disclosures and Presumptively Prohibited Conflicts for Faculty," 2001, p. 3–5).

Several issues related to this policy have been noted previously. These include the somewhat arbitrary use of $10,000 to define a "Significant Financial Interest" and the fact that an institution has to certify that it has a policy in place but does not have to identify specific details of conflicts that are identified or the manner in which they are being addressed. One stumbling block is the policy regarding "Significant Equity Interests." An equity interest in a start-up private company is virtually impossible to value. In many instances, an investigator whose intellectual property has been the basis of a company will hold an equity interest. Since that interest may be impossible to accurately value, the policy would hold that this represents a significant financial interest. It is worth pointing out that nothing forces an investigator to accept equity in a start-up. An alternative is to have equity ownership assigned to the institution and allow the investigator to share in the distribution of future gains in accord with the patent policy. Although not eliminating the conflict, this approach can mitigate it. Another issue worth noting is that an investigator can have a significant conflict of interest if he or she is doing research sponsored by or related to the business of a company that is a competitor of a company with which he or she has a financial connection. We usually think about situations in which bias could lead to an overly positive interpretation of results, but the opposite may also be the case. Thus, a negative result could rebound to the benefit of an investigator who holds equity in a company that is a competitor of the company whose product is being investigated. Conflicts of this type may be difficult to identify, and it is the responsibility of the institution to make investigators aware that an indirect conflict is fully as real as a direct conflict.

Once a conflict has been identified, a faculty committee such as the Conflict of Interest Standing Committee at the University of Pennsylvania is responsible for devising an appropriate management plan. In nearly all cases, a critical part of this plan is full and open disclosure. Disclosure should be made on all publications and presentations and to all coworkers, including, specifically, students and trainees. It is important to emphasize that all of the obligations imposed by the patent policy remain in effect. Even if the work is supported by a commercial entity, the resulting intellectual property remains the property of the university. An entity responsible for technology transfer, such as the Center for Technology Transfer, will work with an investigator to arrange for licensing, including licensing to the sponsor. Finally, although not directly related to conflict of interest, it is important to note that no agreement should be entered into that in any way restricts or abridges the right and the responsibility of a member of the faculty to publish the results of his or her work. In most cases, a significant conflict of interest is managed by disclosure. One situation that is not managed by disclosure arises when an investigator has a fiduciary role with a company. A faculty member who is an officer of a company would not usually be permitted to receive research support from the company.

FINANCIAL DISCLOSURE AND PRESUMPTIVELY PROHIBITED CONFLICTS FOR FACULTY PARTICIPATING IN CLINICAL TRIALS AT THE UNIVERSITY

CLINICAL TRIALS ARE recognized as a special area in which research is carried out. The vulnerability of patients, complicated by the fact that they may be desperate, which, in turn raises questions about the meaning of informed consent, together with the nature of new therapies, which, almost by definition, bring with them indefinable risks, requires additional special precautions. The specific guidelines enumerated previously to identify a significant financial interest are the same for clinical research as for nonclinical research. However, in the case of nonclinical research, the usual management plan will include requirements for disclosure on publications and presentations and to students or fellows who might participate in the research. In the case of clinical research, the holding of equity greater than $10,000 or representing more than 5% of the stock of a publicly traded company would represent a presumptive prohibition for participation in a clinical trial (see "Financial Disclosure Policy for Research and Sponsored Projects," 2003).

One approach frequently used by the Conflict of Interest Standing Committee at the University of Pennsylvania is to determine whether there is a compelling circumstance that justifies a particular investigator's participation in a trial despite having a significant financial interest. Not infrequently, the trial in question represents a test of a particular hypothesis that the investigator was instrumental in developing. A company may have been formed around the technology in question, and the investigator may be highly motivated to be involved and may have uniquely valuable insights. The criterion currently used to justify a determination of so-called compelling circumstance is that the investigator, despite being conflicted, is uniquely able to carry out the proposed research. A possibly less arbitrary rationale for approving an investigator's participation would be to give explicit credit to an investigator who is doing clinical research in an area that he or she has pioneered. The advantage of allowing a specific exception for this circumstance is that it would explicitly acknowledge the value of the expertise of an academic investigator who has made a meaningful discovery, and it would relieve the investigator and the Conflict of Interest Standing Committee of the burden of trying to construct a compelling argument for a unique capability.

Another issue that occurs with clinical trials relates to the extent and level of participation permitted for a conflicted investigator. This specifically excludes an investigator from serving as Principal Investigator (PI) and excludes a role in preparing protocols, recruiting patients, obtaining informed consent, analyzing the data, and preparing manuscripts and reports. The policy as currently interpreted excludes essentially any contact with the subjects in the trial. One possible amendment to current policy would be to permit routine clinical care. In outcomes research, for example, it may be overly restrictive to prohibit a good clinician from providing routine care to a population of patients being treated with an experimental procedure or drug.

Once a conflict is determined to be manageable, a plan needs to be put in place. As discussed above, disclosure is a critical part of any management plan. Depending on the specifics of the situation, a monitoring committee may be required. In some cases, existing relationships between an investigator and a sponsor can make it impossible to devise a plan to make the conflict of interest manageable. An option may be for the investigator to renounce consulting fees, future royalties, or an equity share. Alternatively, an investigator can withdraw from the proposed study and retain his or her involvement with the company.

OTHER ISSUES

TWO OTHER ISSUES deserve mention. The first of these relates to the possibility that the Public Health Service will move to regulate or eliminate conflicts of interest on the part of academic investigators in much the same way that these issues have been addressed for employees of the NIH. As noted previously, the change in policy as applied to NIH employees followed the death of a subject involved in a clinical trial when it was discovered that an employee with critical responsibility for the trial was also a highly remunerated consultant for the trial sponsor. This has led to dramatic restrictions on the level of permitted interactions between NIH employees and commercial entities. The question is what changes, if any, should be imposed on the academic community? The Inspector General of the Department of Health and Human Services issued a report with the following findings (Department of Health and Human Services, Office of the Inspector General, National Institutes of Health, 2008, p. 3–13).

1. NIH could not provide an accurate count of the financial conflict-of-interest reports that it received from grantees during fiscal years 2004 through 2006.
2. NIH is not aware of the types of financial conflicts of interest that exist within grantee institutions because details are not required to be reported and most conflict-of-interest reports do not state the nature of the conflict.
3. Many Institutes' primary method of oversight is reliance on grantee institutions' assurances that financial conflict-of-interest regulations are followed.

In light of these findings, the Inspector General made the following specific recommendations:

1. Increase oversight of grantee institutions to ensure their compliance with Federal financial conflict-of-interest regulations.
2. Require grantee institutions to provide details regarding the nature of financial conflicts of interest and how they are managed, reduced, or eliminated.
3. Require Institutes to forward to OER (Office of Extramural Research) all financial conflict-of-interest reports that they receive from grantee institutions and ensure that OER's conflict-of-interest database contains information on all conflict-or-interest reports provided by grantee institutions. (Department of Health and Human Services, Office of the Inspector General, National Institutes of Health, 2008, p. 16–18)

The first and third of the recommendations call, in essence, for the NIH to work with the academic community to improve the database to be better able to track the types of issues that have been identified. These recommendations would also result in improved internal administrative systems at the NIH to provide oversight of conflict of interest. The NIH and the AAMC have come out in support of the first and third recommendations, but against the second recommendation. This second recommendation would likely lead the NIH to become directly involved in the oversight and adjudication of conflict-of-interest issues that arise at grantee institutions. The responsibility for monitoring and managing conflicts of interest has historically been delegated to individual grantee institutions. They have, in most cases, behaved responsibly, and effective conflict-of-interest management programs have been developed.

The second issue that deserves mention relates to what is called institutional conflict of interest. Institutional conflicts of interest "exist when academic institutions or their senior officials have a financial relationship with or a financial interest in a public or private company" (Ehringhaus et al., 2008, p. 665). These are issues that have only recently begun to be seriously addressed. In a survey of responses, Ehringhaus et al. (2008) reported that about 70% of institutions have policies applicable to financial interests of senior and mid-level officials. The need for policies of this type has become obvious, as evidenced, for example, by the consulting agreements that some administrative officials responsible for student financial aid have had with the companies providing this aid. A significantly smaller percentage of institutions (about 30%) have policies related to financial interests of the institution. It turns out that devising a reasonable approach to handle institutional conflict of interest is far from trivial. The intellectual property that is generated in academic laboratories tends to be at a relatively early stage. In practice, it is unusual for a large company to be willing to pay cash for a license to a university following negotiations with an office of technology transfer. More commonly, a license is taken that gives the university a share in the equity of a start-up company. When this happens, the university has become a partner, and there is an inherent conflict of interest. Banning the taking of equity doesn't appear to be a viable solution because it would significantly inhibit technology transfer. This would not be in the best interest of the investigator, the university, or the welfare of the public. Some institutions have taken the approach of appointing a committee of trustees to approve each instance of institutional conflict. This seems cumbersome, and it is unlikely that trustees would be willing to commit the amount of time that this approach would entail. A compromise might be to have a trustee committee approve general guidelines and be asked to specifically approve licensing agreements that rise to a high level of prominence.

CONCLUSION

CONFLICT OF INTEREST has become a high priority issue. More attention has been given to issues of individual conflict, but concern about institutional conflict has been increasing. A recent report by the AAMC-AAU Advisory Committee on Financial Conflicts of Interest in Human Subjects Research (Association of American Medical Colleges, 2008) made detailed recommendations about policies on individual conflict of interest as well as on the more challenging issues of institutional conflict of interest. The report also provided detailed recommendations on the implementation of policies to manage conflict of interest. Clearly the goal cannot be to eliminate conflict of interest altogether. That would be impossible given the complex world in which we live and the continuously increasing scope and depth of the interactions between the private sector and the academy. The formal aspects of identifying and managing conflict of interest have been growing and are likely to continue to do so. On the other hand, codes of conduct and sensitivity to the appearance of a conflict of interest can go a long way in maintaining and increasing the trust that the public has in the academic university and medical center.

REFERENCES

Association of American Medical Colleges. (2008). *A report of the AAMC-AAU Advisory Committee of Financial Conflicts of Interest in Human Subjects Research, protecting patients, preserving integrity, advancing health: Accelerating the implementation of COI policies in human subjects research.* Author.

Association of American Medical Colleges, Task Force on Financial Conflicts of Interest in Clinical Research. (2001). *Protecting subjects, preserving trust, promoting progress–Policy guidelines for the oversight of individual financial interests in human subject research.* Author.

Association of American Universities, Task Force on Research Accountability. (2001). *Report on individual and institutional financial conflict of interest.*

Bayh-Dole Act. (1980). P.L. 96-517, Patent and Trademark Act Amendments of 1980.

Bekelman, J. E., Li, Y., & Gross, C. P. (2003). Scope and impact of financial conflicts of interest in biomedical research, a systematic review. *Journal of the American Medical Association, 289*(4), 454–465.

Code of Federal Regulations. (2000). Title 42, Vol. 1, parts 1–399, cite 42CFR50.

Department of Health and Human Services, Office of the Inspector General, National Institutes of Health. (2008). *Conflicts of interest in extramural research, Daniel R. Levinson, Inspector General.* OEI-03-06–00460. Author.

Ehringhaus, S. H., & Korn, D. (2004). *US medical school policies on individual conflicts of interest. Results of an AAMC survey.* Washington, DC.

Ehringhaus, S. H., Weissman, J. S., Sears, J. L., Goold, S. D., Feibelmann, S., & Campbell, E. G. (2008). Responses of medical schools to institutional conflicts of interest. *Journal of the American Medical Association, 299,* 665–671.

Financial disclosure policy for research and sponsored projects. (2003). *Almanac of the University of Pennsylvania, 49*(32), 8–9.

Financial disclosures and presumptively prohibited conflicts for faculty. (2001). *Almanac of the University of Pennsylvania, 47*(21), 3–5.

Health and Human Services. (2005, August 21). *Federal Register, 70*(168). CFP Parts 5501 and 5502, RIN 3209-AA15 p. 51559.

Part V

Reproductive Technologies

26

Regulating Assisted Reproductive Technology: Avoiding Extremes

JENNIFER L. ROSATO

FOR OVER 25 years, infertile couples have sought the assistance of technology to create families of their own. During this period, a number of technologies have become available to couples who can afford them. In vitro fertilization (IVF) made it possible to unite a sperm and egg outside the uterus. Intracytoplasmic sperm injection (ICSI), a procedure in which sperm is injected into an egg, initially was used when male infertility was indicated and now is used extensively in IVF cycles to increase the probability of fertilization. Preimplantation genetic diagnosis (PGD), which allows the provider to detect genetic mutations in an embryo before implantation, improves the probability of giving birth to a healthy baby. Embryos are cryopreserved as part of standard fertility practice, and egg freezing is developing as an alternative for women who desire pregnancy later in life or after medical treatments that could cause sterility (such as chemotherapy).

Also during this period the population of prospective parents served by these technologies has not only increased in number but also has broadened to include single parents as well as gay and lesbian parents. The number of assisted reproductive technology (ART) cycles has doubled in the last 10 years, and the live birth rate continues to increase (CDC, 2005).

What has remained the same is an unsatisfying holding pattern in the level of regulation over these practices in the United States. Some regulation of ART exists, but it lacks coherence and direction. It also consciously fails to address the ethical implications of these practices, even though many of these implications are well-known and incorporated into the laws of other countries (Parens & Knowles, 2003). Overall, the law in the United States has fallen woefully behind emerging technologies, providing insufficient guidance to providers and inadequate protection to adult participants and children born of ART.

At the federal level, the primary legislation governing ART essentially takes a consumer protection approach by requiring fertility centers to provide information regarding the success of these practices. Such information—published in annual reports by the Centers for Disease Control—includes the percentage of IVF cycles resulting in a pregnancy or live birth and the average number of embryos transferred in a cycle (CDC, 2005). Federal agencies also have been involved in efforts to improve the quality of certain ART practices: for example, the FDA (Food and Drug Administration) oversees the safety of fertility drugs used and the quality of donated gametes and embryos, and the CMA (Centers for Medicare and Medicaid Services) is charged with overseeing standards for laboratories in which ART practices are performed (President's Council on Bioethics, 2004).

Some states have regulated a limited assortment of ART issues through statutes, such as those that determine parentage and set forth limits on surrogacy practice. And when disputes inevitably arise in this unregulated environment, judges need to step in. For example, judges determine parentage in family law when no statute resolves the issue, or they determine whether recovery should be permitted under tort law when harm occurs (Rosato, 2004). Through this incoherent approach, we have continued to avoid the difficult core ethical issues that need addressing, including protection of the health and well-being of the children created by ART and the women participating in these procedures.

Principled regulation is possible. Regulation has been recommended by the President's Council on Bioethics as well as numerous experts in bioethics and in law (President's Council on Bioethics, 2004). Canada's recently enacted Assisted Human Reproduction Act provides a model for comprehensive, principled regulation. The act implements the country's core values, including protection of the health and well-being of the children created by and the women participating in ART, as well as reducing commodification and exploitation. Based on

297

*Regulating
Assisted
Reproductive
Technology:
Avoiding Extremes*

these core values, Canada has banned some practices, such as human reproductive cloning, and is regulating others, such as gamete donation (Assisted Human Reproduction Act, 2004).

Although meaningful regulation of ART in the United States is possible, it remains unlikely. ART, like stem cell research, has been caught in the crossfire of abortion politics that has stalled any meaningful development in the law—thus contributing to the existing paralysis of inaction. Additional barriers to regulation are the strong desires of intended parents to create a family, the determination of doctors to make technology available and protect the doctor-patient relationship from outside interference, and the strong protection given to individual rights under the United States and state constitutions (Rosato, 2004). None of these barriers are insurmountable, however, and they need to be taken into account when considering any comprehensive approach.

Consistent with my prior work in this area (Rosato, 2004), this chapter advocates a continued, steady push toward principled regulation. First, the chapter identifies a unifying theory for regulation. Second, the chapter describes the ineffectiveness of existing approaches that guide existing practices. Third, it proposes a more centered approach that is both principled and incremental. Regulation would be guided by a desire to avoid a significant risk of physical and emotional harm to the children of ART or any adult involved in the process (usually women whose health is directly affected). Success would require collecting information regarding existing practices; collaborating across disciplines at the federal and state levels to provide guidance to lawmakers, providers, and parents; and controlling high-risk practices at the state level. This chapter considers how existing priorities would change with such an approach, particularly regarding PGD and implantation of multiple embryos.

A NEED FOR GUIDING PRINCIPLES

ONE REASON **ART** is not effectively regulated is that there is no unifying set of principles that guides lawmakers. The range of possibilities includes protecting the embryo, protecting children of ART, protecting the health of participants, protecting relationships, and protecting other societal values such as justice and equality. Some of these principles are difficult to articulate, and others are difficult to realize because of the lack of societal consensus in this area. For example, it may be difficult to agree on what "protection of human dignity" means (President's Council on Bioethics, 2004, p. xli) or to articulate how best to further "the well-being of our society" (Parens & Knowles,

2003, p. 53). And such broadly worded values would have a tendency to be expanded by those seeking more protective laws, causing pushback from those concerned with any expansion, thus perpetuating the legal paralysis we are trying to avoid. Any policy that would seek to protect preembryos would run head-on into our contentious culture clash over abortion and related issues (Malinowski, 2006).

In order to effectively move forward, I suggest regulation rooted in two related core values: protecting the health and welfare of the children of ART and of the adult participants in ART, particularly women. The safety of children and adults should be paramount, and they are core values likely to be shared by most members of society. These values form the basis for our child abuse and domestic violence laws, which are well-established and broadly supported at the state and federal levels.

In the context of ART, the protection of children and of adults has also been consistently asserted as paramount values by a number of authorities. Specifically, I propose that regulation of ART be designed to prevent a significant risk of serious physical harm to children or to adult participants. It is anticipated that this standard would move the law out of its existing holding pattern and make it more consistent with international norms. It would allow us to avoid making excuses for inaction and instead act on the values we can agree on. Thus far, the proposed approaches to limiting ART practices have been either not enough or too much.

EXISTING REGULATION: NOT ENOUGH OR TOO MUCH

THE EXISTING RANGE of regulatory responses is not desirable. This section highlights three approaches and concludes that none are appropriate models for limiting ART on a broader scale. A degree of recklessness is embodied by the current hands-off approach to PGD and preimplantation genetic screening (PGS), whereas excessive paternalism is evidenced by states that have equated or will equate the rights of embryos with the rights of children already born. Even the current "wait and see" approach taken by professional organizations to prevent high-order multiple births insufficiently balances the competing interests involved.

HANDS-OFF: PGD AND PGS

PGD INVOLVES GENETIC testing of a cell from an embryo that is a few days old to determine the existence of mutations that result in

299

*Regulating
Assisted
Reproductive
Technology:
Avoiding Extremes*

disease. It allows the provider to select embryos for implantation that are free of mutations (Baruch et al., 2006). A related procedure, PGS, tests the embryo's chromosomes for abnormalities to improve the likelihood of a successful pregnancy (Mastenbroek, 2007).

Introduced as an experimental procedure in 1990, PGD gradually became a part of infertility practice in the 1990s; in 2006, 74% of IVF clinics offer and provide PGD to their patients (Baruch et al., 2006). Even though it is estimated that thousands of IVF cycles have included this technology, this widespread use has not been accompanied by additional oversight. The CDC does not require reporting about the procedure, and the FDA has not asserted jurisdiction over it (Hudson, 2006). American Society for Reproductive Medicine (ASRM) recently has begun to address meaningfully the ethical and efficacy issues raised by PGD and PGS.

A 2006 study conducted by the Genetics and Public Policy Center shows that most clinics offer PGD to their patients for a variety of purposes: for detecting disease—including congenital diseases such as Tay-Sachs and late-onset diseases such as Alzheimer's—and for Human Leokocyte Antigen (HLA) matching, which allows a child to be born as a donor match to an ill sibling requiring a compatible donor. PGD is also offered for nonmedical sex selection in almost half of the clinics offering PGD and IVF, even though such a practice has been discouraged by ASRM (Baruch et al., 2006).

We still do not know whether the PGD and PGS procedures are safe for resulting children (possibly numbering in the thousands), as they have not been studied following birth. We also do not know if these procedures are helpful, as recent studies have revealed that PGS may not be effective in increasing the probability of pregnancy or live birth (Mastenbroek, 2007).

This hands-off approach to regulating PGD and PGS is far from exemplary and borders on reckless. It should not have taken 16 years to study these techniques, particularly because of their widespread use in fertility centers, potential harm to children, and the vexing ethical issues they pose. However, we need to be careful about moving to the opposite end of the spectrum and overregulating in the name of protecting children.

EXCESSIVE PATERNALISM: EMBRYO AS CHILD

CURRENT LAW RELATED to ART rarely demonstrates excessive paternalism. However, a few examples of such paternalism do exist. Notably, in Louisiana the legislature has established that an embryo, from the moment of fertilization, is a juridical person. Under this law, the embryo can sue or be sued and can be appointed a curator to protect its rights; it also provides for the physician to serve as temporary guardian when no intended parents are identified. As a juridical person, an embryo cannot be intentionally destroyed, which infers that cryopreserved embryos should either be used by the intended parents or placed for adoption whenever possible (La Rev. Stat. Ann, 2007).

Other states have introduced similar initiatives to protect the sanctity of life in the ART context. For example, one state recently introduced legislation to treat embryo donation as an adoption of a child, which would have required that all embryo donations in the state include a court's determination that the placement with the intended parents satisfies the best interests of the embryo (Texas H. B., 2007). Another state is considering a referendum to define life from the moment of conception (Colorado Human Life Amendment, 2007), and similar protective legislation is likely be proposed by other states.

This approach is certainly principled, as it expresses a strong value to protect human embryos. However, such an approach is unnecessary to protect the interests of children and is intended to further a value that may not be shared by the majority of the citizenry in the state. This approach also would cause slippery slope problems by arguably limiting current abortion and contraception practices in violation of federal or state constitutional law.

WAIT AND SEE: PREVENTING MULTIPLE BIRTHS

MULTIPLE BIRTHS HAVE been considered an unavoidable consequence of assisted reproductive technology, as it has been standard fertility practice to implant multiple embryos to maximize the probability of a live birth. More births have resulted because of these multiple transfers, including more twins and high-order multiples such as triplets and quadruplets.

It is well-established that multiple births pose significant health risks not only to the pregnant woman but also to the resulting children. Mortality rates for multiple births are significantly higher than for singletons, as are rates of preterm birth and low birth weight. Children born as multiples have a significantly higher risk of serious congenital birth defects such as cerebral palsy (Rosato, 2004).

The need to decrease the number of multiple births—particularly triplets and higher—has resulted in initiatives to increase the probability of a healthy singleton birth. The CDC reports that the number of singleton births continues to increase. In the most recent CDC report, when fresh nondonor eggs or embryos are used, the percentage of singleton live births is 68%, twins 30%, and triplets and above 2%. Just this year the CDC has begun to report the risk for preterm birth and low birth weight in ART (CDC, 2005).

301

*Regulating
Assisted
Reproductive
Technology:
Avoiding Extremes*

In addition, ASRM has continued to revise its guidelines on the number of embryos transferred. The 1998 and 1999 revisions to these guidelines, recommending limits to these transfers, have been correlated to a decrease in the birth of high-order multiples (triplets and above) from 1997 to 2003, with the greatest decrease documented in 1998–1999 (Stern et al., 2007). The most recent guidelines revision in 2006, recommending further limits, includes a provision that patients under 35 with a favorable prognosis should be implanted with a single embryo, with no more than two for any patient in this age group (unless extraordinary circumstances exist), and not more than two embryos for a patient between 35 and 37 who has a favorable prognosis (Practice Committee of the Society for Assisted Reproductive Technology & Practice Committee of the American Society for Reproductive Medicine, 2006). It is also notable that a major fertility center, concerned with the high rate of twin births, enacted a policy that limited transfer to one blastocyst and (as part of this policy) educated intended parents on the risks of twin births (Ryan et al., 2007).

Although laudable, these affirmative voluntary efforts have been insufficient to remedy the negative consequences of multiple births, especially the twin rate. The twin rate has not decreased since reporting began. And the new ASRM guidelines do not impose clear lines, still allowing the provider to consider individual circumstances. The consequences of compliance remain ineffectual. The guidelines state that providers be audited by the professional organization Society for Assisted Reproductive Technology (SART) if the multiple gestation rate for a center is more than two standard deviations from the mean rate for all SART reporting clinics for 2 consecutive years (Practice Committee of the Society for Assisted Reproductive Technology & Practice Committee of the American Society for Reproductive Medicine, 2006); however, these guidelines (like others) are voluntary, and noncompliance does not appear to result in meaningful consequences.

Realistically, providers are less likely to implant only one embryo because reducing transfer from two to one embryo is also likely to result in a decreased pregnancy rate; consequently, multiple implantations may be a risk the provider is willing to take to ensure that its success rate is not affected. This choice is particularly likely when it is the intended parents who insist on multiple implantations and choose to ignore the negative health consequences of having twins.

In the end, these voluntary efforts do not go far enough. They are not rigorous enough to improve the welfare of children, especially since each multiple pregnancy threatens the life and health of the resulting children—even twins. Moreover, such efforts are not part of a thoughtful, comprehensive approach guided by a collective desire to prevent harm to children and adult participants.

A CENTERED APPROACH TO REGULATING ART

IN ORDER TO regulate ART effectively, any standards should be reflective of the broader policies that guide intervention in this field. As discussed previously, these policies should be the protection of the health and welfare of children and adult participants in the ART process, and the standard of intervention articulated is to prevent a significant risk of serious harm. With this approach, we need to be careful not to define or apply the standard for intervention too broadly. For example, protecting the quality of the child's future relationships or the child's right to an open future are not sufficiently focused or agreed-on as directions for regulation.

For many reasons, it is unlikely that the United States will adopt a comprehensive approach to regulation or appoint a centralized authority to oversee ART, as Canada and Great Britain have done (Parens & Knowles, 2003). Instead, we need to consider a realistic approach that protects participants and children while valuing the doctor-patient relationship, scientific progress, consumer choice, and familial privacy. Three initiatives should be pursued in the near term: collecting more information about ART practices that have been and will be developed, collaborating across disciplines, and controlling high-risk practices.

COLLECTING INFORMATION

MUCH OF THE existing ART practice and its regulation are not based on current information because that information is not available. Before extensive regulation of ART practices is undertaken, much more information about these practices is needed. Studies such as the survey of PGD practices conducted by the Genetics and Public Policy Center provide a model for future inquiries (Baruch et al., 2006). Additional evidence is needed about specific practices, such as ICSI, egg donation, egg freezing, and selective reduction of embryos. Specifically, more information is needed about the impact of these practices on the physical and emotional health of women participants and the children of ART.

Some efforts to collect information have been recommended and should be implemented as soon as possible. For example, the President's Council on Bioethics proposed that children of ART be included in a national longitudinal study and that comprehensive studies be federally funded to determine the adverse effects of practices (such as PGD) on women and children (President's Council on Bioethics, 2004). A comprehensive PGD registry is being planned: this registry should be created as quickly as possible and be made part of mandatory CDC reporting to maximize accountability and communication of the information (Baruch et al., 2006). Another area for additional study was

303

*Regulating
Assisted
Reproductive
Technology:
Avoiding Extremes*

suggested by the Genetics and Public Policy Center: the short- and long-term effects of egg donation so that donors can assess the risks before they participate (Farrell et al., 2006). Overall, effective regulation can not be implemented without accurate data about the effects of these practices.

COLLABORATING ACROSS DISCIPLINES

ONCE ACCURATE DATA is collected regarding the use of ART and its effects, collaboration is necessary to determine directions for change. This collaboration should occur at both the national and state levels, with interdisciplinary advisory committees on ART existing at both levels. These advisory committees can expertly evaluate the data received and make recommendations for more studies, greater ethical oversight, or needed regulation. The representation of the committees should include a broad representation of interests, including fertility doctors, ob-gyns and pediatricians, ethicists, government representatives, and other policy makers. For the immediate future, the committees need to remain focused on the specific risks of serious harm, so there should be no litmus test related to a member's position regarding the status of the embryo or similar issues.

CONTROLLING HIGH-RISK PRACTICES

NOT ALL ISSUES that arise from collection of data and professional collaboration will require regulation. Some high-risk practices, however, require immediate governmental attention to reduce the risk to participants or to children of ART.

One area needing such attention because of the negative health effects on the children of ART is that of multiple gestations caused by transfer of multiple embryos. The health risks of multiples (even twins) are undisputed. Consequently, transferring multiple embryos (especially three and above) is a practice that poses a significant risk of serious harm and needs to be limited, even though it currently accounts for close to 50% of the ART cycles. The law should limit the maximum number of embryos transferred to three per cycle. In addition, we need to begin to move to a standard of one-embryo transfer. SART needs to more actively enforce its current standards that limit transfer to one or two embryos. There is an emerging consensus in favor of one healthy baby that needs to be enforced consistently.

Other practices, such as allowing older women (e.g., over 50 years old) to bear children or nonmedical sex selection, pose a risk of harm that is serious, but the probability of such harm is not yet known. Allowing older women to bear children could pose risks to the health of the mother and resulting children and raises concerns about children being orphaned by the death of an older parent. Nonmedical sex selection could lead to broader societal harm through discrimination and stereotyping, limited expectations of children based on gender, and manipulation of the male/female birth rates. One of the reasons for collecting data is to become aware of both the seriousness and likelihood of harm from these and other practices.

CONCLUSION

THE GAP BETWEEN the practice of ART and its regulation needs to be narrowed. Neither extreme—either a hands-off or an overly paternalistic approach—is desirable. Instead, what is needed is a centered approach that advances this technology and creates families while still adequately protecting the participants and especially the tens of thousands of children born with the assistance of ART each year.

REFERENCES

Assisted Human Reproduction Act, c.2. Retrieved November 23, 2007, from http://laws.justice.gc.ca/en/ShowFullDoc/cs/A-13.4///en

Baruch, S., Kaufman, D. J., & Hudson, K. (2006). *Genetic testing of embryos: Practices and perspectives of U.S. IVF clinics*. Retrieved November 23, 2007, from http://www.dnapolicy.org/resources/PGDS.pdf

Centers for Disease Control and Prevention. (2005). *Assisted reproductive technology success rates: National summary and fertility clinic reports*. Retrieved December 24, 2007, from http://www.cdc.gov/ART/ART2005/508PDF/2005ART508.pdf

Colorado Human Life Amendment. (2008). Amendment 48: Formerly Proposed Initiative 38, Colorado, Secretary of State. Retrieved September 9, 2008, from http://www.elections.colorado.gov/DDefault.aspx?tid=1047

Ethics Committee of the American Society for Reproductive Medicine. (1999). Sex selection and preimplantation genetic diagnosis. *Fertility and Sterility, 72*, 595–598.

Farrell, R., Baruch., S., & Hudson, K. (2006). *IVF, egg donation and women's health*. Retrieved December 2, 2007 from www.DNApolicy.org/resources/IVF_Egg_Donation_Womens_Health_final.pdf

Hudson, K. L. (2006). Preimplantation genetic diagnosis: Public policy and public attitudes. *Fertility and Sterility, 85*, 1638–1645.

La. Rev. Stat. Ann. (2007). §§ 9: 121–133.

Malinowski, M. (2006). A law-policy proposal to know where babies come from during the reproductive revolution. *Journal of Gender, Race, and Justice*, 549–568.

305

Regulating
Assisted
Reproductive
Technology:
Avoiding Extremes

Mastenbroek, S., Twisk, M., van Echten-Arends, J., Sikkema-Raddatz, B., Korevaar, J. C., Verhoeve, H. R., et al. (2007). In vitro fertilization with pre-implantation genetic screening. *The New England Journal of Medicine, 357,* 9–17.

Parens, E., & Knowles, L. P. (2003). Reprogenetics and public policy: Reflections and recommendations. *The Hastings Center Report, 33,* S1–S24.

Practice Committee of the Society for Assisted Reproductive Technology & Practice Committee of the American Society for Reproductive Medicine. (2006). Guidelines on number of embryos transferred. *Fertility and Sterility, 86,* S51–S52.

Practice Committee of the Society for Assisted Reproductive Technology & Practice Committee of the American Society for Reproductive Medicine. (2007). Preimplantation genetic testing: A practice committee opinion. *Fertility and Sterility, 88,* 1497–1504.

President's Council on Bioethics. (2004). *Reproduction and responsibility: The regulation of new biotechnologies.* Washington, DC: Author.

Rosato, J. (2004). The children of ART (assisted reproductive technology): Should the law protect them from harm? *Utah Law Review,* 57–110.

Ryan, G. L., Sparks, A. E. T., Sipe, C. S., Syrop, C. H., & Dokras, A., & Van Voorhis, B. J. (2007). A mandatory single blastocyst transfer policy with education campaign in a United States IVF program reduces multiple gestation rates without sacrificing pregnancy rates. *Fertility and Sterility, 88,* 354–360.

Shannon, T. A. (Ed.). (2004). *Reproductive technologies: A reader.* Lanham, Boulder, New York, Toronto, Oxford: Rowman & Littlefield Publishers.

Stern, J. E., Cedars, M. I., Jain, T., Klein, N. A., Beaird, C. M., Grainger, D. A., et al. (2007). Assisted reproductive technology practice patterns and the impact of embryo transfer guidelines in the United States. *Fertility and Sterility, 88,* 275–282.

Texas H. B. 1703. (2007). Relating to prohibiting the transfer of an embryo Except in an adoption proceeding: Providing a penalty. Retrieved September 9, 2008, from http://www.legis.state.tx.us/BillLookup/Text.aspx?LegSess=80R& Bill=HB1703

27

Choosing Future People: Reproductive Technologies and Identity

MARK GREENE

WHO WILL EXIST?

MY **MOTHER TELLS** the story of a high school friend who was teased because she was adopted. The friend retorted, "My parents chose me. Yours just had to put up with whoever came along." Back when my mother was in high school that pretty much closed the debate. At that time, the lottery of human reproduction was such that the only way to parent a specific individual was to take on the guardianship of someone who already existed. However, at about the time of this exchange, Francis Crick, Rosalind Franklin, James Watson, and Maurice Wilkins were laying the foundations of the field of molecular genetics (Watson & Crick, 1953). Subsequent advances in that field, in combination with the emergence of assisted reproductive technologies, may be changing the parameters of a debate that seemed so elegantly to have been won by my mother's friend in the middle of the last century.

For some time now, in vitro fertilization (IVF) and chromosomal analysis have allowed couples to screen for the sex of the embryo and for chromosomal abnormalities such as trisomy 21 (Down syndrome). More recently, preimplantation genetic testing has begun giving the means to detect an expanding range of genetic diseases, such as cystic fibrosis and Huntingdon's disease, and even to identify genetic markers indicating predispositions to diseases such as breast cancer. Early detection of chromosomal and genetic characteristics makes it possible for prospective parents to select embryos on the basis of those characteristics. Looking beyond embryo selection, scientists and ethicists have started to consider the possibilities of genetic manipulation and human reproductive cloning. Could advances in reproductive technologies make it possible to fix the reproductive lottery so that biological parents need no longer simply put up with "whoever comes along"?

According to Heyd, scientific advances suggest that "[w]e are getting closer to the power to choose at least some elements in the genetic character of future children, and hence their identity" (Heyd, 2003, p. 205). Does this mean that parents may soon enjoy some control over who comes along? We must be careful; there are multiple senses of *identity*, and this makes it difficult to interpret and evaluate claims about the potential of reproductive technologies to influence identity. This chapter will distinguish three notions of identity: qualitative identity, cultural identity, and numerical identity. Each notion raises distinct, though interrelated, ethical challenges.

QUALITATIVE FEATURES

IDENTICAL TWINS ARE identical in the qualitative sense; although they are distinct individuals, they may be nearly indistinguishable in their physical characteristics and may even share striking similarities of character. When Heyd talks about "designing the genetic identity of future children" (Heyd, 2003, p. 205), he is, presumably, thinking about interventions that will affect the genetic sequence, something that is a qualitative feature of individuals at the molecular level. At both the molecular level and the macroscopic level, the language of qualitative identity is apt to lead to confusion with other senses of identity. For this reason, it is better to talk about the *genetic sequence* rather than *genetic identity*, and about *qualitative features* or *exact similarity* rather than *qualitative identity*.

If there ever was a time when reproductive technologies were aimed only at the treatment of infertility, it did not last long. Even fertile couples might have reason to use reproductive technologies as a means of exerting some control over qualitative features of their future children. The possibility of embryo selection on the basis of chromosomal or genetic features and, even more pointedly, the possibility of embryonic genetic manipulation, raises concerns about what parents might do with the ability to influence specific qualitative features of their future children.

Some uses of embryonic selection, while not free of controversy, already enjoy broad acceptance in actual medical practice. The most widely accepted uses involve screening for serious genetic or chromo somal disorders. For example, couples may choose to undergo genetic testing before attempting to conceive. If testing reveals that prospective parents risk passing, say, cystic fibrosis on to their future children, then the couple will have the option to use IVF and preimplantation genetic diagnosis to select embryos free of cystic fibrosis.

More troubling is selection for nondisease-related characteristics. The most widely debated example of this is sex selection. While sex selection may be used to avoid certain genetic diseases such as hemophilia, it could also be used to serve straightforward parental preferences to have a boy or a girl. Some critics worry that allowing such practices may lead to an entrenchment of existing sexual prejudices and discrimination (Moazam, 2004; O'Neill, 2006; Warren, 1999). Others charge that such practices undermine an essential value in reproduction, namely that of acceptance and unconditional love of one's children whoever they may turn out to be (McDougall, 2005). Defenders of such reproductive choice tend to be more sanguine about the alleged threats to social justice. Stressing the value of reproductive freedom, they argue that since parents frequently do have strong preferences about such matters as the sex of their future children, allowing them to exercise the choices that reproductive technologies offer can actually promote acceptance of children (Heyd, 2003; Savulescu, 1999).

The ability not just to screen for genetic features but to manipulate the genetic sequence might extend the reach of reproductive technologies beyond disease prevention to genetic enhancement. It is easy to imagine parents being tempted by the hope of boosting IQ, sporting abilities, or physical attractiveness in their future offspring. Two kinds of issues make genetic enhancement seem especially problematic (Allhoff, 2005). One set of issues concerns the balance of risks and potential benefits. Characteristics likely to be of interest for enhancement are influenced by multiple genes in complex interaction with each other and environment. This complexity will make it especially difficult to predict either the impact of a genetic manipulation on a desired characteristic or its potential for untoward side effects. Adding to concerns about risk is the fact that adverse effects are likely to be especially far-reaching because they may be passed on to future generations.

The second kind of issue concerns the intuitive distinction between therapy and enhancement. Genetic enhancement would appear to overstep the bounds of what some regard as the proper province of medicine, the treatment and prevention of disease (Pellegrino, 2001). However, it proves surprisingly difficult to draw an ethically substantive therapy-enhancement distinction. Consider Henrietta, who has a normal IQ of 100. Imagine there is a synthetic drug that might boost Henrietta's IQ to 110 with no ill effects. If the drug substitutes for slightly low thyroid hormone levels, it would be considered therapy, but if there is no underlying abnormality it would be enhancement. It is hard to believe that this distinction could make a decisive difference in the moral permissibility of taking the drug.

CULTURAL IDENTITY

A N INDIVIDUAL'S CULTURAL identity is constituted by those cultural groups with which that individual identifies and that accept that individual as a member. Cultural identity is not fixed by matching objective features of individuals with the unifying features of cultural groups. For example, one does not have to be deaf to identify with and to be accepted by the Deaf community, and a deaf individual need not identify with Deaf culture. Notice, also, that an individual may have many cultural identities, some of which may overlap, others of which may be in tension with each other; for example, one person may consider herself an academic, Scottish (but not British), a woman, a Celtic fan, a socialist, and so on.

We have seen that reproductive technologies already give parents some influence over qualitative features of future children. Qualitative features can affect cultural identity both by influencing the likelihood that the future individual will identify with a particular cultural group and by affecting that individual's chances of acceptance by that group. For example, couples will often seek gametes from donors with whom they share a racial or ethnic background. Features such as skin color have historically been treated, and continue to be treated, as relevant for certain aspects of cultural identification and acceptance. However, physical appearance is not the only relevant consideration in this context. In Jewish law there is ongoing debate concerning the status of children born using donor semen. According to some authorities, the child of a Jewish couple who conceive using semen from a Jewish donor will be illegitimate whereas a child conceived using semen from a non-Jewish donor would not be (Schenker, 1992; Wahrman, 2005). Such distinctions may have profound implications for the future child's acceptance within some Jewish communities.

Discussion of issues raised by genetic screening is especially advanced within the Deaf community. The culturally Deaf community is not simply the community of those with hearing loss. Deaf

311

*Choosing
Future People:
Reproductive
Technologies
and Identity*

culture is characterized, amongst other things, by its own language, its own customs and mores, and its own history, all of which are distinct from those of the hearing community and not simply a subset of it. Many deaf people identify primarily with the hearing community, and there are active members of the Deaf community who are not themselves deaf. However, being deaf is certainly relevant to the probability that a child will grow up identifying with, and being accepted by, the Deaf community. Many members of the Deaf community see technical advances, such as cochlear implants and genetic selection against deafness, as threats to their community and culture. Middleton, Hewison, and Mueller (1998) report that a significant number of delegates at a conference focused on cultural Deafness would prefer to have deaf children. This illustrates both the significance of qualitative features for cultural identity and the fact that considerations of culture and community may be experienced as more important than some of the clinical criteria that are the focus in medical contexts.

NUMERICAL IDENTITY AND THE NONIDENTITY PROBLEM

A COMMON THREAD of concern with reproductive technologies is that the control they offer may be used to satisfy the whims of prospective parents more than to advance the best interests of their future children, in breach of parental duties to those future children. However, it has been argued, most prominently by Parfit, that there is a fundamental problem with standard accounts of our duties to future people; this is the so-called nonidentity problem (Adams, 1979; Kavka, 1982; Parfit, 1982, 1984). The nonidentity problem is a problem of numerical identity. No matter how alike identical twins may be genetically, physically, and even psychologically, they are distinct people. Identical twins are not identical in the numerical sense; if one twin commits a crime it would make no sense to punish the other, if one is harmed it would make no sense to compensate the other. Such basic ethical notions turn on numerical identity.

Imagine that Adam and Eve want to have a baby but Adam is infertile. Eve could conceive using donor sperm, but the couple decides they'd rather keep genetics inside the family. Adam and Eve consider an experimental reproductive cloning procedure: the nucleus of one of Adam's cells will be transferred into one of the Eve's enucleated eggs, which will then be stimulated to get it dividing, and implanted into Eve's uterus for what they hope will be a normal pregnancy. Adam and Eve are warned that a child cloned in this way is likely to have a shorter than normal life expectancy and will be more prone to health problems than a child conceived using donor sperm.[1] They sign up anyway, the cloning procedure is successful, and Seth is born. Although Seth is a happy child there are, as expected, problems; in preschool his mobility starts to be hindered by mild arthritis, he struggles intellectually, and is hit harder than his peers by the usual childhood diseases.

It seems clear to many people that Adam and Eve have done wrong. Perhaps the most straightforward way to justify that intuition is to appeal to a duty of care to future children that is breached by such risky reproductive choices. The intuition is that, just as present parents are duty-bound to set their own immediate interests aside in favor of the well-being of their *present* children, prospective parents' reproductive preferences are constrained by duties to promote the well-being of their *future* children. The President's Council on Bioethics places safety concerns at the core of its case against cloning to produce children, asserting that "concerns regarding the safety of the human cloning procedure ... are widely, indeed nearly unanimously, shared" (President's Council on Bioethics, 2002, p. 87) and that "risks to the cloned child-to-be must be taken especially seriously" (President's Council on Bioethics, 2002, p. 89). Even beyond the child-to-be there are possible grandchildren and great grandchildren-to-be who may inherit the ill effects of today's careless reproductive choices.

The attempt to ground an account of Adam and Eve's wrongdoing on a duty of care to future children runs into the nonidentity problem. Have they breached a duty of care to Seth? It is hard to see how Adam and Eve could have done any better by him. The choice was between having a child by cloning and having one by artificial insemination using donor sperm. A child conceived by artificial insemination might have been healthier and happier than Seth, but he or she would not have been Seth. Seth owes his existence to his parents' choice of cloning. The choice of artificial insemination would not have discharged a duty of care to Seth by making *him* healthier and happier, instead it would have ensured that Seth never existed. It is a strange duty of care that demands we should have ensured the nonexistence of someone who has a happy life.

The nonidentity problem is not confined to cases of cloning or embryo selection. Once noticed, the nonidentity problem appears to be ubiquitous in reproductive decisions and not only those involving reproductive technologies. Because of the facts of human biology, the identities of people are fragile. The slightest difference in the circumstances of conception can change the gametes that are involved, and hence can change who exists.

313

*Choosing
Future People:
Reproductive
Technologies
and Identity*

RESPONSES TO THE NONIDENTITY PROBLEM

I WILL NOW outline four strategies for responding to the non-identity problem. The first two responses share the intuition that nonidentity precludes personal wrongdoing. The third and fourth responses attempt to identify personal wrongdoing despite nonidentity, one by questioning assumptions about the notion of harm and the other by arguing that one can be personally wronged without being harmed.

One response to the nonidentity problem is to adopt a no-harm-no-foul view. Richard Adams takes this line in his nonidentity-based defense of God against the charge of permitting evil. Supposing that, if we cannot show a personal harm then we have no grounds to complain of having been personally wronged, Adams infers that "God has not wronged any created person [with a life worth living] by allowing evils that were necessary for that person's existence" (Adams, 1979, p. 56). While reproductive technologies do not make us gods, they do give us some influence over the evils that may be suffered by future people. If a reproductive choice gives rise to someone with a life of such profound suffering as not to be worth living, there may be a sense (though this is controversial) in which that individual has suffered a personal harm; her life of suffering makes her worse off than she would have been had she not existed. But most reproductive choices are not like this. In particular, Adam and Eve's decision to take a chance on cloning is not expected to result in a life not worth living. If their choice had harmed Seth, then he might have grounds to complain of a breached duty of care. But, since Seth is no worse off than *he* would have been had his parents chosen the more reliable option of artificial insemination, he has no such grounds for complaint. On the no-harm-no-foul view, the nonidentity problem shows that many of the duties we may have thought we had to future people must be illusory.

The second response to the nonidentity problem retains the intuition that we do have ethical duties to future people by denying the intuition that ethical duties must be owed to some particular person. Parfit himself is the most prominent defender of an impersonal response to the nonidentity problem. Parfit points out that we object to the wanton depletion of natural resources on grounds of the adverse consequences for our grandchildren and great grandchildren, but we find ourselves no less convinced of the wrongness of such policies when we reflect and realize they will change who our grandchildren and great grandchildren will be. To accept this is to accept what Parfit calls the "no difference view," the view that nonidentity makes no moral difference (Parfit, 1984, pp. 361–371). If we accept both the wrongness of wanton depletion and the no difference view, we must drop the assumption that duties are owed to particular people. Parfit suggests dropping the idea of owing personal duties to specific future people in favor of some impersonal comparative principle that it is worse if people are worse off, regardless of who they are (Parfit, 1984, p. 360). In this view, wrongdoing need not be personal. Seth has not been personally wronged by his parents, but Adam and Eve have done an impersonal wrong in that the person they bring into existence is worse off than the distinct person who would have existed had they chosen an alternative means of reproduction.

Noting that the nonidentity problem arises from the attempt to assess harm by comparison to nonexistence, the third response seeks an alternative notion of harm that allows us to identify personal wrongdoing, despite nonidentity, to Seth and to other progeny of careless reproductive choices. One way to do this is to defend an alternative basis for the welfare comparison, one that does not rely on the existence of any particular person. Candidates for an alternative baseline include identifying a so-called normal or a minimally decent level of well-being; Seth is wrongly harmed on such accounts if his welfare predictably falls short of that of a normal child or below standards of minimal decency (Archard, 2004; Steinbock & McClamrock, 1994). The great challenge for such accounts is to set a level of normality or minimal decency that is not morally arbitrary. Also, a standard of normality seems to frown on the reproductive freedoms of those whose children, though likely to be loved and happy, are likely to suffer greater than normal welfare limitations through genetic misfortune or social circumstances. Shiffrin (1999) takes a different direction in rethinking the notion of harm. She suggests a noncomparative notion, characterizing harms as conditions that obstruct or frustrate a person's efforts in life and that are experienced as things to be endured. The experience of illness or injury, for example, is one of endurance and frustration. Thus, even if Seth's arthritis does not make him worse off than he might otherwise have been, it is a harm on Shiffrin's account because Seth endures it as a frustration of his rational aims in life. However, as Shiffrin acknowledges, all children will endure obstructions and frustrations in life, and it is, therefore, a consequence of this view that all parents harm their children by bringing them into existence. It remains controversial whether an alternative notion of harm can do defensible moral work.

The final kind of response also attempts to identify personal wrongdoing in the face of nonidentity, arguing that there can be personal wrongdoing in the absence of any harm. Kavka offers, as an example, the case of lying to a terminally ill patient who wants to know the severity of his condition. A physician who lies wrongs the patient, even if lying is certain to ease the burden of his last few days (Kavka, 1982, p. 97). Kavka claims there is a "common intuition that there is something seriously wrong with people living restricted lives," that is, lives that are

315

*Choosing
Future People:
Reproductive
Technologies
and Identity*

"significantly deficient in one or more of the major respects that generally make human lives valuable and worth living" (Kavka, 1982, pp. 105–106). People who, like Seth, have shortened lives or significant handicaps, have restricted lives in Kavka's sense, even if they have lives that are, overall, worth living. If Kavka's intuition is correct, Adam and Eve might be held accountable for avoidably bringing Seth into existence with a restricted life; just as in the case of the lying physician, Kavka does not consider having done no harm to be a reliable ethical defense.[2]

CONCLUSION

BOTH PRACTICAL AND theoretical debate over reproductive ethics will continue. It may seem dispiriting that firm answers are so hard to find, but the careful search for ethical understanding has a value in itself. It is by struggling with difficult issues that we come to a deeper understanding of moral fundamentals and of our own nature. New reproductive technologies are an especially rich area of bioethical inquiry in this regard. Techniques such as embryonic selection, genetic manipulation, and human cloning force us to face practical ethical questions about the limits of permissible conduct in the area of reproduction. These advances also raise fundamental questions regarding ethical theory, human identity, and, especially in the context of the nonidentity problem, require that we rethink some widely shared ethical intuitions about personal harm and wrongdoing.

Nevertheless, there are some fundamental points that should inform continuing debate. Reproductive technologies do give prospective parents choices that influence qualitative features of future children. Thus, reproductive decisions can have great impact on our children's lives and well-being, both directly and indirectly via the contingencies of cultural identification. However, as identical twins demonstrate, qualitative features must not be confused with numerical identity. The prospects for genetic control of qualitative features are often exaggerated, and, in any case, no amount of control would enable parents to choose to conceive a specific future individual: despite technological advances, parents will continue to have to put up with whoever comes along.

NOTES

1. The first mammal cloned using adult cells, Dolly the sheep, was euthanized at an early age after suffering from health problems that may have been cloning-related. Other cloned animals have been found to have cloning-related abnormalities (Wells, 2005).

2. Kavka does not make entirely clear whether Adam and Eve would be violating a personal duty to Seth—suggested by framing the issue as one of harmless personal rights violations and in the modified Kantian duty (Kavka, 1982, pp. 97, 110)—or a more general duty to avoid the intrinsically undesirable societal conditions of more people living restricted lives (Kavka, 1982, p. 105).

REFERENCES

Adams, R. M. (1979). Existence, self-interest and the problem of evil. *Noûs, 13,* 53–65.

Allhoff, F. (2005). Germ-line genetic enhancement and Rawlsian primary goods. *Kennedy Institute of Ethics Journal, 15,* 39–56.

Archard, D. (2004). Wrongful life. *Philosophy, 79,* 403–420.

Heyd, D. (2003). Male or female, we will create them: The ethics of sex selection for non-medical reasons. *Ethical Perspectives, 10,* 204–214.

Kavka, G. S. (1982). The paradox of future individuals. *Philosophy and Public Affairs, 11,* 93–112.

McDougall, R. (2005). Acting parentally: An argument against sex selection. *Journal of Medical Ethics, 31,* 601–605.

Middleton, A., Hewison, J., & Mueller, R. F. (1998). Attitudes of deaf adults toward genetic testing for hereditary deafness. *American Journal of Human Genetics, 63,* 1175–1180.

Moazam, F. (2004). Feminist discourse on sex screening and selective abortion of female foetuses. *Bioethics, 18,* 205–220.

O'Neill, O. (2006). "Reproductive autonomy" *versus* public good? *Prenatal Diagnosis, 26,* 646–647.

Parfit, D. (1982). Future generations: Further problems. *Philosophy and Public Affairs, 11,* 113–172.

Parfit, D. (1984). *Reasons and persons.* Oxford, UK: Clarendon Press.

Pellegrino, E. D. (2001). The internal morality of clinical medicine: A paradigm for the ethics of the helping and healing professions. *Journal of Medicine and Philosophy, 26,* 559–579.

The President's Council on Bioethics. (2002). *Human cloning and human dignity: An ethical inquiry.* Washington, DC: Author.

Savulescu, J. (1999). Sex selection: The case for. *The Medical Journal of Australia, 171,* 373–375.

Schenker, J. G. (1992). Religious views regarding treatment of infertility by assisted reproductive technologies. *Journal of Assisted Reproduction and Genetics, 9,* 3–8.

Shiffrin, S. V. (1999). Wrongful life, procreative responsibility, and the significance of harm. *Legal Theory, 5,* 117–148.

Steinbock, B., & McClamrock, R. (1994). When is birth unfair to the child? *The Hastings Center Report, 24,* 15–21.

Wahrman, M. Z. (2005). Fruit of the womb: Artificial reproductive technologies and Jewish law. *The Journal of Gender, Race and Justice, 9,* 109–136.

Warren, M. A. (1999). Sex selection: Individual choice or cultural coercion? In H. Kuhse & P. Singer (Eds.), *Bioethics: An anthology* (pp. 137–142). Oxford, UK: Blackwell.

Watson, J., & Crick, F. (1953). A structure for deoxyribose nucleic acid. *Nature, 171,* 737–738.

Wells, D. N. (2005). Animal cloning: Problems and prospects. *Revue Scientifique et Technique (International Office of Epizootics), 24,* 251–264.

28

Ethical Aspects of Egg Donation

Luigi Mastroianni, Jr.

A S THE METHODS for harvesting fertilizable human eggs have been refined, the use of egg donors has become standard practice. In the initial phases of the development of in vitro fertilization (IVF) techniques, eggs were removed via laparoscopy or even laparotomy, usually requiring general anesthesia. Although hormonal treatment was used to induce the development of multiple follicles, the methods of egg recovery have long been refined to increase efficiency and safety. Present day methods for precise timing of the procedure to ensure accessibility of mature but preovulatoy eggs were still under development. These considerations resulted in low IVF success rates by today's standards but a ratc that the infertile couple was willing to accept because alternative methods of treatment were either not available or even less successful than IVF.

Given the complicated protocols involved, recruitment of volunteers to donate their eggs was problematic. In the present day climate, hormonal treatment allows predictable timing of egg recovery, and the recovery itself is carried out using ultrasound-guided needle aspiration under minimal sedation. These modifications reduced risks and substantially improved success and economic feasibility. As egg donation became increasingly practical, indications for its use have been expanded, and guidelines for the management of ovum donors have been refined. The American Society for Reproductive Medicine (ASRM) and its functioning component, the Society for Assisted Reproductive Technology

(SART), presented their first guidelines on ovum donation in 1998 (Practice Committee Report, 1998). These include recommendations for evaluating ovum donors as well as for testing of the embryo recipient.

INDICATIONS FOR THE USE OF DONOR EGGS

A T THIS POINT in time, women who have diminished ovarian reserves or premature ovarian failure are the principal candidates for donor eggs. These include patients who for a variety of reasons fail to develop a cadre of healthy eggs, as well as those who display evidence of persistently poor oocytes or embryo quality in prior IVF attempts. The indications for donor eggs have been expanded to include those women with a significant genetic defect or those recovering from surgery or chemotherapy for cancer, which would seriously impair ovarian function. Additionally, programs now accommodate same-sex male couples. This does, of course, require the availability of an embryo carrier but provides the comfort of genetic identification of at least one of the partners.

At the extreme end of the spectrum, donor eggs allow women to reproduce well beyond the normal age of menopause. The oldest successfully treated woman of record was 67. The use of donor eggs in recipients who are well beyond the age of natural menopause has been extensively reviewed. The major reason cited as justification to proceed in these cases is respect for a woman's autonomy. After all, men reproduce with seemingly no age limit and no societal restrictions. Most pregnancies involving older men, however, do not require the aid of assisted reproductive technology and occur naturally. Admittedly, there is a difference in attitude when a male in his 70s produces a pregnancy as compared with his female counterpart who is asking her body to sustain a pregnancy. The issue here is the ability to evaluate the safety of pregnancies among women in their late 50s, early 60s and beyond. On ethical grounds, these cases can easily be classified as human experiments, which, in my judgment, would require the input and evaluation of an ethics advisory committee, and in most institutions, discussion and approval of an institutional review board. Those cases that have received publicity and substantial press attention, by and large, were not explored in this manner. At the very least, women considering pregnancy at the extreme end of the age spectrum require the most meticulous of medical and psychological evaluations. There is no way to predict a woman's response to pregnancy, but clearly with advancing age comes increasing exposure to the risks associated with atherosclerosis and chronic hypertensive disease. In addition to consideration of the health issues facing the recipient of the donor eggs, one must also consider the impact on placental function, and hence, on the embryo and fetus as it matures. Clearly, uterine circulation is potentially less efficient as women mature into the menopausal years. Finally, there are the societal implications of intentionally producing a pregnancy well beyond menopausal age. There is more than a subtle difference between a pregnancy produced naturally and one that occurred after extensive medical intervention, including the use of donor gametes.

One can make a good case for seriously discouraging this use of reproductive technology. At the very least, the donor should be apprised of the fact that her eggs will be utilized to produce a pregnancy in a recipient of advanced age, and the IVF program should make every effort to abide by the highest standards of informed consent including meticulous evaluation of safety issues associated with human experimentation.

ADDRESSING ASPECTS OF SPERM AND EGG DONATION

WHEN REPRODUCTIVE RIGHTS are concerned, gender issues surface immediately when donor gametes (egg or sperm) are under consideration. The gender differences are striking. The use of donor sperm has been part and parcel of the practice of reproductive medicine for almost a century, although it has been refined in recent years. Standards have been codified and guidelines for efficient availability of properly screened specimens for infertility treatment applied. The standards for donor specimen screening have been modified. The most recent revised ASRM Practice Committee Report governing sperm donation was released in 2004 (Practice Committee Report, 2004). A potential donor is screened for genetic diseases and urinary tract infections. Specimens are frozen and quarantined so that the donor can be retested for HIV at 6 months. This protocol was arranged because the virus may not be detected at the time of initial screening. The semen specimen is divided into aliquots, which can be thawed at intervals for multiple uses.

We have a great deal of experience with sperm freezing in clinical settings, and numerous studies have confirmed its safety. Freezing allows much wider flexibility in terms of donor selection. Increasingly candidates for donor sperm turn to carefully monitored commercial laboratories, except in special circumstances in which a known donor has been identified. Whether or not the donor is known, the rigorous requirements that have long been recommended by the ASRM apply, and testing procedures used for anonymous donors should be applied equally rigorously to a known donor. It is the responsibility of the clinic to ensure safety measures and screen donors completely and without exception.

The differences between sperm and egg donation are striking. There are relatively few eggs produced in a given treatment cycle in contrast to the millions of spermatozoa in each donor semen specimen. The ability to freeze sperm is another substantive difference inasmuch as it allows repeat testing for HIV. Methods are emerging for direct testing of the initial semen specimen for HIV, which eventually may supersede the required double testing of male donors. The number of healthy eggs available for donation is influenced by age and hormonal status of the egg donor. This is a major factor that is obviously less important in the male, who continues to produce spermatozoa into old age.

The overall screening process for egg donors has been patterned on that used for sperm donors, but it is significantly more complicated. By and large, the male donor has less of an emotional involvement in the process, and his interaction with the agent/physician/clinic is limited as compared with the preparation required for a standard ovum retrieval cycle. The limited fertility span in women is also a factor in donor selection. An age range between 21 and 35 for donors has been recommended in the ASRM guidelines, and additional evaluation of this aspect is standard, including a measurement of follicle stimulating hormone (FSH) level on day 3 of the woman's cycle in addition to a general evaluation of menstrual function.

The emotional interplay between reproduction and the hormonal changes that precede it is quite different in the male and in the female and certainly warrants discussion during the selection process. The potential donor needs to be made especially aware of the possibility that success in the recipient results in a genetically related offspring. This aspect is all the more important in the event that the donor, unrelated to the process of donation, subsequently becomes infertile. Meticulous informed consent is all the more critical in donor egg screening and evaluation. The pressure to maintain an adequate supply of screened ovum donors can be substantial. Clinicians should be reminded at intervals of the importance of separating themselves from the practicalities of direct service. The most rigorous standards, including an extensive psychological evaluation, not generally required in male donors, must be applied in egg donor selection.

One source of donor eggs or spermatozoa is the known donor. Often this is a sibling or a friend. In these situations, it is all the more important as part of the screening process to evaluate the possibility of coercion or excessive reward. Psychological evaluation or counseling should be a part of the overall management. The potential impact of the relationship between the donor and recipient needs to be thoroughly explored. We at PENN Fertility Care (the IVF program of the University of Pennsylvania's Health System) have been approached on more than one occasion by patients who have established a new

relationship and whose daughter from her first marriage has supposedly volunteered to donate eggs. In these circumstances, the possibility
of coercion is significant. In each case, after extensive counseling, the
patient recognized the complicated set of relationships that would result and decided not to pursue this option.

The ASRM committee stresses the importance of the clinic maintaining permanent records on each donor including the genetic workup. In
addition, there should be some formal mechanism to link this information to each gamete (egg or sperm) donation and to retrieve the information as needed.

FINANCIAL COMPENSATION OF DONORS

PAYMENT IN RETURN for services, and specifically for the time
and effort that is involved in preparation and procurement of eggs,
has been the subject of vigorous controversy worldwide. In some parts
of Europe, monetary compensation is forbidden by law. This policy
has led to a marked slowdown in egg donation procedures (Heng, 2007;
Spaar, 2007). It was designed to mimic a similar ruling on sperm donation. In the United States, reproductive medicine has generally not been
the subject of legislation and regulation. The impetus toward legislation
covering aspects of IVF and embryo management has been blunted by
the efforts to provide guidelines by the ASRM and its affiliated society,
SART. As egg donation has been incorporated into standard practice, a
tradition of compensation has emerged. The ASRM Ethics Committee
has issued guidelines specifically addressing the financial incentives
and recruitment of egg donors (Ethics Committee of the ASRM, 2004).
The two ethical questions that have surfaced are: (a) Are the interests
of the egg donors protected in the course of the recruitment practices?
and (b) Do financial incentives treat eggs as property or commodities
and therefore devalue human life? Those providing donor eggs include
women undergoing IVF who are willing to share any excess eggs. This
option became less available when techniques were developed for reliable frozen storage of their fertilized eggs for their own future use. For
a woman undergoing IVF who expresses willingness to share excess
eggs with another person, the provision of a discounted fee has been
utilized by some centers. The ethical dilemmas raised by a two-class
system of medical care, especially in reproductive services, remain a
major source of concern. Egg-sharing programs have been reported
to exist in a number of countries including the United Kingdom,
Israel, Denmark, Australia, Spain, and Greece (Ahuja, Simons, Mostyn, &
Bowen-Simpkins, 1998). Such programs and their proponents should
consider the distress that would occur if the donor failed to conceive

knowing that another woman might have successfully established a pregnancy using her eggs. This approach has been criticized as an indirect form of egg and ultimately child buying (National Advisory Board on Ethics in Reproduction, 1996).

Justification for financial incentives for egg donors is based on the idea that although egg donation is an act of giving, women who donate ought to benefit in a tangible way (Ahuja, Mostyn, & Simons, 1997). Certainly, it would be inappropriate to allow compensation of males for providing spermatozoa and not of females for providing eggs. The compensation ought to be for the time and effort involved in a procedure that is more complicated than obtaining a semen specimen. Every effort should be made to minimize the possibility of undue influence and exploitation. This can usually be accomplished by appropriate psychological evaluation and counseling (Braverman, 1993). Informed consent ought to be carried out, and the donor should be adequately counseled as to the potential risks of the procedure including the psychological risk, especially if later the donor herself suffers infertility. In general, it is essential that donors receive accurate and clearly spelled out information on the psychological and physical effects of the whole process of egg retrieval and donation. That makes it all the more important to limit donors to women who are at least 21 years of age so that one can be reasonably sure they have the emotional maturity required for such a decision. The ASRM Ethics Committee suggests that donors be given the opportunity to decide how their eggs should be used—that is, would they be willing to provide them for same-sex couples or unmarried persons?

It is generally agreed that financial compensation should reflect the time, inconvenience, and the physical and emotional demands associated with egg donation. The ASRM Ethics Committee finally concluded that sums of $5,000 or more require some justification. Amounts over $5,000 were in 2004 adjudged inappropriately excessive. The amount of compensation should not be based on the number and quality of eggs retrieved or on the donor's ethnic or other personal characteristics. In a 2006 survey of the United States, the national standard of donor compensation was $4,217, highest in the east/northeast at $5,018 (Covington & Gibbons, 2007).

DONOR ANONYMITY

THE ISSUE OF donor anonymity surfaces repeatedly in couples who use both sperm and egg donations. Since the earliest experience with donor sperm, common practice was to maintain secrecy. After conception, it remained a never-to-be-discussed matter out of concern that such knowledge would somehow alter the relationship between the child and the social/legal father. The importance of genetic status accompanied by an increased openness in reproductive matters has been the major impetus behind re-exploring this approach. Increasingly, couples have elected to inform offspring regarding the method by which their conception occurred. When considering the appropriate timing of sharing this information, it is important to take into consideration the age of the offspring, as well as their level of understanding.

In general, ovum donation programs have tended to encourage open discussion. A firm roadmap providing guidelines to this approach is not often available during this interchange between counselors and prospective parents. This is a very individual matter heavily dependent on the emotional makeup of those involved. The wishes and feelings of the donor must play an important role in this decision. The donor must agree to the disclosure in advance, and the specific level of disclosure must be acceptable to her. Standard systems have been worked out to ensure that the interests of both the recipient couple and the donor are respected.

In recent times, it has been suggested that the parental relationships following pregnancies resulting from the use of donor gametes are no different than those observed in adoption. Many argue that the similarities justify firmly held positions that disclosure should not only be encouraged but required (McGee, Brakman, & Gurmankin, 2001). The experience with adoption disclosure has been, by and large, positive. Others, however, take the position that adoption and donor gamete pregnancies are sufficiently dissimilar as to allow parental discretion in this matter (Patrizio, Mastroianni, & Mastroianni, 2001). With donor gamete pregnancy, one parent is in fact the biological parent and the other the social parent. In the case of adoption, neither parent has a biological link to the child. The adopted child was relinquished by his or her genetic parents. A child conceived through the use of a donor gamete faces different psychological issues. This offspring does not face a psychological sense of rejection by biological parents that is implied by adoption. Most critical is the fact that the mother of the child conceived with gamete donation usually has carried the pregnancy, which in and of itself establishes a psychological bond. Furthermore, intimate maternal-infant interaction continues postpartum, including breast feeding.

Finally, the matter of parental responsibility on the part of the donor comes into play. In the United States, there is no legal requirement for disclosure in contrast to the arrangements in several other countries in which systems for disclosure are prearranged, so that in each case the donor is willing to be identified in the future. Such arrangements encourage some to seek out reproductive services in countries that have less restrictive guidelines (Spar, 2007). In a large survey, in less than 15% of cases was the information shared with the offspring. Forty percent shared it with no one. Eighty-seven percent reported that were they to do it again, they would not tell anyone (Klock & Maier, 1991).

THE DONOR EGG PROGRAM AT PENN

ALTHOUGH THE IVF program at Penn was initiated in 1982, a comprehensive egg donor component was not organized until 2003. There were many reasons for this delay. PENN Fertility Care is an integral component of the University of Pennsylvania Medical Center. It is structured within the Division of Reproductive Endocrinology and Infertility of the Department of Obstetrics and Gynecology. It addresses the traditional missions of an academic medical center with its emphasis on teaching and research as well as patient care. The financial and interpersonal relations in such an arrangement have been extensively reviewed and debated (Reindollar, 2005; Soules, 2005a, 2005b). Fertility programs that include a donor egg program demand substantial departmental and institutional commitment. They require both administrative flexibility and the enthusiastic and selfless personal commitment of the clinic staff. They are labor intensive and generate significant overhead expenses. As procedures were refined with decreased risks and sacrifice on the part of the donor, as well as increased success rates for the recipient, it soon became clear that a program such as ours was not complete without offering this service. This decision was reinforced by the increasing numbers of patients in our practice for whom a donor egg procedure was the only realistic option. A structure has been designed to allow the IVF team to provide uncompromising patient care while maintaining its academic integrity in an increasingly complex marketplace.

CONCLUSION

ARTIFICIAL INSEMINATION WITH sperm from a third party has long been looked on as acceptable in clinical practice, at least for those who have no religious or ethical objections. More recently, development of techniques to recover functional eggs, which are then fertilized and transferred to a recipient uterus, has also become increasingly utilized. Although obtaining eggs requires greater manipulation and planning than that required for sperm, the ethical and social issues surrounding their use are remarkably similar. Some situations are, however, unique to eggs. Chronological age of the recipient has a direct affect on the quality and availability of eggs. Indeed, one of the principal indications for donor egg use is failure of the recipient's ovaries to produce healthy eggs. Accessibility of eggs and ease of manipulation is adversely affected by our current inability to freeze and store them for later clinical use. This will change as frozen storage methods are developed in the laboratory. In spite of these constraints, there has been an increased use of donor eggs. Indications for their use have, in some cases, been explored without carefully considering their ethical ramifications. One example of the premature application of donor eggs is their use in recipients who are well beyond the age of actual menopause. Those in influential positions should be mindful of the larger picture as these remarkable advances in infertility treatment mature.

REFERENCES

Ahuja, K. K, Mostyn, B. J., & Simons, E. G. (1997). Egg sharing and egg donation: Attitudes of British egg donors and recipients. *Human Reproduction, 12,* 2845–2852.

Ahuja, K. K., Simons, E. G., Mostyn, B. J., & Bowen-Simpkins, P. (1998). An assessment of the motives and morals of egg share donors: Policy of "payments" to egg donors requires a fair review. *Human Reproduction, 13,* 2671–2678.

Braverman, A. M. (1993). Survey results on the current practice of ovum donation. *Fertility and Sterility, 59,* 1216–1220.

Covington, S. N., & Gibbons, W. E. (2007). What is happening to the price of eggs? *Fertility and Sterility, 87,* 1001–1004.

Ethics Committee of the ASRM. (2004). Financial incentives in recruitment of oocyte donors. *Fertility and Sterility, 82*(Suppl.), S240–S244.

Heng, B. C. (2007). Should fertility specialists refer local patients abroad for shared or commercialized oocyte donation? *Fertility and Sterility, 87,* 6–7.

Klock, S., & Maier, D. (1991). Psychological factors related to donor insemination. *Fertility and Sterility, 56,* 489–495.

McGee, G., Brakman, S. V., & Gurmankin, A. D. (2001). Gamete donation and anonymity: Disclosure to children conceived with donor gametes should not be optional. *Human Reproduction, 16*(10), 2033–2036.

National Advisory Board on Ethics in Reproduction. (1996). Report and recommendations on oocyte donation. In C. B. Cohen (Ed.), *New ways of making babies: The case of egg donation* (pp. 233–247). Bloomington: Indiana University Press.

Patrizio, P., Mastroianni, A. C., & Mastroianni, L. (2001). Disclosure to children conceived with donor gametes should be optional. *Human Reproduction, 16*(10), 2036–2038.

Practice Committee Report. (1998). Guidelines for oocyte donation. *Fertility and Sterility, 70*(3 Suppl.), S5–S6.

Practice Committee Report. (2004). Guidelines for sperm donation. *Fertility and Sterility, 82*(1 Suppl.), S9–S11.

Reindollar, R. H. (2005). Assisted reproductive technology has been detrimental to academic reproductive endocrinology and infertility: Depth of the problem and possible solutions. *Fertility and Sterility, 84*, 580–582.

Soules, M. R. (2005a). Assisted reproductive technology has been detrimental to academic reproductive endocrinology and infertility. *Fertility and Sterility, 84*, 570–573.

Soules, M. R. (2005b). Reflections on the differences between academic medicine and private practice. *Fertility and Sterility, 84*, 583.

Spar, D. (2007). The egg trade—making senses of the market for human oocytes. *New England Journal of Medicine, 356*, 1289–1291.

29

Ethical Aspects of Male Infertility

GEORGIOS KARNAKIS AND PASQUALE PATRIZIO

INFERTILITY IS DEFINED as the inability to conceive after a year of regular unprotected intercourse, and in about 50% of the cases, the male is identified as responsible for the reproductive malfunction (Galan et al., 2006), either exclusively (about 30%) or as coresponsible (about 20%; Oehninger & Kruger, 2007). Physicians who care for infertile couples must thus know how to perform a basic evaluation of the male reproductive function and, furthermore, need to recognize men who require more extensive evaluation by fertility specialists. The initial screening relies on at least two semen analyses performed at 6-week intervals. Of note, although far from being ideal, the results of the semen analysis are still universally used as indicators of male fertility. Currently, the reference values for normal males include a minimum volume of 2.0 ml, a pH between 7.2 and 7.8, a concentration of 20×10^6 spermatozoa/mL or greater, and a total sperm number of at least 40×10^6 spermatozoa per ejaculate (Payne & Lamb, 2004). Additional parameters are motility of 50% or more, vitality of at least 50%, and white blood cell count of fewer than 1×10^6/mL. Sperm morphology is also considered part of the standard semen analysis and can be assessed according to the World Health Organization manual or to other strict criteria. In absence of an absolute specific value, it is accepted that when sperm-normal morphology falls below 30%, the rate of fertilization in vitro decreases.

TABLE 29.1   Commonly Used Definitions of Male Infertility

1. *Azoospermia*, which means no sperm in the ejaculate, affecting 25% of infertile males.
2. *Oligoasthenozoospermia*, which means low sperm count and low motility, affecting 60% of infertile males.
3. *Teratozoospermia*, which means all sperm are non viable or with severe abnormal morphology, affecting 5% of infertile males.
4. *Coital factors,* including men with paraplegia, men with retroperitoneal lymph node dissection because of prostatic cancer, and men with retrograde ejaculation, affecting 10% of infertile males.

Although it is widely recognized that a number of definitions are responsible for male infertility, a considerable percentage of cases are still of unknown etiology. Table 29.1 is a summary of the most commonly known causes of male infertility, reported according to the results of the semen analysis and categorized into four groups.

The field of male infertility, as with its corresponding female counterpart, is constantly adjourning policies and guidelines to keep reproductive options open. These strategies are subject to ethical debates. One example is the ongoing ethical challenge raised by fertility preservation of cancer patients. As survival rates of patients stricken by cancers during their reproductive years increase, fertility preservation by sperm banking is becoming a reasonable and effective option for men who require chemotherapy or radiation treatment. It can serve as a backup in the event that spermatogenesis does not rebound after treatment. However, it is important to discuss, at the time of sperm banking, what will be the directives regarding the specimens, should a patient die. It is equally important to recognize experimental approaches versus established practices, particularly when children are the subjects of research studies aiming at protecting their future reproductive options. Other examples are the use of donor sperm and parental ambivalence regarding disclosure to future offspring, potential limitations on the number of offspring each sperm donor should be allowed to sire, and some issues surrounding posthumous conception.

USE OF DONOR SPERM TO PROCREATE

IN THE LAST few years, thanks to the advent of intracytoplasmic sperm injection (ICSI) for the treatment of infertile males with very low sperm counts and motility, the requests for donor sperm insemination (DI) have been drastically reduced. In fact, while in 1987 there were about 170,000 inseminations per year, in 2004 there were only 80,000 inseminations with donor sperm (Payne & Emmet, 2004).

Nonetheless, these figures translate into about 30,000 births per year due to DI.

The practice of donor sperm insemination raises two major ethical issues:

1. Should donor sperm identity be kept anonymous and should disclosure to children conceived with donor sperm be optional or mandatory?
2. Should there be a maximum number of pregnancies achieved by the same donor?

SHOULD DISCLOSURE TO CHILDREN CONCEIVED WITH DONOR SPERM BE OPTIONAL OR MANDATORY?

IN THE UNITED States most, if not all, sperm banks and DI programs offer recipients of donor sperm the option of using open-identity donors (i.e., donors who consent to have their identities revealed to a future child resulting from the use of their sperm). In other countries, such as Sweden and the United Kingdom (Scheib, Riordan, & Rubin, 2005), recipients are required to use open-identity donors. An immediate consequence of open donor identity has been a sharp decrease in the availability of donors. In addition, there has been a shift in the characteristics of men donating sperm: they are more senior and already have a family of their own; they have become more aware of the consequences of their donation and are accepting this increased responsibility.

An important factor in deciding whether donor anonymity should be removed is the well-being of the child. For parents who plan to tell their child about his or her conception origins, having as much information as possible may help answer a child's questions as they arise. For example, about half the children in a sample of lesbian-headed families wanted more information about their donor (American Society for Reproductive Medicine, 2007).

Testimonials from DI youths and adults who learned of their origins before adulthood also indicate that individuals feel less resentment toward their family than those that found out on their own, but the desire and need to know more about the donor remains. Some have argued that, for the well-being of the children, disclosure should be mandatory and that children resulting from gamete donation should be compared to children from adoption (who are almost universally told of their origin). At the moment, however, there is no conclusive evidence to support a forced disclosure. Furthermore, it is incorrect to compare the practice of gamete donation to adoption. In the case of sperm donation, one of the parents—the mother—is the biological parent, while the father is the social parent. In the case of adoption, both parents are nonbiological, social parents.

In addition, if a policy requiring disclosure has to be truly effective, various conditions need to be satisfied. These include: (a) a couple willing to reveal the origin of the gametes to their offspring; (b) a donor who is willing to donate his spermatozoa knowing that later he may be identified, as a segue to mandatory disclosure of gamete origin; (c) a system of enforcement to ensure that the couple will reveal the source of the gamete (perhaps through the use of a special notation on the birth certificate); (d) health providers who will restrict reproductive services only to couples who agree to sign a consent for disclosure; (e) assurance that the provider of obstetric care, usually a different physician, is informed by the couple of the means by which reproduction was achieved and made aware of the existence of consent to disclose in order to complete the birth certificate.

This list, by no means complete, makes the issue of disclosure quite complicated. Requiring potential parents to tell their child of his/her genetic origin as a condition for admission into a infertility program may be seen as discriminatory (Patrizio, Mastroianni, & Mastroianni, 2001). Actually, forced disclosure, rather than protecting the child's interest, may have the outcome of not creating a child at all, because potential parents and clinics may find the burden of controlling disclosure too heavy and may forgo the process altogether. In countries where the identification of the donor is required by law, such as the Netherlands, Sweden, and the United Kingdom (U.K. legislation in April 2005 imposed mandated disclosure), the pool of sperm donors has substantially decreased, and many clinics have ceased using this option or have such long waiting lists that couples are giving up.

A BBC survey in September 2006 found that 90% of U.K. sperm donors were recruited in just 10 of 87 licensed clinics for donor insemination and that after the removal of donor anonymity, the cost of purchasing sperm rose very substantially—about an eight-fold increase. Between 2004 and 2006 there was a 30% reduction in patients requiring donor insemination but a much larger, about 45%, reduction in the number of treatment cycles using donor sperm.

A 2008 survey of DI services by the British Fertility Society found that:

- 37 per cent of clinics are finding it harder to recruit donors
- 94 per cent of clinics are finding it harder to buy in donor sperm
- 74 per cent of clinics have increased waiting lists for DI treatment
- 86 per cent of clinics are able to offer less choice of donors and are only able to match for racial group.

‹ 60 per cent have introduced rationing of treatment cycles
‹ 9 per cent have closed their DI service
‹ 89 per cent charge more for treatment because of the increased cost of the sperm they are able to purchase. (Wardle & Skew, 2008)

The impact of the legislation to remove donor anonymity has confirmed those concerns expressed by the opponents of a mandatory disclosure law (Patrizio, Mastroianni, & Mastroianni, 2001). A possible solution to this problem would be to review and amend the current legislation to give donors the choice of retaining complete anonymity, disclosing only nonidentifying information, or being identified in the way the law currently requires. Couples needing DI treatment would then, at the very least, have the choice of deciding whether they want sperm from a donor who is prepared to be identified in the future.

SHOULD THERE BE A MAXIMUM NUMBER OF PREGNANCIES ACHIEVED BY THE SAME DONOR?

IT IS VERY important to maintain detailed medical records of the number of pregnancies for which a given donor is responsible and to try to establish a limit. It is difficult, however, to provide a precise number of times that a given donor can be used because one must take into consideration the population base from which the donor is selected and the geographic area that may be served by a given donor. According to ASRM guidelines it has been suggested that in a population of 800,000, limiting a single donor to no more than 25 births (ASRM, 2006) would avoid any significant increased risk of inadvertent consanguineous conception. This suggestion may require modification if the population using donor insemination represents an isolated subgroup or if the specimens are distributed over a wide geographic area. In the future, keeping in mind the issues of patient confidentiality, providers of reproductive care and sperm banks should devise a database tracking system to avoid the recruitment of the same sperm donor in excess of the limit set for pregnancies within a particular geographic area.

FERTILITY PRESERVATION

THE CONTEMPORARY USE of powerful chemotherapeutic and radiotherapy protocols are procuring a cure for, or significantly extending the survival of, many patients with cancer. As a result of this progress, quality of life issues after cancer are emerging, including the protection of future fertility from the toxicity of cancer treatments. Five-year survival rates with testicular cancer, hematology malignancies, and other cancers (sarcoma) that strike young people may be in the 90%–95% range. However, treatment of these cancers is often highly detrimental to male reproductive function, and as a consequence 20%–25% of these patients become irreversibly sterile (The Ethics Committee of the American Society for Reproductive Medicine, 2005). The testis is highly susceptible to the toxic effects of radiation and chemotherapy at all stages of life. Cytotoxic chemotherapy and radiotherapy may produce long-lasting or persistent damage to spermatogonial (primordial) cells, leading to oligo- or azoospermia. One of the most effective and established methods for preserving fertility in males affected by cancer is sperm banking by cryopreservation. However, in some other circumstances, such as prepubertal boys or adolescents unable to produce a sample by ejaculation, gonadal tissue biopsy may also help to preserve fertility. Surveys of cancer patients reveal a very strong desire to be informed of available options for fertility preservation and future reproduction (Oehninger, 2005).

THE ROLE OF CANCER SPECIALISTS IN PRESERVING FERTILITY

PHYSICIANS TREATING YOUNGER patients for cancer should be aware of the adverse effects of treatment on fertility and of ways to minimize those effects. If gonadal toxicity is unavoidable, they should also be knowledgeable about options for fertility preservation and offer referrals to patients (Lee et al., 2006).

Oncologists traditionally have focused on providing the most effective treatments available to help prolonging life, but in cases of younger persons with treatable cancers they need to consider fertility preservation as well. This involves informing patients and/or their families of options, benefits, and risks, and referring them to fertility specialists, if appropriate. Unless patients are informed or properly referred before treatment, options for later reproduction may be lost. Fertility specialists and patient organizations should work with cancer specialists to promote awareness of this issue.

THE ROLE OF FERTILITY SPECIALISTS IN PRESERVING FERTILITY

FERTILITY SPECIALISTS ARE constantly involved in developing and using procedures to preserve gametes, embryos, and gonadal tissue before cancer treatment. Their role is to assist cancer survivors in understanding the limits of each technology and to counsel patients while providing hopes and assistance to protect future fertility.

Consultation with the patient's oncologist often is essential. The specialists must ask about the patient's health and prognosis, and decide with the patient when and how to undergo a fertility preservation procedure (Robertson, 2005).

From an ethical standpoint, the key reason for pursuing fertility protection is to restore personal autonomy to those who are unable to conceive. However, since many of the technologies are innovative but experimental, it is difficult to design clinical trials: how to provide a proper informed consent and respect for autonomy? Who to include or exclude in the trials? How to assess the risks? Can the moral principle of beneficence be upheld if testicular tissue cryopreservation poses future risks to any children who might result from this technique? Ideally the decision about who is a candidate for fertility preservation should be rendered by a team including a medical oncologist, reproductive endocrinologist, a pathologist, and a psychologist, all guided by written protocols that can be shared with patients. Patients should not be provided with false hopes, and at times the best recommendation is that of no intervention. It is reasonable in absence of grant funds to seek reimbursement from patients to cover the expenses of the research, but there should be no charge for clinical fees. Finally, for the time being, fertility preservation involving testicular harvesting for freezing should be performed only in a few specialized centers working with proper consents approved by institutional review boards (IRBs).

PRESERVING FERTILITY IN CHILDREN WITH CANCER

UNFORTUNATELY, THE MODALITIES that are available to children to preserve their fertility are limited by their sexual immaturity and are essentially experimental. For boys who cannot produce mature sperm, harvesting and cryopreservation of testicular stem cells with the hope of future autologous transplantation or in vitro maturation represents a promising method of fertility preservation. Although it is difficult for children to conceptualize impaired future fertility as another potential consequence of exposure to cancer therapies, it may be potentially traumatic to them as adults. In addition, given the uncertainty of predicting fertility outcomes and the experimental nature of the options available, it is also difficult to counsel parents.

Care and tact should be taken in discussing all the options with parents and child, and with the child alone. If children cannot ejaculate or are too young, then testicular biopsy for sperm extraction or biopsy to use as germ cell repository can be done under IRB experimental conditions. Child assent and parental consent should always be sought. If the child is too young to give assent, no procedure involving more than minimal risk and not for their proven benefit should be permitted. The consent should cover the possible use of the reproductive tissue, the duration of storage, and the disposal of the tissue in the event of mental incapacitation or death. According to regulation of the Human Fertility Embryology Act (HFEA) (in the United Kingdom) parental control over the stored gametic material is restricted to storage only, thus allowing the patient greater control over their genetic material. It is anticipated that transition of absolute control would normally occur at the point of the child's maturity (Bahadur, Chatterjee, & Ralph, 2000).

Additional risks associated with fertility preservation are more difficult to assess because of the lack of data to quantify them. For instance, the potential risk of reintroduction of malignant cells to the patient when gonadal tissue is retransplanted cannot be estimated because only limited animal data exists. Moreover, potential risks to offspring conceived through such technologies, such as inheritance of genetic predisposition to cancer or other unforeseen genetic conditions, are currently unknown.

POSTHUMOUS CONCEPTION

STORING REPRODUCTIVE TISSUE AND GAMETES

THE LEGAL SYSTEM has recognized that a person's prior wishes about disposition of reproductive material after death in a consent form, advance directive, or another reliable indicator of consent before death, should be honored. The law permits gametes and embryos to be used after death if the person has given such directions or if the partner or next of kin has control of them. Some courts have also accepted that children born after posthumous conception or implantation are the legal offspring of the deceased if he gave instructions that gametes or embryos may be used after his death for reproduction. Whether offspring conceived posthumously will be recognized under the deceased's will or state inheritance laws depends on the law of the state where the event occurs (Pennings et al., 2006).

Programs that are storing gametes, embryos, or gonadal tissue for cancer patients inform patients of the options for disposition of those materials at a future time when depositors are (because of death, incompetence, or unavailability) unable to consent to disposition themselves. Interestingly, sperm cryopreservation has also been utilized recently by soldiers going to war (Iraq and Afghanistan), and specific directives about sperm disposal issues have been left in the hands of their spouses.

Postmortem Sperm Retrieval: What Are the Guidelines and Who Can Consent?

SPERM CAN BE retrieved after the death of a man. The decision to perform a postmortem sperm retrieval (PMSR) usually has to occur within a short time frame (within 24 hours of death), because recovery of viable sperm appears relatively uncommon at a later time unless the body has been cooled. There are significant questions to consider prior to performing PMSR. Consideration of postmortem conception is rarely anticipated and thus prospective authorization or consent is not likely to occur. A reasonable expectation that the recently deceased would have consented to having his sperm used for procreation would best be determined by his actions and discussions prior to death with respect to intended pregnancy. Therefore, only men undergoing fertility treatment, actively attempting conception, or who had specifically expressed their plans to attempt conception in the immediate future would be suitable candidates for retrieval. For this reason, the person most capable of determining the intentions of the deceased man and to give procedural consent regarding conception is his wife (Tash et al., 2003). The wife must understand that assisted reproduction would be required to use these specimens. Regardless of the expressed wishes of the deceased, the wife may decide not to proceed with an attempted conception.

CONCLUSION

WHILE MANY MALE fertility disorders remain poorly understood, the field is in continuous evolution. New technologies create new options for patients and their families. These new options raise the need for formulating guidelines to address ethical concerns around issues such as disclosure to children born of sperm donation, fertility preservation of adults and children, which requires consenting children to experimental protocols, and, finally, posthumous reproduction.

REFERENCES

American Society for Reproductive Medicine. (2006). 2006 guidelines for gamete and embryo donation. *Fertility and Sterility, 86*, 38–50.

American Society for Reproductive Medicine. (2007). Open identity donor insemination in the United States: Is it on the rise? *Fertility and Sterility, 88*, 231–232.

Bahadur, G., Chatterjee, R., & Ralph, D. (2000). Testicular tissue cryopreseva-
tion in boys. Ethical and legal issues. *Human reproduction, 15*, 1416–1420.

The Ethics Committee of the American Society for Reproductive Medicine.
(2005). Fertility preservation and reproduction in cancer patients. *Fertility and Sterility, 83*, 1622–1628.

Galan, J. J., De Felici, M., Buch, B., Rivero, M. C., Segura, A., Royo, J. L., et al.
(2006). Association of genetic markers within the *KIT* and *KITLG* genes
with human male infertility. *Human Reproduction, 21*, 3185–3192.

Lee, S. J., Schover, L. R., Partridge, A. H., Patrizio, P., Wallace, W. H., Hagerty, K.,
et al. (2006). American Society of Clinical Oncology recommendations
on fertility preservation in cancer patients. *Journal of Clinical Oncology,
24*(18), 2917–2931.

Oehninger, S. (2005). Strategies for fertility preservation in female and male
cancer survivors. *Journal of the Society for Gynecologic Investigation, 12*,
222–231.

Oehninger, S., & Kruger, T. (2007). *Male infertility diagnosis and treatment*. London: Informa Healthcare.

Patrizio, P., Mastroianni, A., & Mastroianni, L. (2001). Disclosure to children
conceived with donor gametes should be optional. *Human Reproduction,
16*, 2036–2038.

Payne, M., & Lamb, E. J. (2004). Use of frozen semen to avoid human immunodeficiency virus type 1 transmission by donor insemination: A cost-
effectiveness analysis. *Fertility and Sterility, 81*, 81–92.

Pennings, G., De Wert, G., Shenfield, F., Cohen, J., Devroey, P., & Tarlatzis, B.
(2006). ESHRE Task Force on Ethics and Law 11: Posthumous assisted
reproduction. *Human Reproduction, 21*, 3050–3053.

Robertson, J. A. (2005). Cancer and fertility: Ethical and legal challenges. *Journal
of the National Cancer Institute Monographs, 34*, 104–106.

Scheib, J. E., Riordan, M., & Rubin, S. (2005). Adolescents with open-identity
sperm donors: Reports from 12–17 year olds. *Human Reproduction, 20*,
239–252.

Tash, J. A., Applegarth, L. D., Kerr, S. M., Fins, J. J., Rosenwaks, Z., & Schlegel,
P. N. (2003). Postmortem sperm retrieval: The effect of instituting guidelines. *The Journal of Urology, 170*(5), 1922–1925.

Wardle, P., & Skew, B. (2008, February 18). The real impact of the removal of
donor anonymity. *BioNews.Org.UK*. Retrieved August 30, 2008, from
http://www.bionews.org.uk/commentary.lasso?storyid=3731

30

Preimplantation Genetic Diagnosis: Ethical Considerations

Frances R. Batzer and Vardit Ravitsky

PREIMPLANTATION GENETIC DIAGNOSIS (PGD) is a procedure performed on eggs or embryos following in vitro fertilization (IVF) for the purpose of obtaining genetic information prior to uterine implantation. The polar bodies of the egg or one or two cells from the embryo are obtained by biopsy and genetically tested. The rest of the cells continue to develop normally. PGD is an alternative to prenatal genetic diagnosis, which takes place after implantation. It can be provided to infertile couples who use IVF to conceive, or to fertile couples who are willing to go through the invasive process of IVF to use PGD in order to prevent or ensure a specific genotype in their future child.

The first successful reported application of PGD in humans occurred in 1989 when Handyside and colleagues (Handyside, Kontogianni,

The authors would like to thank Andrea Kalfoglou for her helpful comments and Krystene Boyle for her help with this chapter.

Hardy, & Winston, 1990; Handyside et al., 1989) used a technique of Y chromosome identification that allowed parents to choose female embryos for implantation, thus avoiding the risk of a boy suffering from certain X-linked genetic diseases. Since then, advances in the technology have resulted in an ever-increasing list of genetic diseases for which PGD may be applied (Handyside, 1998; Lissens & Sermon, 1997) as well as increasing concern for potential nonmedical uses of the technology. Studies of PGD outcomes have concluded that the risk of birth defects is no greater for PGD babies than for those conceived naturally, indicating that neither IVF nor embryo biopsy pose a serious threat to embryos (Harper et al., 2008; Verlinsky et al., 2004).

Potential uses of PGD range from medical (disease oriented) to nonmedical. On one end of the spectrum are uses such as testing for lethal childhood diseases (e.g., Tay-Sachs) or chromosomal abnormalities (e.g., Down syndrome), for susceptibility to late-onset diseases (e.g., Huntington's disease and breast cancer), or for traits that are considered by most people to be a disability (e.g., deafness). Another medical use is the selection of an embryo that would be a genetic match to a sick child (a *savior sibling*) in order to obtain stem cells or tissue for transplantation. We consider this to be a medical use because it has a therapeutic purpose, even though it is performed not for the medical benefit of the prospective child, but rather for that of another. On the other end of the spectrum are nonmedical uses such as sex selection and—potentially in the future—selection for desired physical phenotypes (e.g., eye color, hair color, and height) or even cognitive and behavioral traits (e.g., intelligence and sexual orientation). In addition, PGD can be used to select for a genetic trait that is generally perceived as undesirable but is preferred by a certain population. For example, parents who are proud members of the Deaf community might wish to select a deaf embryo.

This chapter explores some of the ethical issues raised by these different uses of the technology. We put forward two considerations that are relevant to the ethical analysis of PGD: gradual respect for the developing human embryo and privacy in matters related to reproduction, often referred to as reproductive freedom,[1] and we argue that these considerations need to be appropriately balanced. Because PGD requires the potential creation of more embryos than will be implanted and carried to term, some embryos—both abnormal and normal—may be discarded in the process.[2] Respect for the developing embryo (i.e., refraining from creating it only to discard it without justification) thus needs to be balanced against parental freedom.

ETHICAL CONSIDERATIONS

THE MORAL STATUS OF THE IN VITRO HUMAN EMBRYO

A SPECTRUM OF positions exists in the bioethical and the religious literature regarding the moral status of the in vitro–created human embryo. These positions range from treating the embryo as a person from the time of conception, through treating it with varying degrees of respect, all the way to treating it as a biological entity that has not yet attained human status. For example, conservative Catholic positions hold that in vitro embryos deserve full respect from the time of conception (O'Hara, 2003), whereas the traditional Jewish position holds that the status of embryos outside the uterus is comparable to that of gametes, namely, they should not be wasted in vain but may be manipulated for therapeutic purposes that would benefit human beings. According to this tradition, even in utero the embryo acquires the status of a *formed* human only after 40 days (Bioethics Advisory Committee of the Israel Academy of Sciences and Humanities, 2001).

The ethical framework of this chapter does not embrace either of these extreme positions. Rather, we hold an approach of gradual respect, which is the position consistently maintained by the Ethics Committee of the American Society of Reproductive Medicine (2004) and by the American College of Obstetrics and Gynecology (Committee Opinion ACOG Committee on Ethics, 2006). This position holds that as a biological entity that has the potential to become a human being, "the human embryo is entitled to profound respect; but this respect does not necessarily encompass the full legal and moral rights attributed persons." Even though the in vitro embryo "cannot achieve its potential to become a fetus and thus potentially a child unless and until it is transferred into the uterus" it still deserves special respect as a "symbol of future human life" (European Society of Human Reproduction and Embryology [ESHRE] Task Force on Ethics and Law, 2001, p. 1046). This special respect means that one needs justification for creating human embryos and then discarding them.

We argue that the use of PGD should not be a trivial choice. The reasons behind each type of use and the circumstances of each clinical situation should be evaluated. Couples and clinicians should be encouraged to pause and consider the ethical implications of their choices. This approach is in line with the results of a recent study that looked at public opinions regarding the use of new reproductive genetic technologies, including PGD (Kalfoglou et al., 2005), and revealed that the destruction of human embryos is indeed of concern to most Americans.

REPRODUCTIVE FREEDOM

THE POSITION THAT endorses the unfettered reproductive freedom of potential parents is prevalent in the American bioethical literature. It holds that individuals are entitled to decide not only whether and when to have children, but also what kind of children to have, using any type of available technology (Robertson, 1994). The use of PGD for any reason is thus perceived as yet another expression of parental reproductive freedom that should not be proscribed. The importance of this freedom is emphasized by the fact that PGD allows prospective parents to avoid the extreme physical and psychological burden of prenatal genetic testing followed—potentially—by the termination of a pregnancy due to an unfavorable diagnosis.

While recognizing reproductive freedom as an important value and acknowledging its cultural significance in the United States, we also recognize that it should be balanced against a certain degree of respect due to in vitro–created embryos. Moreover, while parents' freedom to choose is of paramount value, another important consideration is the autonomy of clinicians to decide in which cases they do not wish to provide services, based on their own values. Clinicians should not be forced to participate in procedures under circumstances that they consider unethical, although they should be willing to refer patients to others (see chapter 14 of this volume).

MEDICAL USES OF PGD

SINGLE-GENE DISORDERS AND CHROMOSOMAL ABNORMALITIES

PGD WAS FIRST implemented as an alternative to prenatal diagnosis for the identification of single-gene disorders known to be highly penetrant and to cause significant morbidity (such as cystic fibrosis, fragile X, beta thalassemia, Tay-Sachs, and sickle cell anemia),[3] in order to prevent the heartache of birth of a sick child or abortion (The ESHRE Ethics Task Force et al., 2003). Parents of an affected child or parents who carry a significant risk are often highly motivated seekers of PGD. PGD offers couples who wish to avoid being confronted with an abortion decision an alternative that may be physically, emotionally, and ethically realistic for them, without which they might have chosen not to conceive at all. Selected embryos that are transferred into the uterus are genetically unaffected by the disorder for which they have been tested. PGD for highly penetrant single-gene disorders is considered by most clinicians to be an acceptable reason to subject a potentially fertile couple to the inconvenience, the cost, and the risk of going through IVF, because it is meant to prevent significant suffering and premature death.

PGD is also used to test for a change in the number of chromosomes (known as aneuploidy), which can lead to a chromosomal abnormality, such as Down syndrome, or to chromosomally related recurrent miscarriages, as in the case of couples with balanced translocation in one or both partners (Gianaroli, Magli, Ferraretti, & Munné, 1999). Translocation means that a portion of one chromosome is transferred to another chromosome. When the translocation is balanced, there is an even exchange of material and there is no missing or extra genetic information, so the individual is not affected. However, any attempt at conception may result in recurrent miscarriage as the chromosomes are unable to divide evenly to achieve the haploid state necessary for fertilization.

Testing for aneuploidy has long been one of the most common reasons to consider prenatal testing. Originally offered to women over the age of 35, it has become clear that while incidence increases with maternal age, all maternal ages and pregnancies can be affected. The current chromosome testing panel for PGD includes the most common aneuploidy abnormalities routinely found with prenatal testing.

LATE-ONSET DISEASES

PGD PROVIDES AN option for avoiding the transmission of a late-onset disease (e.g., Huntington's disease [HD] or early-onset Alzheimer's disease). Some diseases (e.g., HD and Duchenne's muscular dystrophy) have a 100% penetrance with no known treatment or cure to date (Sermon et al., 1998). The case of testing for HD has received ample attention in the literature (Greenamyre, 2007), partly because the onset of the disease is relatively early. The progressive neuropsychiatric deterioration begins at the mean age of 40 years with a 15-year progression toward death.

The more controversial use of PGD is testing embryos for *susceptibility* to late-onset disease, which means that penetrance is uncertain and a carrier may even live a full healthy life and never develop the disease. An example would be embryos that carry a BRCA mutation, which involves an increased risk of developing breast or ovarian cancer later in life (Braude, 2006). Many couples requesting PGD for such conditions have lived through the anguish of watching a loved one die of the disease. For them, prevention is desirable at all costs, even though treatments exist and new treatments may become available in the future.

When addressing the ethical implications of PGD for late-onset diseases, one should balance the ethical cost of creating surplus embryos against the benefit of preventing the suffering associated with the disease and also with carrying the burden of knowledge of potential or pending disease onset, which can have major psychological implications throughout life (Harmon, 2007). Considering the significance of disease prevention in such cases, we argue that reproductive freedom should override other considerations and that parents' choices to use PGD for this purpose is ethically appropriate. This argument is particularly strong with regard to imminent diseases with a relatively early age of onset.

PGD for susceptibility to late-onset diseases has been ongoing in the United States since 2001 (Rechitsky et al., 2002), and the Human Fertilization and Embryology Authority (HFEA) in the United Kingdom recently authorized its use for this purpose (Braude, 2006). According to the HFEA, however, only severe genetic conditions with a single identified gene that would dramatically affect the offspring's quality of life are appropriate for such testing.

SELECTING AGAINST DISABILITY

DISABILITY IS A physical or a mental impairment that substantially limits activity, in relation to the standard in society. Using PGD to select a nondisabled embryo is considered by many to be ethically unproblematic. Parents' choice to have a hearing rather than a deaf child or a sighted rather than a blind child are based on their wish to bring into the world a child that would be able to enjoy a wide range of opportunities and thus—arguably—a better life. Yet, such choices do raise certain ethical challenges.

First, defining *disability* is conceptually challenging because it requires an agreement regarding what is considered to be *normal* or *typical* for human beings versus what is considered to be a *deviation* from the norm (see chapter 17 of this volume). Second, the history of the 20th century carries the shadow of eugenics, and selections that echo a desire for a *perfect baby* can arguably promote eugenic social attitudes (Buchanan, Brock, Daniels, & Wikler, 2000). Some even argue that "fostering the notion that only a 'perfect baby' is worthy of life threatens our solidarity with and support for people with disabilities, and perpetuates standards of perfection set by a market system that caters to political, economic and cultural elites" (Darnovsky, 2001, p. 134). Thus, selecting against disabled embryos is considered by some to be ethically problematic because it emphasizes the fact that the children born of these embryos are deemed to have a life *not worth living*. Such choices, it is argued, "express a hurtful attitude about and send a hurtful message to people who live with those same traits"

(Parens & Asch, 1999, p. 2) and might negatively influence attitudes toward them.

However, we argue that the choice to use PGD to select against disability should be protected under the umbrella of reproductive freedom. The burden of raising a disabled child and caring for her special needs would fall on the shoulders of the parents and they are, therefore, entitled to decide whether or not they are willing to take such a risk or cope with such an outcome. Considering the momentous impact of having a disabled child on the lives of all family members, the choice to select against disability should be viewed as ethically acceptable and remain at the discretion of prospective parents. Different families hold different value systems and possess different types of resources for dealing with challenging circumstances. It would thus be ethically inappropriate to deprive families of the freedom to make choices that align with their values and capabilities, particularly in a social reality that provides only partial support systems to individuals living with disabilities.

SELECTING A SAVIOR SIBLING

THE USE OF PGD to screen for an embryo that would be a matching donor for an affected child who might benefit from bone marrow, umbilical cord stem cells, tissue, or even an organ, is considered ethically controversial by some (Boyle & Savulescu, 2001; Wolf, Kahn, & Wagner, 2003). This use is sometimes referred to as creating a *savior sibling*. When there are no obvious living donors, intentionally creating a donor through PGD is among a short list of possible treatment options (Wagner, Davies, & Auerbach, 1999). Human leukocyte antigen (HLA) matching enables the couple's next child to serve as a matched hematopoietic donor for their existing sick child (Spriggs & Savulescu, 2006) and can also ensure that the new sibling will not suffer from the same genetic disease. PGD for HLA matching has received media attention since the so-called Nash Case (de Wert 2005; Kahn & Mastroianni, 2004). The parents of Molly Nash who suffered from Fanconi anemia opted for PGD to prevent the birth of another affected child and to select HLA-matched embryos that at birth could provide donor stem cells from the umbilical cord blood.

Statistically, in the context of a recessive trait, one in four embryos conceived via sexual intercourse will be a noncarrier (Wasserman, 2003), but the chance of an HLA match in addition to that is much lower (3 in 16) (Robertson, Kahn, & Wagner, 2002). In addition, natural conception followed by prenatal diagnosis to establish the HLA type and genetic status of the fetus is complicated. First, it would require the termination of a nonmatching pregnancy. For many couples there is a major physical, emotional, and ethical difference between aborting an already established normal pregnancy and not transferring certain embryos in the first place. Second, it is a longer process, and time can be a critical factor when a family is attempting to save the life of a sick child. IVF plus PGD for HLA typing can accomplish the goal more directly and within a shorter time frame.

However, PGD for HLA typing has raised moral concerns. During childhood, HLA-identical siblings have no autonomy to choose whether or not to donate. This decision is made by their parents or guardians. There is an implicit expectation that brothers and sisters would want to act in their sibling's best interest, but in fact these children have no say in the matter. Since HLA-matched siblings may serve as the best possible donors for any kind of tissue or organ transplant for a lifetime, concerns arise regarding future coercion or exploitation of one child for the benefit of another (Pennings, Schots, & Liebaers, 2002). A recently published fictional novel explores these ethical complexities and brings them to life by telling the story of a family's struggle to keep one child alive at the expense of making her younger sister an ongoing donor throughout her childhood (Picoult, 2004).

Concerns have also been raised regarding parents' unconditional acceptance of their new child, because this child is *designed* for the benefit of another child. Some have argued that it is ethically acceptable to treat a child as a means to a worthwhile end, as long as the child is also respected as an end in itself (Robertson et al., 2002). However, parents of a seriously ill child who learn that stem cell donation from an HLA-matched sibling could provide significant benefits may feel pressured to opt for another pregnancy even if they did not initially plan to have another child (Fost, 2004). Such scenarios raise speculative concerns regarding the psychological impact on the child. Since PGD was first used for HLA typing in 2000, the eldest children born through this procedure have yet to reach adolescence. The psychological effects of having been conceived specifically through HLA typing PGD are yet to be studied (Pennings et al., 2002; Wasserman, 2003).

Although the ethical concerns described here are not without merit, considering their speculative nature in comparison to the urgent need to save the life of an existing child leads us to argue that here, again, parents' reproductive freedom should be protected. Moreover, when the use of IVF with PGD is essential in order to prevent the birth of another child with the same disease, the additional testing for HLA typing can be seen as a part of the process. The choice to use PGD to select a savior sibling is ethically acceptable, providing mechanisms are in place to protect the interests of the future child and prevent any type of coercion until the child reaches adulthood and is able to make her own decisions. Indeed, considering the intricate nature of family dynamics, it would be extremely challenging to establish such mechanisms, but this is a worthwhile endeavor that would enable great benefits.

NONMEDICAL USES OF PGD

SEX SELECTION

USING PGD TO select the sex of the embryo is legally permissible in the United States but considered by many to be ethically controversial. A recent survey of public attitudes found that most Americans disapprove of this use of PGD (Hudson, 2006). A couple of distinctions should be made to clarify the ethical debate on this complex issue.

The first distinction is between using PGD to select the sex of the first child and that of subsequent children. It has been argued that selecting the sex of the first child inherently expresses sexist and discriminatory attitudes, whereas selecting the sex of a second child to be the opposite to that of the first expresses a legitimate parental desire for variety in rearing experiences (Nisker & Jones, 1997). The differences in the rearing experiences of boys and girls are widely acknowledged and support the argument that such parental preferences are not necessarily grounded in discriminatory attitudes that privilege one sex over another (Steinbock, 1992). We argue that in this specific context, reproductive freedom should prevail because parental preference for a certain sex is an expression of parents' autonomy to shape an important aspect of family life, considering the profound influence that children's sex has on family dynamics.

A second relevant distinction is between sex selection in Western countries that exhibit no dominant cultural or social preference for boys, and in countries where the cultural preference for boys is overwhelming. Arguments are often made against the use of PGD for sex selection on the grounds that it strengthens discriminatory attitudes, devalues women, and exacerbates the demographic imbalance between males and females in countries such as India and China (Oomman & Ganatra, 2002). Such arguments are, in fact, not against sex selection per se, but rather against male preference. A recent survey has shown that in the United States there is no dominant preference for males over females (50% wished to have a family with an equal number of boys and girls, 7% with more boys than girls, 6% with more girls than boys, 5% with only boys, 4% with only girls, and 27% had no preference) (Dahl et al., 2006).

In a cultural climate that exhibits no sex preference and in a society in which equal opportunities are available—at least theoretically—to both sexes, arguments based on discrimination and demographic concerns are not as relevant because they only apply to certain cultural minorities. We therefore argue that in such societies, reproductive freedom may prevail even after balancing parental preferences against the respect for the in vitro human embryo that will be created and discarded to allow this choice.

TRAIT SELECTION

THE USE OF PGD to select physical, personality, or behavioral traits, sometimes pejoratively referred to as creating a *designer baby,* is not currently available to parents because the genetic basis of such complex traits has not been identified and such tests do not exist. Some believe that "our knowledge of human genetics is not likely to make it possible to choose alleles for high intelligence, athletic ability, musical genius, and so on" (Greely, 2006, p. 1632), because according to our understanding at present, most traits are influenced by more than one chromosome. Others, however, see such uses as possible future developments. Whatever the future holds, the academic and public debate regarding the ethical issues surrounding such scenarios is already in full swing.

This ethical debate addresses a range of potential uses, from relatively simple physical or cosmetic traits such as eye color and hair color, through more complex traits such as probable adult height and male pattern baldness, all the way to extremely complex traits such as intelligence, sexual orientation, aggressiveness, or novelty-seeking. Currently in the United States there are no legal limits on which tests may be used for PGD, and no mechanism is in place to regulate future possible tests. This regulatory vacuum may raise ethical concerns for the future. A recent survey showed that 72% of Americans disapprove of the use of PGD to ensure a child has desirable characteristics (Hudson, Scott, & Kalfoglou, 2002).

Some are concerned that the cumulative effect of many individual choices made by parents will result in the strengthening or the creation of eugenic attitudes on a social level. If a critical mass of wealthy parents uses PGD to *up the ante* by ensuring their children are equipped with the best genetic makeup, others will have to follow in order to compete, and our society may find itself on a eugenic track. To date, these arguments are empirically weak because the cost and the burden of IVF with PGD ensure their use will not be prevalent.

Another concern has to do with the cost of PGD and the issue of access. If only the better-off will be able to afford access to this technology, the gaps between the haves and the have-nots will widen over time. Some social critics have even warned about the gradual creation of two different species. Others have voiced concerns about the loss of genetic diversity, arguing that most parents will follow similar cultural norms and that their choices will thus create a more homogeneous population than that created by the *genetic lottery*. Yet another concern revolves around the possible influence of such genetic choices on the relationship between parents and children. Parents may be more critical or demanding of a child that has been carefully *designed* for certain types of achievements, or even come to perceive children as *commodities* rather than *gifts*.

The use of PGD for trait selection is deeply controversial (Hudson, 2006). It would require the creation of multiple embryos solely for the sake of choosing a child with specific traits over another, while paying the ethical price of discarding embryos that could develop into healthy individuals. Balancing the special respect they deserve against parental desires for certain traits is a complex undertaking. While some proponents of reproductive freedom have no ethical qualms about such uses of PGD, others have voiced concerns, as outlined previously. Although a full analysis of each of these speculative uses is beyond the scope of this chapter, we would like to emphasize an important point: the discussion of trait selection and *designer babies* is often popularized, conflating many different traits and addressing them as one. A thoughtful bioethical analysis would require an examination of each of these uses separately, highlighting the unique context of each choice. A desire to select against homosexuality is not similar to a desire to select against blue eyes. Each of these parental preferences ought to be examined within its unique context.

SELECTING *FOR* DISABILITY

USING PGD TO choose an embryo that carries what most would consider a *genetic disorder* may be the most controversial potential use of the technology. In such cases, what seems particularly disturbing to some is the fact that the selected embryos are precisely those carrying the trait that is typically screened out, while multiple nonaffected embryos are discarded. For many, this means that parental choice in this case harms the future child and is therefore ethically unacceptable. The two examples usually raised in this context are the choice of an embryo that would develop into a deaf rather than a hearing child, and the choice of an embryo with achondroplasia (dwarfism) rather than one that would develop into a person of average height (Davis, 2001).[4]

Deafness, for some deaf parents, is a cultural identity that they wish to pass on to their children. The Deaf community has developed a rich culture that provides unique and valuable opportunities and benefits to its members. Some claim a *birthright of silence,* a right to their own culture. They see the Deaf way of life as something to be cherished rather than eliminated (Tucker, 1998).[5] Within this framework, deaf people reject the suggestion that they suffer from impairment or disability. When expecting a baby, they "characteristically hope to have children with whom they can share their language, culture, and unique experiences—that is, deaf children" (Lane & Bahan, 1998, p. 298). For such parents, a deaf baby is a *special blessing* (Mundy, 2002), and some have argued that they believe that they can be better parents and have a stronger family unit raising a *child like themselves* (Sanghavi, 2006).

Does this position justify the use of PGD to ensure the birth of a deaf baby? Much of the bioethical literature on this issue focuses on the possible ethical obligation to protect the prospective child's *open future*. Such arguments revolve around the idea that parents' choices for their children are unethical if they trap children in a life in which they have very limited opportunities (Davis, 1997). The major challenge in defending these arguments is that almost any intentional parental choice narrows down the child's future range of opportunities to some degree (e.g., which language is taught or what type of education is chosen). Defining the particular choices that would *close* the child's future to such an extent that they become unethical is a challenging conceptual task (Ravitsky, 2002).

Such scenarios require an ethical analysis that addresses the interests of the future child, which raises the nonidentity problem (see chapter 27 of this volume). However, one straightforward point should be made here: clinicians may be particularly reluctant to participate in such procedures if they are not comfortable with assisting in the creation of a child that they perceive as disabled. Clinicians' autonomy should be respected and their choice to not participate is ethically acceptable.

CONCLUSION

P GD WAS INITIALLY developed as an alternative to prenatal diagnosis with potential subsequent pregnancy termination, thus mitigating the physical and the emotional hardship of aborting an otherwise wanted fetus. While our current knowledge indicates no identifiable problems for children conceived through IVF with PGD, experience is limited. While the Ethics Committee of ASRM (American Society for Reproductive Medicine, 1994) found "a strong ethical justification for PGD in the prevention of inherited diseases that severely deplete the quality of human life or longevity" (p. 66S)—a position that reflects a wide ethical consensus—other uses remain ethically controversial. We have argued that when exploring the ethics of PGD, parents' reproductive freedom should be balanced against the appropriate degree of respect for the in vitro–created embryos. This call for balance emphasizes the notion that the choice of PGD should not be trivial and that all involved parties should consider the ethical implications of their choices.

NOTES

1. We do not discuss the value of preventing pain and suffering from the prospective child because this consideration raises the nonidentity problem, and the scope of this chapter does not allow for a discussion of this complex issue. For a comprehensive discussion of the nonidentity problem see chapter 27 of this volume.

2. Another alternative is to freeze all leftover embryos, but this cannot be done indefinitely and therefore does not solve the problem.

3. *Penetrance* refers to the likelihood of a condition manifesting in an individual if they carry a faulty copy of the gene. The higher the penetrance, the greater the chance that the condition will actually develop.

4. While being homozygous for a deafness gene usually affects only hearing, the same is not true for dwarfism. Achondroplasia is devastating in its homozygous form, leading to an early death from breathing failure due to restricted chest size and neurologic issues related to hydrocephalus. Thus, PGD for achondroplasia serves a medical purpose, preventing loss of a wanted child.

5. Similar arguments have been made regarding the short-stature community. "There is a common feeling of self-acceptance, pride and community that has been compared to more traditional disability groups and the deaf community. The concept of a dwarf community is illustrated in part by the dozens of dwarf children from all over the world adopted by Little People of America members" (Ricker, 1995).

REFERENCES

American Society for Reproductive Medicine. (1994). Preimplantation genetic diagnosis. *Fertility and Sterility, 62,* 64S–66S.

Bioethics Advisory Committee of the Israel Academy of Sciences and Humanities. (2001). *Report on the use of embryonic stem (ES) cells for therapeutic research.* Retrieved August 9, 2008, from http://www.academy.ac.il/bio ethics.html

Boyle, R. J., & Savulescu, J. (2001). Education and debate. Ethics of using preimplantation genetic diagnosis to select a stem cell donor for an existing person. *Australian Medical Journal 323,* 1240–1243.

Braude P. (2006). Preimplantation diagnosis for genetic susceptibility. *New England Journal of Medicine, 355,* 541–546.

Buchanan, A., Brock, D. W., Daniels, N., & Wikler, D. (2000). *From chance to choice: Genetics and justice.* Cambridge, UK: Cambridge University Press.

Committee Opinion, American College of Obstetrics and Gynecology Committee on Ethics. (2006). Using preimplantation embryos for research. *Obstetrics and Gynecology, 108,* 1305–1317.

Dahl, E., Gupta, R. S., Beutel, M., Stoebel-Richter, Y., Brosig, B., Tinneberg, H. R., et al. (2006). Preconception sex selection demand and preferences in the United States. *Fertility and Sterility, 85,* 468–473.

Darnovsky, M. (2001). The case against designer babies: The politics of genetic enhancement. In B. Tokar (Ed.), *Redesigning life? The worldwide challenge to genetic engineering* (pp. 133–149). London: Zed Books.

Davis, D. S. (1997). Genetic dilemmas and the child's right to a open future. *Rutgers Law Journal, 28*(3), 561–570.

Davis, D. S. (2001). *Genetic dilemmas: Reproductive technology, parental choices, and children's futures.* New York: Routledge.

de Wert, G. (2005). Preimplantation genetic diagnosis: The ethics of intermediate cases. *Human Reproduction, 20*(12), 3261–3266.

The ESHRE Ethics Task Force, Shenfield, F., Pennings, G., Devroey, P., Sureau, C., Tarlatzis, B., et al. (2003). Taskforce 5: Preimplantation genetic diagnosis. *Human Reproduction, 18,* 649–761.

The Ethics Committee of the American Society for Reproductive Medicine. (2004). Donating spare embryos for embryonic stem-cell research. *Fertility and Sterility, 82,* S224–S227.

European Society of Human Reproduction and Embryology (ESHRE) Task Force on Ethics and Law. (2001). I. The moral status of the pre-implantation embryo. *Human Reproduction, 16,* 1046–1048.

Fost, N. C. (2004). Conception for donation. *Journal of the American Medical Association, 291,* 2125–2126.

Gianaroli, L., Magli, M. C., Ferraretti, A. P., & Munné, S. (1999). Preimplantation diagnosis for aneuploidies in patients undergoing in vitro fertilization with a poor prognosis: Identification of the categories for which it should be proposed. *Fertility and Sterility, 72,* 837–844.

Greely, H. T. (2006). An introduction and some conclusions. *Fertility and Sterility, 85,* 1631–1632.

Greenamyre, J. T. (2007). Huntington's disease–making connections. *New England Journal of Medicine, 356,* 518–529.

Handyside, A. H. (1998). Clinical evaluation of preimplantation genetic diagnosis. *Prenatal Diagnosis, 18,* 1345–1348.

Handyside, A. H., Kontogianni, E. H., Hardy, K., & Winston, R. M. L. (1990). Pregnancies from biopsied human preimplantation embryos sexed by Y-specific DNA amplification. *Nature, 344,* 768–770.

Handyside, A. H., Penketh, R. J. A., Winston, R. M. L., Pettinson, J. K., Delhanty, H. A. D., & Tuddenham, E. G. D. (1989). Biopsy of human preimplantation embryos and sexing by DNA amplification. *The Lancet, 1*(8634), 347–349.

Harmon, A. (2007, March 18). Facing life with a lethal gene. A young woman's DNA test reveals an inevitably grim fate. *The New York Times,* retreived September 29, 2008, from http://www.nytimes.com/2007/03/18/health/18huntington.html

Harper, J. C., de Die-Smulders, C., Goossens, V., Harten, G., Moutou, C., Repping, S., et al. (2008). ESHRE PGD consortium data collection VII: Cycles from January to December 2004 with pregnancy follow-up to October 2005. *Human Reproduction, 23*(4), 741–755.

Hudson, K. L. (2006). Preimplantation genetic diagnosis: Public policy and public attitudes. *Fertility and Sterility, 85,* 1638–1645.

Hudson, K., Scott, J., & Kalfoglou, A. (Eds.). (2002). *Public awareness and attitudes about reproductive genetic technology.* Washington, DC: Genetics and Public Policy Center.

Kahn, J. P., & Mastroianni, A. C. (2004). Creating a stem cell donor: A case study in reproductive genetics. *Kennedy Institute of Ethics Journal, 14,* 81–96.

Kalfoglou, A. L., Doksum, T., Bernhardt, B., Geller, G., Le Roy, L., Mathews, F. J. H., et al. (2005). Opinions about new reproductive genetic technologies: Hopes and fears for our genetic future. *Fertility and Sterility, 83,* 1612–1621.

Lane, H., & Bahan, B. (1998). Ethics of cochlear implantation in young children: A review and reply from a Deaf-World perspective. *Otolaryngology—Head and Neck Surgery, 119,* 297–308.

Lissens, W., & Sermon, K. (1997). Preimplantation genetic diagnosis: Current status and new developments. *Human Reproduction, 12,* 1/56–1/61.

Mundy, L. (2002, March 31). A world of their own. *Washington Post,* W22.

Nisker, J. A., & Jones, M. (1997). The ethics of sex selection. In F. Shenfield & C. Sureau (Eds.), *Ethical dilemmas in assisted reproduction* (Vol. 7, pp. 41–50). New York: The Parthenon Publishing Group.

O'Hara, N. (2003). Ethical consideration of experimentation using living human embryos: The Catholic Church's position on human embryonic stem cell research and human cloning. *Clinical and Experimental Obstetrics and Gynecology, 30*(203), 7–81.

Oomman, N., & Ganatra, B. R. (2002). Sex selection: The systematic elimination of girls. *Reproductive Health Matters, 10*(19), 184–188.

Parens, E., & Asch, A. (1999). The disability rights critique of prenatal genetic testing—reflections and recommendations. *A Special Supplement to the Hastings Center Report, 29*(Suppl.), 1–22.

Pennings, G., Schots, R., & Liebaers, I. (2002). Ethical considerations on preimplantation genetic diagnosis for HLA typing to match a future child as a donor of haematopoietic stem cells to a sibling. *Human Reproduction, 17*(3), 534–538.

Picoult, J. (2004). *My sister's keeper*. New York: ATRIA Books.

Ravitsky, V. (2002). Genetics and education: The ethics of shaping human identify. *The Mount Sinai Journal of Medicine, 69*(5), 312–316.

Rechitsky, S., Verlinsky, O., Chistokhina, A., Sharapova, T., Ozen, S., Masciangelo, C., et al. (2002). Preimplantation genetic diagnosis for cancer predisposition. *Reproductive Biomedicine Online, 5*(2), 148–155.

Ricker, R. E. (1995). *Do we really want this? Little people of America Inc. comes to terms with genetic testing*. Retrieved January 30, 2003, from http://home.earthlink.net/~dkennedy56/dwarfism_genetics.html

Robertson, J. A. (1994). *Children of choice—Freedom and the new reproductive technologies*. Princeton, NJ: Princeton University Press.

Robertson, J. A., Kahn, J. P., & Wagner, J. E. (2002). Conception to obtain hematopoietic stem cells. *Hastings Center Report, 32*(3), 34–40.

Sanghavi, D. M. (2006, December 5). Wanting babies like themselves, some parents choose genetic defects. *New York Times*. Retrieved September 7, 2008, from http://www.nytimes.com/2006/12/05/health/05essa.htm

Sermon, K., Goossens, V., Seneca, S., Lissens, W., De Vos A., Vandervorst, M., et al. (1998). Preimplantation diagnosis for Huntington's disease (HD): Clinical application and analysis of the HD expansion in affected embryos. *Prenatal Diagnosis, 18*, 1427–1436.

Spriggs, M., & Savulescu, J. (2006). In Victoria, Australia, some parents are now able to select embryos free from genetic disease which will provide stem cells to treat an existing sibling. *Journal of Medical Ethics, 28*, 289.

Steinbock, B. (1992). Sex selection: Not obviously wrong. *Hastings Center Report, 32*(1), 23–28.

Tucker, B. P. (1998). Deaf culture, cochlear implants, and elective disability. *Hastings Center Report, 28*, 6–14.

Verlinsky, Y., Cohen, J., Munne, S., Gianaroli, L., Simpson, J. L., Ferraretti, A. P., et al. (2004). Over a decade of experience with preimplantation genetic diagnosis. *Fertility and Sterility, 82*(2), 302–303.

Wagner, J. E., Davies, S. M., & Auerbach, A. D. (1999). Hematopoetic stem cell transplantation in the treatment of Fanconi anemia. In S. J. Forman, K. G. Blum, & E. D. Thomas (Eds.), *Hematopoetic stem cell transplantation* (2nd ed., pp. 1204–1219). Malden, MA: Blackwell Science.

Wasserman, D. (2003). Having one child to save another: A tale of two families. *Philosophy and Public Policy Quarterly, 23*(1–2), 21–27.

Wolf, S. M., Kahn, J. P., & Wagner, J. E. (2003). Using preimplantation genetic diagnosis to create a stem cell donor: Issues, guidelines and limits. *Journal of Law, Medicine and Ethics, 31*, 327–339.

31

The Influence of Language on the Beginning of Life Debate

Thomas A. Marino

Words mean more than what is set down on paper. It takes the human voice to infuse them with deeper meaning

—*Maya Angelou*

N A **MARCH** 11, 2007, article in the *Baltimore Sun,* Tricia Bishop reported that legislators in Maryland had replaced the word *embryo* with *certain material* so that stem cell legislation might pass. This is a strategy, as noted by Bishop, "That has led both supporters and opponents of various stem cell work to wield often ambiguous—or particularly pointed—words in the hopes it will help sell certain messages to one another and the public" (Bishop, 2007, p. 1C). Halfway across the country, and 10 days later, Jonathan D. Moreno and Sam Berger, in an editorial for the *Wichita Eagle,* noted that opponents of stem cell research altered scientific terminology to gain political advantage in the Kansas legislature. They stated that "Efforts to politically define complicated biological terms, however, often result in ill-conceived laws that satisfy neither opponents nor supporters, confuse scientists attempting to pursue research in the state, and may even create legal problems for those attempting to conduct cooperative studies across state lines" (Moreno & Berger, 2007, p. 9A).

Jane Maienschein, in an article titled "What's in a Name: Embryos, Clones, and Stem Cells" (Maienschein, 2002), questioned whether legislators, reporters, the lay public, or indeed any of us know what we are talking about when participating in the beginning of life debates. Perhaps even more to the point: even if we do know what we are talking about, do the people we are debating with know what we are talking about? Are we all using the same language and are we using it correctly?

This chapter explores the use of language over the last 28 years to promote various political points of view in the beginning of life debate. I argue that while the stages of human development have not changed during those years, the politics surrounding abortion, reproductive technologies, and stem cell research have prompted many to use language in attempts to redefine the process of early development. Both conservatives and liberals have revised the language used to describe early embryology. Furthermore, it is speculated that underlying motivations for the redefinition of the early embryonic period have to do with emotional manipulation meant to trigger anger and disgust and thereby to mold the nature of the debate.

EARLY EMBRYOLOGY

THE PROCESS OF embryonic development has been elegantly and quite carefully described and catalogued in the Carnegie Collection of Embryology now housed in the Human Developmental Anatomy Center (HDAC) part of the Research Collections division of the National Museum of Health and Medicine (HDAC, n.d.). The Carnegie Collection of Embryology divides the early development of the human into 23 stages. These stages describe the first 8 weeks after fertilization. Stage 1 is the 24 hours over which fertilization takes place. This includes the penetration of the sperm into the oocyte, the formation of the male and female pronuclei, the re-establishment of 46 chromosomes, and the initiation of cleavage. These events take place in the uterine tube. Stage 2 takes place over the next 2 days and consists of a series of reduction divisions. The cells of the embryo get progressively smaller and become a morula. During Stage 3, the morula undergoes a series of changes as the embryo becomes an outer shell of cells called the trophoblast and an inner group of cells called the inner cell mass. These events occur from day 4 to day 5 of development as the embryo is leaving the uterine tube to enter the uterus. The embryo at this time is also referred to as the blastocyst. The blastocyst attaches to the uterine epithelium during Stage 4, which occurs between days 5 and 6 of gestation.

Stage 5 of gestation sees the proliferation of the fetal components of the placenta, and the trophoblast differentiates into a cytotrophoblast and a syncytiotrophoblast, which invade the endometrium of the uterus. The inner cell mass becomes a bilaminar disc composed of the epiblast and the hypoblast. Stage 6 occurs as the second week of development ends. The embryo is now an oval bilaminar disc.

The main change seen at Stage 7 is the development of the primitive streak, primitive node, and the notochordal process. The embryo at this time is beginning gastrulation and going to transform from a bilaminar disc into a trilaminar disc. By Stage 8 the primitive node and pit have continued to develop, and the body axis is formed. This is occurring around day 18 of gestation. At the end of the third week of development Stage 9 has the embryo as a trilaminar disc, and the ectoderm, mesoderm, and endoderm are present. The paraxial mesoderm has already developed into 1–3 somites.

As the fourth week of development begins, the embryo is at Stage 10. The heart tube is present and beginning to beat. The neural tube is fusing and on either side there are 4–12 somites. Stage 11 sees the closure of the anterior neuropore in the embryo. The urogenital system is beginning to appear. Evidence of the development of the eyes is present as well. By the end of the fourth week of development the vertebrate body plan is nearly complete. Stage 12 has the embryo with ear and eye primordia present. The arm buds are beginning to appear. The embryo has undergone lateral body folding and head and tail folding and is attached to the placenta via the umbilical cord.

During the fifth week of development the embryo is in stages 13 and 14. The heart septates and assumes its four-chamber morphology, with embryonic circulation taking place. The kidneys begin to form. The arm and leg buds are present and developing. The trachea and lung buds grow caudally to develop in the future pleural cavity.

Carnegie stages 15 and 16 are found during week 6 of development. During these stages of embryogenesis the face is beginning to develop. The upper and lower limbs are beginning to have distinct segments and shoulder and hand regions are apparent. The seventh week of development finds Carnegie stages 17–19. The embryo now is producing urine from mesonephric kidneys. The face is developing, with a nose present and external ears visible. Eyelids are now visible, and the hands exhibit the formation of the fingers.

Week 8 of embryogenesis marks the end of the embryonic period of development and the beginning of the fetal period. Carnegie stages 20–23 occur at this time, and the embryo now has most of the organs developed. The fingers and toes are present. The face is developed. The gastrointestinal organs are developing and the midgut will soon return to the abdominal cavity. The gonads are present and the external genitalia will begin to differentiate over the next month. The heart and lungs continue to develop but the lungs can not support oxygen exchange. The fetal period will last until birth.

THE POLITICS OF SCIENTIFIC TERMINOLOGY: EMBRYOS, FETUSES, AND CHILDREN

IN THE LATE 1970s, a scientific landmark occurred when the first baby was born as a result of in vitro fertilization (IVF). This turned a page in the debate over the status of the embryo. Since the egg was fertilized and developed outside the female reproductive tract for a short period of time, a new question emerged: is this embryo different from an embryo that was fertilized in vivo? Questions arose as to the status of the in vitro embryo, who owned the embryo, and what might become of the embryo if it was not returned to the reproductive tract for development. Stenger (2006) pointed out that when the possibilities of human cloning and the potential of human stem cells became apparent, rancor and division were added to the discussion. Other elements of the debate ranged from eugenics to creating human/animal clones.

In 1979, Clifford Grobstein correlated the first attempts of IVF, or *external* human fertilization, as he called it, with the first several weeks of normal human development (Grobstein, 1979). Grobstein described the early embryology and then began to discuss personhood. His interpretation of when, during development, a person appears became the focus of his article. He chose to use what he called "external signs" (Grobstein, 1979, p. 64) to redefine human development. He decided to take the embryonic period and divide it into two segments: the cellular or pre-embryonic period and the embryonic phase. His argument was that "the properties of human beings (as well as the properties of life) are not the same as the properties of persons. The pre-embryonic and embryonic stages are alive and are human, but they are not externally recognizable as to personhood. (The same is of course true of cells and tissues that are separated from an adult: they remain alive and human, but they do not constitute a person.)" (Grobstein, 1979, p. 66). This was the first attempt to redefine early embryonic development so that the embryo became "cells and tissues"—a *pre*-embryo.

In order to describe IVF, those involved began to redefine early development and the language used to describe it. In 1986, the Ethics Committee of the American Fertility Society was charged by the board to "take a leadership position in addressing ethical issues in reproduction and providing disseminated knowledge of these positions" (The Ethics Committee of the American Fertility Society, 1986, p. iii). The focus was on IVF, and in this case the committee decided to define a pre-embryo as "a product of gametic union from fertilization to the appearance of the embryonic axis" (The Ethics Committee of the American Fertility Society, 1986, p. 3S), implying that the pre-embryo is a "product" and conveying the notion that it is an object or property. The committee decided that the pre-embryo might have some moral status, but the status could be outweighed by other moral considerations. As they addressed these issues they chose to not only address the "ethical issues in reproduction," but also decided they had to change the terminology at the same time.

In 1994, an ad hoc group of consultants to the advisory committee to the director of the National Institutes of Health issued a report on funding for research on preimplantation human embryo research. The committee considered both single-criterion views as well as the pluralistic approach to defining the moral status of embryos. "The Panel determined that formation of the primitive streak at approximately 14 days of development (Carnegie Stage 8) and the beginning of cell differentiation and individual organization marks a stage of development that merits an enhanced degree of protectability" (*Report of the Human Embryo Research Panel*, 1994, p. 51). Thus this group added further to the subdivision of the embryonic period by defining a preimplantation embryo and also another stage of development that occurred after implantation and prior to gastrulation. They took a developmental stage and accorded it moral meaning, as if changing the language describing the early stages of embryogenesis changes the moral status of the embryo.

In 1997 Eisenberg and Schenker (1997a, 1997b) reviewed the literature on the use of so-called pre-embryos for medical and scientific research. They noted the ethical and moral considerations and discussed the potential benefits for this research including preventing early pregnancy loss and improving IVF technology. They also pointed out that this research would aid in understanding early human development and would lead to better preimplantation diagnosis and perhaps gene therapy as well. They explored the legal and religious views of pre-embryo research and concluded that for most groups in society there was a measure of acceptability in performing research on the pre-embryo.

An editorial in *Fertility and Sterility* came out in 2002 written by Jones and Veeck. In it they put forth five reasons why the period between fertilization and formation of the primitive streak should be segregated and called the pre-embryonic period. Their reasons included the fact that large numbers of the fertilized eggs do not form normally and many do not implant. Second, most of the development at this time revolves around implantation and the formation of the placenta. Third, they cited the fact that twinning can occur during this period. Hence they supported the idea that only after day 14 of gestation did the embryos attain special moral status.

Two responses to this editorial elicited opposite points of views. Tacheva and Vladimirov (2002) supported the views of Jones and Veeck and gave several other reasons for the special status of the pre-embryonic period. However, Thorne and Kischer (2002) rebutted that the embryonic stage from fertilization onward is a continuum and should not be subdivided based on assigning moral value.

In 2004, President George W. Bush's Council on Bioethics issued a report called "Monitoring Stem Cell Research." In that report they defined stems cells, reviewed current federal law, discussed recent ethics debates including the moral standing of human embryos, and then examined the current findings in stem cell research and therapy (President's Council on Bioethics, 2004). One of the most interesting statements they make is the opening paragraph in the section on terminology. The council states:

> In considering complicated or contested public questions, language matters—even more than it ordinarily does. Clear thinking depends on clear ideas, and clear ideas can be conveyed only through clear and precise speech. And fairness in ethical evaluations and judgments depends on fair framing of the ethical questions, which in turn requires fair and accurate description of the relevant facts of the case at hand. (President's Council on Bioethics, 2004, p. 12).

Two paragraphs later in the council's report, language became the issue. In this paragraph, the council states:

> Strictly speaking, there is no such thing as "the embryo," if by this is meant a distinctive being (or kind of being) that deserves a common, reified name—like "dog" or "elephant." Rather, the term properly intends a certain stage of development of an organism of a distinctive kind. Indeed, the very term comes from a Greek root meaning "to grow"; and embryo is, by its name and mode of being, an immature and growing organism in an early phase of its development. (President's Council of Bioethics, 2004, p. 12)

However, this is confusing in light of statements made in the glossary:

> [The embryo is] (a) In humans, the developing organism from the time of fertilization until the end of the eighth week of gestation, when it becomes know as a fetus. (NIH) (b) The developing organism from the time of fertilization until significant differentiation has occurred, when the

organism becomes known as a fetus. An organism in the early stages of development. (President's Council of Bioethics, 2004, p. 149)

The terms *embryo, fetus, child,* and *adolescent* define periods of development. However, the topic becomes confusing to the reader and open to various interpretations when first "there is no such thing as the embryo" and then it is clearly defined. The council then further obfuscates the issue. Later in the report, in the section "Moral Standing of Human Embryos," it goes on to ask:

> What are early human embryos, and how should we regard them morally?...Thus to many observers, some of the central questions in this arena would appear to be those that surround human embryos: How ought we to think about and act toward human embryos? (President's Council of Bioethics, 2004, pp. 62–63)

This framing demonstrates the importance of language. Biologically speaking, we know what embryos are; what is at issue here is their moral status. As the council notes in its section "Preambles to the Bills—Hype Versus Doom":

> Legislators are currently considering bills that govern the technologies of cloning or embryo stem cell research. But even when the provisions of those bills are narrowly tailored to deal with those specific technologies, lawmakers include extensive preambles that include sweeping pro-life or pro-biotechnology language. (President's Council of Bioethics, 2004, p. 205)

In 2004, the *Connecticut Law Review* published a commentary forum called "What Is an Embryo?" The stated goal was to have a discussion in the hope that "attempts to eradicate biological ambiguity and attempts to eradicate lexical ambiguity converge" (Sirois, 2004, p. 1049). The forum is a compilation of much of the literature that involves the terminology surrounding the first 2 weeks of development. The scientific, state, and federal as well legal perspectives are summarized and reviewed in this publication, which very clearly demonstrates that the term *embryo* is not consistently used by any of these communities. Inconsistency exists in federal laws as well as the state laws, in governmental offices, and even among scientists.

The forum begin with an article titled "What Is an Embryo?," which suggested that the confusion around the term *embryo* has much to do with what the egg is "asked to do" (Kiessling, 2004). Kiessling pointed out that prior to the advent of IVF technology, eggs were only fertilized by sperm, and this process occurred in vivo. However, Kiessling suggests that the term *embryo* be used for eggs fertilized by sperm, but only after blastocysts have implanted. Kiessling goes on to advocate that other eggs developing for other reasons be called *parthenotes* and *ovasomes*. In this way embryos destined for stem cell research could be called something besides embryos. She also wanted to dissociate embryos during the first week of development from implanted embryos by calling the embryos prior to implantation pre-embryos.

In contrast, Latham and Sapienza took a much different approach. They stated:

> The solution is not to coin new terms, such as "pre-embryo" or "ovasome," or redefine existing terms, thus repeating past errors. The solution lies, instead, in education and the demystification of early stages of embryogenesis so that societal concerns can be addressed openly and without artifice. (Latham & Sapienza, 2004, p. 1171)

WHY REDEFINE SCIENTIFIC TERMINOLOGY DURING POLITICAL DEBATE?

I N T H E *CONNECTICUT* Law Review forum, the two lawyers speaking made very salient points about the terminology surrounding the first 2 weeks of development. Crockin stated:

> Lawyers know that language matters and is often outcome determinative. Nowhere is this more readily apparent than in legal matters involving reproductive technologies and reproductive genetics—where contract, family, and constitutional law; genetics; and intentionality all come into play. (Crockin, 2004)

In his article, Noah (2004) included a section titled "Playing Word Games Out of School." In this section he says:

> Consider the following statement by one of the most well-known eggs in English literature: "'When I use a word,' Humpty Dumpty said in a rather scornful tone, 'it means what I choose it to mean—neither more nor less.'" (Noah, 2004, p. 1152)

So language is important, and how words are used is critical in the political debate over issues surrounding the beginning of life. The real question involves what the words are trying to convey. Just why is it important to call the embryo during the first week of development a pre-embryo? Noah (2004, p. 1153) quotes Silver saying that this terminology debate is "political."

The words used and misused in these political debates may actually be ways to consciously or unconsciously influence others by evoking emotions, especially the emotions of disgust and anger. Jones examines the scientific literature on the emotion of disgust in a recent news feature in *Nature* (Jones, 2007). He asks whether the emotion of disgust is or should be used to direct ethical decision-making, he suggests that recent evidence shows it may not be a reliable compass to navigate through ethical issues. This is in contrast to Kass (1997) and Midgley (2000), who both suggest that there is importance in at least paying attention to emotions and especially the emotion of disgust or repugnance when considering ethical issues.

In terms of the use and misuse of language involved in beginning of life ethical debates, there may be another way to look at this. Rozin, Lowery, Imada, and Haidt (1999) put forth the CAD triad hypothesis, which maps the emotions contempt, anger, and disgust (CAD) to the moral codes community, autonomy, and divinity (CAD). Autonomy involves those issues such as individual rights and freedoms. The core values revolve around an individual's right to choose and his or her liberty. Violations of these rights trigger the emotion of anger. The core values that characterize the ethics of autonomy are particularly important to liberals and progressives (Rozin et al., 1999). The moral code that is important to conservatives is the ethics of divinity. Divinity involves the respect of a higher authority or deity and respect for oneself and others. Violations of this code maps to the emotion disgust. Disgust, as defined by Haidt, Rozin, and McCauley (1997), involved threats to an individual that cannot be escaped. Taken even further, disgust is the emotion generated when there is a feeling of meaningless in an individual's perception of their own self worth (Haidt et al., 1997). Disrespect for oneself or others in more general terms results in disgust. The idea that coming into contact with death elicits disgust was expanded by the same authors (Rozin, Haidt, & McCauley, 2000). If the actions taken disrespect the human community, they are perceived as disgusting. Violations of an individual's rights and autonomy would elicit anger, whereas removing or not including an individual in the community is an inhumane act and would generate disgust.

So those who espouse a pro-choice philosophy try not to use language that would give the embryo the status of human personhood. They do not want the embryo to be part of the human community. Those supporting a pro-life philosophy would always use language to describe the embryo from fertilization as a human life with all community rights conferred. What is interesting to note is that Turner suggests that not all individuals respond to the same stimulus with the same level of disgust if they even have any emotional reaction at all (Turner, 2004). Inbar, Pizarro, and Bloom (in press) have recently found that conservatives respond to issues with disgust more than liberals do. This is especially true for sociomoral issues. They found issues that elicited disgust from conservatives included abortion. This makes sense in light of the CAD hypothesis and provides insight into the use and misuse of language in the beginning of life debates. Liberals are more concerned with autonomy, freedom, and an individual's right to choose. For them, violations lead to anger. Conservatives think more about society, hierarchy, deity, and respect for oneself and others. Violations would generate a disgust reaction.

Those in favor of IVF, preimplantation genetic diagnosis, stem cell research, a woman's right to choose, and cloning, want to use language that supports their position without eliciting disgust. Hence, they would prefer calling a 5-day-old embryo, a pre-embryo, *certain material,* or a product of fertilization. At the Planned Parenthood Web site, the ethics of autonomy is seen in the language that is used to argue for abortion rights. When describing early pregnancy, the Web site incorrectly uses language to avoid suggesting that the first week of embryonic development is part of pregnancy or involves an embryo. The Web site states:

> Medical and scientific experts agree that pregnancy begins with implantation. It happens several days after fertilization when the developing pre-embryo is implanted in the wall of the uterus. Implantation begins the release of hormones that are necessary to support a pregnancy. In short, a woman is not pregnant until the developing pre-embryo is attached to her and gets nutrients from her. For example, a fertilized egg in a petri dish does not represent a pregnancy. (Planned Parenthood, n.d.)

Here language is misused to have the reader believe one is not pregnant until the blastocyst implants into the uterus and the fetal components of the placenta are in place. In fact, Bernstein and Weinstein (2007) state in *Current Diagnosis and Treatment Obstetrics and Gynecology* that "The human conceptus from fertilization through the eighth week of pregnancy is termed an **embryo;** from the eighth week until delivery, it is a **fetus**" (Bernstein & Weinstein, 2007, p. 187).

In contrast, those who adopt the conservative view and promote the politics of the right to life movement take a different tact when approaching the issues of right to life, abortion, cloning, and stem cell research. They actually try to elicit disgust. For example, on the main page of the National Right to Life Web site is a series of medical illustrations that show a partial birth abortion (National Right to Life, n.d.). These graphic diagrams are designed to evoke the emotions that are most associated with ethics of divinity. When discussing early embryology, the National Right to Life Web site also misuses language to promote its political perspective and says:

> The life of a baby begins long before he or she is born. A new individual human being begins at fertilization, when the sperm and ovum meet

to form a single cell. If the baby's life is not interrupted, he or she will someday become an adult man or woman. Worldwide, millions of un-born babies are killed each year. In the United States over 40 million unborn babies have been killed in the 29 years since abortion was legal-ized and more than 1.3 million are killed each year. (National Right to Life, n.d.)

Note that the embryo now becomes a baby at fertilization and that abortions kill babies. Here again language is misused to elicit the emo-tions that conservatives believe will convince others to adopt their viewpoint. Disgust and contempt are primary emotions displayed on the conservative Web sites. The ProLife Action League Web site de-scribes their sidewalk counseling:

> Thousands of children are alive today because the Pro-Life Action League was there at the moment of crisis. We care about the women being exploited by the abortion industry as well as the innocent babies being killed. That's why we're there on the sidewalk outside abortion facilities. (Pro-Life Action League, n.d.)

Finally, Nightlight Christian Adoptions is a nonprofit adoption agency that has started the Snowflakes program, which allows indi-viduals and couples to "adopt" frozen embryos. The misuse of the term *adoption* when considering embryo donation or transfer lies in the language that incorrectly implies the status of personhood has been approved for embryos. As Mercer (2006) and even the Snowflakes' Web site (*Snowflakes Program,* n.d.) point out there are no laws governing embryo transfer. So the language used is political and used to confer a status to the embryo—one not legally binding. However the term *do-nation* is also problematic because this term implies that the embryo is an object, and hence property. So language becomes critical to the debate.

CONCLUSION

THE EVENTS FROM fertilization through birth have been char-acterized, and the Carnegie Collection of Embryology has docu-mented the developmental stages and the language used to describe them from fertilization on. When IVF became possible and early stages of embryo development took place in a petri dish, some sci-entists began to change the language used to describe the embryo and the terms *preimplantation embryo* or *pre-embryo* came into use. When the politics of the beginning of life debate began to acceler-ate, language became an important tool. Liberals tried to promote autonomy while depersonalizing the embryo—calling it a product of fertilization. Conservatives attempted to use language to advance their views on the divinity of life and its importance to the community. Thus their language was personal and their viewpoint was put forth in the language of disgust—who wants to kill babies? The debate continues, and both sides try to use language to win support for their views, which makes communication more difficult. The early stages of development have been defined, and the proper terminology should be used. The debate can then focus not on the science but on the moral question of when human life and personhood begins. Science cannot tell us that.

REFERENCES

Bernstein, H. B., & Weinstein, M. (2007). Normal pregnancy and prenatal care. In A. H. DeCherney & L. Nathan (Eds.), *Current diagnosis and treatment obstetrics and gynecology* (10th ed., pp. 187–202). New York: McGraw Hill.

Bishop, T. (2007, March 11). In the high-stakes world of stem cell research, success or failure can hinge on the turn of a phrase. *The Baltimore Sun*, p. 1C.

Crockin, S. L. (2004). "What is an embryo?" A legal perspective. *Connecticut Law Review, 36*(4), 1177–1132.

Eisenberg, V. H., & Schenker, J. G. (1997a). The ethical, legal and religious aspects of pre-embryo research. *European Journal of Obstetrics and Gynecology and Reproductive Biology, 75,* 11–24.

Eisenberg, V. H., & Schenker, J. G. (1997b). Pre-embryo research: Medical aspects and ethical considerations. *Obstetrical and Gynecological Survey, 52*(9), 565–574.

Ethics Committee of the American Fertility Society. (1986). Ethical considerations of the new reproductive technologies. *Fertility and Sterility, 46*(Suppl. 1), 1S–93S.

Grobstein, C. (1979). External human fertilization. *Scientific American, 240,* 57–67.

Haidt, J., Rozin, P., & McCauley, C. (1997). Body, psyche and culture: The relationship between disgust and morality. *Psychology and Developing Societies, 9,* 107–131.

The Human Developmental Anatomy Center. (n.d.). *The Carnegie Collection of Embryology.* Retrieved May 29, 2007, from http://nmhm.washingtondc.museum/collections/hdac/Carnegie_collection.htm

Inbar, Y., Pizarro, D. A., & Bloom, P. (in press). Conservatives are more easily disgusted. *Cognition and Emotion.*

Jones, D. (2007). The depths of disgust. *Nature, 447,* 768–771.

Jones, H. W., & Veeck, L. (2002). What is an embryo? *Fertility and Sterility, 77,* 658–659.

Kass, L. R. (1997). The wisdom of repugnance. *New Republic, 216,* 17–26.

Kiessling, A. A. (2004). What is an embryo? *Connecticut Law Review, 36*(4), 1051–1092.

Latham, K. E., & Sapienza, C. (2004). Developmental potential as a criterion for understanding and defining embryos. *Connecticut Law Review, 36*(4), 1070–1176.

Maienschein, J. (2002). What's in a name: Embryos, clones and stem cells. *American Journal of Bioethics, 2*(1), 12–19.

Mercer, B. S. (2006). Embryo adoption: Where are the laws? *Journal of Juvenile Law, 26,* 73–83.

Midgley, M. (2000). Biotechnology and monstrosity: Why we should pay attention to the "yuk factor." *The Hastings Center Report, 30,* 7–15.

Moreno, J., & Berger, S. (2007, March 21). Stop politicizing scientific terminology. *The Wichita Eagle,* p. 9A.

National Right to Life. (n.d.). *Abortion: Some medical facts.* Retrieved June 7, 2007, from http://www.nrlc.org/abortion/ASMF/asmf3.html

Noah, L. (2004). A postmodernist take on the human embryo research debate. *Connecticut Law Review, 36*(4), 1133–1161.

Planned Parenthood. (n.d.). *How pregnancy happens.* Retrieved August 19, 2008, from http://www.plannedparenthood.org/health-topics/pregnancy/how-pregnancy-happens-4252.htm

President's Council on Bioethics. (2004). *Monitoring stem cell research.* Retrieved June 16, 2007, from http://www.bioethics.gov/reports/stemcell/index.html

Pro-Life Action League. (n.d.). *Sidewalk counseling.* Retrieved October 12, 2007, from http://www.prolifeaction.org/sidewalk/

Report of the Human Embryo Research Panel. (1994). Bethesda, MD: National Institutes of Health.

Rozin, P., Haidt, J., & McCauley, C. R. (2000). Disgust. In M. Lewis & J. M. Haviland-Jones (Eds.), *Handbook of emotions* (2nd ed., pp. 637–653). New York: Guilford Press.

Rozin, P., Lowery, L., Imada, S., & Haidt, J. (1999). The CAD triad hypothesis: A mapping of three emotions (contempt, anger, disgust) and three moral codes (community, autonomy and divinity). *Journal of Personality and Social Psychology, 76,* 574–586.

Sirois, J. I. (2004). Commentary introduction: Brave new words. *Connecticut Law Review, 36*(4), 1049–1050.

Snowflakes program. (n.d.). Retrieved July 29, 2007, from http://www.nightlight.org/snowflakeadoption.htm

Stenger, R. L. (2006). Embryo, fetuses, and babies: Treated as persons and treated with respect. *Journal of Health and Biomedical Law, 1,* 33–68.

Tacheva, D. M., & Vladimirov, I. K. (2002). Embryos, preembryos and stem cells. *Fertility and Sterility, 78,* 1354–1355.

Thorne, R., & Kischer, C. W. (2002). Embryos, preembryos and stem cells. *Fertility and Sterility, 78,* 1355.

Turner, L. (2004). Is repugnance wise? Visceral responses to biotechnology. *Nature Biotechnology, 22,* 269–270.

Part VI

Genetics

32

Eugenics

MARK B. ADAMS

SINCE **WORLD WAR** II, *eugenics* has become a dirty word. To accuse some idea, procedure, or policy of being eugenic or reminiscent of eugenics is to call forth images of inhuman medical experiments or Hitler's death camps. Far from the simple name of a historically interesting movement, *eugenics* has become an accusatory term of invective charged with political and ideological import, and suggestive of sexism, racism, right-wing extremism, and brutality. There are few terms in the bioethical lexicon that call forth such knee-jerk emotional affect, disdain, or outrage.

In fact, this post–World War II construct has very little relation to *historical* eugenics: that is, to the ideas set forth by its founder, or the characteristics of the international movement they led to. In recent decades, historians have begun to reconstruct the eugenics movements in dozens of countries, and what has emerged is a varied and interesting picture that requires us to reconsider our understanding of the term.

GETTING OUR TERMS STRAIGHT

THE TERM *EUGENICS* (which comes from Greek and means "wellborn") was coined by Charles Darwin's cousin, Francis Galton, in 1883. Galton had come to believe that many features of human beings—their physiology, constitution, and behaviors—were based on heredity and were passed from parents to children. In his view, society could not improve, and indeed might well degenerate, if current generations did not freely choose to adjust their reproductive behavior in the interests of humanity.

Galton suggested two ways that future generations could be improved. Policies and behaviors *increasing* the reproduction of the fittest constitute *positive eugenics*. Galton worried that upper- and especially middle-class professionals were tending to have fewer children than the under-classes, and that this would adversely affect the character of the next generation. Another way to increase the quality of further generations would be *negative eugenics,* that is, *decreasing* the reproduction of the unfit to future generations—including those with hereditary diseases, debilitating physical anomalies, and forms of behavior (prostitution, criminality, violence, aggression, schizophrenia, and so forth), which he and other contemporaries regarded as having a hereditary basis.

How could such results be brought about? Galton believed foremost in education: once people had learned what their hereditary constitution was and how their reproductive behavior could affect the future of humanity, he felt, they would want to adjust their behavior accordingly. Compliance was to be voluntary, and informed. In this sense, Galton can be seen as an early founder of both sex education and genetic counseling.

At the turn of the century, thinkers in other countries were developing ideas similar to Galton's but derived from their own national traditions and agendas. In Germany, Wilhelm Schallmayer became concerned about the demographic future of his nation and, along with Alfred Ploetz and others, developed the notion of *racial hygiene*. Hygiene was an important international movement at the turn of the century in many countries, centered on immunization, sanitation, cleanliness, exercise, health, nutrition, and the prevention of disease. Schallmayer and others believed that the health of the race was also important, and the racial hygiene movement emphasized reproductive policies aimed at increasing the numbers, health, and fitness of future German generations. Some associated with the German movement became concerned about the degeneration of the Aryan race. With the coming together of the German state in the late 19th century, the idea of race provided a way of understanding German identity across confused geographical and political boundaries.

German thinkers brought with them a statist tradition, in which the interests of the nation overrode and governed individual behavior, especially in matters related to public health. In 18th-century Prussia, for instance, the State Health Police had wide powers over immigration, quarantine, and disease control in the interests of keeping its population (and its military) strong and healthy. As a result of German statist traditions, and in contrast to Galton and other English-speaking thinkers, German thinkers tended to emphasize statist solutions involving state agencies, bureaucracies, and medical panels in determining and applying reproductive policy. Indeed, in Weimar Germany, *Eugenik* and *Rassen-Hygiene* were competing ideas: Hermann Muckermann (Jesuit activist) proposed adopting the term *Eugenik,* reorienting the German movement along more Galtonian lines, de-emphasizing race, and focusing on education and voluntary compliance; but ultimately, it was *race hygiene* that won out. Contributing to these German developments was a persistent fear of German underpopulation by comparison to France, which would then have the numerical advantage in any future wars. Ironically, France had similar fears with respect to Germany. There, neither eugenics nor race hygiene made much headway, but analogous French fears about future generations led to the development of analogous movements: *euthenics* emphasized the use of environmental amelioration (education, exercise, public health, sanitation, immunization) as a way to improve future generations; *puericulture* emphasized motherhood and scientific child-rearing as a means to the same end.

Another term often confused with eugenics is *social Darwinism,* but that association can be misleading. Unlike *eugenics,* which was a term coined by Galton and embraced by its advocates, *social Darwinism* was principally a pejorative term used by its opponents to castigate thinkers and ideas they opposed. Those so castigated tended to emphasize intraspecific competition for resources between individuals, groups, populations, and nations. Indeed, although both emphasized the biological fitness of future generations, their varying perspectives sometimes led to conflicts over important issues. One such issue was war: social Darwinists tended to see warfare as part of the Darwinian struggle for existence, with the fittest emerging victorious. By contrast, many advocates of eugenics regarded war as *dysgenic* in that many of the fittest members of each warring population would end up dying on the battlefield.

SETTING THE RECORD STRAIGHT: MYTHS AND MISCONCEPTIONS

B Y 1935, EUGENICS and other related ideas had spread widely, and eugenics societies and movements had been founded in more than 40 countries. Although most national societies were members of an international eugenics federation, their individual activities and character were largely based on local or national traditions, conditions, and configurations. Understandably, then, stereotypes based on one particular nation or figure or movement have often led to misimpressions about eugenics as a whole that persist, despite the vast amount of recent historical research that have shown them to be misleading.

WAS EUGENICS BASED ON THE BIOLOGICAL DETERMINISM OF MENDELIAN GENETICS?

IT HAS SOMETIMES been argued, and is often assumed, that the development of Mendelian genetics beginning in 1900 and the subsequent development of the chromosomal theory of heredity by T. H. Morgan's group were somehow crucial to the efflorescence of eugenics, in that it embodied a hard concept of heredity according to which traits were determined by genes that could not be altered by their environment (as opposed, for example, to neo-Lamarckianism, according to which acquired traits can be inherited). This argument often sees both eugenics, and the genetics on which it was ostensibly based, as forms of reductionistic biological determinism. While such a characterization may be true of some eugenicists and geneticists in some movements, it hardly applies to eugenics as a whole. For one thing, Galton had already coined the word *eugenics* and worked out his eugenic ideas some 17 years before the work of Mendel was rediscovered. Furthermore, many of Galton's most influential followers in Britain—such as Karl Pearson and the so-called biometric school—were dubious of the validity and generality of Mendel's pea laws and based their strong advocacy of eugenics on a more statistical approach to inheritance. Indeed, a number of national eugenics societies (for example, the Brazilian society) were founded by Lamarckians, and influential Lamarckians in Europe and elsewhere were eugenicists.

WAS EUGENICS SEXIST?

SOME MAY BE under the impression that eugenics was essentially sexist, that it represented a way for the male establishment to control women's bodies, that it was somehow antagonistic to feminism. Such an impression finds little support in the historical record. Data on various eugenic societies and research institutions suggests that women scientists were more heavily represented in eugenics work than in most other contemporary scientific fields. From Galton on, eugenicists regarded women as equal partners in contributing to the hereditary constitution of their offspring, so many eugenicists believed that for any eugenic program to be effective, it was vital for all women to receive education so that their physical and mental potential could be fully realized. Indeed, Margaret Sanger and other feminist birth control advocates of the day were strong supporters of eugenics.

WAS EUGENICS RACIST?

LIKE MOST OTHER fields at the time, eugenics recognized race as a reality and an appropriate analytical category, although the number of human races, their origins, and their characteristics continued to be matters of disciplinary dispute. Eugenicists noted that the frequency of blood types, as well as certain genetic diseases, differed in various ethnic populations. Certainly, in certain movements (notably the German movement), it was commonly believed that certain races were superior to others in certain characteristics, and many German race hygienists wished to protect the Aryan stock from dilution by supposedly inferior racial groups. However, this was by no means universal, and eugenic science provided conflicting paradigms concerning the issue of racial interbreeding. Animal and plant breeders were well aware of both hybrid sterility (the tendency of distant hybrids to be less viable) and also hybrid vigor (the tendency of certain distant hybrids to be more robust than either parent stock). Those predisposed against racial mixing could point to the former as a reason to restrict interracial marriage; those advocating it could point to the latter. For example, in certain Latin American countries, eugenicists urged racial mixing between European and native populations as a way to produce a more perfect race, the people of the Sun. Again, the attitude toward issues revolving around race tended to be dominated by local issues and traditions, not eugenics, which was often selectively appropriated as scientific justification for actions otherwise motivated.

WAS EUGENICS RIGHT WING?

FOLLOWING WORLD WAR II and the revelation of Nazi death-camp atrocities, many people have tended to associate eugenics with right-wing political groups and especially fascism. In actuality, eugenics as a movement comfortably incorporated members of a wide range of political stripes, ranging from the extreme right wing to the extreme left, and everything in the middle. For example, many American eugenicists in the early 20th century identified with the progressive movement, and eugenicists were often allied with such causes as the preservation of the American wilderness, conservation, birth control, women's suffrage, child labor laws, and other contemporary campaigns that could hardly be characterized—then or now—as right wing. And there were strong advocates of eugenics on the far left as well.

The proponents of what historian Dan Kevles (1995) has labeled *reform eugenics* (including J. B. S. Haldane, H. J. Muller, and Julian Huxley) were distinctly left wing in orientation. In 1920s Britain, Haldane proposed eugenic *ectogenesis* (eugenically bred bottled babies) as a way to save humanity from degeneration, an idea later satirized by Aldous Huxley (Julian's brother) in *Brave New World* (1932); elsewhere, Haldane had advocated genetic experimentation on human beings—this by the same Haldane who in the 1930s was a member of the central committee of the British Communist Party. For his part, Muller would spend the period of 1933–1937 in Soviet Russia, agitating for Stalin to establish eugenic communes using artificial insemination to speed the development of communism. Yes, some influential eugenicists and movements were indeed right wing—but some were left wing, and many others were neither.

VARIETIES OF EUGENICS

IN 1929, RUSSIAN geneticist and eugenicist Alexander Serebrovsky distinguished between *human genetics,* which was a science, could be illuminated by research, and was universal, and *eugenics,* which was the social policies concerning human reproduction put into place in society, and which therefore would differ from country to country depending on that country's situation, conditions, traditions, and values, as well as its social, economic, and political system. This is a useful distinction to keep in mind in evaluating the incredible diversity of worldwide eugenics.

The spread of eugenic ideas was related to the popular ideas and ideologies of the time and, like those movements, eugenics took many different forms in different national settings. Those various movements also understandably became involved in the national issues and agendas of the day, including immigration, disease control, colonialism, race relations, political power, and economic development. Quite understandably, then, the various eugenics-related movements in various countries assumed different forms. It should, therefore, not surprise us in the least that the eugenics movement in Romania was quite different from that in Sweden or China. Depending on each country's ethnic makeup, economic character, political structure, professional traditions, educational system, and current concerns, eugenics movements adapted a common international aspiration to a host of local realities.

Often, the form the eugenics movement took in any given country depended on the professional background of its membership. Different configurations of disciplines often reflected local interests and tilted the movement's activities. In Germany, for example, the large representation of anthropologists reinforced the preoccupation with race. In France, pediatricians and demographers were more heavily involved, and those physicians in other countries who got their medical training in France often reflected those interests. The foreign associations and training of the membership also played an important role. A good illustration of this is Japan. In the 1920s and 1930s, there were two distinct societies in Japan: the Eugenics Society, whose membership consisted of Japanese zoologists and agricultural scientists who had trained in Britain or the United States (often at Cornell), and took more Galtonian approaches; and the Race Hygiene Society, consisting largely of bacteriologists and physicians who had received their medical training in Germany, and took a more racialist approach.

Among the ways countries differed were in their religious traditions, make-up, and values. It should not surprise us, then, that the way ethical issues relating to eugenics were seen and understood also differed at different places and times.

EUGENICS AND ETHICS

ACCORDING TO THE common misinformed stereotypes (hopefully dispelled above), eugenics might seem to be inherently unethical. As we have seen, however, those stereotypes are false and misleading. Assuming for the moment that the important bioethical issues concerning eugenics arise not by virtue of what eugenicists may have said, advocated, or published, but by the actions they took or supported, let us consider the bioethical dimensions of eugenics that seem most closely associated with it. These center around the eugenic research that was conducted, and the social policies supported by eugenicists that were put into effect. Another important distinction to be made is the degree to which eugenics conformed to the ethical standards of its time and place, and how those standards compare to those of today.

ETHICS AND EUGENICS RESEARCH

COMPARED TO THE research undertaken in most biomedical fields, most of the research undertaken by eugenicists was tame indeed and ethically uncomplicated. Early eugenicists sought to establish which human traits were hereditary, and how they were passed down in families. Beginning with Galton, such research most often involved collecting family histories and carrying out twin studies. Often such research involved compiling and analyzing vast quantities of records (hence, the title of the leading American eugenics research institution, the Eugenics Record Office). Thus, records of family histories of color blindness, height, weight, physiological or anatomical anomalies, hair and eye color, and so forth were compiled in order to single out the hereditary basis and transmission of those traits.

Although measuring and recording human traits and analyzing vast amounts of such data were essential to eugenic research, they do not present any ethical issues that are not present in most fields involving human subjects—notably, the issue of privacy and of informed consent. In most cases, this did not present any systemic problem. Family history data was most often coded, so as to keep the personal identities of the individuals and families from whom data had been collected confidential, and was reported only in general terms, and, in most cases, the data was volunteered. Indeed, given the persistent Galtonian emphasis on eugenics as a civic religion, and the priority most eugenicists placed on educating the population, the informed consent given by most of those volunteering such data was probably considerably more informed than the consenter would have cared it to be.

ETHICS AND EUGENIC POLICIES: STERILIZATION

THE MOST PRESSING bioethical issues associated with eugenics concern sterilization. In many U.S. states, legislation was passed, often with strong rhetorical support from eugenicists, to provide compulsory sterilization to certain members of the population regarded as hereditarily defective. Often the political motives for such actions went beyond eugenics: legislatures were often concerned with the future costs of having to institutionalize large numbers of mentally incompetent, criminal, or ill wards of the state, and the burdens on social resources such incarceration would necessitate. But there is no doubt that eugenicists often strongly supported such legislation, in the United States and elsewhere.

In eugenic terms, sterilization was a form of *negative eugenics*—that is, a way of decreasing the contribution of the less fit to the next generation by making it impossible for them to reproduce further (since most of those sterilized had already begotten children). As objectionable as it may seem to us today, in the early 20th-century compulsory sterilization was regarded by many as a humane scientific solution far preferable to the alternatives. Consider the matter as contemporaries may have understood it: how could society keep someone from reproducing who refused to stop having children? In the absence of sterilization, the only other option seemed to be incarceration. With the development of such surgical techniques as the vasectomy, it appeared that a relatively simple medical procedure could achieve the desired result at considerably less cost, and with less violation of the rights of the patient. Indeed, at the time, there was a large body of scientific opinion that such procedures as castration could actually improve mental and physical health. The contemporary endocrinological research of Eugen Steinach on rejuvenation suggested that x-ray sterilization of the gonads left those organs free to rejuvenate the body with internal secretions that would help keep the body young and fit. By the end of the 1920s, "getting Steinached" became a fashionable rejuvenation technique, undergone gladly by such figures as Sigmund Freud, Pablo Picasso, and W. B. Yeats. Clearly, the issue is not sterilizations per se: most have been voluntary. The bioethical issue concerns those compulsory sterilizations performed by the state without the informed consent of the patient.

Another curious ethical feature of this form of negative eugenics is that it was relatively uncontroversial among geneticists and eugenicists of the time. Today, it might seem that the ethically questionable form of eugenics would be negative eugenics, since it would involve limiting the reproduction of the unfit; encouraging the fit to have more children would seem ethically unproblematic. Yet, as historian Diane Paul has established, historically it was just the reverse. Geneticists, eugenicists, and even Lamarckians seemed to have no qualms about the sterilization of the unfit: eliminating genetic diseases seemed a no-brainer. What they found ethically problematic was positive eugenics, because there was no consensus as to which human characteristics were so desirable that humans should be bred for them. (Among those traits variously proposed were altruism, strength, leadership, intelligence, height, sociability, musicality, longevity, cooperativeness, friendliness, and luck.)

Ultimately, however, the bioethical issues related to compulsory sterilization have less to do with eugenics than with human rights and legitimate state powers. Is having as many children as one wishes a human right? Does the state have any rights regarding the reproduction of its citizens? What if the state has the obligation to provide for the welfare of its children? What if the state feels its vital interests are at stake? Ultimately, the question boils down to this: Under what circumstances, if any, is it ethical for the state to compel someone to be sterilized?

CONCLUSION

CERTAINLY, GOVERNMENTS HAVE been involved in influencing the reproduction of their citizens for many hundreds of years, by providing incentives, maternal support, and other inducements to reproduce, as well as disincentives for others. What are the ethical limits of such state behavior? Historically, the answers to these questions have varied with time and place. But the central determinant has little to do with the theory of heredity one believes in, or the character of one's politics: rather, it has to do with one's willingness or wish for the state to do things to people without their consent or against their will.

The tantalizing ethical complexities of eugenic history can be seen in the case of M. V. Volotskoi—a Jew, an ardent Bolshevik, a Lamarckian, and, in the early 1920s, the secretary of the Russian Eugenics Society. Volotskoi had the dubious distinction of being the chief proponent of eugenic sterilization in postrevolutionary Russia, and urged the government to adopt a truly Bolshevik approach by sterilizing large numbers of the unfit in order to hasten socialism and improve society. As it happens, postrevolutionary Russia was undergoing a population implosion at the time (the result of wartime devastation, disease, famine, and civil war), and the proposal was not well received. Iurii Filipchenko, head of the Academy of Sciences's Eugenics Bureau, criticized Volotskoi on the grounds that compulsory sterilization was unethical; state officials failed to see how his proposal would help to repopulate a ravaged country; medical officials argued it would be a waste of limited resources. The proposal was soon dropped.

The Volotskoi example is informative precisely because of the many stereotypes about eugenics it confounds: sterilization, stereotypically associated with right-wing, racist Mendelians, is being advocated by a Bolshevik Jewish Lamarckian. Volotskoi was not the only Lamarckian advocate of compulsory sterilization: indeed, since Lamarckians believed that traits acquired during one's lifetime could become hereditary, it was actually easier to justify sterilization from a Lamarckian than from a Mendelian point of view. Although his timing was unfortunate, Volotskoi was not completely wrong: with a new activist Bolshevik government in charge, and its own statist traditions (derived in part from Germany), Russian society was a natural venue for statist solutions. By the 1930s, under Stalin, such involuntary statist solutions would take other, darker forms that had nothing to do with eugenics. So too would they, at roughly the same time, in Nazi Germany.

The primary bioethical issue relating to the history of eugenics, then, is not really about eugenics, not about race or politics or science. The issue, rather, is this: under what circumstances, and in what ways, can the state legitimately act to control the reproductive behavior of its citizens? Today that question is being answered quite differently in the United States, India, Singapore, and China. Whether any international ethical consensus will emerge remains to be seen. Failing that, as in the past, each country will have to work out its own version of what it finds ethically acceptable under current circumstances, and we will all have to live with the consequences.

FURTHER READING

THERE IS A vast literature on eugenics and its history, but it is uneven in quality, and much of it is specialized, focusing on one particular country or issue. For those wishing to learn more about eugenics, three works provide a good place to begin: Daniel J. Kevles, *In the Name of Eugenics: Genetics and the Uses of Human Heredity* (Cambridge, MA: Harvard University Press, 1995); Diane B. Paul, *Controlling Human Heredity: 1865 to the Present* (Atlantic Highlands, NJ: Humanities Books, 1995); and Mark B. Adams, ed., *The Wellborn Science: Eugenics in Germany, France, Brazil, and Russia* (New York: Oxford University Press, 1990).

33

Human Gene Patents

Jon F. Merz

O N **December 7,** 2006, Dr. Francis Collins, director of the U.S. National Human Genome Research Institute was asked by Steven Colbert on *The Colbert Report* whether human genes could be patented, expressing concern that someone might want a copy of his genes. Dr. Collins, after acknowledging the legitimacy of Colbert's concerns, answered:

> Any genes that haven't already been patented can't be because we put all of the DNA sequence in the public domain and now it's called prior art and nobody can claim it. That was one of the goals of the Human Genome Project, to stop all this patenting of fundamental information about our own genome. It didn't seem to be a good thing. (Collins, 2006)

Data from the same period suggested that roughly 20% of the more than 23,000 known human genes were claimed in a set of 4,258 U.S. utility patents issued up until April 5, 2005 (Jensen & Murray, 2005). However, publication of the consensus sequence of the human genome by Craig Venter and his many collaborators most certainly did *not* stop the patenting of human genes. Some evidence suggests that the rate of filing slowed at least initially, and what is being patented may have been significantly narrowed by applicants to meet tighter U.S. and international patentability thresholds (Hopkins, Mahdi, Patel, & Thomas, 2007), but patenting human genes clearly continues apace.

A search of the U.S. Patent and Trademark Office's database of patents and published applications (typically published 18 months after filing) shows that there are thousands of patents issued, and thousands of patents pending, many of which having filing dates after Venter's *Science* paper in early 2001 presenting the sequence of the human genome (Venter et al., 2001). Just searching U.S. Class 435/6 (molecular biology, involving nucleic acid sequence) for patents that include "Seq." in their claims yields 5,643 U.S. patents issued through April 15, 2008, and 15,069 open applications through April 10, 2008. Restricting this search to the post-Venter publication period, we find 1,643 issued patents and 14,559 published applications filed after February 1, 2001. Indeed, in class 435/6 alone, 385 now-published patent applications including sequence claims have been filed since Dr. Collins made his previously quoted statement. According to the data compiled by Jensen and Murray, some 19% of patented human gene sequences have been classified in 435/6 (K. Jensen, personal communication, May 23, 2008), so this single subclass appears to capture a relatively large fraction of human gene patents.

In 1996, shortly after coming to the University of Pennsylvania, I met with a Penn neurologist, Kenneth Fischbeck. In the course of the discussion, Dr. Fischbeck pulled out a copy of U.S. Patent No. 5,306,616 that claimed, among other things, the diagnosis of Charcot-Marie-Tooth disease (CMT-1A) by examining a patient's DNA. The patent claim was poorly worded, but it claimed exclusivity to the use of well-established molecular biology techniques to characterize whether a patient has a particular genetic anomaly that the inventors had associated with the phenotype of CMT. Dr. Fischbeck was particularly aggrieved by this patent, because while he himself had collaborated with the Baylor inventors who cloned the gene and got the patent, this patent could be used to inhibit his own research as well as the clinical care of his patients. This conversation spurred a look into these types of diagnostics, and we declaimed:

> Making associations of genetic differences and phenotypic expressions has a long history. For example, Stevens discovered the correlation of the X and Y chromosomes with gender in 1905, LeJeune discovered the association of trisomy 21 with Down's syndrome in 1959, and Nowell discovered the Philadelphia chromosome (t(9;22)) and its association with chronic myeloid leukemia in 1960. The technology used to make those discoveries was the microscope. Today, there is a wide variety of tools used in molecular biology, including Southern analysis, PCR and other amplification methods, and DNA sequencing. Simply, our "microscopes" have gotten much better, enabling us to "see" not only trisomies and translocations, but subchromosomal mutations. Yesterday's discoveries of chromosomal anomalies and disease are similar in kind to

today's discoveries of disease-associated mutations. But unlike today's discoveries, none of these past discoveries was patented. (Merz, Cho, Robertson, & Leonard, 1997, p. 299, citations omitted)

Clearly, what had changed since those early discoveries was not merely advances in technology but also the market-driven economic environment of academia (spurred on as it was by the propitiously timed 1980 Bayh-Dole Act) combined with the resplendent growth of the biotechnology industry.[1] Indeed, the CMT-1A patent had been licensed by Baylor exclusively to a company called Athena Diagnostics, and there were concerns that Athena would use this patent to capture the molecular testing market. Baylor itself learned a painful lesson when Athena, probably using the blood samples it received for testing for CMT-1A, discovered and patented an X-linked CMT and purportedly debarred Baylor from testing for this allele.[2] Around the same time (1997), other cases were brought to our attention, including Myriad Genetics and the breast and ovarian cancer gene BRCA1, Miami Children's Hospital and the gene that causes Canavan disease, the Apo-E gene and Alzheimer's disease (which had been licensed exclusively for clinical testing purposes by Duke University to Athena), and SmithKline Beecham and the gene for hemochromatosis.

STUDIES OF GENE PATENTS IN THE MARKETPLACE

To GET A sense of the scope of this emerging patent landscape, a pilot survey was performed on a convenience sample of molecular pathologists attending a national meeting of the Association for Molecular Pathology and the American Association for Clinical Chemistry. We left questionnaires to be picked up and filled out by willing attendees, and we received 74 responses (representing about 30% of meeting attendees). Roughly a quarter of respondents reported being blocked from performing some genetic testing services, and nearly half reported that they had refrained from developing a known test because of patent concerns (Cho, 1998).

In addition, we performed a search for gene patents that had extremely broad diagnostics claims. We identified a set of 37 U.S. patents, 33 of which were current and owned by U.S. entities. Seventeen technology transfer or licensing officials from entities that owned 27 of these patents were interviewed. Fourteen of the patents had been licensed, all exclusively to one firm. Older patents and those known to have clinical utility were more likely to have been licensed (Schissel, Merz, & Cho, 1999). We perceived that the problem was not so much in the patenting itself but in the granting of market exclusivity to testing firms that could block molecular pathologists from developing tests, from training fellows on how to perform tests, and from performing research to find new genetic disease alleles (Merz, 1999).

Indeed, to flesh out what was occurring in one high-profile case (identified as a current problem by respondents in our pilot survey), we performed an analysis of the diffusion of testing, in light of its patenting, for the gene HFE, which causes hemochromatosis. Three years after the discovery, we attempted to identify and interview all U.S. laboratories capable of performing such testing, and we documented when the labs had begun testing. As suspected, testing was offered clinically quite rapidly upon publication of the research, with 58 of 119 capable labs performing the test at the time of our study. Sixty percent of the labs offering the test had begun doing so before the key patent had even issued. About 20% of the labs reported that the patent was the reason they had refrained from developing the HFE test. Interestingly, HFE was not discovered in a university or a hospital but by a startup biotech firm, Mercator Genetics (although the firm collaborated with an academic clinician who clearly had provided access to patients and blood to facilitate the research—he is not included as an inventor, which is not an atypical product of academic-industry collaborations! Ducor, 2000). HFE was used as a platform for the development of the firm's proprietary positional cloning methods; the gene was difficult to find because it is in a highly conserved part of the human genome. Soon after its discovery, Mercator was merged into Progenitor, which licensed the patents on exclusive terms for clinical testing (but not sale of kits) to SmithKline Beecham Clinical Laboratories (SBCL). SBCL then began enforcement of the patents against the molecular pathology community, and many of our interviewees reported that they had received letters from SBCL threatening to pursue legal action if they use the test. In epilogue, SBCL was sold off to Quest Diagnostics, which then sold its patent interests to Bio-Rad Laboratories, which used the patents to bolster its proprietary test kit in the marketplace (Merz, Kriss, Leonard, & Cho, 2002).

We later broadened this study by again surveying molecular pathologists across the United States, asking broader questions about patent constraints on their clinical and research activities. Significantly, and consistent with our pilot survey and HFE study, of 122 laboratorians interviewed, 25% reported that they had stopped at least one test, and 53% reported that they had not developed at least one clinical or research test because of their concerns about patents. Respondents uniformly believed that patents restricted patients' access to clinically useful tests and constrained research activities. We felt this was ironic, given that some 60% of the patents these laboratories reported having to deal with had resulted at least in part from research sponsored by the federal government (Cho, Illangasekare, Weaver, Leonard, & Merz, 2003).

This led us to perform a more systematic study of gene patent licensing. With NIH funding, we identified 48 firms and 62 nonprofits (e.g., universities or hospitals) each owning more than three patents classified in 435/6 and issued since 1990. We then attempted to interview technology transfer and licensing executives from these entities about their licensing strategies. This study showed some marked differences between firms and nonprofits regarding patenting and licensing practices. Firms were much more likely to seek patent protection for inventions, which serve to round out a patent portfolio, which may earn royalties as well as ensure the firm the freedom to operate within a technology domain. Nonprofits were more likely to carefully assess the value of an invention before seeking patents, going so far as to license an invention early to get a licensee to pay patent prosecution costs (which can run to several hundred thousand dollars for world-wide rights). Firms reported that they were unlikely to grant exclusive licenses to their patents, unless they were to simply sell off the patents when they no longer would work on a particular technology; nonprofits, however, were highly likely to report granting exclusive licenses, which they perceived as being easiest to negotiate and often reported this was necessary to give the licensee the incentive to invest further in downstream development toward bringing a useful product to market. (Of course, we argued long and strenuously that this is not the case in diagnostics, which anyone can practice as soon as the locus of a clinically useful marker is identified; Henry, Cho, Weaver, & Merz, 2002, 2003.)

THE MARKETPLACE RESPONDS

THESE STUDIES OBVIOUSLY did not ingratiate us in the biotechnology (business) community. Indeed, after the publication in *Nature* of our survey on the diffusion of HFE testing, several of us were interviewed by a purported news writer for *Nature Biotechnology*. This individual turned out to also be the vice president for intellectual property at a gene therapy company. His news piece was libelous, conveying unsubstantiated and clearly false accusations that our survey methodology was biased, "lacks credible evidence and scientific rigor," and even somehow violated "IRB guidelines" (Chahine, 2002, p. 419). Interestingly, until this attack took place, we were not apprised by anyone of such concerns about our work. We appropriately wrote a letter to *Nature Biotechnology,* and, as of the day before the deadline for our letter, the editor told us that no replies had been submitted to our letter. Thus, we were again surprised when the issue appeared with two replies, one from Chahine (the aforementioned purported news writer) and one from the Biotechnology Industry Organization (BIO), with the editor backing up Chahine's attack. Interestingly, Chahine in this reply cited a "detailed multipage outline" generated by an "industry representative" to support his assertions that we violated ethical guidelines for human subjects research. I made various requests for this outline, but both Chahine and the editor of *Nature Biotechnology* refused to provide it to me. I have yet to ever see it. This raises the troubling thought that *Nature Biotechnology* is captive to the industry it covers, and academic standards of honesty and transparency have been sacrificed to financial expediency (Correspondence, 2002, p. 657).

Later on, when we sought to perform our study of licensing practices, the National Human Genome Research Institute (NHGRI) was fortuitously seeking to fund such a study. However, I was told in rather blunt terms by an NHGRI analyst that, inasmuch as I had been so long and so vocally critical of gene patents, I was biased and thus incapable of performing such a study. Instead of seeking this funding, we secured instead a supplement to our NIH grant studying cases of gene patenting, to perform the licensing substudy, which we performed relatively quickly. Although our sampling methods were slightly different, there was substantial overlap between our sample and that of the group that did get the NHGRI award. Admittedly, their methodology was much more detailed than was ours, and their work contributed usefully to our understanding of current university gene patent licensing practices. It is interesting, however, that when this group's paper appeared in *Nature Biotechnology* in early 1996, some 3.5 years after our *Science* paper appeared and more than 2 years after our more thorough exposition in the *Journal of Law, Medicine and Ethics,* the authors somehow failed to cite this antecedent work (Pressman et al. 2006).

CONCLUSION

D**ID OUR WORK** have any impact on the policies and practices surrounding gene patents, besides earning industry ire? We like to think so. We have presented our work to the U.S. Congress, the Department of Health and Human Services Secretary's Advisory Committee on Genetic Testing, and the Secretary's Advisory Committee on Human Research Protections; Representative Rivers proposed legislation back in 2002 that would have exempted from infringement research and certain clinical uses of genetic diagnostics, but this bill went nowhere (and Rep. Rivers was redistricted out of Congress in 2002).

The NIH published licensing guidelines in 2005 that strongly supported a default of nonexclusive, broad licensing of human gene patents, with exclusivity reserved for fields of use and applications that required large investments for the development of useful products. Overall, the market for gene patents has evolved over the last dozen years, as licensors and licensees have come to understand the complexities of the technology and its patent landscape. Of course, there have been bumps in the road, but the unwise licensing program pursued by Miami Children's Hospital was the exception (Merz, 2002), not the rule, and the bad actors in the diagnostics world have been limited to a handful of companies.

NOTES

1. The Bayh-Dole Act gave U.S. universities, small businesses, and nonprofits intellectual property control of inventions that resulted from research funded by the federal government.
2. U.S. Patent Nos. 5,691,144 and 6,001,576.

REFERENCES

Bayh-Dole Act, Public Law 96-517, U.S. Code § 35, (1980).

Chahine, K. (2002). Industry opposes genomic legislation. *Nature Biotechnology, 20,* 119.

Cho, M. (1998). Ethical and legal issues in the 21st century. In *Preparing for the millennium: Laboratory medicine in the 21st century* (pp. 47–53). Orlando: AACC Press.

Cho, M. K., Illangasekare, S., Weaver, M. A., Leonard, D. G. B., & Merz, J. F. (2003). Effects of patents and licenses on the provision of clinical genetic testing services. *Journal of Molecular Diagnostics, 5,* 3–8.

Collins, F. (2006, December 7). *The Colbert report* [Television interview]. Retrieved April 4, 2008, from http://www.comedycentral.com/colbertreport/videos.jhtml?videoId=79237

Correspondence. (2002). *Nature Biotechnology, 20,* 657.

Ducor, P. (2000). Coauthorship and coinventorship. *Science, 289,* 873, 875

Henry, M. R., Cho, M. K., Weaver, M. A., & Merz, J. F. (2002). DNA patenting and licensing. *Science, 297,* 1279.

Henry, M. R., Cho, M. K., Weaver, M. A., & Merz, J. F. (2003). A pilot survey on the licensing of DNA inventions. *Journal of Law, Medicine and Ethics, 31,* 442–449.

Hopkins, M. M., Mahdi, S., Patel, P., & Thomas, S. M. (2007). DNA patenting: The end of an era? *Nature Biotechnology, 25,* 185–187.

Jensen, K., & Murray, F. (2005). Intellectual property landscape of the human genome. *Science, 310,* 239–240.

Merz, J. F. (1999). Disease gene patents: Overcoming unethical constraints on clinical laboratory medicine. *Clinical Chemistry, 45,* 324–330.

Merz, J. F. (2002). Discoveries: Are there limits on what may be patented? In D. Magnus, A. Caplan, & G. McGee (Eds.), *Who owns life?* (pp. 99–116). Amherst, NY: Prometheus Press.

Merz, J. F., Cho, M. K., Robertson, M. A., & Leonard, D. G. B. (1997). Disease gene patenting is a bad innovation. *Molecular Diagnosis, 2,* 299–304.

Merz, J. F., Kriss, A. G., Leonard, D. G. B., & Cho, M. K. (2002). Diagnostic testing fails the test: The pitfalls of patenting are illustrated by the case of haemochromatosis. *Nature, 415,* 577–579.

Pressman, L., Burgess, R., Cook-Deegan, R. M., McCormack, S. J., Nami-Wolk, I., Soucy, M., et al. (2006). The licensing of DNA patents by US academic institutions: An empirical survey. *Nature Biotechnology, 24,* 31–39.

Schissel, A., Merz, J. F., & Cho, M. K. (1999). Survey confirms fears about licensing of genetic tests. *Nature, 402,* 118.

Venter, J. C., Adams, M. D., Myers, E. W., Li, P. W., Mural, R. J., Sutton, G. G., et al. (2001). The sequence of the human genome. *Science, 91,* 1304–1351.

34

Genetics Research and Race: Whither Bioethics?

Pamela Sankar

THE EMERGING SALIENCE of race in genomic research represents a serious challenge facing bioethics today. Genetic research that uses race, especially research aimed to alleviate common chronic conditions such as heart disease, diabetes, and cancer, raises all of the issues usually associated with genetic research, such as informed consent, confidentiality, ownership of genetic information, and future use of genetic samples. But raised against a backdrop of race, these issues become all the more troublesome. This is the case especially in the context of disparities in health status, which in the United States are most serious among racial minorities. This context heightens concern because the combination of race and genetics can activate essentialist thinking that deflects attention away from the social conditions that foster most health disparities and makes them appear instead as the inevitable result of a natural fact, that is, of race.

Essentialist thinking treats race and ethnicity as innate, salient, and immutable differences among people. The degree to which scientists and others actually endorse essentialist thinking about race is unclear and cannot be assumed. Nonetheless, using race in the context of genetic research is more likely to encourage this conceptualization than in other settings, because of a second line of essentialist thinking, which is that genes determine outcomes, such as health or behavior, more than do environmental factors. And, in the reductionist logic of essentialist thinking, if race is innate, or genetic, and if genetics is responsible for health and illness, then racial differences in health status cause themselves. This framing is certainly not consciously endorsed by researchers, but the likelihood that genetic research concerning race could encourage such thinking makes it an important topic for bioethics.

Bioethics has engaged these issues extensively, drawing attention to various problems caused by failing to account conceptually and methodologically for the complexity of race and the confusion that surrounds its use in genetic research and in biomedicine generally (Altman, 2002; Kahn, 2006; Neil & Craigie, 2004; Sharp & Foster, 2002). Nonetheless, despite the intensity of interest, this topic has not found an obvious home in one of the established areas of interest within bioethics and so finds itself without an obvious analytic framework or critical foundation in bioethics.

Several possible homes exist for work on race and genetics in bioethics, such as social justice theory (Knoppers & Joly, 2007; Lee, 2003) or recent work on public health ethics (Lindegren et al., 2004). Another line of thinking suggests situating these questions in research ethics. An advantage of this move is that it not only could help to situate inquiries into the implications of race and genetic research more centrally in bioethics but also could contribute to an expanded and more socially grounded approach to research ethics. Several commentaries have noted recently the need to develop a new approach to research ethics, one that moves beyond the current prescriptive approach to a broader framework that incorporates accounts of social context and consequence (Buchanan & Miller, 2006; Jones, 2007; Kitcher, 2004).

TRADITIONAL RESEARCH ETHICS

THE CURRENT RESURGENCE of genetic research, and its use of the concept of race, has been some two decades in the making. Over this period, regulations governing the ethical conduct of biomedical research have focused on two broad areas. The first is human subjects protections, which focuses on assessing benefits and harms of research participation and assuring that people interested in participating do so voluntarily and with sufficient understanding of the implications of doing so (Ryan et al., 1979). The second area on which research ethics has concentrated is assurance of scientific integrity. Referred to often as the responsible conduct of research, these concerns focus more directly on investigators and scientific inquiry and address issues such as data management, authorship, peer review practices, conflict of interest, and research misconduct, meaning deliberate interference with the research process or results.

Two related features of these regulations are important to highlight. First, they focus on the research protocol itself, its possible side effects for the subject, and the setting in which the work is conducted and reported (Kimmelman & Levenstadt, 2005). With the notable exception of community consultation in emergency research and in some genetics research, regulations are directed at the individual subject, not at groups of subjects or people associated with subjects (Baren & Biros, 2007; Richardson, Quest, & Birnbaum, 2005; Sharp & Foster, 2007). Second, consonant with this narrow focus, regulations govern only the research means, not its ends. In other words, ethical review is restricted to the conduct of science, not the consequences of its conduct.

Research ethics regulations have not changed much over the recent period of intensified interest in genetics. However, attention to the regulations and concern with assuring their dissemination and strengthening acceptance of the norms on which they are based have increased dramatically, in part inspired by concern with research that was fostered by the Human Genome Project (HGP) (Dettweiler & Simon, 2001; Fox, 2000; Smaglik, 2000). This attention led to reforms that encouraged increasingly elaborate and institutionally based guidelines and more comprehensive training requirements. Coupled with greater oversight, these reforms have encouraged more consistent enforcement and probably more consistent practice (Kimmelman & Levenstadt, 2005). Whether these changes have resulted in more ethical research, even as narrowly defined within traditional research ethics, is difficult to determine, although considerable research suggests that specific innovations, such as simpler informed consent forms, are effective at least under study conditions (Ibrahim, Ong, & Taylor, 2004; Sorenson, Lakon, Spinney, & Jennings-Grant, 2004).

EXPANDED RESEARCH ETHICS

RESEARCH ETHICS REGULATIONS often draw complaints that they are impractical or have not kept pace with changes associated with the increasing commercialization of science and closer ties between science and industry (Dresser, 2006; Hampson, Joffe, Fowler, Verter, & Emanuel, 2007; Wolf, Walden, & Lo, 2005). A stronger claim, of interest here, is that the scope and focus of current guidelines are wrong (Buchanan & Miller, 2006; Jones, 2007; Kitcher, 2004).

This challenge has been framed in several ways, often inspired at least in part by a growing unease with the global and national imbalance of biomedical research that leads to what one author refers to as the "10/90 gap" (Kitcher, 2004). This gap, the author explains, is created by the fact that "10 percent of the world's resources are directed toward diseases that afflict 90 percent of the population" (p. 335), and, by implication, that 90% of the resources is directed toward the needs of a mere 10%. He goes on to suggest that a revised research ethics could help to reduce this imbalance by incorporating attention to the values that encouraged decisions that allowed such an imbalance to develop in the first place and that allow it to continue. Another suggestion is to apply a public health perspective to research ethics, broadening concern from the welfare of individuals to the health of the whole population (Buchanan & Miller, 2006). Such a new research ethics could attend not only to a physician's or an investigator's obligations to individual patients or subjects, but would be "guided by giving due consideration to the risks and benefits to society in addition to the individual research participants" (Buchanan & Miller, 2006, p. 729). Yet another proposal suggests a more comprehensive code of ethics for the life sciences (Jones, 2007). What unites these proposals is that they all state the need to rethink the purpose of scientific inquiry and to bring an expanded research ethics to bear on this exercise.

Three points distinguish this revised framework: First, attention to the consequences of research extends beyond research participants to the whole population. Second, that attention extends beyond possible benefit or harm of the actual protocol to include possible social implications of the reporting and use of the results of the research. In other words, the new research ethics rejects the premise that what *can* be done justifies what *is* done and asks instead what *should* be done (Jones, 2007). These moves beyond the direct consequences of the protocol imply a third difference, which is that scientists have a contract with society through which the *should* of research gets negotiated. These negotiations do not address the actual design of research, which remains the realm of scientific expertise. Rather, the negotiations are envisioned as broadly inclusive exchanges about the direction and impact of scientific inquiry (Kitcher, 2004).

RACE, GENETICS, AND THE HUMAN GENOME MAP

GENETIC RESEARCH LENDS itself to this revised research ethics framework better than do some fields of research, in part because the shared nature of the human genome makes genetics a topic of broad social concern (Knoppers & Joly, 2007). In addition, genetic research has introduced a new paradigm of health and illness for which it must gain public acceptance, that of personalized medicine. This approach bases diagnosis and treatment on a patient's genotype and proposes to deliver care that is safer and more efficient because it is more precisely calibrated to the individual patient. It promises considerable benefit to people but also introduces or heightens certain risks, such as stigmatization, loss of privacy, and worsening restriction of access to health resources. Already considerable effort has been dedicated to explaining genetic research and treatment to the public and to getting buy-in to this new paradigm (Petersen, 2005; Rotimi et al., 2007). Such efforts imply, albeit modestly, that some kind of contract exists between the researchers and the public. The fact that the recent surge in genetic research leading to this new paradigm was funded by the HGP, a highly publicized, taxpayer-sponsored effort costing billions of dollars, and that genetic research funding continues at public expense, also contributes to this sense of contract. One more feature of the HGP makes it a useful example to examine the meaning of contracts between investigators and the public: its relationship to race.

During the many press conferences and interviews announcing the completion of the human genome map in 2000, a common remark concerned the existence of races in the human species. Specifically, experts addressed the map's potential to settle definitively the controversy whether race has a genetic basis. If it does, then the purported differences should appear on the map as distinct, divergent allelic patterns. Indeed, the map showed nothing of the sort, and instead led speakers, such as President Clinton, to proclaim that one of the "great truths" to emerge from the human genome map is that

> in genetic terms, all human beings, regardless of race are more than 99.9 percent the same...modern science has confirmed what we first learned from ancient faiths. The most important fact of life on this Earth is our common humanity. (United States Office of the Press Secretary, 2000)

HGP leadership likely assumed that one person's genome would be largely identical to another's, regardless of race or ethnicity, well before the mapping project began because research and theorizing over the preceding half century had repeatedly shown as much. Nonetheless, although the claim's proof was no surprise to participants, they still chose to highlight it in press conferences and publications announcing the map's completion. However, such claims and their celebration notwithstanding, even before the human genome map's final features were filled in, investigators started using its insights to design research that relied on race (Lin, Hwang, & Tzeng, 2006; McEvoy, Beleza, & Shriver, 2006; Powell et al., 2001). This trend grew over the next several years as results became available from the HapMap,

a follow-up project that provided volumes of genetic data easily categorized into racial groups.

The contradiction that a project characterized as invalidating race
instead reinvigorated the concept raised concern almost immediately,
and funding initiatives, articles, and conferences soon followed (American Anthropological Association, 2007; ELSI Research Into Human
Genetic Variation RFA HG-99-002, 1999; Gates, 2006). Several excellent
articles appeared that examine the ensuing debate over whether race
was or was not genetic (Bamshad, Wooding, Salisbury, & Stephens,
2004; Fausto-Sterling, 2004; Jorde & Wooding, 2004). They suggest that
the scientists who use race in genetic research often do so based on the
argument that race acts as a proxy for genetic variation. The reasoning
behind this argument is based on current understanding of the history
of human population migration, which suggests that groups of people
living near one another are more likely to share certain genetic patterns than those who live at a distance. These similarities are considered by some to mirror population distributions across the continents.
Because continents map roughly to popular notions of race, researchers have found that racial identity can act as a proxy for continental
ancestry, which in turn reflects somewhat predictable patterns of
genetic variation.

This explanation for the persistence of the use of race as a variable
in genetic research, despite the human genome map's declaration that
there is no genetic evidence for race among humans, is strengthened
by claims that at least among population geneticists, the word *race*
has a narrow, well-established meaning that differs from the 19th-
century typological, hierarchical race. This meaning defines race as "a
population of varying individuals freely mating among each other but
different in average proportions of various genes from other populations" (Lewontin, Rose, & Kamin, 1984, p. 120). Existence of this narrow definition clarifies the motivation for some genetic research uses
of race. Still, even critics who accept these arguments are likely to respond that continued use of race terms in genetic research is at best
dated or naïve.

Onlookers who see it as something more troublesome reject claims
that population geneticists have constructed a different concept of
race, and some argue that the use of race as a variable in genetic research belies continued acceptance of 19th-century typological race
(Fausto-Sterling, 2004; Gannett, 2003). Alternatively, some critics suggest that while population geneticists might well have theorized a different concept of human difference represented by the word *race,* in
practice they slip from using race in this technical sense to using it in
a popular sense. This use carries mixed connotations, some of which
suggest a genetic or natural basis to race (American Anthropological

Association, 2007; Appiah, 1996; Stevens, 2002). Further, as critics point out, when geneticists, as representatives of a science that earlier in the 20th century explicitly supported eugenics, fall into such carelessness it means something different (see chapter 38). This slippage, while unintentional, might contribute to the inference that long-repudiated theories of typological race are being rejuvenated.

WHAT IS AT STAKE

THE POSSIBLE CONSEQUENCES of such trends are, at least initially, likely to be subtle and dispersed. For example, it is hard to know now what influence on beliefs about race might result from the approval of BiDil, the first race-specific drug, or from the growing popularity of genetic ancestry testing companies. Two recent research projects, however, demonstrate what is potentially at stake. They are useful examples because they touch on sensitive issues yet were published in prominent journals, suggesting some level of acceptance in the scientific community.

The first was reported in a 2005 *Science* article titled, "Microcephalin, a Gene Regulating Brain Size, Continues to Evolve Adaptively in Humans," written by a researcher at the University of Chicago, Bruce Lahn (Evans et al., 2005). Lahn's research seeks to determine whether brain size continued to evolve after the emergence of anatomically modern humans. Analysis of the global distribution of the microcephalin gene, located in what is called *haplotype D* and known to be associated developmentally with brain size in humans, shows a greater presence among populations in Europe, Asia, and the Middle East, than among sub-Saharan African populations. This pattern is consistent with the hypothesis that the brain continued to evolve after human populations began to migrate out of Africa, which, Lahn notes, occurred around 40,000 years ago. Lahn suggests that selection might have acted positively on one or more of several brain-related phenotypes, including cognition, personality, or susceptibility to psychiatric disease. Lahn supports his inferences about continued brain evolution with additional analysis that points out that these changes would have coincided with the advent of the Upper Paleolithic period in human history, which witnessed the introduction of symbolic practices such as art and funerary rituals. Putting these events together, Lahn proposes a scenario whereby the genetic mutations required to support the cognitive leap represented by the Upper Paleolithic are evident most everywhere, except among populations living in sub-Saharan Africa.

The second research project was reported in a 2007 article by Lisanne Palomar in the *American Journal of Obstetrics and Gynecology,* titled, "Paternal Race Is a Risk Factor for Pre-Term Birth." The article re-ports on research that examined over 500,000 birth records collected between 1989 and 1997 in the state of Missouri. The objective was to test the hypothesis that paternal race is associated with risk for pre-term birth. Based on chart review data that includes the race of the mother and father, as either Black or White, and a handful of demo-graphic variables such as parental age, maternal education, smoking, and body mass index, the authors conclude that the race of the fa-ther, when Black, accounts for the greatest amount of variation in the likelihood of preterm birth if the mother is White. On this basis, the comment section of the paper opens with the statement: "The findings of our study are that genetic determinants, as reflected by race, may influence birth timing" (Palomar, DeFranco, Lee, Allsworth, & Muglia, 2007, p. 152).

TRADITIONAL VERSUS EXPANDED RESEARCH ETHICS

ASSESSING THESE ARTICLES using a traditional versus a re-vised research ethics framework highlights different issues. Some of the issues specified by traditional research ethics, such as authorship practices, cannot be assessed based on the article alone. Others, how-ever, can. Relying as both studies did on secondary data analysis, the research itself posed no direct harms to subjects. Both articles report receiving approval from the relevant ethics boards to use the data they analyzed. The most probable immediate harm—breach of the subjects' confidentiality—was avoided as no identifying information about subjects appears in the articles. In other words, within the traditional research ethics framework, the research reported in each article ap-pears to pass muster.

Some commentary concerning these articles focused on method-ological flaws, such as Lahn's failure to identify phenotypic corre-lates to the identified genetic variation or Palomar's assumption that variation not accounted for by a limited set of demographic vari-ables (including only one explicitly associated with the father, age) must per force be explained by genetics (Montoya & Howard, 2008; Woods et al., 2006). Such issues have been identified in other genetic research (Altman, 2002; Brandt-Rauf, Raveis, Drummond, Conte, & Rothman, 2006; Joseph, 2004) but, important as they are, their cor-rection would not eliminate ethical concern about these studies. The question that needs to be asked here is not whether these studies were conducted correctly—although that is important—but why they were conducted at all. Expanded research ethics helps to frame this question generally by asking: What kind of research *should* be done? (Jones, 2007).

CONCLUSION

Aᴺˢᵂᴱᴿᴵᴺᴳ ᴛʜᴇ ǫᴜᴇˢᴛᴵᴏɴ "What kind of research *should* be done?" requires not only evaluating whether the conduct of the research itself harms or benefits subjects but also how the use of its results harms or benefits society. What might be the social consequences of conducting such research? Would the benefits outweigh the harms? Indeed, what are the full range of harms and benefits? The benefits include advancing knowledge about human evolution and increased understanding of factors influencing preterm births. Harms that have been mentioned include one critic's suggestion that Lahn's article was "doing damage to the whole field of genetics" (Regalado, 2006, p. A1), while a letter to the editor of *American Journal of Obstetrics and Gynecology* suggested that Palomar's research "reinforce[s] racial stereotypes about the black body" (Montoya & Howard, 2008, p. 483). Recalling the 10/90 gap, another question is at what expense is this research being done while other urgent biomedical questions are left unexamined?

Such questions are beyond the scope of research ethics traditionally conceived, but they are important and do fall within the purview of an expanded research ethics. Pursuing them accomplishes several goals at once. It provides a site for practical debate over what an expanded research ethics would look like and it engages bioethics directly in efforts to mitigate its traditional overemphasis on individual rights at the expense of social consequences. Further, it provides a basis for formalizing efforts to encourage genetics researchers interested in race to see their research in a social context and to take responsibility for its consequences in that context.

REFERENCES

Altman, D. G. (2002). Poor-quality medical research: What can journals do? *Journal of the American Medical Association, 287*(21), 2765–2767.

American Anthropological Association. (2007). *Race: Are we so different?* Retrieved October 21, 2007, from http://www.understandingrace.org/home.html

Appiah, K. A. (1996). Race, culture, identity: Misunderstood connections. In Grethe B. Peterson (Ed.), *The Tanner Lectures on Human Values* (Vol. 1, pp. 51–136). Salt Lake City: University of Utah Press.

Bamshad, M., Wooding, S., Salisbury, B. A., & Stephens, J. C. (2004). Deconstructing the relationship between genetics and race. *Nature Reviews Genetics, 5*(8), 598–609.

Baren, J., & Biros, M. (2007). The research on community consultation: An annotated bibliography. *Academic Emergency Medicine, 14*(4), 346–352.

Brandt-Rauf, S. I., Raveis, V. H., Drummond, N. F., Conte, J. A., & Rothman, S. M. (2006). Ashkenazi Jews and breast cancer: The consequences of linking ethnic identity to genetic disease. *American Journal of Public Health, 96,* 1979–1988.

Buchanan, D. R., & Miller, F. G. (2006). A public health perspective on research ethics. *Journal of Medical Ethics, 32*(12), 729–733.

Dettweiler, U., & Simon, P. (2001). Points to consider for ethics committees in human gene therapy trials. *Bioethics, 15*(5–6), 491–500.

Dresser, R. (2006). Private-sector research ethics: Marketing or good conflicts management? *Theoretical Medicine and Bioethics, 27*(2), 115–139.

ELSI Research Into Human Genetic Variation RFA HG-99-002. (1999). *Studies of the ethical, legal and social implications of research into human genetic variation.* Retrieved May 12, 2008, from http://www.genome.gov/10001017

Evans, P. D., Gilbert, S. L., Mekel-Bobrov, N., Vallender, E. J., Anderson, J. R., Vaez-Azizi, L. M., et al. (2005). Microcephalin, a gene regulating brain size, continues to evolve adaptively in humans. *Science, 309*(5741), 1717–1720.

Fausto-Sterling, A. (2004). Refashioning race: DNA and the politics of health care differences. *Journal of Feminist Cultural Studies, 15*(3), 1–37.

Fox, J. (2000). Investigation of gene therapy begins. *Nature Biotechnology, 18*(2), 143–144.

Gannett, L. (2003). Making populations: Bounding genes in space and in time. *Philosophy of Science, 70,* 989–1001.

Gates, H. L. J. (2006, February 1, 8). *African American Lives* [Television series]. Chappaqua, NY: Kunhardt Productions.

Hampson, L. A., Joffe, S., Fowler, R., Verter, J., & Emanuel, E. J. (2007). Frequency, type, and monetary value of financial conflicts of interest in cancer clinical research. *Journal of Clinical Oncology, 25*(24), 3609–3614.

Ibrahim, T., Ong, S. M., & Taylor, G. J. S.C (2004). The new consent form: Is it any better? *Annals of The Royal College of Surgeons of England, 86*(3), 206–209.

Jones, N. L. (2007). A code of ethics for the life sciences. *Science and Engineering Ethics, 13*(1), 25–43.

Jorde, L., & Wooding, S. (2004). Genetic variation, classification and "race." *Nature Genetics, 36*(11 Suppl.), S28–S33.

Joseph, J. (2004). *The gene illusion: Genetic research in psychiatry and psychology under the microscope.* New York: Algora Publishing.

Kahn, J. (2006). Genes, race, and population: Avoiding a collision of categories. *American Journal of Public Health, 96*(11), 1965–1970.

Kimmelman, J., & Levenstadt, A. (2005). Elements of style: Consent form language and the therapeutic misconception in phase 1 gene transfer trials. *Human Gene Therapy, 16*(4), 502–508.

Kitcher, P. (2004). Responsible biology. *BioScience, 54*(4), 331–336.

Knoppers, B. M., & Joly, Y. (2007). Our social genome? *Trends in Biotechnology, 25*(7), 284–288.

Lee, S. (2003). Race, distributive justice and the promise of pharmacogenomics: Ethical considerations. *American Journal of PharmacoGenomics, 3*(6), 358–392.

Lewontin, R., Rose, S., & Kamin, L. J. (1984). *Not in our genes: Biology, ideology, and human nature.* New York: Pantheon Books.

Lin, E., Hwang, Y., & Tzeng, C. (2006). A case study of the utility of the HapMap database for pharmacogenomic haplotype analysis in the Taiwanese population. *Molecular Diagnosis & Therapy, 10*(6), 367–370.

Lindegren, M. L., Kobrynski, L., Rasmussen, S. A., Moore, C. A., Grosse, S. D., Vanderford, M. L., et al. (2004). Applying public health strategies to primary immunodeficiency diseases: A potential approach to genetic disorders. *Morbidity and Mortality Weekly Report Recommendations and Reports, 53*(RR-1), 1–29.

McEvoy, B., Beleza, S., & Shriver, M. (2006). The genetic architecture of normal variation in human pigmentation: An evolutionary perspective and model. *Human Molecular Genetics, 15*(2), 176–181.

Montoya, M. J., & Howard, B. M. (2008). Dangerous implications of racial genetics research. *American Journal of Obstetrics and Gynecology, 198*(4), 483.

Neil, D., & Craigie, J. (2004). The ethics of pharmacogenomics. *Monash Bioethics Review, 23*(2), 9–20.

Palomar, L., DeFranco, E. A., Lee, K. A., Allsworth, J. E., Muglia, L. J. (2007). Paternal race is a risk factor for pre-term birth. *American Journal of Obstetrics and Gynecology, 197*(2), 152–159.

Petersen, A. (2005). Securing our genetic health: Engendering trust in UK Biobank. *Sociology of Health & Illness, 27*(2), 271–292.

Powell, I., Carpten, J., Dunston, G., Kittles, R., Bennett, J., Hoke, G., et al. (2001). African-American heredity prostate cancer study: A model for genetic research. *Journal of the National Medical Association, 93*(12 Suppl.), S25–S28.

Regalado, A. (2006). Scientist's study of brain genes sparks a backlash: Dr. Lahn connects evolution in some groups to IQ; debate on race and DNA "speculating is dangerous." *Wall Street Journal.* Retrieved May 15, 2008, from http://online.wsj.com/public/article/SB115040765329081636-T5DQ4 jvnwqOdVvsP_XSVG_lvgik_20060628.html?mod=blogs

Richardson, L., Quest, T., & Birnbaum, S. (2005). Communicating with communities about emergency research. *Academic Emergency Medicine, 12*(11), 1064–1070.

Rotimi, C., Leppert, M., Matsuda, I., Zeng, C., Zhang, H., Adebamowo, C., et al. (2007). Community engagement and informed consent in the international HapMap project. *Community Genetics, 10*(3), 186–198.

Ryan, J. K., Brady, J. V., Cooke, R. E., Height, D. I., Jonsen, A. R., King, P., et al. (1979). *Belmont Report: Ethical principles and guidelines for the protection of human subjects of research.* Washington, DC: The National Commission for the Protection of Human Subjects of Biomedical and Behavioral Research.

Sharp, R., & Foster, M. (2002). Community involvement in the ethical review of genetic research: Lessons from American Indian and Alaska native populations. *Environmental Health Perspectives, 110*(2 Suppl.), 145–148.

Sharp, R., & Foster, M. (2007). Grappling with groups: Protecting collective interests in biomedical research. *Journal of Medicine and Philosophy, 32*(4), 321–334.

Smaglik, P. (2000). NIH tightens up monitoring of gene-therapy mishaps. *Nature, 404*(6773), 5.

Sorenson, J., Lakon, C., Spinney, T., & Jennings-Grant, T. (2004). Assessment of a decision aid to assist genetic testing research participants in the informed consent process. *Genetic Testing, 8*(3), 336–346.

Stevens, J. (2002). Symbolic matters: DNA and other linguistic stuff. *Social Text, 20*(1), 105–136.

United States Office of the Press Secretary. (2000, June 26). *Remarks by the President, Prime Minister Tony Blair of England (via satellite), Dr. Francis Collins, director of the National Human Genome Research Institute, and Dr. Craig Venter, President and Chief Scientific Officer, Celera Genomics Corporation, on the completion of the first survey of the entire human genome project.* Delivered at the White House East Room.

Wolf, L. E., Walden, J. F., & Lo, B. (2005). Human subjects issues and IRB review in practice-based research. *Ann Fam Med, 3*(1 Suppl.), S30–S37.

Woods, R. P., Freimer, N. B., De Young, J. A., Fears, S. C., Sicotte, N. L., Service, S. K., et al. (2006). Normal variants of microcephalin and ASPM do not account for brain size variability. *Human Molecular Genetics, 15*(12), 2025–2029.

35

Biobanks

Bernice S. Elger

MANY COMMON DISEASES are believed to result from defects in multiple genes in combination with lifestyle, biographical, or other environmental factors. In 2003, the Human Genome Project completed the entire sequencing of the human genome. The challenge is to match genotypes against phenotypes and to analyze genetic variations related to susceptibility to diseases. The technical possibilities of automated data analysis of DNA samples and their bioinformatic processing have developed dramatically over the last few years and are constantly being improved. They provide important new possibilities for this type of medical research. The combination of health and genetic data on large populations in so-called biobanks has become an important research tool (Kaiser, 2002; Swede, Stone, & Norwood, 2007). Three-quarters of the clinical trials drug companies submit to the FDA for approval include provision for sampling and storing blood for any genetic analysis that may be required in the future (Abbott, 2003).

According to the most common use of the term, a biobank is composed of tissue and data about the individuals from whom those tissues have been taken. The storage of the tissue samples should be distinguished from the storage of the data linked to the samples or obtained from the samples. Such information concerning the donor of the material may include demographic characteristics, type of disease, outcome of disease, treatment, and so forth. Because DNA can be considered by itself a form of information, many use the term *genetic database* more or less synonymously with the term *biobank*. Biobanks may vary in size from those consisting of only a few samples to those storing human material and data from entire populations. Research involving biobanks, especially when genetic tests are involved, has stirred an enormous debate about the adequate ethical framework that should govern the operation and use of biobanks. The main goal of this debate is to ensure the protection of the rights of those who have provided the human material, without unduly hampering research.

CONSENT

A MAJOR ETHICAL CONCERN related to biobanks is that of informed consent. The doctrine of informed consent is fundamental in classical research ethics (World Medical Association [WMA], 2000). Because biobanks are typically established for long-term use, the details of future research projects are not known. Obtaining new informed consent for each new project is in most cases difficult, if not unfeasible. However, many believe that general consent to future research projects is not sufficient. One proposed solution to this dilemma is to accept general consent for future research if participants have the option of opting out and if future research projects are approved by an institutional review board (IRB). Adopting a somewhat lower standard than that of a classical informed consent could be justified because the risks to individuals resulting from research on their human biological material do not involve physical harm, as is the case for clinical trials. Another still largely unresolved issue concerns research that will provide information on a family, group, or population (including those who may have refused to participate, but are indirect subjects of research). Is individual consent a meaningful concept in this context? Different models of group consent or group consultation have been proposed in addition to the individual informed consent of the sample donor (Kaye, 2004).

In light of the ethical controversies, informing participants about the details of storage and research involving their samples is crucial. It is widely agreed that sample donors must be informed about:

- The circumstances of sampling, including the risks and benefits of the procedure;
- The circumstances of the storing (length, location, person responsible for the biobank);
- The measures taken to protect confidentiality (who will have access to the samples and information and what are the risks for individual donors and for groups);

- The aims of the storage (clinical purpose, research purpose);
- The type of consent used (informed consent for the primary clinical or research purpose, or also a general consent for future research);
- The right to opt out and which person should be contacted in such a case;
- The use of biobank samples for commercial purposes (patents planned, benefit sharing planned, and if so in which form);
- Whether individual or aggregated research results will be disclosed to sample donors.

RIGHT TO WITHDRAW

THE DEBATE ABOUT biobanks highlights the question of whether research participants may withdraw not only themselves but also biological material and personal data that they have already provided to researchers. Researchers fear that the destruction of data and samples mandated by withdrawal could bias research results. The right to withdraw was originally formulated as a means of ensuring that research participants remain free to stop their participation based on their suffering in an experiment. Some argue that this right does not exist in the context of biobanks because donors are not physically involved in the research. However, adverse effects could be caused if researchers do not respect donors' wishes to avoid violations of privacy or other nonphysical harms that might arise from their material or data being part of a biobank. Respect for autonomy means that donors have to receive adequate information about factors that might influence their decision to remain in the study, such as additionally discovered risks that have not been specified in the consent form.

Another ethical controversy is whether samples and data need to be destroyed in the case of withdrawal and whether the destruction should include only material stored in the biobank or also those samples already given out to researchers. If withdrawal is intended to protect against harms to privacy, it could be justified to limit the right to withdraw to a request for irreversible anonymization of one's samples and data. However, others argue that the principle of respect for autonomy implies that research participants should be able to mandate the destruction of their DNA samples (Harlan, 2004) and even of all unpublished data generated from them, because anything less than this means that participants are still (involuntarily) involved in the research.

CONFIDENTIALITY

SAMPLE DONORS AND the public are increasingly worried about the sensitivity of genetic information and the management of samples and data (Hoeyer, Olofsson, Mjorndal, & Lynoe, 2004). The public is concerned about unauthorized electronic access to biobank data files and the use of stored information for illicit purposes (Clayton, 2005) and is apprehensive of the risk of personal genetic information being transmitted to third parties, such as insurers and employers. In consequence, a central question in the ethical debate is which form of anonymization or coding should be chosen for the storage and use of samples and data. Protection of confidentiality is achieved through two types of laws: those that declare the violation of confidentiality a punishable act and those that proscribe genetic discrimination. It is well known that legal protection is limited. For example, it is difficult to prove that employees have been dismissed because of genetic discrimination. Therefore, anonymization plays an important role in protection.

Coding and anonymization are practically and ethically challenging. Irreversible anonymization is obtained by removing identifiers linked to samples (Swede, Stone, & Norwood, 2007), although the concept of absolute anonymity has been found to be theoretically unachievable for DNA: specifying DNA sequence at only 30 to 80 statistically independent SNP (single nucleotide polymorphisms) positions will uniquely define a single person (Lin, Owen, & Altman, 2004). The problem with irreversible anonymization is that it greatly decreases the scientific and clinical utility of most biobanks, because no longitudinal study could function without adding health data to the biobank—for example, data on the future development of diseases, their progress and outcome—with or without treatment. As an alternative, double coding has been proposed, which has the advantage of adding another layer of protection of privacy. Two codes are required to link the sample and the donor, and one of them is often put into the hands of an independent key-holder who is supposed to defend the interests of participants in an impartial way.

ANONYMIZATION AND CONSENT

THE DEBATE ABOUT anonymization and coding is framed by the *Declaration of Helsinki,* which states that "Medical research involving human subjects includes research on identifiable human material or identifiable data" (WMA, 2000). It could be concluded that any research using nonidentifiable samples does not need to meet the ethical and legal requirements of medical research, such as informed consent and IRB approval. However, the meaning of *identifiable* is all but clear. A multitude of different terms exist (Elger & Caplan, 2006). Examples for terms used frequently are: *anonymous, anonymized, completely anonymized, unlinked* or *linked anonymized, reversibly* or *irreversibly anonymized, linked* or *unlinked to an identifiable person, irretrievably unlinked to an identifiable person, de-identified, permanently de-linked, not traceable, identifiably linked, pseudonomisiert* (important German term meaning that personal identifiers of the data are replaced by a pseudonym), *encoded, encrypted, confidential, identified, nominative, directly identified,* and *fully identifiable.* Communication barriers are the unavoidable consequence where the same terms are used with a different meaning in the discussion, as is presently the case. In addition to the semantic controversy, at present the United States and Europe are pursuing contradictory approaches concerning anonymization and consent. In the United States, coded material is regarded as nonidentifiable in certain circumstances (Office for Human Research Protections, 2004) and its use does not require the consent of the sample donor. However, according to the guidelines of the Council of Europe (COE), both coded and linked anonymized materials are considered identifiable and the consent standards of the declaration of Helsinki apply (Elger & Caplan, 2006).

OWNERSHIP

ADVANCEMENTS IN GENETIC research and biotechnology have heightened the debate regarding ownership of human material and its commodification (Charo, 2006). A biobank is of scientific and economic value that largely exceeds the value each single donor might claim for his or her individual sample. The presence of linked medical records and other data regarding the donor of the sample increases the value of the biobank. This aggregate value is one factor leading to contested ownership rights. The legal and ethical controversy is further accentuated by the conflicts between the interests of sample donors, biobank holders, researchers, and the public. Traditionally, geneticists have acknowledged that sample donors own their DNA, but on the other extreme, biobanks have claimed to own samples, referring to the concept of a gift; as the term *donor* implies, samples are given away. Between both extremes lies the approach that the concept of ownership is composed of different rights attributed to different stakeholders. For example, the COE established that no financial gain is permitted from human tissue (COE, 1997), and it has been proposed that biobanks are custodians (Comité Consultatif

National d'Ethique, 2003), not owners, of data and samples, which are considered a form of common good (like the ocean). The classical notion of ownership seems insufficient to provide a solution to the ethical issues. A more promising approach to balancing the various interests is to define more specifically the autonomy rights maintained by sample donors (for example, the right to withdraw samples from a biobank) and the acquired rights of biobank holders and researchers to use samples under specified circumstances. In both cases, rights are limited and do not amount to the equivalent of full ownership.

TRANSFER OF SAMPLES AND SHARING OF RESULTS WITH THE BIOBANK

MOST BIOBANKS PROVIDE samples and data to a variety of researchers who are often not directly affiliated with the biobank holders. The transfer of samples and sharing of data raises a certain number of ethical problems. If samples and data are physically transferred outside of the biobank, the recipient might use the material for purposes other than those to which sample donors have consented, or transfer the samples to third parties, thus putting at risk the privacy of donors. If recipients use samples for their own purposes, the investment and effort of the original biobank holder could be threatened. Biobank material is a valuable resource, and the ethical issue of just allocation emerges if the samples and data are misused. On the other hand, if transfer of samples is too restrictive because of transfer agreements that include complex and costly control mechanisms, the resulting inaccessibility of biobank material does not allow a large number of researchers to use this resource in the interest of science and public good.

Another ethical issue is the question of whether researchers should have an obligation to disclose research results in the form of raw data to the biobank. This data would help increase the value of the biobank and would facilitate future research. On the other hand, researchers might claim the right to use their results solely for their own purposes, including patents and commercialization, based on the idea that results are considered intellectual property and that such practice is supposed to stimulate research efforts.

Overall, in questions related to transfer and sharing of results, the protection of the privacy interests of the sample donors must be balanced against the interest in advancing research and providing sufficient encouragement and facility to researchers in order to assure broad use of precious biobank resources.

BENEFIT-SHARING AND REMUNERATION OF SAMPLE SOURCES

Q<small>UESTIONS CONCERNING BENEFIT</small> sharing and remuneration, although not limited to research involving biobanks, have caused considerable ethical debate in this context. Traditionally, research participants have agreed to take part in medical studies for altruistic reasons without receiving any economic compensation. Coercion is avoided when research participants do not expect any reward and provide material to biobanks for the sole reasons of advancing human knowledge and benefiting mankind. However, the Human Genome Project and the Human Genome Organization (HUGO) stressed the notion of the human genome as a common heritage of humanity and concluded from this that all of humanity should share in the benefit resulting from its use.

Different concepts of just sharing of the benefit resulting from biobanks have been proposed. Benefits to humanity can be understood in various ways. One approach is that the benefits of research involving collections of human biological material should be distributed predominantly to the least well-off (Simm, 2007) in order to compensate for global inequity in biomedical research. Inequity is a problem in particular if commercial entities in highly developed countries profit from the use of biobanks established in developing countries (Schulz-Baldes, Vayena, & Biller-Andorno, 2007). To carry out compensation, HUGO proposed that profit-making entities dedicate a percentage (e.g., 1%–3%) of their annual net profit to health care infrastructure and/or to humanitarian efforts (HUGO, 2000). Another concept of benefit sharing relies on compensation understood in a more reciprocal way as providing benefit to either those who agreed to provide samples to a biobank or to the entire population to which donors belong. Pharmaceutical companies have proposed free genetic tests (Iceland) or free information about individual genetic profiles (Estonia) for donors.

Both benefits provided to groups and those provided to individuals are at risk of creating unjustified material inducement to participation. Particular problems of balancing the risk of inducement against the principle of justice are raised if sample donors from different countries in an international study are receiving different amounts of compensation. Although the principle of equity seems to require that all receive the same compensation for the same service (the donation of samples to a biobank), the risk of inducement might require defining compensation in a relative way, for example as the average wage in the country for several hours of work. While the idea of buying human material from participants is often rejected as contrary to the dignity of human material and therefore ethically inappropriate, reimbursement for lost earnings, travel costs, or other expenses in-curred in providing samples and data to a biobank are in general considered acceptable. The idea of providing a small sum of money for inconvenience to those who contributed samples without receiv-ing any direct medical benefit from the future studies is acceptable to many. Sample donors may also receive medical services unrelated to the biobank research or have procedures and tests performed free of charge (Council for International Organizations of Medical Sciences, 2002).

INFORMING DONORS ABOUT
RESEARCH RESULTS

RESEARCH INVOLVING POPULATION biobanks commonly aims to study the relationship between genetic and environmen-tal determinants of common diseases. Biobanks collect samples from patients suffering from a particular disease and often generate infor-mation about the genetic determinants of this disease or the efficiency of treatment. This information could improve the health of the stud-ied population and its members by providing the opportunity of pre-vention or specific early treatments for those donors with a particular identified genetic or environmental predisposition.

Informing donors about aggregate scientific results should be distin-guished from providing individualized information of relevance to the health of a given individual. In order to honor altruistic sample donations for research, it seems ethically appropriate to offer donors feedback regarding aggregate results. Providing individual results to donors is clearly more controversial. Although the ethical foundations of the right to know and not to know are well established in international guidelines, practical as well as ethical problems impede wide imple-mentation of this practice in research involving biobanks. Some un-resolved issues include who should inform donors and what type of counseling should be obligatory to protect donors from potential harm resulting from the disclosure. Individual benefit from disclosure is often balanced against the benefit expected from research, because the significant costs of disclosure procedures might take resources away from important additional research. Legal concerns further complicate the issue. For example, in the United States only laboratories certified under the Clinical Lab Improvement Act (CLIA) are authorized to disclose results to individuals. Personal interests might influence the decision of a research laboratory not to seek CLIA certification, especially when informing donors about individual research results could imply various legal liabilities for researchers. Respect for the autonomy of donors implies that the consequences of any chosen disclosure approach should be explained clearly to them. The principle of beneficence justifies establishing disclosure procedures for incidental findings that have important health consequences and informing donors about these procedures.

CONCLUSION

CONTROVERSIAL ETHICAL ISSUES raised by biobanks cause ample disagreement. Hardliners defending classical research ethics and patients' rights advocates disagree with those who want to advance research and fear practical problems arising from high standards of sample donor protection. However, it would be an oversimplification to reduce the ethical controversy surrounding biobanks to a conflict between the interests of different stakeholders, such as sample donors expecting protection and respect of their rights, biobank holders, or researchers who wish to avoid costly ethical safeguards. In the long run, society, research participants, and researchers will all benefit from simple procedures that do not impose undue burden on research, as well as trustworthy protection of sample security and donors' rights. The controversies most difficult to resolve concern questions related to justice, and this explains why approaches to benefit sharing vary widely. Finally, disagreement on empirical questions is an important factor that shapes the ethical debate, and one should be vigilant not to confound genuinely different ethical standpoints with those differences that are caused only by uncertainty regarding empirical questions, such as the protective value and practical burden of double coding or the frequency and costs of withdrawal policies.

REFERENCES

Abbott, A. (2003). With your genes? Take one of these, three times a day. *Nature, 425*(6960), 760–762.

Charo, R. A. (2006). Body of research—ownership and use of human tissue. *New England Journal of Medicine, 355*(15), 1517–1519.

Clayton, E. W. (2005). Informed consent and biobanks. *The Journal of Law, Medicine, and Ethics, 33*(1), 15–21.

Comité consultatif national d'ethique pour les sciences de la vie et de la santé. (2003). *Avis No. 77. Problèmes éthiques posés par les collections de matériel biologique et les données d'information associées: "biobanques," "biothèques"* [Opinion No. 77. Ethical problems raised by collections of biological

material and associated information: "biobanks," "biocollections"].
Retrieved August 15, 2006, from http://www.ccne-ethique.fr/francais/
pdf/aviso77.pdf

Council for International Organizations of Medical Sciences. (2002). *Inter-national ethical guidelines for biomedical research involving human subjects.*
Retrieved August 15, 2007, from http://www.cioms.ch/frame_guide
lines_nov_2002.htm

Council of Europe. (1997). *Convention for the protection of human rights and dignity of the human being with regard to the application of biology and medicine: Convention on human rights and biomedicine.* CETS No. 164. Retrieved September 2, 2008, from http://www.hrni.org/files/instruments/HRNi_EN_214.
html

Elger, B. S., & Caplan, A. L. (2006). Consent and anonymization in research involving biobanks: Differing terms and norms present serious barriers to an international framework. *European Molecular Biology Organization Reports, 7*(7), 661–666.

Harlan, L. M. (2004). When privacy fails: Invoking a property paradigm to mandate the destruction of DNA samples. *Duke Law Journal, 53,* 179–219.

Hoeyer, K., Olofsson, B. O., Mjorndal, T., & Lynoe, N. (2004). Informed consent and biobanks: A population-based study of attitudes towards tissue donation for genetic research. *Scandinavian Journal of Public Health, 32*(3), 224–229.

Human Genetics Organization Ethics Committee. (2000). *Statement on benefit-sharing.* Retrieved September 20, 2007, from http://www.hugo-inter
national.org/Statement_on_Benefit_Sharing.htm

Kaiser, J. (2002). Biobanks. Population databases boom, from Iceland to the U.S. *Science, 298*(5596), 1158–1161.

Kaye, J. (2004). Abandoning informed consent: The case of genetic research in population collections. In R. Tutton & O. Corrigan (Eds.), *Genetic databases: Socio-ethical issues in the collection and use of DNA* (pp. 117–138). London: Routledge.

Lin, Z., Owen, A. B., & Altman, R. B. (2004). Genetics. Genomic research and human subject privacy. *Science, 305*(5681), 183.

Office for Human Research Protections. (2004). Guidance on research involving coded private information or biological specimens. Rockville, MD: Author.

Schulz-Baldes, A., Vayena, E., & Biller-Andorno, N. (2007). Sharing benefits in international health research. Research-capacity building as an example of an indirect collective benefit. *European Molecular Biology Organization Report, 8*(1), 8–13.

Simm, K. (2007). Benefit-sharing and biobanks. In M. Häyry, R. Chadwick, V. Arnason, & G. Arnason (Eds.), *The ethics and governance of human genetic databases: European perspectives* (pp. 159–169). Cambridge, UK: Cambridge University Press.

Swede, H., Stone, C. L., & Norwood, A. R. (2007). National population-based
biobanks for genetic research. *Genetics in Medicine, 9*(3), 141–149.

World Medical Association. (2000). *Declaration of Helsinki, adopted by the 52nd
World Medical Association General Assembly, Edinburgh, Scotland.* Retrieved
August 15, 2008, from http://www.wma.net/e/policy/b3.htm

36

Prenatal Choices: Genetic Counseling for Variable Genetic Diseases

Curtis R. Coughlin II

PEMBREY AND ANIONWU (1996) have defined the aim of medical genetics as enabling people and families with a genetic disadvantage to live and reproduce as normally as possible. Although an admirable definition, it fails to clarify important concepts that are central to the understanding of reproductive genetics. First, one needs to define genetic disadvantage. Obviously, not any variation of the genetic code constitutes a disadvantage. Genetic mutations do not always translate into clinically evident disease. While this becomes apparent as a newborn develops and becomes a child and then an adult, it is difficult to determine what lies ahead of a developing fetus. In addition, the natural history of a genetic disease may be significantly altered through treatments and social policies that minimize the burdens associated with it.

Second, what is *normal* reproduction? Despite the effective treatment available for a handful of inherited disorders, such as dietary treatments for inborn errors of metabolism and enzyme replacement therapy for lysosomal storage diseases, the vast majority of genetic disorders have few therapeutic options. Prenatal diagnosis allows families who are at risk for a genetic or hereditary disorder to have a child free from that specific genetic disease. For these families, recurrent risks and prenatal testing are a part of routine obstetrical care and perceived as *normal* reproduction.

Since the 1970s, invasive prenatal diagnosis has been available to detect a number of genetic disorders from chromosomal differences such as Down syndrome to inherited disorders such as Tay-Sachs disease (Atkins, Milunsky, & Shahood 1974; Milunsky & Littlefield, 1972; Nadler & Gerbie, 1970). Invasive prenatal testing is performed through either chorinoic villi sampling (CVS) in the first trimester of pregnancy or amniocentesis during the second and third trimester of pregnancy. Invasive prenatal testing has an innate risk of miscarriage or preterm labor regardless of the genetic status of the fetus. The important ethical question that has emerged is this: Which genetic conditions are serious enough to warrant offering to those at risk invasive prenatal testing and the option of pregnancy termination?

PRENATAL TESTING FOR GENETIC DISEASE

PRENATAL TESTING WAS originally offered based on an identified risk, such as maternal age, a history of a previous pregnancy with a chromosomal disorder, or a history of an inherited disorder. Families experienced the disease in question and formed personal feelings about living with a genetic disorder before the option of prenatal diagnosis was ever discussed. In 1984, Merkatz, Nitowsky, Macri, and Johnson (1984) identified a biochemical marker that, when measured during the appropriate time in pregnancy, could screen for structural anomalies and chromosomal disorders. Subsequently a myriad of serum screening tests, accompanied by ultrasound, have become available, resulting in sensitive screening programs for chromosomal disorders (American College of Obstetrics and Gynecology, 2007). As a result of the screening programs, prenatal testing has become available to a larger proportion of the population, and the discussion of prenatal testing has become a routine part of obstetrical care.

Historically, prenatal screening programs and invasive prenatal diagnosis have been available for chromosome anomalies or specific genetic disorders. Since prenatal testing was aimed at one specific disease, it allowed for comprehensive counseling and informed consent that focused on the specific disease in question. However, prenatal testing for even one disease may result in ambiguous results and counseling difficulties.

Gaucher disease is a case in point. It is the most common lyso-somal storage disorder in the White population, with an incidence of approximately 1 in 50,000. Like sickle cell disease or cystic fibrosis, Gaucher disease is inherited in an autosomal recessive pattern, which means that two copies of the abnormal gene must be present in order for the disease to develop (both from the father and from the mother). Approximately 6% of individuals of Ashkenazi Jewish ancestry and 1% of individuals of non-Jewish populations are carriers for a Gaucher disease mutation (Horowitz et al., 1998; Meikle, Hopwood, Clague, & Carey, 1999). Gaucher disease is the result of a deficiency in one enzyme, glucocerebrosidase. The storage of this enzyme within lysosomes can cause multisystem involvement including, but not limited to, hepatosplenomegaly, skeletal system involvement, and hematologic findings (Charrow et al., 2000). Gaucher disease is classified into three distinct types, based on central nervous system involvement. Type I is the most common and is nonneuronopathic. Type II has an early or infantile onset with severe neurologic consequences and early death. Type III involves milder central nervous system involvement with an onset in adolescence or early adulthood (Beutler & Grabowski, 1995).

Prenatal testing for Gaucher disease invokes concern because Gaucher disease type I is both a variable and a treatable genetic condition. As many as 50% of individuals with the N370S/N370S genotype, which is the most common mutation found in Gaucher disease type I, will remain asymptomatic or at least never require treatment (Azuri et al., 1998; Zuckerman et al., 2007), and approximately 20% of individuals with this same genotype will have significant clinical symptoms of Gaucher disease before 8 years of age (Garbowski, 2000). It is difficult to determine whether a fetus with a genetic diagnosis of Gaucher disease will develop into a child or an adult with a clinical diagnosis of Gaucher disease. This highlights the fact that even when prenatal testing is targeted at a specific genetic disorder based on a single gene, genetic results can be ambiguous, resulting in difficult prenatal decisions.

Gaucher disease is also a treatable disease. For those individuals with Gaucher disease type I who do develop clinically recognizable signs of disease, effective treatment exists through the use of enzyme replacement therapy (ERT). ERT utilizes a recombinant human enzyme (imiglucerase) to treat those individuals who have a deficiency in glucocerebrosidase. Treatment has been shown to reduce liver and spleen size, decrease bone pain while increasing bone mineralization, and resolve anemia and thrombocytopenia (Charrow et al., 2000, 2004). Therefore, even those who will show clinical symptoms will have an effective treatment to ensure that they do not continue to exhibit symptoms.

The example of Gaucher disease demonstrates the significant hurdles to prenatal testing even for a single genetic disease. Although the disease is well described and the genetic basis is well known, prenatal testing results may be ambiguous, forcing couples to make difficult choices regarding pregnancy termination. Significant ambiguity remains regarding whether the child (or adult) would ever exhibit physical symptoms, and questions arise regarding the necessity of a prenatal diagnosis when effective treatments are available. Moreover, future advances in treatment strategies may redefine the course of the disease over that child's lifetime. However, couples at risk for Gaucher disease do undergo invasive prenatal testing, and pregnancies that are diagnosed with Gaucher disease type I have been terminated as a result. The statistical nature of the genotype/phenotype correlations, the uncertainty about the natural history of the disease, and the scope of available treatment options, make prenatal counseling difficult and time consuming, which may add to a family's stress during pregnancy (Garbowski, 2000).

Despite these challenges, genetic counseling remains extremely important. Both lay press and scientific papers have noted that families who have undergone prenatal counseling by a Gaucher disease expert are less likely to terminate a pregnancy as compared to those who do not receive such counseling. One study examined multiple screening programs in Israel, in which 16 pregnancies were identified with Gaucher disease type I. Couples who did not receive counseling from a Gaucher disease expert had a high rate of pregnancy termination (3 of 3 pregnancies were terminated), whereas in couples who did receive such counseling only 1 of 13 pregnancies was terminated (Kaplan, 2007; Zuckerman et al., 2007). These findings are similar to findings of other studies that examined abortion rates in cases of various genetic disorders and found that rates differ significantly when counseling is provided by a genetic professional or experienced expert (Hall, Abramsky & Marteau, 2003; Marteau et al., 2002). It is evident that the type of counseling and disease information a couple receives may significantly alter the family's perception of the disease and the decision to continue or terminate the pregnancy.

THE CHALLENGES RAISED BY LARGE-SCALE GENETIC SCREENING

A S TECHNOLOGY ADVANCES it will become increasingly possible to change our screening strategy from identifying risk for a single disease or genetic disorder to large-scale genetic screening. Barriers of technology and economic cost are eroding, and the promise of full genome sequencing appears to be eminent (Service, 2006). Opponents of large-scale genetic screening believe that testing will provide ambiguous results regarding a range of conditions, from serious disorders to conditions that many consider a *normal* genetic variation, and that it might also stigmatize individuals.

Microarray-based comparative genomic hybridization (CGH) may be the next step toward comprehensive genetic testing. Microarray CGH analyzes copy number variation throughout the human genome and can detect small deletions or duplications of genetic material (Kallioniemi et al., 1992). There are a number of well-defined microdeletion syndromes that correlate with conditions such as learning disabilities or mental retardation. Microarray CGH allows large-scale screening for these recognized microdeletion syndromes but also detects deletions or duplications that have never before been described. Although variation of copy number has been associated with certain conditions, it is often still difficult to predict the impact of a novel copy number repeat result (Shaw-Smith et al., 2004).

Historically, prenatal testing provided chromosome analysis and testing for a single genetic disorder. Prenatal microarray CGH testing provides families information about a myriad of known genetic syndromes (Rickman, Fiegler, Carter, & Bobrow, 2005; Roa, Pulliam, Eng, & Cheung, 2005; Sahoo et al., 2006). Microarray technology also allows for this information to be provided within a few days as opposed to the week or more that is required for traditional cytogenetic techniques. This is beneficial because decisions to continue or terminate a pregnancy are typically time sensitive and because the decrease in time may help alleviate anxiety that is associated with the uncertainty of prenatal diagnosis (Rickman et al., 2005).

Large-scale screening with microarray CGH has invoked concerns about the amount of information obtained as well as the uncertainty that may arise when a copy number variation is identified that is not well defined (Grody, 2003; Shuster, 2007). Copy number variation throughout the human genome has been found in individuals who do not exhibit any disease, or at least an identifiable disease (Sebat et al., 2004). As seen with the example of Gaucher disease, uncertainty in prenatal diagnosis is common even when a specific and well-delineated disease is identified. Enigmatic chromosome results are not unique to microarray CGH or advanced technology, and even traditional cytogenetic techniques reveal novel translocations, marker chromosomes, and mosaicism, which leave significant uncertainty in the outcome of a pregnancy.

However, microarray's ability to examine a large number of genetic syndromes has intensified the debate about what should and should not be tested for during a pregnancy (Grody, 2003). The traditional model of invasive prenatal testing for a single genetic disorder is still problematic. Significant variation exists even within a single genetic disorder and as treatment options expand, whether enzyme replacement, transplantation, gene therapy, or social and environmental improvements, the natural history of a genetic disorder changes. Large-scale genomic testing will intensify the ethical aspects of determining which conditions warrant or justify prenatal testing.

The debate concerning prenatal testing centers on which diseases present severe physical or emotional hardship. In the past, advisory committees reviewed specific disorders to evaluate whether population screening was deemed appropriate. Prenatal testing was often justified based on economic analysis as well as a narrow definition of severity (Hagard & Carter, 1976; Watson et al., 2004). The use of prenatal microarray CGH testing and the completion of the Human Genome Project promote the notion of large-scale testing for genetic disease as well as genetic variability. This leads to the heart of the ethical difficulty, which is the distinction between disease and normal variation.

The difficulty in making this distinction raises the important issue of who should be responsible for making it: the medical genetics community? philosophers and bioethicists? or perhaps the disability community? Past efforts made by major medical genetic societies to define "serious genetic disorder" were characterized by disagreement. Wertz and Knoppers (2002) asked genetic professionals to rank disorders as lethal, serious but not lethal, and not serious. No consensus was reached about which disorders were in which category. Another study included participants from various fields of study (philosophy, disability community, genetics, genetic counseling, law, social science, and economics) and demonstrated that they could not agree on which genetic disorders should warrant prenatal testing (Parens & Asch, 1999). In addition, individuals with disabilities caution against paternalistic social attitudes toward those who have disabilities and the way they influence definitions of severity (Munger, Gill, Ormond, & Kirschner, 2007; Parens & Asch, 1999).

Limiting prenatal testing to diseases that are considered *severe* raises concerns about social attitudes towards those who live among us with the same conditions (Parens & Asch, 1999; Shakespeare, 1998). Moreover, severity cannot be clearly defined. It is rather an ever-evolving part of a continuum, since genetic mutations do not always lead to genetic disease, treatments for disease continue to evolve, and personal views of disability vary. Rather than focusing the debate on the issue of which genetic variations justify prenatal testing, we should focus on the process of decision-making following the identification of a genetic variation.

GENETIC COUNSELING FOR PRENATAL TESTING

INVASIVE PRENATAL TESTING raises ethical concerns whether performed for a single, well-defined genetic disorder or for a large number of genetic syndromes and chromosomal variations. As new technologies are developed, results of uncertain significance will multiply. Prenatal testing also invokes concern about the definition of disease, as many disagree what constitutes disease and what is considered normal variation.

Nondirective counseling has been a central theme since the inception of genetic counseling, which emphasized the support of a patient's values, beliefs, and personal decision-making (Weil, 2003). One of the earliest definitions of genetic counseling also emphasized helping an individual or family choose the decision that is appropriate to them (Ad Hoc Committee on Genetic Counseling, 1975). Ideally, genetic counseling for prenatal testing occurs prior to the decision to pursue invasive prenatal diagnosis and upholds the importance of voluntary and informed consent (National Society of Genetic Counselors, 1993; Wustner, 2003). Voluntary and informed consent, which is based on the ethical principle of respect for autonomy (Beauchamp & Childress, 2001), ensures decisions are free from coercion. It is the fundamental element that distinguishes personal decisions about prenatal testing from eugenic practices that involve coercive social forces that determine what constitutes disease and disability versus normal genetic variation.

Concern has been voiced about whether it is possible for a patient to make autonomous decisions when faced with results of unclear significance (Grody, 2003; Shuster, 2007). However, to exercise autonomy, a person is not required to know the exact outcome of her decision. Rather, autonomous decisions must only involve the knowledge that exists and the options that are available at the time of decision-making (Hodgson & Spriggs, 2005).

CONCLUSION

NORMAL REPRODUCTION MAY be impossible to define, but it arguably includes the possibility of having children who are free from serious and lethal diseases. However, the definition of *serious disease* is rapidly changing as treatment options continue to expand. While it is challenging to understand the implications of being diagnosed with one disease, the challenge of coping with a multitude of diagnoses is daunting. Considering the difficulty of distinguishing serious diseases from treatable diseases, and treatable diseases from normal variation, it seems that rather than focusing on whether a disease is worthy of prenatal testing, we should focus on whether it is possible for a family to understand the true implications of a prenatal diagnosis. A prenatal diagnosis should include counseling by professionals who understand the spectrum of disease as well as practicalities of treatment, and counseling that respects the family's beliefs and values as well as patient autonomy. Without the support of counseling, families do not have with the option of a true prenatal choice.

REFERENCES

Ad Hoc Committee on Genetic Counseling. (1975). Genetic counseling. *American Journal of Human Genetics, 27*, 240–242.

American College of Obstetrics and Gynecology. (2007). ACOG practice bulletin no. 77: Screening for fetal chromosome abnormalities. *Obstetrics and Gynecology, 109*, 217–227.

Atkins, L., Milunsky, A., & Shahood, J. M. (1974). Prenatal diagnosis: Detailed chromosomal analysis in 500 cases. *Clinical Genetics, 6*, 317–322.

Azuri, J., Elstein, D., Lahad, A., Abrahamov, A., Hadas-Halpern, I., & Zimran, A. (1998). Asymptomatic Gaucher disease implications for large-scale screening. *Genetic Testing, 2*, 297–299.

Beauchamp, T., & Childress, J. (2001). *Principles of biomedical ethics* (5th ed.). New York: Oxford University Press.

Beutler, E., & Grabowski, G. A. (1995). Gaucher disease. In C. R. Scriver, A. L. Beaudet, W. S. Sly, & D. Valle (Eds.), *The metabolic and molecular basis of inherited disease* (pp. 2641–2669). New York: McGraw-Hill.

Charrow, J., Andersson, H. C., Kaplan, P., Kolodny, E. H., Mistry, P., Pastores, G., et al. (2000). The Gaucher registry: Demographics and disease characteristics of 1698 patients with Gaucher disease. *Archives of Internal Medicine, 160*, 2837–2843.

Charrow, J., Andersson, H. C., Kaplan, P., Kolodny, E. H., Mistry, P., Pastores, G., et al. (2004). Enzyme replacement therapy and monitoring for children with type 1 Gaucher disease: Consensus recommendations. *The Journal of Pediatrics, 144*, 112–120.

Grabowski, G. A. (2000). Gaucher disease: Considerations in prenatal diagnosis. *Prenatal Diagnosis, 20*, 60–62.

Grody, W. (2003). Ethical issues raised by genetic testing with oligonucleotide microarrays. *Molecular Biology, 23*, 127–138.

Hagard, S., & Carter, F. A. (1976). Preventing the birth of infants with Down's syndrome: A cost-benefit analysis. *British Medical Journal, 27*, 753–756.

Hall, S., Abramsky, L., & Marteau, T. M. (2003). Health professionals' reports of information given to parents following the prenatal diagnosis of sex chromosome anomalies and outcomes of pregnancies: A pilot study. *Prenatal Diagnosis, 23*, 535–538.

Hodgson, J., & Spriggs, M. (2005). A practical account of autonomy: Why genetic counseling is especially well suited to the facilitation of informed autonomous decision making. *Journal of Genetic Counseling, 14*, 89–97.

Horowitz, M., Pasmanik-Chor, M., Borochowitz, Z., Falik-Zaccai, T., Heldmann, K., Carmi, R., et al. (1998). Prevalence of glucocerebrosidase mutations in the Israeli Ashkenazi Jewish population. *Human Mutation, 12,* 240–244.

Kallioniemi, A., Kallioniemi, O. P., Sudar, D., Rutovitz, D., Gray, J. W., Waldman, F., et al. (1992). Comparative genomic hybridization for molecular cytogenetic analysis of solid tumors. *Science, 258,* 818 821.

Kaplan, K. (2007, September 19). Genetic tests offer knowledge, not wisdom. *The Los Angeles Times,* p. A1.

Marteau, T. M., Nippert, I., Hall, S., Limbert, C., Reid, M., Bobrow, M., et al. (2002). Outcomes of pregnancies diagnosed with Klinefelter syndrome: The possible influence of health professionals. *Prenatal Diagnosis, 22,* 562–566.

Meikle, P. J., Hopwood, J. J., Clague, A. E., & Carey, W. F. (1999). Prevalence of lysosomal storage disorders. *Journal of the American Medical Association, 281,* 249–254.

Merkatz, I. R., Nitowsky, H. M., Macri J. N., & Johnson W. E. (1984). An association between low maternal serum alphafetoprotein and fetal chromosome abnormalities. *American Journal of Obstetrics and Gynecology, 148,* 886–894.

Milunsky, A., & Littlefield, J. W. (1972). The prenatal diagnosis of inborn errors of metabolism. *Annual Review of Medicine, 23,* 57–76.

Munger, K. M., Gill, C. J., Ormond, K. E., & Kirschner, K. L. (2007). The next exclusion debate: Assessing technology, ethics, and intellectual disability after the human genome project. *Mental Retardation and Developmental Disabilities Research Reviews, 13,* 121–128.

Nadler, H. L., & Gerbie, A. B. (1970). Role of amniocentesis in the intra-uterine diagnosis of genetic defects. *New England Journal of Medicine, 282,* 596–599.

National Society of Genetic Counselors. (1993). Code of ethics. In D. M. Bartles, B. S. LeRoy, & A. L. Caplan (Eds.), *Prescribing our future: Ethical challenges in genetic counseling* (pp. 169–171). New York: Aldine de Gruyter.

Parens, E., & Asch, A. (1999). The disability rights critique of prenatal genetic testing—reflections and recommendations. *A Special Supplement to the Hastings Center Report, 29*(Suppl.), 1–22.

Pembrey, M. E., & Anionwu, E. N. (1996). Ethical aspects of genetic screening and diagnosis. In D. L. Rimoin, J. M. Connor, & R. E. Pyeritz (Eds.). *Emery and Rimoin's principles and practice of medical genetics* (3rd ed.). New York: Churchill Livingstone.

Rickman, L., Fiegler, H., Carter, N. P., & Bobrow, M. (2005). Prenatal diagnosis by array CGH. *European Journal of Medical Genetics, 48,* 232–240.

Roa, B. B., Pulliam, J., Eng, C. M., & Cheung, S. W. (2005). Evolution of prenatal genetics: From point mutation testing to chromosome microarray analysis. *Expert Review of Molecular Diagnostics, 5,* 883–892.

Sahoo, T., Cheung, S. W., Ward, P., Darilek, S., Patel, A., del Gaudio, D., et al. (2006). Prenatal diagnosis of chromosomal abnormalities using array-based comparative genomic hybridization. *Genetics in Medicine, 8,* 719–727.

Sebat, J., Lakshmi, B., Troge, J., Alexander, J., Young, J., Lundin, P., et al. (2004). Large-scale copy number polymorphism in the human genome. *Science, 305*, 525–528.

Service, R. F. (2006). The race for the $1000 genome. *Science, 311*, 1544–1546.

Shakespeare, T. (1998). Choices and rights: Eugenics, genetics and disability equality. *Disability and Society, 13*, 665–681.

Shaw-Smith, C., Redon, R., Rickman, L., Rio, M., Willatt, L., Fiegler, H., et al. (2004). Microarray based comparative genomic hybridization (array-CGH) detects submicroscopic chromosomal deletions and duplications in patients with learning disabilities/mental retardation and dysmorphic features. *Journal of Medical Genetics, 41*, 241–248.

Shuster, E. (2007). Microarray genetic screening: A prenatal roadblock for life? *Lancet, 369*, 526–529.

Watson, M. S., Cutting, G. R., Desnick, R. J., Driscoll, D. A., Klinger, K., Mennuti, M., et al. (2004). Cystic fibrosis population carrier screening: 2004 revision of American College of Medical Genetics mutation panel. *Genetics in Medicine, 6*, 387–391.

Weil, J. (2003). Psychosocial genetic counseling in the post-nondirective era: A point of view. *Journal of Genetic Counseling, 12*, 199–211.

Wertz, D. C., & Knoppers, B. M. (2002). Serious genetic disorders: Can or should they be defined? *American Journal of Medical Genetics, 108*, 25–35.

Wustner, K. (2003). Ethics and practice: Two worlds? The example of genetic counseling. *New Genetics and Society, 22*, 61–87.

Zuckerman, S., Lahad, A., Shmueli, A., Zimran, A., Peleg, L., Orr-Urteger, A., et al. (2007). Carrier screening for Gaucher disease: Lessons for low-penetrance, treatable diseases. *Journal of the American Medical Association, 298*, 1281–1290.

37

Ethical Issues in Animal Biotechnology

Autumn Fiester

ANIMAL BIOTECHNOLOGY IS the use of scientific principles and techniques to produce or modify animals for research or commercial purposes. Types of animal biotechnology include the following: cloning (the use of somatic cell nuclear transfer to make a near-identical genetic copy of an animal), transgenics (the introduction of a foreign gene into an animal's genome), and gene knock-out projects (the use of technology to inactivate a particular gene in an animal). One of the most dramatic achievements of this science was the cloning of Dolly the sheep in 1996, but there has been an explosion of the technology since then, with projects ranging from biopharming (the manufacture of pharmaceuticals in the milk of transgenic animals) and the production of milk and meat from cloned animals to the creation of novelty transgenic pets (like the Glofish), xenotransplantation research (using knock-out technology to try to make pig organs compatible with a human host), and the creation of animal models for human diseases.

Animal biotechnology raises two different types of ethical concerns or arguments that need to be addressed as this science progresses: on the one hand, projects in animal biotechnology may generate adverse consequences to animals, human beings, or the environment; on the other hand, various projects in animal biotechnology may violate important moral prohibitions or principles (Fiester, 2005). The first type of critique employs consequence-based arguments to assess the merits of this technology; the second type of critique employs principle-based arguments.

CONSEQUENCE-BASED ARGUMENTS AGAINST ANIMAL BIOTECHNOLOGY

THE MOST WIDELY cited concern about animal biotechnology is the direct consequences it has for animals, that is, the pain and suffering animals experience in the research process and in the commercial applications of this technology. There are three main areas of concern with regard to the pain and suffering of animals: the suffering they experience as new techniques, such as cloning, are developed; the overall health of cloned or transgenic animals; and the suffering of animals specifically created to exhibit certain diseases and pathologies for medical research.

Cloning research offers a good case study for this type of ethical argument. Early data on the success rates of cloning procedures and the health and survival statistics of animal clones presented a fairly grim picture. There is a large body of literature citing high rates of miscarriage, stillbirth, early death, genetic abnormalities, and chronic diseases among the first generations of cloned animals. These problems occur against a backdrop of what in biotechnology science has been called *efficiency,* the term used to talk about the percentage of live offspring from the number of transferred embryos. The efficiency of animal cloning has often been as low as 1%–2%, so for every 100 embryos that are implanted in surrogate animals, about 98 of the embryos fail to produce a live animal offspring. These numbers have serious consequences for both the donor and surrogate being impregnated: surgery must be used to remove the donor animal's eggs and then another surgical technique used to implant the embryos into the surrogate. Cloned fetuses often exhibit a very high birth weight, frequently necessitating a c-section delivery, again causing pain and suffering to the surrogate animal. Of the live clones born, many have experienced compromised health status or early death. These adverse effects have prompted national animal welfare organizations to take a strong stance against animal biotechnology. The Humane Society of the United States (HSUS), for example, has called for a ban on products coming from cloned animals or their offspring (HSUS, 2003).

Although proponents of cloning argue that efficiency rates and health outcomes for cloned animals have improved dramatically, they acknowledge that such problems still exist. But they also argue that any criticism of the pain and suffering involved in animal biotechnology must be viewed in the context of standard, accepted practices involving animals, such as conventional medical research, companion animal breeding, or agriculture, which also involve a certain measure of suffering. Defenders of this science argue that animal biotechnology should not be held to a higher standard of preserving animal welfare than is the current practice in the various areas of animal use. Of course, the assumption in this argument is that those practices are morally acceptable, but if the pain and suffering involved in traditional breeding, factory farming, or medical and pharmaceutical research is not morally acceptable, then animal biotechnology is as morally suspect as those practices (though, arguably, no worse than those practices).

Defenders of animal biotechnology also note that a consequence-based analysis of this science requires that the pain and suffering of animals be weighed against the potential good that may result from this technology. It seems reasonable to argue that if the cost to research animals is small enough and the gain for human beings is large enough, then certain projects in animal biotechnology may well be worth pursuing. On the other hand, while the pain and suffering that animals endure in this research might be justified by noble ends (such as curing human or animal diseases, for example, or preserving endangered species), animal welfare issues are harder to ignore when biotechnology is undertaken for ends that seem frivolous—for example, the creation of novelty pets.

Two other consequence-based arguments have been made against animal biotechnology in general: it may have negative consequences for the environment, and it may have negative consequences for human beings. The environmental concern focuses on potential adverse effects from the interaction of genetically modified (GM) animals with non-GM animals, or the release of GM animals into a natural ecosystem. Regulators demand tight control over such animals, but some fear that regulatory policy cannot be foolproof.

The most pressing concern about the way that animal biotechnology could have untoward consequences for human beings is through the slippery slope of reproductive biotechnology progress. Many express concern that once cloning techniques are developed in nonhuman primates, for example, it will be a very short time until those techniques are applied to human beings. While this prospect is troubling, it is not an attack on animal biotechnology per se but is clear evidence for the need to establish an international ban on human reproductive cloning.

A final concern about the effect of animal biotechnology on human beings involves the safety of food produced from cloned livestock. The

FDA has determined that milk and meat from cloned animals is safe, though many people want such products labeled in order to give consumers a choice about whether or not to eat them. Consumers are already suspicious of GMO (genetically modified organism) foods, and food producers might struggle to convince consumers that these agricultural products are appealing to eat. With the majority of Americans believing that animal biotechnology is morally wrong, it won't be surprising if Americans resist products made from cloned animals.

In summary, the consequentialist arguments against animal biotechnology raise important concerns, but they do not constitute a justification for a blanket rejection of animal biotechnology. In the case of adverse effects to human beings and the environment, the solution appears to be tight regulation of the industry as opposed to a banning of animal biotechnology. In the case of adverse effects to animals, consequentialist arguments show that projects are morally permissible if the costs in animal suffering are small and the benefits are large.

PRINCIPLE-BASED ARGUMENTS AGAINST ANIMAL BIOTECHNOLOGY

A PART FROM THE ethical issues that arise because of the potential consequences of animal biotechnology, there is a significant set of ethical concerns about biotechnology that are based on principle-based, or deontological, considerations. Critiques of animal biotechnology that use this approach will claim that this science violates an important moral prohibition or duty, making the activity objectionable in and of itself, irrespective of the consequences.

The most well-known of these deontological arguments, and quite possibly the prime source of the public's condemnation, is the "playing God" problem: ought we to be creating life in this manner? On this view, animal biotechnology is a hubristic attempt by human beings to be divine. Cloning and transgenics cross an important moral line between facilitating the creation of life (as in assisted reproduction) and engineering life. In the first case, human beings are the builders using a God-given blueprint; in the second, they are the architects. While many individuals making this type of argument come from a religious tradition, thus anchoring their arguments in theology, not all of them do. There is also a secular version of this moral concern. According to this objection, we dehumanize ourselves and devalue the natural world by engaging in such activity. For these opponents of biotechnology, there is a reverence due the natural world that is violated when we manipulate living organisms in this manner. The sense that something is being lost or something profound is being compromised by biotechnology is part of what lends credence to Leon Kass's famous, but underdeveloped, "wisdom of repugnance" claim (Kass, 1997). Individuals in this camp emphasize the widespread intuition that something is deeply wrong with this enterprise, however difficult it is to say precisely what the moral prohibition is.

Proponents of animal biotechnology respond to this critique by arguing that we have been modifying organisms throughout human history and that only the means of modification has changed. But if the modifications of the past were morally permissible, what is the morally relevant difference in the current science? This is a powerful critique of the "playing God" argument because the onus is on the antibiotech camp to explain what's different about animal biotechnology. On the other hand, until this argument is adequately addressed by biotechnology proponents, it will likely be the central impasse in garnering widespread public support for this kind of work.

A second principle-based critique of animal biotechnology is that this science negates the intrinsic value of animals through both objectification and commodification. On this view, biotechnology treats animals as mere things, rather than living, breathing, sentient subjects. While biotechnology opponents admit that animals are already considered property and products, they argue that biotechnology takes this objectification to new levels. If animals are simply objects that we can create, then how different are they from disposable products like automobiles, telephones, and so forth? Of course, the argument of the defenders is already made by the opponents: animals are now and have historically been considered objects, both legally and in practice, so biotechnology science simply reaffirms the status quo; this constitutes no argument specific to animal biotechnology.

By extension of the objectification argument, opponents of this technology argue that it further commodifies animals. Biotechnology connotes so-called pure product and implies that no attention need to be paid to them as subjects. Opponents ask where this ultracommodification will take us in terms of animal welfare. Again, the obvious response by proponents is that human beings have always bartered and traded animals as commodities, but, they add, at no time in human history has more concern been paid to the pain and suffering of food and research animals as is being paid to them today. That response may not be the end of the debate. It does not defeat the objection to argue that animals have always been a means for human beings. The distinction opponents are making is one between being a pure means and a means while also at the same time an end (Fiester, 2007). If, for example, traditional farmers argued that they cared about their animals, then, even if they sold them or had them butchered for food, they could plausibly have been described as treating the animals as subjects or ends in themselves—while at the same time being a means for the farmer to sustain his life, physically or economically. This treatment of food animals as ends in themselves may have ended with the rise of factory farming, but does biotechnology exacerbate this trend? Does it delude us into believing that animals are no different from machines? Parallel to the problems with the consequentialist arguments about animal suffering, these deontological arguments attack many forms of contemporary use of animals and are not specific to animal biotechnology. But that does not necessarily undermine their efficacy or seriousness. The success of these arguments rests with the public's perception of the moral status of animals, and it may someday become the most compelling antibiotechnology argument. For now, biotechnology proponents must at least take seriously this type of objection.

A NOVEL APPROACH TO EVALUATING ANIMAL BIOTECHNOLOGY: THE PRESUMPTION OF RESTRAINT

BOTH THE CONSEQUENTIALIST and principle-based approaches to evaluating animal biotechnology are problematic and inadequate, for different reasons. Consequentialist-based critiques of animal biotechnology raise important moral concerns about risks, costs, and benefits, and they have the advantage of allowing us to weigh certain concerns against others, but they fail to capture some of the most deeply held reservations about this science: Does it go too far? Does it alter the world in ways that are inappropriate? Is this the right use of such powerful technology? On the other hand, the principle-based critiques are all-or-nothing: they either entirely prohibit or permit the use of this technology, without being able to make distinctions between various projects.

To overcome the weaknesses in the two approaches, I argue for a position that attempts to merge the set of concerns about animal biotechnology into a framework I call the presumption of restraint: a default position of wariness that must be overcome by morally compelling reasons in order to justify a particular project's moral legitimacy or permissibility (Fiester, 2008). This is not an argument for the prohibition of animal biotech research and commercialization that follows from the principle-based antibiotech arguments, nor is it simply a weighing and balancing of consequences. The presumption of restraint amounts to a "proceed with caution" stance that can be overcome when all of the relevant considerations are taken into account, but it stands in direct contrast to the no-holds-barred approach to animal biotechnology that currently prevails. Rather than condemn or embrace all animal biotechnology projects, this approach constitutes a middle-of-the-road position that escapes the all-or-nothing character of the debate as it now stands. The presumption of restraint is a justificatory *process*—a gate-keeping mechanism—to determine which projects should move forward and which ought to be rejected based on a set of moral considerations that extends well beyond concerns merely about safety to the environment or human health or concerns about animal welfare.

A presumption, philosophically speaking, is a default principle that guides action in the absence of compelling, overriding reasons that speak in the action's favor. A presumption is not a prohibition; it is a set of conditions that must be met in order to trump the default position. The creation of a default position of restraint in animal biotechnology begins with a review of the ordinary facts that form a backdrop to all projects in this science. First, living organisms and the ecosystem are vastly complex and nuanced. Second, we didn't put life on this planet; we are not the causal agent of life being here. In fact, we are just two-bit manipulators compared to nature or evolution or God. Whatever or whoever is responsible for life being here, we know it was not the agency of human beings. Third, not only are human beings not the creators of life on the planet, we can barely even blueprint certain aspects of some forms of life. The complexity is beyond both our comprehension and mastery. Fourth, we depend on the natural world, and our interventions in it can threaten our existence in more and less profound ways that mirror the threat to (or destruction of) other forms of life that we have caused. Add to this set of facts another specifically relevant to the case of the novelty pet or animal-as-art-object. First, these creatures are alive: they are sentient, they can feel pain, and they can feel something like fear (maybe even terror). Second, like all research animals, they are dependent on human beings for their subsistence and have no control over their treatment (not only how they will fare, but what they will become), and this makes them vulnerable.

Where do these uncontroversial facts get us? On my approach, they lead to a set of criteria that must be met in order to overcome a presumption of restraint. Specifically, a project must demonstrate: (a) a pressing reason to take the dramatic step of genetically altering life; (b) careful consideration of the potential consequences of the project, including the big picture concerns of how we are radically, possibly irreversibly, altering our world; (c) a recognition that unbridled animal biotechnology could create a world we no longer recognize or want to live in, which means that our animal biotechnology projects must be carefully, reflectively chosen; (d) a clear regard for the basic tenet of animal research, that is, that the benefit must far outweigh the cost; and (e) a strong resistance to the debasement and adulteration of sentient life.

Presumptions—and the considerations for overriding them—are not algorithms: they do not provide a definitive diagnostic to determine which projects we ought to support and which we ought to condemn. The purpose of a presumption is to set the terms of the discussion, not to provide an algorithmic decision procedure. This means that reflective participants in the debate might legitimately disagree in their determinations of moral permissibility on any particular project. But the presumption of restraint in animal biotechnology accomplishes an important framework for structuring the debate: it provides a collection of moral reasons that can be used to evaluate specific projects in animal biotechnology, allowing us to benefit from the enormous potential of the science while also recognizing the radical harm it could cause if left unbridled and unrestrained.

CONCLUSION

ADVANCES IN ANIMAL biotechnology raise many ethical concerns that need to be addressed as this technology develops. Serious arguments against this science have been made from both a principle-based and a consequence-based perspective, although both critiques have shortcomings that make an assessment of individual research projects difficult. As a possible assessment tool for the moral permissibility of animal biotechnology projects, I propose the framework of a presumption of restraint, placing the onus of justification on the proponents of the individual projects. This "proceed with caution" approach has the merit of distinguishing projects that truly serve the human good from projects that have less serious purpose and import.

REFERENCES

Fiester, A. (2005). A review of the ethical issues in animal cloning. *Perspectives in Biology and Medicine, 48*(3), 328–343.

Fiester, A. (2007). Casuistry and the moral continuum: Evaluating animal biotechnology. *Politics and the Life Sciences, 25*(1–2), 15–22.

Fiester, A. (2008). Justifying the principle of restraint in animal biotechnology. *American Journal of Bioethics, 8*(6), 36–44.

Humane Society of the United States (HSUS). (2003). HSUS asks the FDA to ban sales from cloned farm animals. Retrieved September 3, 2008, from http://www.hsus.org/ace/15431

Kass, L. (1997). The wisdom of repugnance: Why we should ban the cloning of humans. *New Republic, 216*, 17–26.

FURTHER READING

Burkhardt, J. (1998). The inevitability of animal biotechnology: Ethics and the scientific attitude. In A. Holland & A. Johnson (Eds.), *Animal biotechnology and ethics* (pp. 114–131). London: Chapman and Hall.

Midgley, M. (2000). Biotechnology and monstrosity. *Hastings Center Report, 30*(5), 7–15.

Robert, J. S., & Baylis, F. (2003). Crossing species boundaries. *American Journal of Bioethics, 3*(3), 1–13.

Rollin, B. (1995). *The Frankenstein syndrome: Ethical and social issues in the genetic engineering of animals.* New York: Cambridge University Press.

Thomson, P. (1997). *Food biotechnology in ethical perspective.* London: Chapman and Hall.

38

Ethical and Social Aspects of Transgenic Plants

David C. Magnus

MUCH IS AT stake in the development of transgenic plants. Genetic engineering has the potential to both positively and negatively affect a host of vital issues including food security, consumer rights, environmental protection, human health, trade laws, and our relationship to the natural world. Because of its vast significance, the genetic modification of plants has been widely debated both in the United States and internationally. Dissension and rancor dominate in discussions among various stakeholders in the debates. On one side, proponents—industry, scientists, and regulatory bodies— hail the 21st century as the era of biotechnology and champion a future that includes foods with far greater nutritional and pharmaceutical benefit and high-yield and drought resistance crops. They point to future possible products such as so-called golden rice as a way to help solve problems of food scarcity and nutritional and medical problems throughout the world. Critics of genetically modified (GM) food—some small farmers, environmentalists, and consumer groups—dismiss this optimistic vision as misguided and point to a wide range of food safety and environmental concerns. Both the advocates and opponents of GM food appear equally intransigent, with the prospect of reconciling the two sides seemingly bleak.

RISK ASSESSMENT FRAMEWORK

MUCH OF THE debate has tended to focus on several risks associated with biotechnology. First, there is concern about food safety. What impact will genetically modified organisms (GMOs) have on the health of those who eat them? Will some individuals develop allergic reactions? The new technology makes it possible to cross species barriers with impunity. Will a shellfish gene placed in a tomato lead to allergic reaction? This worry is exacerbated by the challenges involved in segregating parts of the food supply that are approved for human consumption from parts that are not. The difficulty of segregating commodity crops was made apparent in the case of StarLink corn. StarLink produced the *Bacillus thuringiensis* (Bt) toxin protein Cry9C. In 1998, the U.S. Environmental Protection Agency (EPA) approved Star-Link corn for animal consumption and for industrial production of ethanol. Human consumption was not approved because Cry9C resists both heat and digestion, and those traits are associated with allergens. Thus, the EPA determined that the protein was itself a potential allergen. In September 2000, several newspapers reported that StarLink corn had been detected in Taco Bell–brand taco shells sold in grocery stores. The Genetically Engineered Food Alert, a coalition of environmental groups, had sent the shells to the Iowa-based company Genetic ID for testing. That independent laboratory reported that the sample taco shells contained at least 1% StarLink corn. Kraft Foods, which distributed the taco shells, responded the next day with a press conference and a special report posted on its Web site. Kraft stated that it was conducting its own tests to confirm the results and would voluntarily recall the taco shells if Cry9C was detected.

Kraft later confirmed that Cry9C was in the taco shells, and it recalled the nearly 3 million boxes. Subsequently, hundreds of corn-based products were recalled because of concern about StarLink contamination. In late September 2000, Aventis—the company that developed and produced the seed—suspended sales. That was the first time a biotechnology company had frozen sales of a genetically engineered seed. By agreement with the U.S. Department of Agriculture (USDA), Aventis bought back all the remaining StarLink corn to ensure that it would be used only for animal feed and ethanol production (at a cost of roughly $100 million). There is no conclusive evidence that StarLink produced an allergic reaction in any person.

As development of transgenic plants continues, newer applications include plant-made pharmaceuticals (PMPs) and crops that are used in production of industrial compounds. Given the large start-up costs of factories that produce biologics such as human monoclonal antibodies, for example, PMPs represent a potentially lucrative market. But the developments also heighten worries about the escape of certain plant products and transgenes into the food supply. Among the first companies to come to public attention was Prodigene, a leader in PMP development. In 2001, Prodigene planted corn genetically engineered to produce pharmaceutical products at various field sites. The next year, at one of the Nebraska sites, a conventional crop—soybeans—was grown on the land that had been used for the experimental crop. Seed from the experimental crop germinated among the soybean plants. Although volunteer corn initially went undetected, eventually, inspectors from the USDA Animal and Plant Health Inspection Service identified the plants. Nonetheless, the plants were subsequently harvested with the soybeans. Pieces of transgenic corn plants ended up with the soybeans in a grain elevator. The USDA imposed a quarantine of 500,000 bushels of soy. Some commentators hold that this demonstrates success of the current U.S. regulatory system; others argue that it shows that companies cannot be trusted to apply adequate protection. In either case, the importance of confinement methods has been demonstrated as have their potential weaknesses (Taylor & Tick, 2003).

A second set of concerns arises over the environmental impact of transgenic plants. First, there are worries about gene flow. The same genes that may one day make it possible for plants to grow in poor, salty soil or in relatively arid regions could create an ecological nightmare if those same genes should be introduced to other plants. This can happen through out-crossing between the transgenic plants and other closely related plants. For example, although the risk is low, some have expressed concerns that genetically engineered wheat could cross with native grasses to alter the make-up of the ecosystem and potentially create so-called super-weeds and that even in the absence of gene flow, the transgenic plants themselves could become super-weeds as a result of the traits that make them better suited to new habitats. In certain circumstances the environmental trade-off for technology that makes it possible to produce sustainable agriculture in regions where greater productivity is required is the risk of loss of biodiversity. In addition to these concerns over the ecosystem and the creation of super-weeds, there is a worry over the potential impact of some transgenic plants on nontarget organisms. Cornell researchers found that pollen from Bt corn could kill the larvae of monarch butterflies who ingested it. This raised the fear that these engineered crops could kill butterflies and other nontarget organisms in addition to the corn borer the Bt corn was meant to protect against. Subsequent field research to determine whether the Bt corn really represents a threat outside of the lab *has been mixed, though most scientists do not believe Bt represents a serious threat* (Hansen Jesse & Obrycki, 2000; Sears et al., 2001).

What has often been missed in the biotechnology debate is an adequate discussion of the moral and cultural issues associated with conducting genetic engineering responsibly. Biotechnology is not an isolated scientific process but a social practice that involves different contexts, actors, relationships, and dynamics of power. The complex web of relationships that make up biotechnology requires that the ethical obligations human beings have to one another, the environment, and future generations, both human and nonhuman, be central in discussions about GMOs.

One major philosophical tradition embodies the approach that has largely dominated policy discussions: consequentialism. The weighing of risks (and sometimes benefits) has tended to dominate the discussion. This is unsurprising given the controversy and, in some cases, uncertainty surrounding many of the applications of GMOs. So most GM food discussions focus almost exclusively on risk—risk to the ecosystem, risk to endangered species, risk to future generations, and risk to the food supply. In these discussions, risk is understood and evaluated in purely quantitative, cost/benefit terms. For example, disputes about risk frequently center on the efficacy of the so-called precautionary principle as a means to minimize risk to the environment.[1] Regardless of an individual's or organization's position regarding the precautionary principle, however, all those engaged in controversy typically accept its underlying assumption: that risk is solely a scientific phenomenon. One consequence of this way of framing the debate is that it circumscribes the role of values and transforms the debate into what seems to be mainly a matter of getting the facts straight and the importance of educating an ignorant public. At the extreme, some have claimed that the acceptability of GMOs is entirely a scientific matter and one in which nonexperts should play no role (Nestle, 2003). Scientists and only scientists can tell us what the benefits and risks of GMOs are and thus whether GMOs are worthwhile.

Critics often try to respond to the narrowing of the debate into risk/benefit terms by noting that science is not the last word when it comes to food. This places the critics in the position of constantly appearing to be antiscientific or indifferent to the findings of science. The GMO debate takes on the appearance of being a pro- and antiscience battle.

Ethicists will note that the consequentialist framework that is typically operational is actually a very crude form of utilitarianism. Needless to say, this is not at all an adequate framework for capturing the full range of moral considerations in debates over GMOs.[2]

While there are dozens of issues and possible topics, I will illustrate the broader concerns at stake in a fairly narrow issue: confinement or containment of GMOs (including the use of biotechnology as a tool to better contain GMOs).

CONFINEMENT OF GMOs

THERE ARE A number of social values bound up with the need for adequate confinement of GMOs. When the USDA initially sought comments for proposed rules defining organic products, it included the recommendation that GMOs could potentially be included. The result was a massive public response (Nestle, 2003). Prior to this issue, the USDA had never received more than 8,000 public comments, yet by the close of the comment period, the USDA had received 275,603 comments, most of them complaining about the idea of including GMOs under the organic rubric (Lambrecht, 2001; Nestle, 2003). While at least part of the massive nature of this response can probably be attributed to the development of the Internet as a new method for grassroots activism on this topic (Priest, 2001), the scale of the response was sufficient to ensure that organics would be GMO free. Many commentators have pointed out that there is no scientific evidence that organic foods are safer or more nutritious than nonorganic foods. However, there are a number of values that are captured by organic production, including views about globalization, corporate control of the food supply, and the meaning of food and its relationship to nature. Clearly, GMOs are presently incompatible with many of these values. The problem that arises is that there is little confinement effort aimed at preventing gene flow from conventional GM crops into organics. Physical separation requirements reduce gene flow but do not eliminate it. Organisms vary in pollination ranges. For example, the degree of physical separation commonly used for rapeseed is inadequate to prevent a significant degree of gene flow (McHughen, 2000, p. 235). Herbicide-resistant genes have been found in neighboring canola fields (Rieger, Lamond, Preston, Powles, & Roush, 2002). The economic and social problem that this represents can be handled by allowing a certain amount of GM crop to be included without loss of the organic label. However, this response fails to adequately address the values that were expressed by the strong response to the initial USDA suggestion on organics. The decision to allow GMOs into labeled organics represents a compromise with the value systems of those opposed to modern, large-scale, industrial agricultural practices. The decision about how much should be tolerated (5%, 1%, or .1%) and how this challenges socially constructed notions of the purity of organics is a difficult one and may require a stronger set of biological confinement measures than would be required from a point of view that focused exclusively on safety and risk. It also highlights the need for transparency and participation of the public in these sorts of determinations.

Similar considerations are involved in the controversy over the discovery of transgenes in Mexican landraces of maize. Researchers at

University of California, Berkeley, reported in *Nature* that they had discovered transgenes in supposedly pristine landraces in Oaxaca (Quist & Chapela, 2001). While they made other claims about GMOs that became the focus of controversy (and resulted in a politically charged debate that culminated in the repudiation of the article by the editors of *Nature* who published it), the existence of the transgenes was never questioned. Subsequent analysis confirmed that GMOs had invaded Mexico on a surprisingly large scale (Mann, 2002). It is now clear that these invasions represent little or no threat to human health. But the significance of rare forms of maize, especially in Mexican culture, may not be adequately captured by considerations of risk or safety. Again, this may require greater consideration of the need for adequate biological confinement methods, as well as highlighting some of the weaknesses in any confinement system—particularly human intervention.

Given the cultural significance of food, it is unsurprising that there is a close connection between food and religion. There are numerous dietary restrictions that are observed by different groups. GMOs that may be perfectly safe may be nonetheless forbidden because of these dietary restrictions. For example, if porcine genes are placed into conventional crops, will those crops be permissible to religious individuals who are enjoined from eating pork? Different answers to this type of question are emerging. The majority position within Judaism seems to be that such foods can be kosher (Chaudry & Regenstein, 1994). The discovery of the existence of microorganisms represented a challenge to Kashrut if they were found to violate the dietary laws. Several prominent rabbis permitted eating them on the grounds that Kashrut only applies to things that can be seen by the naked eye. Using this as a basis, since porcine genes cannot be seen, they are not relevant to whether or not a food is kosher. Islam, in contrast, considers that any kind of mixing of forbidden foods (haram) with permitted foods (halaal) results in forbidden foods. Hence, porcine genes would render any foods haram. To date, Catholics have not publicly addressed the issue of whether it is permissible to eat foods with animal genes in them on Fridays during Lent. Each of these cases raises interesting issues for confinement. The degree of confinement necessary to satisfy religious sanctions is likely to be stringent indeed. Allowing a small percentage of crops with porcine genes in them may not be a viable option for many religious groups. To satisfy such stringent demands, it may be necessary to avoid putting certain genes into common commodity crops—the most stringent bioconfinement method.

These examples are illustrations of a more general point. The products of genetic engineering are organisms that may have social significance or be infused with value for any number of reasons. Trees have important symbolic, social, and aesthetic value that represents important challenges for biotechnology (McQuillan, 2000, 2001). The desire for natural (and even wild) forests will likely require far stricter confinement methods than simple safety considerations would dictate. The purity of certain kinds of culturally significant foods may similarly necessitate stringent confinement to ensure that these values are preserved.

In summary, beyond risk assessment, broader social and ethical values of society must play a role in determining the level of biological confinement necessary for various organisms. Justice will require that attention is paid not merely to the level of risk but also to who is exposed to it, who benefits from it, and who makes the ultimate decisions about it. The values of transparency and participation follow from the consideration of informed consent that is grounded in the principle of respect (like justice, a fundamental principle of the Belmont Report). The values of specific groups and communities must likewise be respected and taken into account in the choice of biological and physical confinement methods.

BIOETHICAL DEBATE OVER CONFINEMENT METHODS: THE CASE OF TERMINATOR TECHNOLOGY

JUST AS THERE are ethical values involved in decisions about the degree to which confinement methods are required, there are a number of ethical issues at stake in the use of some of the bioconfinement methods that may affect their social acceptability. So-called terminator technologies are methods for restricting the use of genetically modified plants by causing second-generation seeds to be sterile. Public opposition to such technology led to widespread opposition and the eventual demise of the technology in common usage. Can terminator-related technologies such as genetic use restriction technologies (GURTs) be resuscitated? GURT produces sterile seeds, which means that farmers who purchased seeds containing the technology cannot save the seed from a current crop for future planting. There are several issues that need to be distinguished. First, it is important to distinguish the technical problems and uncertainties surrounding these technologies from the ethical acceptability of utilizing the technologies. The ethical issues in turn are related to, but distinct from, the issue of the social acceptability of the technology. A second important set of distinctions involves the purposes of the technology. Use of the technology to protect intellectual property (IP) interests of private companies, while potentially legitimate, is nonetheless morally different from use of the technology as a bioconfinement method to avoid environmental harm.

The primary objections to terminator-type technology revolve around the fact that it seems to undermine a traditional farming practice that remains important in many developing countries and also has symbolic significance in the United States even if it is not widely practiced. Seed saving from year to year has historically been an integral part of agricultural practice. It continues to be important in some parts of the world. There is a fear that the loss of the ability to save seed will lead to worsening food security problems and create a terrible dilemma in which less-developed nations must either forgo the benefits of biotechnology or run the risk of economic hardship through a reliance on yearly purchases of new seed. Given that one of the key moral justifications of biotechnology is its potential role in improving food security, terminator technology represents a clear problem if it is regularly linked to food crops.

In the United States, many farmers have grown used to annual seed purchases, as the hybrids that they desire typically lack significant characteristics in the next generation. However, even here there is an important argument. Though the development of hybrids in the past few decades has largely eliminated seed saving in practice, it remains a historically important and symbolically significant part of the understanding that many have of the meaning of farming. When new biotechnology makes it possible to produce some of the same benefits that crossbreeding produces without the loss of value in the next generation, there is the presumption that this benefit should accrue to the farmers. Farmers have always had the right to save their seeds even if (because the seeds had little value) they didn't do so. Purchasing seed is purchasing a living organism—and reproduction is an essential part of what living organisms do (Boorse, 1975). This helps to explain why the use of terminator technologies in the context of intellectual property protection is so morally problematic. When one purchases a product, it is usually understood that one is entitled to the full, normal functioning of the product (Cummins & Perlman, 2002; Eaton, van Tongeren, Louwaars, Visser, & Van der Meer, 2001; Halweil, 2000). If reproduction were understood as part of the normal functioning of an organism, this would seem to imply a claim on the part of those who purchase organisms to the offspring that are produced. The fact that forced sterility is needed to enforce IP rights of the company seems to show something problematic about patents on living organisms. Therefore, it is morally problematic to allow terminator technology to protect IP. (This objection would also render contracts that require annual purchases unethical.)

These arguments mean that the use of GURTs, even as a bioconfinement method, is of moral and social concern. But that concern is especially present in cases of food crops. Morally, the use of GURTs for environmental protection in cases where there is no tradition of seed saving—for example, forest trees and turf grasses—would not raise the same sort of ethical problem.

Socially, GURTs may be difficult to resuscitate with the public. There are several reasons for this. The technology has been closely linked in the public's mind with corporate interests in protecting IP rights (continued legal battles over cases of infringement reinforce this association, even in cases where there are no GURTs) (Priest, 2001). The previously outlined moral arguments certainly contribute to the public response—and concerns about the impact of the technology on less-developed nations are certainly widely cited. The Rural Advancement Foundation International's successful campaign persuaded the public that "life-science companies were bent on controlling the food chain" (Lambrecht, 2001, p. 112) to the detriment of less developed nations. Priest (2001) has argued that the response to Dolly the cloned sheep was also an important part of the backdrop to opposition. But the visceral nature of the response to cloning makes it plausible that a deeper metaphysical unease may be behind the concern as well, a concern that relates to the moral argument against use of GURTs for IP protection.

An important source of the unease that many have with GMOs (and cloning) is the perceived unnaturalness of genetic engineering. While some of this concern is mitigated by recognition that we have altered nature for thousands of years, terminator technology represents a special concern. The connection between life and reproduction is fundamental. Altering an organism to intentionally curtail this function creates a significant "yuck factor." Unpacking this visceral response is challenging. The fact that reproduction is so intimately tied to the nature of life means that the intentional alteration of this trait crosses a very significant boundary. It is a boundary that should not be crossed lightly, and all of the concerns about GMOs in general—anxieties over hubris on the part of the corporate and scientific communities, fears that we are transforming nature and organisms into commodities, and worries that control of the food system rests in the hands of a few powerful corporations—are all issues that GURTs and other technologies that prohibit reproduction heighten. This is especially of concern when the alteration is genetic in character (as opposed to induced sterility) because it is often held to be a more fundamental alteration in the nature of the organism.

CONCLUSION

THE BENEFITS OF the use of GURTs must be taken into account. These technologies represent a potentially powerful bioconfinement tool that will combine with other physical, temporal, and bioconfinement measures to ensure that GMOs will not harm ecosystems or threaten the food supply. From an ethical standpoint, the consequentialist argument would seem to favor the use of GURTs. From a nonconsequentialist perspective, there are two potential issues that must be considered. The justice issues discussed in this chapter must be adequately taken into account. The use of GURTs for food crops where seed saving is commonly practiced (or has a strong history) should not be done if it harms individuals or populations who have little control over the uses of the technology. For aquaculture and forestry, GURTs are far less problematic.

The second issue is the worry over the unnaturalness of genetically engineering organisms to be sterile. This objection is significant for the likely public response to the technology, but it ethically rests on problematic assumptions. The view that genes are more fundamental in determining the true nature of an organism is a highly questionable assumption. Organisms are a result of the complex interplay of environmental, genetic, and epigenetic factors. There is no reason why genetically engineered sterility should be more problematic than physically induced sterility. For such practices to be accepted by the public, it is imperative that we learn from the mistakes and successes of the past (Eichenwald, Kolata, & Peterson, 2001). These technologies should be introduced slowly and carefully; consideration of justice should be paramount; their introduction should be preceded by discussion with stakeholders and parts of the nongovernmental organizations (NGO) community; and the ethical case for their use must be clearly and publicly articulated prior to their use.

NOTES

This work reflects contributions from a number of contributors to a Penn Bioethics Center project on biotechnology. I particularly want to acknowledge the contributions of Art Caplan, Sita Reddy, Pablo Arredondo, and Sarah Eichberg. In addition, some of the material in this chapter was originally prepared for a National Research Council (of the National Academies of Sciences) report (Kirk et al., 2004).

1. For a discussion of the different meanings of the precautionary principle, see Magnus (2008).

2. For a more detailed discussion of the role of nonconsequentialist values in these debates, see Paul Thompson (1997) and Magnus and Caplan (2002).

REFERENCES

Boorse, C. (1975). On the distinction between disease and illness. *Philosophy and Public Affairs, 5,* 49–68.

Chaudry, M. M., & Regenstein, J. M. (1994). Implications of biotechnology and genetic engineering for kosher and halal foods. *Trends in Good Science and Technology, 5,* 165–168.

Cummins, R., & Perlman, M. (Eds.). (2002). *Functions: New essays in the philosophy of biology and psychology.* Oxford, UK: Oxford University Press.

Eaton, D., van Tongeren, F., Louwaars, N., Visser, B., & Van der Meer, I. (2001). Economic and policy aspects of terminator technology. *Biotechnology and Development Monitor, 49,* 19–22.

Eichenwald, K., Kolata, G., & Peterson, M. (2001). Biotechnology food: From the lab to debacle. In M. Ruse & D. Castle (Ed.), *Genetically modified foods: Debating biotechnology* (pp. 31–40). Amherst, NY: Prometheus Press.

Halweil, B. (2000). Monsanto drops the terminator. *World Watch, 13,* 8–9.

Hansen Jesse, L. C., & Obrycki, J. J. (2000). Field deposition of Bt transgenic corn pollen: Lethal effects on the monarch butterfly. *Oecologia, 125,* 241–248.

Kirk, K., Carlson, J. E., Ellstrand, N., Kapuscinski, A. R., Lumpkin, T. A., Magnus, D. C., et al. (2004). *Biological confinement of genetically engineered organisms.* Washington, DC: NAS Press.

Lambrecht, B. (2001). Dinner at the new gene café. New York: St. Martin's Press.

Magnus, D. (2008). Agnotology and the precautionary principle in the GEO debate. In R. Proctor & L. Scheibinger (Eds.), *Agnotology* (pp. 250–265). Stanford, CA: Stanford University Press.

Magnus, D., & Caplan, A. (2002). "Food for thought: The primacy of the moral in the GMO debate." In M. Ruse & D. Castle (Eds.), *Genetically modified foods: Debating biotechnology* (pp. 250–265). Amherst, NY: Prometheus Press.

Mann, C. C. (2002). Has GM corn "invaded" Mexico? *Science, 295,* 1617–1619.

McHughen, A. (2000). Pandora's picnic basket. Oxford, UK: Oxford University Press.

McQuillan, A. G. (2000). Cabbages and kings: The ethics and aesthetics of new forestry. In P. List (Ed.), *Environmental ethics and forestry: A reader* (pp. 293–318). Philadelphia, PA: Temple University Press.

McQuillan, A.G. (2001). Naturalness as a value: How forest biotechnology might be affected by public views of forests and science. *Pew Initiative on Biotechnology and Food Conference on Forestry and Biotechnology.* Retrieved November 4, 2003, from http://pewagbiotech.org/events/1204/presentations/McQuillan2.pdf

Nestle, M. (2003). Safe food: Bacteria, biotechnology, and bioterrorism. Los Angeles: University of California Press.

Priest, S. (2001). A grain of truth. New York: Rowman and Littlefield.

Quist, D., & Chapela, I. H. (2001). Transgenic DNA introgressed into traditional maiz landraces in Oaxaca, Mexico. *Nature, 414,* 541–543.

Rieger, M. A., Lamond, M., Preston, C., Powles, S. B., & Roush, R. T. (2002). Pollen-mediated movement of herbicide resistance between commercial canola fields. *Science, 296,* 2386–2388.

Sears, M. K., Hellmich, R. L., Stanley-Horn, D. R., Oberhauser, K. S., Pleasants, J. M., Mattila, H. R., et al. (2001). Impact of Bt corn pollen on monarch butterfly populations: A risk assessment. *Proceedings of the National Academy of Sciences, 98,* 11937–11942.

Taylor, M. R., & Tick, J. S. (2003). *Post-market oversight of biotech foods.* Washington, DC: Pew Initiative on Food and Biotechnology. Retrieved November 7, 2008, from http://www.pewtrusts.org/uploadedFiles/wwwpewtrustsorg/Reports/Food_and_Biotechnology/hhs_biotech_corn_0403.pdf

Thompson, P. (1997). *Food biotechnology in ethical perspective.* New York: Aspen Publishers.

Part VII

Fetuses and Children

39

The Contested Territory of Medical Decision-Making for Children

WYNNE MORRISON AND CHRIS FEUDTNER

IN THE MEDICAL care of pediatric patients, the health care team typically turns to the child's parents as the most appropriate decision-makers, and then between these parties, therapeutic decisions—small and large—are made. What is the moral justification for how we make such decisions, and what is the best process for doing so? The answer to these questions have great practical importance when physicians, nurses, ethicists, lawyers, advocates, or others question parental decisions regarding the medical care of their children. While some have argued that from the perspective of public policy parents are the best decision-makers because "it is impossible to locate an actor or identify a process that will do the job better" (Rothman & Rothman, 1980, p. 10), more detailed justification regarding the scope and boundaries of parental decision-making authority is needed when specific choices for individual children are contested.

Indeed, from a historical perspective, parental decisions and decision-making authority have been increasingly scrutinized. For most of recorded history, parents were granted nearly absolute power over their children, who were treated legally more as property than as individuals (Cooper & Koch, 1996; Kopelman, 1997). From the mid-19th century onward, Western societies have increasingly recognized that children's interests might not always be in alignment with parents' decisions, an awareness that manifested itself in child labor laws and compulsory public education (Zelizer, 1994), and perhaps culminated in the 1974 federal Child Abuse Prevention and Treatment Act, which provided funds to states for the evaluation and treatment of abused or neglected children (Child Abuse Prevention and Treatment Act, 1974).

In this chapter, we examine ethical and practical issues regarding medical decision-making for children. We will focus mostly on issues quite specific to pediatric health care, passing over many of the debates about appropriate decision-making (especially regarding the appropriate allocation of scarce resources, the use of treatment viewed by some as futile, or whether informed consent/permission is sufficiently informed) that appear in both the pediatric and adult medical realms. Since families come in many different varieties, whenever we use the term *parents* we intend to be inclusive of single-parent decision-makers and other legal guardians. We will first situate some of the core ethical principles within a pediatric framework. We will then introduce into the discussion the concepts, on the one hand, of children's emerging capacity to make increasingly complicated and weighty decisions (with the associated process of seeking the child's assent) and, on the other hand, of children with severe impairments having diminished capacity, perhaps permanently, and how quality of life considerations should (or should not) be assessed. We will then turn to examine processes that guide pediatric decision-making in situations where either there is no apparent conflict or where different types of conflict are manifest. Throughout, we attempt to unify our overview by highlighting several cases that illuminate the interplay of general arguments and specific circumstances in this dynamic and evolving area of medical ethics.

SITUATING ETHICAL PRINCIPLES WITHIN A PEDIATRIC FRAMEWORK

THE AUTHORITY OF medical decision-making for adult patients is typically grounded in the ethical principle of individual *autonomy*, which in turn is situated among political and social concepts of human rights and protections. The principle of autonomy grants a remarkably wide scope of medical decision-making authority, including an inviolable right to refuse treatment, to persons who have the cognitive capacity to understand their situation and the consequences of their choices. This ethical schema is paralleled by the legal framework of decision-making competency, which typically sets 18 years of age as the default threshold for acquiring decision-making authority.

Thus, unlike the situation for competent adults, justifying the standards and procedures of medical decision-making for children cannot be based on the principle of autonomy—or at least not in a literal or legalistic reading of what the concept of autonomy represents. If autonomy is understood, however, as a specific manifestation of a more fundamental *respect for persons*—and in particular as a means to acknowledge and protect human rights—then this set of allied concepts can be as readily applied to children as to adults (see chapters 40 and 41 in this volume). For instance, the 1989 United Nations Convention on the Rights of the Child emphasized that children are deserving of respect, even when they are not legally protected (Goldhagen, 2003; Zawistowski & Frader, 2003). In a similar manner, the concept of *surrogate decision-making*, which is used to justify decision-making for adults who are unable to voice their wishes, can be applied to children. Whereas for adult patients a surrogate decision-maker is often able to base decisions on the previously competent patient's prior expressed wishes, written or verbalized, children typically have never been in a position to be independent decision-makers, cognitively or legally, so that their prior wishes may be either unknown or lack the authority associated with a competent autonomous decision-maker. Nevertheless, many parents attempt to approximate a substituted judgment, in that they attempt to decide what their children would want were they able to speak on their own behalf. Much as surrogate decision-makers for adult patients can feel relieved if they can rely on the guidance of an advance directive rather than bearing the full burden of deciding (Arnold & Kellum, 2003), parents may be more easily able to stop burdensome treatments with little prospect of benefit for their child if they believe that stopping is what the child would want.

The usual decision-making standard applied when deliberating pediatric care focuses on a child's *best interests* (Beauchamp & Childress, 2001; Kopelman, 2007). Under this standard, the parents, as well as the health care team, weigh the potential benefits and burdens of any given treatment and thereby decide what constitutes the best option for the child. Some have argued that the best interests standard is too high a bar to set (Downie & Randall, 1997; Ross, 1998), either because it is impossible to know what is truly the best choice, or because being required to choose the supposed best option for an individual may ignore legitimate competing claims of others such as family members or society.

Given this criticism, several commentators have proposed the *rational parent* or *reasonable parent* standard as an alternative to the best interests standard (Cooper & Koch, 1996; Kopelman, 1997), allowing that parents may choose from a range of potentially acceptable options, consistent with their own family's needs, resources, and values, as long as a threshold of minimum harm is not exceeded. This standard acknowledges that not all individuals, and therefore not all families, would make identical choices given identical circumstances. Instead, this framework—which is allied to a broader principle of *respect for families*—assumes that much of the authority of parental decision-making arises from the family in which the child will grow and develop, as the family will have ongoing responsibility for the care of the child, and the family will bear the lifelong consequences of any decisions made (Ross, 1998). Serious disagreements about what would be in the best interest of the child are therefore required to challenge parents' decisions regarding the care of their child.

In sum, because the authority for pediatric decision-making does not emanate from the autonomous preferences of the child patient, either expressed directly or through a substituted judgment, but rather on one of the other standards of determining what would be best for the child, the term *informed permission* more accurately reflects the complex set of justifications raised than the standard jargon of *informed consent*. The issue then becomes: who is granted the power to provide this permission, and what are the guides for and limits on this authority? An ongoing area of contention regarding decision-making for children—especially when the physical or bodily best interest of the child (as viewed from the medical viewpoint) is pitted against the spiritual or eternal best interest of the child (as viewed from the family viewpoint)—is how to operationally define *serious disagreements,* and what the precise consequences of certain decisions should be. These questions augment the principle of respect for families with the counterbalancing consideration of the *limitations of family autonomy.* Whether the case involves the refusal of immunizations or reliance on prayer rather than antibiotics or insulin, the medical and public health establishments tend to draw the line at the point where the child or the public are placed at significant risk of harm (with usually no precise definition of significant risk offered, although in many instances the risk is quite glaring and substantial). Consequences that ensue when parents do not cede to medical or public health judgments vary considerably (and likely, unjustly), ranging from receiving a cold shoulder to exclusion from daycare or school settings to, at the extreme, court orders, child protective service investigations, removal of children from families, and prosecution of parents. While many of these steps are often fully warranted to protect the physical (and perhaps emotional) well-being of children, the manner in which these measures are targeted and enforced in some instances but not others requires far more scrutiny than currently exists.

EMERGING CAPACITY AND ASSENT

C ERTAINLY, ONE SCENARIO wherein the parental power of permission should both be guided and limited regards older children and adolescents who are maturing in their ability to express preferences and make decisions in their everyday lives. At one extreme, most states have *emancipated minor* or *mature minor* statutes that recognize particular circumstances or decisions where an adolescent is legally allowed to make independent medical decisions (Zawistowski & Frader, 2003). While the specifics vary by state, such circumstances could include a minor who is married, living in financial independence, or in the military, and could also apply to particular types of medical care, such as obtaining birth control or treatment of sexually transmitted infections.

As opposed to a dichotomous concept of decision-making competency, marked by a legally defined age of maturity, a more developmentally appropriate concept of *emerging capacity* acknowledges that the preferences and decisions of children exist across a continuum of moral authority, starting at minimal authority during young childhood and rising potentially to full authority sometime during adolescence. In practice, the authority of a child or adolescent's preferences will vary with age, cognitive ability, prior experience with illness, the complexity of the medical predicament, and the potential consequences of the decision. In keeping with this view, the American Academy of Pediatrics Committee on Bioethics has recommended actively seeking the *assent* of children, when developmentally appropriate, in as many decisions as possible regarding their treatment (Committee on Bioethics, American Academy of Pediatrics, 1995). Nontherapeutic research represents a special circumstance where the assent of a child to participation may be mandatory (see chapter 41 in this volume).

The actual procedure for seeking assent in clinical practice, though, is probably even more variable than that seen in research assent (Kimberly, Hoehn, Feudtner, Nelson, & Schreiner, 2006) and is potentially vulnerable to subtle acts of manipulation or coercion that would undermine the ethical and psychological rationale for the entire undertaking.

CONSIDERATIONS: CURRENT VERSUS LONG-TERM, NARROW VERSUS BROAD

I N DISTINCTION TO most decisions made either by or regarding adult patients, where the time horizon that bounds the decision-making context is usually measured in days to months, many health care decisions made on behalf of children take into account potential consequences several years or even decades into the future. For instance, most immunizations that adults receive protect potentially immediate threats, such as influenza or tetanus, whereas children also receive immunizations in their early youth that aim to protect against diseases that typically occur in late adolescence or early adulthood, such as hepatitis B or human papillomavirus. This general pattern of a longer time-horizon of pediatric medical decision-making reflects a deep-seated and admirable concern for the well-being of the developing child across the trajectory from infancy into adulthood.

The pediatric proclivity for a longer time-horizon of decision-making considerations, however, can increase the complexity and uncertainty of decision-making, as the much-publicized case of Ashley X illustrates (Brosco & Feudtner, 2006; Gunther & Diekema, 2006). At the time that her story came to public attention, Ashley was a 9-year-old girl with severe, irreversible cognitive and developmental delays, never able to walk, sit on her own, feed herself, or speak, functioning at the level of a 3-month-old infant with no prospects of improvement. When she was 6-years-old, her parents had become concerned that with the onset of puberty (of which she was already beginning to show signs) her increasing size would make it difficult for them to care for her, and that at some point in the future (years away) they would have to place her in a long-term care facility. They also feared that developing secondary sexual characteristics would potentially make her more likely in the future to be a victim of sexual abuse, possibly even leading to unwanted pregnancy. After consulting with multiple specialists and a hospital ethics committee, her parents and physicians proceeded with high dose estrogen therapy to attenuate her growth in height, as well as with a hysterectomy (to prevent menstruation and the possibility of pregnancy) and surgical removal of her breast buds (to prevent breast development).

When her story reached the popular press, disability activists decried the surgical procedures, including sterilization, which stirred historical memories of the abuses of the eugenics movement (Committee on Bioethics, American Academy of Pediatrics, 1999), and experimental therapies that aimed to keep her small and in a purportedly gender-neutral state. Her parents vigorously defended their decisions, arguing that keeping her small would enable them to continue to care for her at home in a stable and loving environment with ease of interaction with her family, that she would never be able to have consensual sexual relationships due to her cognitive impairments, that menstruation would only have been uncomfortable and frightening to her, and that they were protecting her future.

455

*The Contested
Territory of
Medical
Decision-Making
for Children*

The desire to protect a child's future—and the difficulty of this quest—are the issues that (among many possible issues) we want to underscore in this case, where all the interventions that Ashley X received were preemptive, tackling problems that lay off somewhere in an uncertain and emotionally charged future. Lest we be misunderstood, we affirm that there is ample ethical justification (based on respect for persons and best interest standards) for this endeavor of thinking well into the future and considering long-term consequences of decisions to intervene or not intervene—indeed, such long-range thinking is imperative in many instances. We do, however, repeat that this is a very arduous and precarious undertaking, especially given what is known about how humans make decisions in the face of uncertainty and risk, and it likely requires forms of decision support that surpass the minimal requirements set forth by informed consent standards, uniting cognitive and emotional support (Feudtner, 2007).

Matters become even more complex when the future involves a protracted or even permanent state of near-total dependency of the child patient on the family. In this regard, children with grave cognitive disabilities represent the antithesis of normal expectations of children developing into independent adults. The fact of this dependency on others for basic care alters—and entwines—the future prospects both for these children and for their families. The key question in such instances is whether the best interests of the child and the course of action endorsed by other family members are aligned (and not whether the motivations of the family members are laudable or not). For instance, in the Ashley X case, extending the range of pertinent decision-making considerations to include the family as well as the patient, one can ask: if the patient benefits by being small and light because the parents benefit by the patient being small and light, is this inherently an ethically problematic situation, or are the child's best interests sufficiently aligned with the parents' (and in this case, the physicians') proposed set of medical interventions (Shannon & Savage, 2007)?

DECISION-MAKING PROCEDURES WHEN THERE IS NO CONFLICT

W E NOW TRANSITION our discussion to evaluate the appropriateness of decision-making for children from a process-based perspective. In the vast majority of circumstances, many signs of mutual affirmation and accord mark the intimate social context between family members and the patient's clinicians. In such cases, most therapeutic decisions are handled informally; when informed permission is sought, the process proceeds in a manner operationally analogous to informed consent: the clinician provides the family members with information about the condition under consideration, the proposed treatment, reasonable alternative courses of action, and the advantages and risks of these possible therapeutic options, and then the family, after mulling over the options, decides whether to accept the proposed intervention and signs a form authorizing treatment.

CONFLICT BETWEEN PARTIES

WHEN BOTH THE parents and the health care team agree on what they all deem to be an acceptable course of action, further inquiry is exceedingly rare. The exceptions arise when parents and the child's physicians jointly make choices that others believe are morally or socially unacceptable. Such a situation occurred in the Baby Doe case of an infant with Down syndrome who was not provided with life-saving surgical intervention; the joint decision by the baby's parents and primary physicians was challenged by other physicians. The subsequent 1984 federal Baby Doe regulations put in place one procedure for initiating such challenges, but these regulations addressed only the care of newborn infants, were extremely unpopular, and ultimately ineffective.

More commonly, when disagreement arises regarding the decision-making by either parents or physicians, individuals sometimes request the involvement of a hospital ethics committee. What percentage of all disagreements reach ethics committees is unknown, and although in theory anyone can request ethics committee consultation, most requests are by physicians or nurses. Although the processes of conducting an ethics consultation vary greatly, most involve information gathering, some process of dialogue and deliberation, and some form of guidance or recommendation, which typically is not binding. As an alternative to the ethics consultation procedure, some hospitals are putting in place more explicit processes of mediation to broker between the disputing parties a mutually satisfactory course of therapeutic action (see chapter 15 in this volume).

Finally, the legal courts are sometimes asked to adjudicate refractory disagreements or other special circumstances. A classic example of an otherwise intractable disagreement would involve a parent who is a Jehovah's Witness who refuses to permit a life-saving blood transfusion for a child. Although not without controversy (Cooper & Koch, 1996), clinicians now routinely obtain a court order to override parents in this circumstance, even while acknowledging that the parents are appropriately advocating what they see as best for their child. Special

457

*The Contested
Territory of
Medical
Decision-Making
for Children*

circumstances include cases, as defined by law, that require a court order to perform a surgical sterilization procedure on a minor.

CONFLICT WITHIN MEDICAL TEAMS

Conflict can also emerge within medical teams, as members of the team may differ regarding what they believe would be in the child's best interest, or external influences may be weighing on their minds. Physicians or administrators may be desperate to open up a hospital bed for another patient, or alternatively have financial incentives to operate on a patient or keep the patient in intensive care to be able to continue to bill. Other physicians may be motivated to pursue an innovative therapy for a patient for the sake of an academic reputation, to get a publication on a résumé, or to improve chances of getting research funding. The staff may be just plain tired of caring for a patient who they think has very little chance of ever recovering. Such conflicts of interest on the part of the health care team are potentially more serious, and probably more common, than those experienced by parents trying to decide for their children, which if true would provide a further empirical justification for the parents being the appropriate surrogates for their children.

Health care teams may have other biases that are less sinister. The ethics committee members who reviewed Ashley's case were undoubtedly moved by an emotional appeal from educated parents who were extremely devoted to Ashley's care and trying their best to find a workable solution for their family. While considering such factors is not wrong, clinicians must make sure they do not lose sight of the patient when trying to help such a sympathetic family. The fact that Ashley's parents are loving caregivers is incredibly important but not sufficient justification for any particular course of action.

CONCLUSION

In summary, parents are in the vast majority of cases the appropriate decision-makers for their children, for decisions ranging from what foods their children are allowed to eat, to where they go to school, to what type of medical care they receive. At the same time, and in contrast to the practice of much of adult medicine, pediatric practitioners are ethically obligated to assess what they deem to be in the child's best interest, to detect cases where this subjective assessment is at odds with the course of action being advocated for by the parents, and in such cases to deepen the processes of collaborative communication, seeking to find common ground and when appropriate pursue a middle path. While most of the time this dialogue and negotiation occurs seamlessly, when conflict arises, clinicians need to proceed with the greatest respect both for the child's place within the family and for the seriousness of our role as advocates for our pediatric patients.

REFERENCES

Arnold, R. M., & Kellum, J. (2003). Moral justifications for surrogate decision making in the intensive care unit: Implications and limitations. *Critical Care Medicine, 31*(5 Suppl.), S347–353.

Beauchamp, T. L., & Childress, J. F. (2001). *Principles of biomedical ethics* (5th ed.). New York: Oxford University Press.

Brosco, J. P., & Feudtner, C. (2006). Growth attenuation: A diminutive solution to a daunting problem. *Archives of Pediatrics and Adolescent Medicine, 160*(10), 1077–1078.

Child Abuse Prevention and Treatment Act, Public Law 93–247 (s. 1191) (1974). *Questions and answers, analysis, and text of the act: Prepared for the subcommittee on children and youth of the committee on labor and public welfare, united states senate.* Washington, DC: U.S. Government Printing Office.

Committee on Bioethics, American Academy of Pediatrics. (1995). Informed consent, parental permission, and assent in pediatric practice. *Pediatrics, 95*(2), 314–317.

Committee on Bioethics, American Academy of Pediatrics. (1999). Sterilization of minors with developmental disabilities. *Pediatrics, 104*(2 Part 1), 337–340.

Cooper, R., & Koch, K. A. (1996). Neonatal and pediatric critical care: Ethical decision making. *Critical Care Clinics, 12*(1), 149–164.

Downie, R. S., & Randall, F. (1997). Parenting and the best interests of minors. *Journal of Medicine and Philosophy, 22*(3), 219–231.

Feudtner, C. (2007). Collaborative communication in pediatric palliative care: A foundation for problem-solving and decision-making. *Pediatric Clinics of North America, 54*(5), 583–607.

Goldhagen, J. (2003). Children's rights and the United Nations convention on the rights of the child. *Pediatrics, 112*(3 Part 2), 742–745.

Gunther, D. F., & Diekema, D. S. (2006). Attenuating growth in children with profound developmental disability: A new approach to an old dilemma. *Archives of Pediatrics and Adolescent Medicine, 160*(10), 1013–1017.

Kimberly, M. B., Hoehn, K. S., Feudtner, C., Nelson, R. M., & Schreiner, M. (2006). Variation in standards of research compensation and child assent practices: A comparison of 69 institutional review board–approved informed permission and assent forms for 3 multicenter pediatric clinical trials. *Pediatrics, 117*(5), 1706–1711.

Kopelman, L. M. (1997). The best-interests standard as threshold, ideal, and standard of reasonableness. *Journal of Medicine and Philosophy, 22*(3), 271–289.

Kopelman, L. M. (2007). The best interests standard for incompetent or incapacitated persons of all ages. *Journal of Law, Medicine, and Ethics, 35*(1), 187–196.

Ross, L. F. (1998). *Children, families, and health care decision making.* Oxford: Clarendon Press.

Rothman, D. J., & Rothman, S. M. (1980). The conflict over children's rights. *Hastings Center Report, 10*(3), 7–10.

Shannon, S. E., & Savage, T. A. (2007). The Ashley treatment: Two viewpoints. *Pediatric Nursing, 33*(2), 175–178.

Zawistowski, C. A., & Frader, J. E. (2003). Ethical problems in pediatric critical care: Consent. *Critical Care Medicine, 31*(5 Suppl.), S407–410.

Zelizer, V. A. R. (1994). *Pricing the priceless child: The changing social value of children.* Princeton, NJ: Princeton University Press.

40

"This Won't Hurt a Bit": Truth-Telling to Children

ALISA A. PADON AND STEVEN D. HANDLER

THE CONTEMPORARY INSTITUTION of health care boasts a robust foundation in beneficence. It has only been recently that autonomy, and its necessary corollary of honesty or truth-telling, have been added to the guiding principles of the doctor-patient relationship. And while this has been widely accepted for adult patients, the debate regarding truth-telling to children is still ongoing. Gazing back to the time of Hippocrates, we can see that a physician's primary guiding principle has been that of acting in the best interest of his patients. This philosophy, until recent times, was delineated through a long history of paternalism. Paternalism, in its simplest conception, is often defined as acting for the benefit of another or to avoid harm to another. As James Childress notes, though, many definitions "omit a crucial element in paternalism: nonacquiescence in a person's wishes and choices" (Childress, 1982, p. 14). Many forms of paternalism involve acts that do not uphold the patients' values. The attitude of *doctor knows best* can be seen in an 1847 American Medical Association (AMA) Code of Medical Ethics:

> The obedience of a patient to the prescriptions of his physician should
> be prompt and implicit. He should never permit his own crude opinions

as to their fitness, to influence his attention to them. A failure in one particular may render an otherwise judicious treatment dangerous, and even fatal. (AMA, 1847, p. 96)

In order to convince patients to comply, physicians may conclude they have been placed in the unsavory position of having to deceive patients in order to administer treatment (Childress, 1982, p. 14). This kind of paternalism is justified today solely when the patient is both at real risk and is deemed incompetent for making her own decisions (Childress, 1982, p. 16). However, up until the mid-20th century, physicians had been looking at every patient, regardless of his mental state, as incompetent to make his own health care decisions.

BACKGROUND

I T WAS IN response to blatant violations of beneficence that came to light in the mid-20th century that the concept of patient autonomy has been given prominence. This evolution can be traced back through a series of key events in medical ethics. The Nuremburg trials introduced the concept of obtaining a patient's consent, and thus requiring telling a patient the full truth about procedures/treatments before they could be performed (De, 2004). Still, this was not a privilege or a right extended to everyone. For example, the first step in the women's health care movement, which begun only in the 1960s, was to promote "'consciousness-raising' to inform women about their anatomy, encouraging self-examination and investigative reporting on medications and procedures harmful to women" (Guest, 2003, p. 67), since providing this information to women before had not been standard. As late as 1971 the infamous Tuskegee syphilis experiment was being conducted on poor, Black men who were deceived about the care they were receiving for four decades (*The Tuskegee Timeline*, 2007). These violations and inequities illuminate what it is about health information that is so crucial to maintaining respect for persons. These examples helped fix in the minds of health care providers the principle that only complete disclosure allows individuals to be free and enables them to make their lives their own.

The growing pains of incorporating the patient as a decision-maker are still especially sharp in child health care. In a recent survey, 74% of clinicians in the United States indicated that they did not believe it is necessary to always inform their young patients about treatment (Lee, Havens, Sato, Hoffman, & Leuthner, 2006). These physicians are assuming that children are both (a) at risk and (b) incompetent and so do not merit partnership in decision-making. The literature, however, provides no definite consensus on when competency develops or how to determine it. Researchers and clinicians propose that children as young as 6 or 7 have been known to make wise, competent decisions about their daily health care (Alderson, Sutcliffe, & Curtis, 2006a). Yet articles in many leading American medical journals propose overriding the child's wishes until the child is at least twice that age, or at most a legal adult at 18 years of age (Nicholson, 1998; Ross, 1997). This may be in part due to the lingering adherence to the theories of Jean Piaget (Nicholson, 1998). While Piaget's scientific contribution to child advocacy and his innovative experimental designs cannot and should not be ignored, it has largely been determined by those in the field that his interpretation of child development as that of a static stage-driven journey is incorrect (Bee, 2000, p. 191; Donaldson, 1978). However, we often still rely on traditional developmental measures, and the methods of these measures usually end up intimidating children, creating a less than ideal experimental environment that confounds results (Alderson et al., 2006b). Additionally, very young children display what is called production deficiency. They are capable of certain tasks or using certain strategies but do not exhibit these capabilities unless prompted (Bee, 2000, p. 182). What is needed is a standardized, age-appropriate assessment for competency (Ross, 1997, p. 43).

The assumption underlying the field of child development is that external factors such as experience vastly influence the rate at which children mature (Penn, 2005, p. 37). Children who suffer from chronic illnesses such as juvenile diabetes or cancer, therefore experiencing an extended exposure to the clinical environment, appear to develop a maturity better suited to handle the full truth regarding their condition and treatment. In this chapter, we argue that children are not only often much more capable of handling the truth than they have traditionally been given credit for but also that full truth-telling is extremely crucial to their ability to cope, cooperate, and recover.

DEVELOPMENT OF SELF-DETERMINATION

THE MENTAL DEVELOPMENT of self-determination can be thought of as involving the development of cognition, including communication and deduction skills, as well as the development of emotion regulation. Accurately assessing self-determination requires an evaluation in each of these dimensions. An individual must first understand what is being asked of her in terms of treatment, but that is not enough if the patient does not also have a sense of what the treatment means for her future. It may be as elementary as understanding that X leads to Y, but this basic ability to reason is essential to one's understanding of her current situation and the foreseeable consequences of her decisions. Last, we have the emotional component of self-determination. The emotions that one will experience as part of coping with a life-altering illness or condition are undeniably valid. However, we recognize that emotions are often ephemeral and that to make decisions that uphold not only our values today but also our values tomorrow we need to be able to regulate our emotions and not allow them to become the sole pertinent factor in our decisions. All of these capabilities are fundamental to the process of competent decision-making, especially in health care, and in order to determine if it would be a violation to deceive a child, we must consider her true level of development within each of these dimensions.

COMMUNICATION

IN TERMS OF cognition and communication, it is important to consider how to appropriately deliver information to an individual of any age so that it is fully understood. It is not enough to provide correct information, because "the affirmative role-based duty of disclosure of information is not discharged by providing information that is not understood" (Childress, 1982, p. 135). Health care providers have a unique obligation to tailor language to the patient's capacity (*The Patient-Physician Relationship,* 2007). A competent patient is often one given a good explanation. For children, therefore, it is not a question of what they understand, but what they *can* understand when given information that is developmentally appropriate (DeRanieri, Clements, Clark, Kkuh, & Manno, 2004; Mahan & Mahan, 1987). In this pursuit, one should consider actual word comprehension, as well as ways of framing information. Children learn new words and new ways of communicating very rapidly. At about age 2 and a half, a child has a vocabulary of around 600 words on average, and that arsenal increases by approximately 10 words per day during the next 3–4 years, and 15–30 words per day during middle childhood (Bee, 2000, pp. 233–234). Between 6 and 10 years of age, children double the number of identifiers they use in speech, which leads to better communication and is an indication of better understanding (Cole & Cole, 1989, p. 426). Of course, for most children these thousands of words have little to do with medicine, unless the child spends enough time in the health care setting. Those who do quickly come to understand and even assign their own simple terms to describe procedures and conditions (Alderson et al., 2006b p. 30). It is important to remember that "the words we choose can be as important as the content they convey" (Stanford, 1991, p. 261). Words with dual meanings, medical jargon, and complex words should be avoided in order to increase specificity, and vivid descriptions and simple comparisons should be utilized. Studies have also shown that when parents are very responsive and speak specifically about objects to their child, language is learned faster (Bee, 2000, p. 235). Children should be encouraged to explore the hospital setting and instruments being discussed during the explanation to increase understanding and lessen anxiety (Leff, Chan, & Walizer, 1991). In taking these measures, we can enhance understanding, and thus coping and cooperation (Stanford, 1991, p. 261).

Communication does not have to be limited to words. The use of additional tools such as cartoons or body-outline dolls can also be very effective in presenting procedures clearly, yet through a medium where the child feels comfortable. A child's affinity for play, fantasy, and story-telling can also enhance communication. "Play techniques have been recognized increasingly as essential to enhancing successful coping and adjustment in work with hospitalized children and families" (Gaynard, Goldberger, & Laidley, 1991, p. 216). Especially in the preschool period, from about 3–5 years, children often tell stories to organize their own thoughts. "Play increases the child's capacity for mental representation by dramatizing in action the child's thoughts and feelings, putting what starts out as an imagined idea into a tangible scenario the child can see in front of her" (Davies, 2004, p. 276). This technique would have to be well managed, because children may also take metaphors literally and thereby create misconceptions (Davies, 2004, p. 324; Stanford, 1991, p. 261), but it is a way of framing complex information so that a child can relate to it and be more emotionally ready for it.

DEDUCTION

A CHILD'S ABILITY TO then use this understanding must include recognition of future implications. Piaget held that this kind of logical thinking first develops during adolescence, during the *formal operational* stage. A teen would begin to be able to "think about possible occurrences...imagining herself in different roles" (Bee, 2000, p. 188). This allows a teen to begin to act in order to pursue future goals. We know the child's progress is highly domain specific. For instance, Alderson writes that even very young children (age 10) with diabetes have shown an understanding of the permanence of their diagnosis and treatment in their lives, and children who were very sick before they were diagnosed tend to better appreciate the risk/benefit analysis of current suffering to avoid future suffering (Alderson et al., 2006b, p. 28). Friedman Ross, however, argues that despite this understanding and competence, because of lack of experience, children do not necessarily have a life-plan yet, and their current, limited value system may not be reflective of their future value system (Ross, 1997, p. 2). Fully disclosing to a child to uphold present-day autonomy then risks losing cooperation at the possible expense of long-term autonomy. While the child's right to an open future is one that must not be violated, this does not necessarily preclude a child from having self-imposed limitations on her own care, even when those limitations may threaten her own life. The fact that the child does not yet know what values he will hold in the future does not make his current experiences any less potent, and his value system any less meaningful to him. For instance, it is not fundamentally any less valid, though certainly more tragic, for a child to refuse a second bone-marrow transplant because of the current and near-future pain and suffering than to decide to undergo chemotherapy even though the child as an adult will not be able to reproduce. Parental partnership in the decision is still extremely important (Aspinall, 2006; Leff et al., 1991). but we cannot ignore how the procedures affect the child today. The most harmful and egregious transgression in these cases is when the child is not told that these are the repercussions (Alderson et al., 2006b, p. 30).

> The doctors never told me the consequences (of cancer drugs). After I started reading about them, I knew what was keeping me from growing and keeping my hair from growing. They also sterilized me. Now I'll never be able to have children. (Leff, et al., 1991, p. 234)

The physician omits information because the child is deemed not able to understand enough of what, for instance, infertility means to her future. But whether or not the child fully grasps what it will mean to not be a biological parent (something many adults may find difficult to understand), this is no excuse for omitting this information and thus excluding the child from the decision-making. Not telling the full truth about a treatment overwhelmingly results in poorer coping, in part because the patient lacks a feeling of trust in her physician and ownership of the consequences (Alderson et al., 2006b, p. 31; *Children's Consent*, 2005). Instead of perceiving the consequences as the result of an inevitable condition, the child perceives them as a result of the doctor's actions and any anger or resentment is thus directed towards the physician (Leff, et al., 1991, p. 234). If future value systems are our focus, we should consider that by forcing the child into treatment we may be negatively and indelibly affecting her future trust in health care and her perception of control over her own body.

It is also important not to equivocate or generalize the types of decisions we are referring to when making broad policy recommendations. Children with chronic conditions are making decisions daily about their health care, and, as such, we must not focus solely on the choices regarding major, life-altering procedures. Most of the time the child's current value system is based on efforts to be a "normal kid" (Alderson et al., 2006a, p. 302; Leff et al., 1991, p. 235). A child can only be expected to make health-related choices with respect to that goal, especially in light of the fact that chronic conditions and frequent hospitalizations pose difficult obstacles. For instance, a child diagnosed with juvenile diabetes has to exercise extremely mature control over a key childhood symbol—sugar. Sugar symbolizes landmark transitions in childhood at birthday celebrations, holiday parties, and so forth, as well as being a prevalent means of positive reinforcement for good behavior (Alderson et al., 2006b, p. 27). A child unable to take part in these events is inevitably going to feel alienated from her peers and may be willing to break rules at the risk of her health in order to be part of the group. The child's health care team and family must remain mindful of these goals and provide ways and alternatives to achieving them that leave room for the child's daily treatment. Developing a healthy sense of autonomy is also highly dependent on an environment in which the child has some control and freedom to make choices (Dix, Stewart, Gershoff, & Day, 2007). As such, much can and must be done to best uphold these choices. This treats the child with respect, nurtures the development of autonomy, and removes the barrier to increased compliance and recovery without deception. Kelman describes a case where doctors deceive a patient who does not want to cooperate because of how the treatment is affecting his life:

> The course of treatment might have been different if the therapists had been prepared to work with the broader motives that the patient brought to the treatment and to draw on the increasing coping capacities that the patient developed as the treatment proceeded—in other words, to deal with him as a whole person. They might have found that deception was not necessary...they might even have concluded that deception was more likely to retard than to advance the treatment process. (Childress, 1982, p. 139)

Childress concludes, "In the justification of deception, whether paternalistic or otherwise, the deception must be *necessary* to obtain the goal" (Childress, 1982, p. 139). It is by no means certain that deception is necessary to circumvent developmental deficiencies in communication or deduction for the child's best interests. On the contrary, we have shown how full truth-telling is extremely necessary for a child to understand her care, to feel at ease in the environment, to take ownership over the outcomes, to develop autonomy, and to feel respected. When these outcomes are achieved, the child is much more likely not only to comply with the treatment regimen but also to best cope with it.

EMOTION REGULATION

THE LAST MAJOR developmental hurdle in a child's readiness to receive the truth is the ability to cope emotionally. "Emotions are elicited when stimuli contain information about the satisfaction status of goals" (Moors, 2007, p. 1238). Almost all of our actions are goal-directed, and we naturally come up against obstacles to achieving these pursued ends. Consequently we may feel a sense of frustrated purpose or unmet expectation of achievement. Often, in order to overcome the obstacle we must attempt to overcome our negative feelings first, or our feelings may become a hindrance to our goals. This is especially important in health, because emotions like fear, depression, and general difficulty dealing with the reality of disease can be real barriers to recovery (Brunnquell & Kohen, 1991). Coping strategies to help us deal with emotional experiences develop as we age, and when unexpected emotional needs arise, adults are able to integrate alternative strategies into their lives and plans to either meet their goals or balance the negative feelings from their loss. For an adult, spoiled plans are often frustrating only until replacement plans are formulated or until temporary relief from negative emotions is found by, for instance, taking time away from a stressful situation while a more sustainable solution is found. For a sick child, dealing with emotional needs can involve the same strategies, such as incorporating favorite games or treats into a daily routine, working health care around the school day, and informing individuals in the child's life to not single him out for treatments. One school rearranged the class's snack time schedule to match that of a boy with juvenile diabetes so as to manage his health needs without drawing attention to them (Alderson et al., 2006b).

Awareness of the reactions of others is also important in self-regulation, as emotional displays may be more or less appropriate based on the surroundings. One anecdotal example showed a little girl who negotiated with her nurses that she could yell during a venipuncture as long as she didn't move, and she took some ownership over her care by rewarding the nurse who needed to only stick her once (Nicholson, 1998, p. 4). Though young children, to a large degree, are inexperienced in these coping strategies, this does not mean they are incapable of coping. They often just need the assistance of parents and others (Bee, 2000, p. 179). We can manage the child's emotional regulation to a point in real-time though, by targeting the child's goals and providing multiple, positive options for the future. This balances the negative tasks and goal interruptions brought on by the child's care. Another factor to consider is how the parents typically respond to the child's emotional expression. If the parents themselves model negative styles of attributing successes and failures, for instance, they should be coached on appropriate responses to emotional reactions in order to minimize negative affect (Thompson, 1994). "If parents are warm, sensitive and noncoercive, children will display willing cooperation at high rates" (Dix et al., 2007, p. 1205). The parents and health care team can both avoid negative suggestions in discussing the procedures and can instead offer positive thoughts and imagery for the child to focus on (Leff et al., 1991, p. 234; Stanford, 1991, p. 262). All of this lends itself to a better present experience for the child and to better cooperation. In addition, an emphasis on the child's choices can help minimize the developmental interference of chronic illness and promote successful integration back into childhood.

CONCLUSION

By withholding the full truth from children who are patients, we eliminate the backdrop of trust that is so necessary to care. This is especially poignant for children with chronic illnesses, who experience frequent and extended interaction with health care providers, but can also be assumed for children with minor or acute illness. Whether the illness is chronic or acute, we should begin with a presumption of competence, thus taking the burden off of the patient and determining competence on a case-by-case basis in real time (Nicholson, 1998, p. 4). Asking the child at the beginning of treatment simple questions about her experiences, her interests, and her fears can be a highly effective way of gaining information and fostering a friendship through which the child's best interests can be achieved. Ultimately, we will protect children by making them aware, not by withholding information. Honesty (truth-telling) should thus be added to beneficence as an important guiding principle in the health care of children.

REFERENCES

Alderson, P., Sutcliffe, K., & Curtis, K. (2006a). Children as partners with adults in their medical care. *Archives of Disease in Childhood, 91*(4), 300–303.

Alderson, P., Sutcliffe, K., & Curtis, K. (2006b). Children's competence to consent to medical treatment. *Hastings Center Report, 36*(6), 25–34.

American Medical Association. (1847). Article II, obligation of patients to their physicians. In *Code of medical ethics*. Chicago: AMA Press.

Aspinall, C. (2006). Children and parents and medical decisions. *Hastings Center Report, 36*(6), 3.

Bee, H. (2000). *The developing child* (9th ed.). Boston: Allyn and Bacon.

Brunnquell, D., & Kohen, D. (1991). Emotions in pediatric emergencies: What we know, what we can do. *Children's Health Care, 20*(4), 240–247.

Children's consent to clinical trial participation. (2005). National Cancer Institute. Retrieved January 11, 2001, from http://www.cancer.gov/clinicaltrials/understanding/childrensassent0101

Childress, J. (1982). *Who should decide?* New York: Oxford University Press.

Cole, M., & Cole, S. (1989). *The development of children.* New York: W. H. Freeman and Co.

Davies, D. (2004). *Child development. A practitioner's guide* (2nd ed.). New York: The Guilford Press.

De, M. (2004). Towards defining paternalism in medicine. *Virtual Mentor: American Medical Association Journal of Ethics, 6*(2). Retrieved December 6, 2007, from http://virtualmentor.ama-assn.org/2004/02/fred1-0402.html

DeRanieri, J. T., Clements, P. T., Clark, K., Kkuh, D. W., & Manno, M. S. (2004). War, terrorism and children. *The Journal of School Nursing: The Official Publication of the National Association of School Nurses, 20*(2), 69–75.

Dix, T., Stewart, A., Gershoff, E., & Day, W. (2007). Autonomy and children's reactions to being controlled: Evidence that both compliance and defiance may be positive markers in early development. *Child Development, 78*(4), 1204–1221.

Donaldson, M. (1978). *Children's minds.* New York: W. W. Norton.

Gaynard, L., Goldberger, J., & Laidley, L. (1991). The use of stuffed, body-outline dolls with hospitalized children and adolescents. *Children's Health Care, 20*(4), 216–224.

Guest, B. (2003). Book review: Into our own hands: The women's health movement in the United States, 1969–1990. *Journal of Public Health Policy, 24*(1), 66–69.

Lee, K. J., Havens, P. L., Sato, T. T., Hoffman, G. M., Leuthner, S. R. (2006). Assent for treatment: Clinician knowledge, attitudes, and practice. *Pediatrics, 118*(2), 723–730.

Leff, P. T., Chan, J. M., & Walizer, E. M. (1991). Self-understanding and reaching out to sick children and their families: An ongoing professional challenge. *Children's Health Care 20*(4), 230–239.

Mahan, C. C., & Mahan, K. T. (1987). Patient preparation in pediatric surgery. *Clinics in Podiatric Medicine and Surgery, 4*(1), 1–9.

Moors, A. (2007). Can cognitive methods be used to study the unique aspect of emotion: An appraisal theorist's answer. *Cognition and Emotion, 21*(6), 1238–1269.

Nicholson, R. (1998). The greater the ignorance, the greater the dogmatism. *Hastings Center Report, 28*(3), 4.

Penn, H. (2005). *Understanding early childhood: Issues and controversies.* New York: Open University Press.

Ross, L. F. (1997). Health care decision making by children. Is it in their best interests? *Hastings Center Report, 27*(6), 41–45.

Stanford, G. (1991). Beyond honesty: Choosing language for talking to children about pain and procedures. *Children's Health Care, 20*(4), 261–262.

The patient-physician relationship: A partnership for better health care and safer outcomes. (2007). American Medical Association. Retrieved December 6, 2007, from http://www.ama-assn.org

The Tuskegee timeline. (2007). Centers for Disease Control and Prevention. Retrieved December 6, 2007, from http://www.cdc.gov/tuskegee/time line.htm

Thompson, R. (1994). Emotion regulation: A theme in search of definition. *Monographs of the Society for Research in Child Development, 59*(2–3, Serial No. 240).

41

Children in Research: Linking Assent and Parental Permission

VICTORIA A. MILLER, WILLIAM W. REYNOLDS, AND ROBERT M. NELSON

THE APPROPRIATE ROLE of children in decisions about treatment and research in medical settings has been a source of debate. Legally, parents (or the child's legally appointed guardian) are required to make such decisions because children are considered incapable of providing informed consent for themselves. The term *parental permission* emerged as a way to distinguish such decisions from informed consent, which applies to decisions that one makes for oneself. However, increasing attention has been paid to whether or not children are capable of being involved in such decisions and, if so, to what extent. Seeking a child's agreement with a particular decision (i.e., assent) is a way to involve children in decision-making, while recognizing that such agreement does not constitute a legally valid authorization. Although obtaining a child's assent is encouraged for a variety of reasons (Committee on Bioethics, 1998), it is not required in the context of beneficial medical treatment. Similarly, the requirement for child assent can be waived for research decisions when the research holds out the possibility of direct benefit that is available only in the research context, or if the child is judged incapable of assent (Federal Policy for the Protection of Human Subjects, 2001).

In this chapter, we will first describe the elements of child assent, followed by a discussion of why these elements vary depending on how one formulates the moral purpose of child assent. We will then present a linked approach to child assent and parental permission and describe the implications of this approach. These implications include attention to developmental factors related to children's understanding, decision-making ability, and voluntariness, as well as the importance of collaborative decision-making for the assent process.

ELEMENTS OF CHILD ASSENT

QUESTIONS ABOUT *WHEN* children are capable of providing assent have permeated the literature. For research decisions, the federal regulations state that the child's age, maturity, and psychological state should be taken into account, but local institutional review boards are left to decide how and when to obtain child assent. The National Commission for the Protection of Human Subjects of Biomedical and Behavioral Research suggested that the elements of assent should include knowledge that procedures will be performed, the choice to freely undergo the procedures, unambiguous communication of this choice, and awareness of the option to withdraw (National Commission for the Protection of Human Subjects of Biomedical and Behavioral Research, 1978). Bartholome (1996) focused more on the process of obtaining child assent and recommended fostering a child's developmentally appropriate awareness of his or her condition, disclosing the nature of the proposed intervention and the child's likely experience, assessing the child's understanding of potential coercive influences, and soliciting the child's willingness to accept the proposed intervention. Bartholome's formulation of assent expands the recommendations of the National Commission, by incorporating the notion of developmentally appropriate understanding and recognizing that children may be more susceptible to undue influence compared to adults (Rossi, Reynolds, & Nelson, 2003). In contrast to this developmentally sensitive approach, some have equated the elements of assent with those of informed consent. For example, one study defined assent as complete understanding of eight of the elements of informed consent (Tait, Voepel-Lewis, & Malviya, 2003). These conflicting views of assent are, at least in part, shaped by different formulations of the moral purpose of child assent.

WHAT IS THE MORAL PURPOSE OF CHILD ASSENT?

MANY WHO HAVE written about child assent do not distinguish between assent and consent and even use the two terms interchangeably (Miller, Drotar, & Kodish, 2004). This confusion has

475

*Children in
Research:
Linking Assent
and Parental
Permission*

implications for how we understand the elements of assent, because the definition will drive conclusions about when and how assent should be obtained (Miller & Nelson, 2006). Part of the confusion rests with the assumption that assent is based on the moral imperative of respect for autonomy (i.e., self-determination). This assumption leads to a formulation of assent that is based on the framework of informed consent for adults. By holding children to the standard of informed consent, this approach may leave younger children out of the decision-making process entirely (Rossi et al., 2003).

However, respect for autonomy is an inappropriate framework for understanding informed consent in pediatric settings (Denham & Nelson, 2002; Kodish, 2003). Respect for autonomy is subsumed under the broader concept of respect for persons, which incorporates two different ethical convictions. The first is that individuals should be treated as autonomous agents, and the second is that persons with diminished autonomy are entitled to protection (National Commission for the Protection of Human Subjects of Biomedical and Behavioral Research, 1979). Although some have criticized the concept of respect for persons as too vague, it contributes to our understanding of informed consent in pediatric settings by recognizing that not all individuals are capable of self-determination. The National Commission for the Protection of Human Subjects in Biomedical and Behavioral Research (1977) acknowledged this when it recommended that both parental permission and child assent be obtained in the context of pediatric research. Parental permission is based on the moral obligation of parents to protect the health and safety of their children, while assent is based on the moral obligation to nurture children's moral growth and developing autonomy. As such, assent is not meant to serve the purpose of self-protection and, consequently, should not be equated to the standards of informed consent. Instead, assent shows respect for children's developing autonomy by involving them in decision-making *to the extent that they are able* (National Commission for the Protection of Human Subjects of Biomedical and Behavioral Research, 1979).

LINKING ASSENT AND PERMISSION

W HEN INFORMED CONSENT in pediatric settings is viewed from the perspective of respect for persons, it becomes clear that assent should not be viewed independently of parental permission. A linked approach to assent and permission ensures that the moral obligations to protect those with diminished autonomy and to nurture children's growing autonomy are both addressed. In addition, this approach allows assent to reflect a range of potential roles that children can play in the decision-making process, rather than a fixed set of standards (Nelson & Reynolds, 2003). This formulation necessitates that assent be understood differently across development, as children's capacities to make their own decisions mature. Furthermore, a linked approach highlights the potential role of collaborative decision-making between parents and children in the assent process.

DEVELOPMENTAL CHANGES IN CHILD ASSENT

UNDERSTANDING

A CHILD'S ROLE in decision-making should depend, in part, on the child's understanding of various aspects of treatment or research, such as the procedures, purpose, risks, and benefits. Prior research has demonstrated that children's understanding of these factors increases with age (Miller et al., 2004). However, age is only a proxy for important developmental variables (Rutter, 1989). For example, increases in cognitive development may underlie the relationship between understanding and age. More cognitively mature children and adolescents may be better able to understand the abstract elements of the decision or aspects of the decision with which they have little or no prior experience (Broome & Stieglitz, 1992). Other developmental variables, such as biological maturation, level of experience, and types of experiences (Rutter, 1989), may also contribute to increases in understanding with age. Although additional research is needed to determine specific guidelines, a developmental approach to assent would allow the child's role in decision-making to vary depending on the child's ability to understand. For example, a child who demonstrates understanding of the purpose or risks of the alternatives could take on a more prominent role in the decision-making process, compared to a child who only understands that certain procedures will be performed.

DECISION-MAKING ABILITY

A CHILD'S ROLE in the informed consent process should also vary according to the child's decision-making ability. While *understanding* typically refers to recall of information, *decision-making* refers to how this information is used to choose among alternatives. Effective decision-making involves identifying the choice to be made, identifying alternatives, weighing costs and benefits, making a decision, and evaluating the effectiveness of the decision. Several elements of effective

477

*Children in
Research:
Linking Assent
and Parental
Permission*

decision-making appear to improve from childhood to adolescence (see Ganzel, 1999; Miller et al., 2004), but there is debate about the extent to which adolescent decision-making abilities differ from those of adults. Although cognitive processes related to decision-making are similar to adults by mid- to late adolescence, several psychosocial factors may shape the actual outcomes of decisions (Steinberg & Scott, 2003). These include self-regulation ability, susceptibility to peer influence, future orientation, and risk perception (Steinberg & Cauffman, 1996).

In our own work, we have examined processes underlying adolescent risk perception and decision-making for research participation (Reynolds & Nelson, 2007). We interviewed adolescents about whether they would participate in hypothetical research studies that involved glucose tolerance and insulin-resistance testing. All adolescents had type 1 diabetes or were at risk for diabetes. Most adolescents quickly evaluated the risks of the research based on past experience with similar procedures and made decisions accordingly. Some participants had an immediate negative affective response to the *magnitude* of the perceived risks (i.e., their subjective perception of severity and tolerability), with the *probability* of the risks playing only a small or negligible role in the decision. This affective response typically was based on an emotionally resonant personal experience that made it unlikely that the adolescent would participate. However, for most adolescents the risk information was affectively neutral, and they decided about participation based on their perception of the overall value of the research to themselves or to others. While normative models of effective decision-making assume a systematic approach characterized by rational choice, participants in our study appeared to use decision-making shortcuts that allowed them to bypass one or more steps in this process. These results raise questions about the extent to which a traditional model of informed consent, which presumes that decisions follow principles of rational choice, can be applied to adolescents.

VOLUNTARINESS

THE NOTION OF voluntariness also arises in discussions about children's assent and is important to examine from a developmental perspective. In a general sense, a voluntary choice is one that is free from undue influence (National Commission for the Protection of Human Subjects of Biomedical and Behavioral Research, 1979). Although several studies have indicated that most children understand that their research participation is voluntary (see Miller et al., 2004), few studies have examined the degree to which children are influenced by factors such as incentives and authority figures. The existing research suggests that

prior parental permission to participate in a research study does not unduly influence children's decisions (Abramovitch, Freedman, Henry, &
Van Brunschot, 1995), that children are more likely to withdraw from a
research study if they are told in advance that the investigator would
not be upset (Abramovitch et al., 1995), and that children's, adolescents',
and young adults' treatment decisions are affected by parental influence (Scherer, 1991). This latter finding is consistent with the developmental literature, which conceptualizes autonomy as a transformation
in parent-child interactions, rather than freedom from parental influence (Hill & Holmbeck, 1986). In fact, parental influence may be an
important component of the transition to greater decision-making independence and effectiveness (i.e., collaborative decision-making; see
the following section of this chapter). A conceptualization of assent
that requires children and adolescents to be free of influence is both
unrealistic and insensitive to the developmental context of assent. For
example, some parents might attempt to persuade their children to
participate in a research study, in an effort to teach them the value of
altruism (Miller, Reynolds, & Nelson, 2008); this persuasion may be appropriate for younger children. Our own work suggests that parents'
willingness to persuade their children to participate in research may
decrease as children cognitively mature (Miller et al., 2008). Future research is needed to clarify the factors that constitute undue influence
during childhood and adolescence.

A COLLABORATIVE APPROACH TO
THE PROCESS OF ASSENT

LINKING CHILD ASSENT and parental permission, rather than
viewing assent independently, also highlights the potential role of
collaborative decision-making between parents and children. The parent-
child relationship provides the foundation for the child's transition to
greater decision-making independence, which occurs gradually and
involves the child or adolescent assuming increased responsibility for
decision-making (Dornbusch et al., 1985). Typically, decision-making
independence is preceded by a period of collaborative decision-
making between children and parents (Dornbusch et al., 1985). The
concept of collaboration underscores the idea that parents often remain important sources of support and advice, even as children and
adolescents become increasingly independent (Fuligni & Eccles, 1993).
It has been hypothesized that collaborative decision-making provides
an opportunity for children to learn what family members take into
account when making decisions, the consequences of decisions, and
the communication skills that are necessary to negotiate and influence

479

*Children in
Research:
Linking Assent
and Parental
Permission*

decisions (Wills, Blechman, & McNamara, 1996). When independent decision-making emerges out of a collaborative process between parents and children, children may be better prepared to make effective decisions on their own. As Geller, Tambor, Bernhardt, Fraser, and Wissow (2003) conclude, "a decision-making paradigm based on an assumption of autonomy obscures the reality of interdependence and masks the possibilities for cooperation" (p. 269).

Approaches to child assent should recognize this normative developmental trajectory and incorporate collaborative decision-making when appropriate (Joffe, 2003). Empirical research has demonstrated that children frequently desire input into treatment and research decisions, even when they believe that the final decision should be their own (Geller et al., 2003; Miller et al., 2008). Our own work suggests that collaborative decision-making between parents and children may increase with the child's cognitive development (Miller et al., 2008). Collaborative decision-making promotes respect for children by facilitating some degree of child involvement for those who are emotionally and developmentally capable of it, while providing support for those who are not. For example, children can be provided with information about the decision, express an opinion about the decision to be made, or engage in a discussion with parents about the benefits and drawbacks of each alternative (Baylis, Downie, & Kenny, 1999; Joffe, 2003; McCabe, 1996). The child's role might also vary according to characteristics of the decision, such as the potential risks and benefits and the availability of alternatives (Miller et al., 2008). A collaborative approach allows children and adolescents to assume greater responsibility for treatment and research decisions over time, as their decision-making skills increase. Ultimately, adolescents who are capable of decision-making according to the framework of informed consent can be given full decision-making authority.

CONCLUSION

THERE HAS BEEN ongoing debate about the appropriate role of children in decisions about medical treatment and research. When child assent is grounded on respect for autonomy, it holds children to a higher standard than what is developmentally appropriate. In contrast, a formulation of assent based on respect for persons incorporates a full range of potential decision-making roles for children and supports a linked approach to assent and permission. A linked approach requires that developmental influences on understanding, decision-making ability, and voluntariness be taken into account when determining the child's role. A developmental approach to assent would seek to understand changes in decision-making with age, taking into account both cognitive and psychosocial influences, and shape the child's role depending on these factors. In addition, linking assent and permission underscores the importance of collaborative decision-making between parents and children for the assent process. Collaborative interactions promote children's developing autonomy while also recognizing that they may not be fully prepared to make certain decisions on their own. By attending to these factors, the assent process can fulfill the goal of respecting children's growing autonomy by involving them in treatment and research decisions to the extent that they are able.

REFERENCES

Abramovitch, R., Freedman, J., Henry, K., & Van Brunschot, M. (1995). Children's capacity to agree to psychological research: Knowledge of risks and benefits and voluntariness. *Ethics and Behavior, 5*(1), 25–48.

Bartholome, W. G. (1996). Ethical issues in pediatric research. In H. Y. Vanderpool (Ed.), *The ethics of research involving human subjects* (pp. 360–361). Frederick, MD: University Publishing Group.

Baylis, F., Downie, J., & Kenny, N. (1999). Children and decisionmaking in health research. *IRB: A Review of Human Subjects Research, 21*(4), 5–10.

Broome, M. E., & Stieglitz, K. A. (1992). The consent process and children. *Research in Nursing and Health, 15*, 147–152.

Committee on Bioethics. (1998). Informed consent, parental permission, and assent in pediatric practice. *Journal of Child and Family Nursing, 1*(1), 57–61.

Denham, J. E., & Nelson, R. M. (2002). Self-determination is not an appropriate model for understanding parental permission and child assent. *Anesthesia and Analgesia, 94*, 1–3.

Dornbusch, S. M., Carlsmith, J. M., Bushwell, S., Ritter, P. L., Leiderman, P. H., Hastorf, A. H., et al. (1985). Single parents, extended households, and the control of adolescents. *Child Development, 56*, 326–341.

Federal Policy for the Protection of Human Subjects, 45 C.F.R. 46.408a (2001).

Fuligni, A. J., & Eccles, J. S. (1993). Perceived parent-child relationships and early adolescents' orientation toward peers. *Developmental Psychology, 29*(4), 622–632.

Ganzel, A. K. (1999). Adolescent decision making: The influence of mood, age, and gender on the consideration of information. *Journal of Adolescent Research, 14*(3), 289–318.

Geller, G., Tambor, E. S., Bernhardt, B. A., Fraser, G., & Wissow, L. (2003). Informed consent for enrolling minors in genetic susceptibility research: A qualitative study of at-risk children's and parents' views about children's role in decision-making. *Journal of Adolescent Health, 32*, 260–271.

481

*Children in
Research:
Linking Assent
and Parental
Permission*

Hill, J., & Holmbeck, G. (1986). Attachment and autonomy during adolescence. *Annals of Child Development, 3,* 145–189.

Joffe, S. (2003). Rethink "affirmative agreement," but abandon "assent." *American Journal of Bioethics, 3*(4), 9–11.

Kodish, E. (2003). Informed consent for pediatric research: Is it really possible? *Journal of Pediatrics, 142,* 89–90.

McCabe, M. A. (1996). Involving children and adolescents in medical decision making: Developmental and clinical considerations. *Journal of Pediatric Psychology, 21*(4), 505–516.

Miller, V. A., Drotar, D., & Kodish, E. (2004). Children's competence for assent and consent: A review of empirical findings. *Ethics and Behavior, 14*(3), 255–295.

Miller, V. A., & Nelson, R. M. (2006). A developmental approach to child assent for non-therapeutic research. *Journal of Pediatrics, 149*(1 Suppl.), S25–S30.

Miller, V. A., Reynolds, W. W., & Nelson, R. M. (2008). Parent-child roles in decision-making about medical research. *Ethics and Behavior, 18*(2–3), 161–181.

National Commission for the Protection of Human Subjects in Biomedical and Behavioral Research. (1977). *Report and recommendations: Research involving children.* Washington, DC: U.S. Government Printing Office.

National Commission for the Protection of Human Subjects of Biomedical and Behavioral Research. (1978). *Research involving those institutionalized as mentally infirm.* Washington, DC: U.S. Government Printing Office.

National Commission for the Protection of Human Subjects of Biomedical and Behavioral Research. (1979). *The Belmont Report: Ethical principles and guidelines for the protection of human subjects of research.* Washington, DC: U.S. Government Printing Office.

Nelson, R. M., & Reynolds, W. W. (2003). Child assent and parental permission: A comment on Tait's "Do they understand?" *Anesthesiology, 98,* 1–2.

Reynolds, W. W., & Nelson, R. M. (2007). Risk perception and decision processes underlying informed consent to research participation. *Social Science and Medicine, 65*(10), 2105–2115.

Rossi, W., Reynolds, W. W., & Nelson, R. M. (2003). Child assent and parental permission in pediatric research. *Theoretical Medicine, 24,* 131–148.

Rutter, M. (1989). Age as an ambiguous variable in developmental research: Some epidemiological considerations from developmental psychopathology. *International Journal of Behavioral Development, 12*(1), 1–34.

Scherer, D. G. (1991). The capacities of minors to exercise voluntariness in medical treatment decisions. *Law and Human Behavior, 15*(4), 431–449.

Steinberg, L., & Cauffman, E. (1996). Maturity of judgment in adolescence: Psychosocial factors in adolescent decision making. *Law and Human Behavior, 20*(3), 249–272.

Steinberg, L., & Scott, E. S. (2003). Less guilty by reason of adolescence: Developmental immaturity, diminished responsibility, and the juvenile death penalty. *American Psychologist, 58*(12), 1009–1018.

Tait, A. R., Voepel-Lewis, T., & Malviya, S. (2003). Do they understand? (Part II): Assent of children participating in clinical anesthesia and surgery research. *Anesthesiology, 98,* 609–614.

Wills, T., Blechman, E., & McNamara, G. (1996). Family support, coping, and competence. In E. M. Hetherington & E. Blechman (Eds.), *Stress, coping, and resiliency in children and families* (pp. 107–133). Mahwah, NJ: Lawrence Erlbaum Associates.

42

Withdrawing and Withholding Life-Prolonging Therapies in Children

Margaret M. Mahon

RECOGNIZING THE NEED to discontinue (or never to start) treatments that can no longer benefit the patient should be a core principle of health care. To take an example completely outside of critical care, consider the case of a 3-year-old whose mother insists that her child needs antibiotics, though the pediatrician believes they are not indicated. Many care providers would acquiesce and prescribe antibiotics; in one study, 44% of children with colds were given a prescription for an antibiotic (Nyquist, Gonzales, Steiner, & Sande, 1998). Many factors other than the physical condition of the patient affect clinical decision-making in the 21st century, including a desire to appease the family or fear of litigation.

PRINCIPLES OF WITHDRAWING AND WITHHOLDING

THE INAPPROPRIATE USE of antibiotics has several important common principles with withdrawing and withholding life-prolonging therapies. Perhaps the most important principle is that a therapy that cannot benefit the patient should not be used (withholding); if a therapy is started but does not accomplish the goals of therapy, that therapy should be discontinued (withdrawing). To make the determination regarding a particular treatment, whether an antibiotic or a ventilator, the health care providers must stipulate the desired outcome of the therapy for a particular patient. The *goals of care* should be determined for each treatment specifically (what should *this* treatment accomplish?), as well as for the overall care trajectory (what is the overall expected outcome for this patient?). Futility, then, is the failure of a specific intervention to accomplish the goals of care (Youngner, 1996).

Decision-making for and about children is distinguished from other clinical decision-making because in most of health care, it is a firm tenet that a patient has the right to determine what shall be done to his or her own body. It is presumed that the patient is in the best position to know what is right for him or her. Most often, however, patient self-determination cannot happen in pediatrics. Most children do not have the knowledge and skills to make the best medical decisions. (How many 5- or 12-year-olds would make an informed consent for a needed immunization?) Because children are often not able to decide, parents are the decision-makers for their children.

Typically, when a patient is unable or chooses not to participate in decision-making, a surrogate is asked to represent the patient's wishes. *Surrogate* comes from the Latin, *surrogatus* (*sur,* from sub, which means *under* or *in the place of,* and *rogare,* which means *to ask* or *propose*), meaning to ask in the place of another. At its best, surrogate decision-making means that someone else will not make decisions *for* the patient but, rather, will represent the *patient's* preferences. This is termed *substituted judgment* and implies that the surrogate knows, or can make an informed decision about, what the patient would likely choose, were she able. In pediatrics, and for certain other patients, preferences were never known. This means that the surrogate, rather than representing the patient's wishes, should act in the *best interest of the patient.* Applying the best interest standard can be one of the greatest challenges in cases of withdrawing or withholding life-prolonging therapies for children, because it is almost impossible to separate the interests of the parents from those of the child (Spence, 2000, p. 1287).

In almost all cases of parents deciding for their children, the best interest of the child dovetails with the best interest of the parents. In

485

*Withdrawing
and Withholding
Life-Prolonging
Therapies in
Children*

the case of withdrawing or withholding a child's life-prolonging treatments, however, the best interest of the child may directly conflict with the best interest of the family.

When there is no potential for cure or likelihood of a good quality of life, the best interest of a child may be to focus solely on the relief of suffering. Therapies that might prolong life can be extremely burdensome. It is almost unfathomable to consider cases in which the death of a child could be in the best interest of the parents or the family. Thus, the best interest of the child may be in direct contradiction to the best interest of the parent and family. Yet parents are able to engage in planning and implementing decisions to limit nonbeneficial therapies. In fact, "parents who engaged in advance care planning for their children intended to create plans that maximized the length and quality of life, while avoiding useless or harmful medical interventions that they felt would have created unnecessary suffering. In this sense advance care planning was not about 'withholding treatment' but rather about creating a thoughtful, informed care plan for the individual child/parent" (Hammes, Klevan, Kempf, & Williams, 2005, p. 771).

In the case of withdrawing and withholding life-prolonging therapies, decision-making is often extremely arduous. Professionals should be involved with parents throughout the process, so that families never feel a decision was made that *caused* the death of a child.

BOX 42.1

Principles of Withdrawing and Withholding Life-Prolonging Therapies

1. There is no moral difference between withdrawing and withholding a life-prolonging therapy.
2. Providers should never start a therapy they are not willing to discontinue.
3. The goals of care both for a specific therapy and for the child's overall treatment should be specified.
4. Medical indications should be considered first when determining clinical options.
5. If the efficacy of a particular therapy is unknown, a trial of that therapy is often reasonable.
6. Though specific therapies may be withdrawn, the child's care should be uninterrupted, often with aggressive attention to symptom management.
7. There is a tremendous moral difference between allowing a death and causing a death.

CAUSES OF DEATH

UNDERSTANDING THE DISEASES from which children die provides a framework for understanding specific issues of withholding and withdrawing nonbeneficial treatments for children. In 2004, more than 2.3 million people died in the United States (Miniño, Heron, Murphy, & Kochanek, 2007). Of these, about 53,000 were children (from live birth to 19 years old; Hamilton et al., 2007; Miniño et al., 2007). The rarity of such deaths and the discomfort they cause means that society, as well as many health care providers, are ill equipped to respond appropriately when decisions must be made about withdrawing and withholding life-prolonging therapies. This may lead to decisions that are not based on the best interest of the child and thereby increase the child's suffering.

BOX 42.2

Causes of Death, Birth to 19 Years of Age, United States Infants (live birth to 1 year of age, 2004; *n* = 27,936; Miniño et al., 2007)

1. Congenital anomalies including chromosomal abnormalities.
2. Issues of prematurity and low birth weight (not specified elsewhere).
3. Sudden infant death syndrome (SIDS).
4. Complications of pregnancy (maternal factors).
5. Injuries (unintentional).
6. Intrauterine hypoxia; hypoxia during delivery.
7. Complications related to placenta, cord, membranes.
8. Bacterial sepsis of the newborn.
9. Neonatal hemorrhage.
10. Diseases of the circulatory system.

Children (1–19 years, 2005; *n* = 25,325; Hamilton et al., 2007)

1. Unintentional injuries.
2. Homicide.
3. Malignant neoplasms.
4. Suicide.
5. Congenital anomalies, including chromosomal abnormalities.
6. Heart disease.
7. Influenza and pneumonia.
8. Chronic lower respiratory diseases.
9. Septicemia.
10. Other neoplasms.

487

*Withdrawing
and Withholding
Life-Prolonging
Therapies in
Children*

Mulder described four trajectories that are likely to lead to decisions about withdrawing or withholding life-prolonging therapies. "The cancer model (healthy, followed by illness, remissions, and death); the cystic fibrosis model (chronic illness since birth with prolonged survival…); progressive fatal disorders, such as mitochondrial and metabolic disorders; and finally 'static' disorders, such as devastating neurologic injury related to drowning" (quoted in Levetown, 2005). With the exception of the final category, each of these types of diseases is a devastating situation and requires a good decision-making process that involves the child (whenever possible) and the family, over time.

About half of the children who die are infants (< 1 year of age). For children 1–19 years of age, three of the four most common causes of death usually result in sudden death. As many as 1,000,000 children in the United States live with potentially life-limiting illnesses (Center to Advance Palliative Care, 2007). It is only during cases of non–sudden death (though this could encompass hours to months to many years) that decisions about withdrawing and withholding life-prolonging interventions can occur.

DECISION-MAKING PROCESSES

Too OFTEN, ETHICS is perceived as separate from, rather than an integral part of clinical decision-making. Clinical ethics involve asking questions that facilitate the integration of ethical dimensions into clinical decision-making. In the case of children, the integration of ethical factors is different than for adults. Too often, the first question asked in medical decision-making is "What do the parents want?" Too often, providers feel bound to acquiesce to a patient's or a parent's preferences. It is only after clinical factors are delineated and clinical options are structured that choices can be made.

The menu from which patients or parents can choose is not limitless. The clinical options should be determined by what is medically indicated. *Respect for autonomy* (Beauchamp & Childress, 1994; Field & Behrman, 2003) means that providers should respect patients' wishes, but they are not always bound by these wishes; professionals' autonomy must also be respected.

Within the context of medical indications, parents' preferences and the child's quality of life should be considered. Decisions about quality of life are perhaps the most controversial dimension of withdrawing and withholding life-prolonging therapies in children (Field & Behrman, 2003). In adults, quality of life decisions are usually based on a comparison with the patient's current or recent quality of life. For children, such decisions are often based on a hypothesis about the future with no reference to the child's quality of life before the illness.

One challenge is *how* to consider cognitive level. The 1970s and 1980s saw many cases in which an expectation of mental retardation led to decisions to withhold a surgical intervention that would have been provided to another child for whom there was an expectation of normal intelligence (Mahon, 1990). It is important to remember that "intolerable" or "unbearable" suffering refers to the proximal physiologic burdens or impending death of a child and *not* to others' reactions to the child or to what others imagine "it must be like to live that way."

DECISIONS FOR NEONATES

DECISION FOR NEONATES tend to fall into two general categories: questions related to gestational age, and questions related to complications of labor and delivery or congenital anomalies. The roles of obstetricians and neonatologists in predicting which infants are likely to survive with a good quality of life are tremendous, and there is great variability between professionals in the messages conveyed to parents (Kaempf et al., 2006). More importantly, accurate prognostication at or near the birth may not be possible, except in cases such as anencephaly (the congenital absence of the brain above the brainstem).

PREMATURITY

SOME PHYSICIANS WILL attempt to resuscitate every infant, regardless of gestational age (Catlin, 2005). The more common current practice is that infants younger than about 23 weeks gestation are not resuscitated because of an expectation of nonsurvival, short-term survival with multiple complications, or longer-term survival with devastating sequelae (Singh et al., 2007). Infants older than 25 weeks are likely to be aggressively resuscitated and treated because of an expectation of better outcomes (Singh et al., 2007). Singh and colleagues (2007) concluded, very appropriately, that the delivery room is often not the place to make decisions about a child's trajectory. "Decisions must never be rushed and must always be made by the team with all evidence available" (Royal College of Paediatrics and Child Health, 2004, p. 11). Starting treatments with the possibility of discontinuing those that were unable to benefit the infants is the recommended course of action (Kaempf, 2007). Singh and colleagues cautioned against an overreliance on numbers. "For 102 infants with birth weights of < 750g, Apgar scores at 1 and 5 minutes and heart rates and 1 and 5 minutes were neither sensitive nor

489

*Withdrawing
and Withholding
Life-Prolonging
Therapies in
Children*

predictive for death before discharge, survival with a neurologic abnormality, or intact neurologic survival" (Singh et al., 2007, p. 519).

Establishment of institutional guidelines for content and process of information about infants at the edge of viability can improve care and satisfaction; "our response to uncertainty need not be automatically either promotion of invasive, elaborate and clinically unproven therapies or withholding of potentially beneficial and life-sustaining therapies" (Kaempf et al., 2006, p. 28). With time, better medical indications for the prognosis for a given child will be clear. At that time, specific decisions about withdrawing or withholding life-prolonging therapies can be implemented.

Whether or not preterm labor is expected, there is likely to be little foundation for decision-making prior to labor. Women and their partners are rarely in a position to make any kind of informed decision *if* information is given, much less if it is not. Discussion about the possibility of prematurity and the sequelae of delivery complications should begin during pregnancy (Catlin, 2005). This can provide at least a rudimentary foundation for informed decision-making if these eventualities do occur.

OTHER NEONATAL CASES

SOME INFANTS ARE born at or near term, but complications of the delivery or the presence of congenital or genetic anomalies threaten the infant's survival. "The most common situation where withdrawal of life support may be contemplated is when a baby is dependent on a respirator because his or her breathing has failed" (Nuffield Council on Bioethics, 2006, p. 35). Just as for extremely premature infants, decisions should not be made in haste. It is almost always better to stabilize the child, even if this means the use of high-tech interventions such as ventilators. This allows time to get the most accurate data about the neonate's condition; "it would generally be regarded as in a baby's best interest for clinicians to continue full intensive care while the prognosis remains uncertain" (Nuffield Council on Bioethics, 2006, p. 99).

At the time of birth, the outcomes for each child often cannot be predicted (Field & Behrman, 2003; Nuffield Council on Bioethics, 2006). Some children will bear no long-term effects of the complications of a premature birth or a birth with other complications. Some children will have minor to severe lifelong effects, such as cerebral palsy or learning disabilities. Some children will not survive infancy. Many infants will spend the entirety of their lives in the neonatal intensive care unit (NICU). It is not until the child's prognosis is clearer that decisions should be made about withdrawing or withholding specific therapies. A decision to discontinue life-prolonging therapies may be considered when it is recognized that the child will never develop enough or heal enough to live free of overwhelming burdens, such as pain or other physical suffering. Because no benefit can be achieved—that is, cure or a life outside of the intensive care unit—the burdens may be deemed not worthwhile.

Other conditions necessitate decision-making, such as the complications of such conditions as Down syndrome. The presence of mental retardation will certainly affect how the child and family live, but the fact of mental retardation should not, in almost every case, affect whether and how comorbidities, such as intestinal obstruction or cardiac defects, should be treated.

DECISIONS FOR OLDER CHILDREN

WHEREAS IN INFANTS much of the discussion about withdrawing and withholding therapies has to do with quality of cognitive life or mental abilities, the decision for older children is often primarily about the degree of physical suffering. While this may seem like an artificial dichotomy, in that both are dimensions of suffering, those involved should be aware of different foci.

FOUR CHILDREN

Seven-year-old Alaina had lived with cancer for 3 years and had undergone repeated courses of chemotherapy and radiation.[1] She had another recurrence of her disease, and another remission seemed unlikely. Her parents were especially excited, then, to tell her that a new protocol for which she was eligible had been found. Everyone was baffled by her adamant refusal to undergo further treatments.

Brad was an 11-year-old who had lived with heart disease his entire life. His death was expected within weeks. His behavior had deteriorated: he was curt and nasty to everyone who interacted with him. One of the nurses asked him about it. Brad explained that he was "being a brat, because that way they won't miss me when I'm gone."

Christina was a 4-year-old who had lived with a neurodegenerative disease her entire life. She was hospitalized in respiratory distress. It had been agreed that she would not be put on a ventilator; the goals of care were palliative and her dyspnea was managed well. The parents and the medical team had agreed that cardiopulmonary resuscitation would not be performed. When Christina's heart did stop, her parents cried, "You have to

491

*Withdrawing
and Withholding
Life-Prolonging
Therapies in
Children*

do something!" The team took this to mean that the parents had changed their minds and wanted CPR. Christina was resuscitated and transferred to the ICU. She died 4 days later.

David was a 16-year-old with cancer. He had been receiving chemotherapy for several months. David had had a sense for many months that his death was imminent. He repeatedly asked his father about it, and his father said, "Absolutely not. If you fight this thing, you're going to win. You're going to live." David's questions became more frequent; his disease continued to advance. He again expressed consternation about dying. The next day David was receiving chemotherapy; his father was at his bedside. David said with great urgency, "I think I'm dying," at which point, he lay back and died.

The cases above indicate opportunities for interventions by providers with families when decisions are being made about whether specific treatments should be withdrawn or withheld. Both Alaina's and David's cases remind us that children should be included in discussions about their diseases, and that they know enough to contribute informed opinions to the discussion. In reality, dying children almost always know that they are dying, and they understand accurately what death means (Beale, Baile, & Aaron, 2005; Bluebond-Langner, 1978). Because parents are decision-makers for their children, however, "it is common for the ill child's perspective to get overlooked" (Levetown, 2005).

Many people would believe that a 7-year-old (or a 16-year-old) is too young to understand her own dying. In reality, a decision not to involve the child in the discussion probably reflects adults' discomfort rather than that of the child. As in David's case, adults' unwillingness to discuss death can isolate the child as he deals with his impending death. Further, it means that children who have salient and informed opinions about treatment decisions are kept out of the discussion. This can hurt all involved.

When parents and providers understand that children are not only aware of their own dying but can also make informed decisions about treatment decisions, they can be unburdened from feelings that they are not "trying for every day that we can get." Parents of children who had died from cancer rated the care of physicians to be higher if that physician had communicated directly with the child (Mack et al., 2005).

Brad's case is illustrative of a different dimension. "Failing to provide children with information and the opportunity to discuss their fears, concerns, and preferences can isolate them and add to their anxiety and other distress" (Field & Behrman, 2003, p. 296). When they recognize their dying, many children take on the responsibility of trying to protect the adults in their lives. "The older children and young adults have never so much feared for themselves but have feared for the sadness and suffering of those they love and leave behind" (Belasco, 2002, p. 749). Brad truly had concerns, but because he had no opportunities to talk about it, he made decisions that were hurtful to those around him, but probably hurt him more.

While almost no one would choose death, there are many cases in which death is less burdensome than ongoing treatments that are unable to achieve the intended goal. Thus, children should be informed about their diseases not just at the time when the inevitability of death becomes clear, but from the time of diagnosis (Hurwitz, Duncan & Wolfe, 2004). This is not to say that information should be forced on children. Rather, children should be given the opportunity to ask questions, and their queries should be answered honestly. This author has a "no secrets" policy, answering children's questions honestly and directly. While this is sometimes initially frightening to parents, they are often relieved to learn what the child knows and not to have to keep secrets.

Whether the decision is to withhold further chemotherapy or CPR, or to withdraw dialysis or ventilator support, the child should be included if she is able and wants to be included. It takes skill and patience to make these determinations, but doing so can unburden the families who will have to live with the death of their child for the rest of their lives.

Although the wishes of the child must be considered (Tournay, 2000), only 16% of children in one study participated in the discussions with the family and health care team about the fact that a cure was not attainable (Wolfe et al., 2000). Though 95% of parents had the discussion with health care providers, "only 38% were very comfortable with the manner in which it was discussed" (Wolfe et al., 2000, p. 2472).

Christina's case reinforces the notion that care is not done once the decision had been made to withhold specific treatments. The decision not to do CPR was clinically the right decision; Christina would not benefit from it, and her brief survival was likely physically burdensome. Her parents were surprised by her death. That should not have happened. The parents seemed unaware of the implications of a DNAR (do not attempt resuscitation) order. Communication was insufficient.

Many people perceive a dichotomy between "doing everything" and "doing nothing." When a treatment is being withheld or withdrawn, the family should be told what the child's trajectory will likely be. As the child's death is imminent, the parents should be told. They should understand the signs the providers see indicating death's proximity. They should be encouraged to touch, to hold, even to plan what they will do when the child dies. If they had understood her dying, Christina's parents would likely have been no less devastated. They could,

493

*Withdrawing
and Withholding
Life-Prolonging
Therapies in
Children*

however, with the support of the team, have understood that not performing CPR was the best decision for their daughter.

Symptoms should be managed aggressively. If a child suffers from a high symptom burden prior to death, parents have reported "lingering anguish" following the death (Hinds, Schum, Baker, & Wolfe, 2005, S/1). Nurses were more likely to report that a child had a higher symptom burden prior to dying than was the child's physician (Andresen, Seecharan, & Toce, 2004). When there is panic, as is neither uncommon nor inappropriate, the health care provider must be willing to follow the plan of care and allow the parents their appropriately intense emotions. Failure to communicate adequately with parents about the child's dying can lead to increased parental suffering after the child dies (Hinds et al., 2005).

THE ROLE OF PARENTS

PARENTS (OR GUARDIANS) remain the ideal surrogate decision-makers for children. While the best interest of the parent (the child being alive) may conflict with the best interest of the child (an end to suffering given no eventual benefit), the parent still is the person most likely to have a vested interest in the child. The challenge, then, is to assist the parent in focusing primarily on the child, the clinical facts of the case, the reality of the child's suffering, and the impossibility of cure. Certainly most parents can do this, though at great personal cost.

It is imperative that health care providers frame the discussion so that parents are not left with the impression that they "killed" or "caused the death" of their child. Many believe this is obvious and does not need to be verbalized. To the contrary: this should be said in every case. "Your child is so lucky to have you. You have been with him during this entire journey. This has cost you so much. You gave him every chance, but we didn't have the medicines or the technology to save him."

Note that the word *fail* was not used in these statements. The child did not *fail* a trial of a medicine or a machine. The disease did not *fail* to respond. There is no failure in cases of withdrawing or withholding life-prolonging therapies. This is not a war. By dying, the child or the family do not lose, nor did anyone not fight hard enough. Communication with patients and families must be clear and direct. Again, the information does not belong to the hospital or the providers. It is the responsibility of the health care team to make the condition and the proposed treatments comprehensible to the patient (even at a very young age) and to the family. Unlike physicians, in addition to clinical excellence, parents of children with end-stage cancer value communication as highly important (Mack et al., 2005).

Meyer, Ritholz, Burns, and Truog (2006) studied parents whose children had died in the ICU following withdrawal of life support. These parents identified six areas that were important in their ICU experiences; however, none of these were that the parents be the decision-maker. Rather, parents wanted honest communication. As one parent said, "Communicate honestly, false hope is unfair" (Meyer et al., 2006, p. 652). Parents wanted the respect of being listened to. They wanted their opinions and their roles to matter, though these and other authors have found that the information that has been provided is often incomplete. As a result, parents do not have the information to understand, much less make informed decisions about their child's care.

Communication can be impeded when too many people are trying to communicate with the family or when there is frequent turnover in physicians (as happens in many teaching hospitals). Parents of children with long-term illnesses, such as certain neurodegenerative diseases, have identified the need for a primary provider. This person should not only provide current and relevant information but should also do so with specific knowledge of this patient and this family (Steel, 2000).

Provider discomfort can also impede the content and timeliness of communication (Hinds et al., 2005). On average, providers recognize the inevitability of a child's death 3 months before the parents do (Wolfe et al., 2000). Parents want prognostic information, but providers often choose to withhold it. Parents will likely be very upset by the information, but they still want and need that information (Mack, Wolfe, Grier, Cleary, & Weeks, 2006). Still, almost half of all pediatric oncologists will not initiate a discussion of advance directives; they wait for the family to ask (Hilden et al., 2001). The information should be shared with the child and the family as it is learned. The focus should be on what this information means for *this* child at *this* time rather than on the functioning of a single organ system.

THE ROLE OF PALLIATIVE CARE

FOR THE LAST 20 years, palliative care has been gaining a foothold across health care settings. Regardless, there are still too many people, including many health care providers, who equate palliative care with end-of-life and hospice care. This misunderstanding is often an impediment to optimal utilization in the care of seriously ill patients, including and perhaps especially children and their families. Only about 10% of pediatric oncologists have formal coursework in palliative care, and less than 3% have a rotation in palliative care

495

*Withdrawing
and Withholding
Life-Prolonging
Therapies in
Children*

(Hilden et al., 2001). Regardless, "the decision to withhold or withdraw life sustaining therapy should always be associated with consideration of the child's overall palliative or terminal care needs. These include symptom alleviation and care, which maintain human dignity and comfort" (Royal College of Paediatrics and Child Health, 2004, p. 11).

Palliative care has three primary foci: aggressive symptom management, assistance with decision-making, and quality end-of-life care. Thus, all of end-of-life care is palliative, but much of palliative care is not end-of-life care.

Withdrawing and withholding life-prolonging therapies involves all dimensions of palliative care. Too often we use the phrase, "There's nothing else we can do." This is wrong for two reasons. First, even if no more curative or life-prolonging measures exist, there are *always* measures that can be taken to maximize comfort, optimize quality of life, and facilitate contact between the patient and family. This dimension of family involvement as death approaches is extremely important to parents (Meyer et al., 2006).

Second, the implication of there being "nothing else we can do" is that, therefore, nothing will be done. This can engender feelings of abandonment for patients and families. Indeed, providers who feel there is nothing else they can do are, in fact, likely to withdraw. *"When Rosario Maria was born with severe brain injury, she was given two days to live. She survived eight years.... It was noticeable that when we finally decided to take the inevitable steps that would lead to her death, the medical staff stopped considering her a priority.* Rosario Avila, parent, 2001" (italics in original; Field & Behrman, 2003, p. 21). Pediatric oncologist Jean Belasco reframed the distinction clearly. "[M]y own physician's oath helps me to focus, to know my limits, to not burn out. My oath is not to cure—which as humans we cannot always do—but the oath is to heal and to relieve suffering—which we can always do" (Belasco, 2002, p. 749). A consultation with the palliative care team can either allow the team that has been caring for the child to learn what more they *can* do or bring a different set of professionals to the bedside to complement the care of the primary team.

CONCLUSION

PATIENTS SHOULD RECEIVE only those treatments that are likely to provide benefit. If a treatment cannot benefit a child, it should either not be started or should be withdrawn when recognition of that futility becomes evident. Decision-making with and about children should focus on the goals of care for a specific child, which should be identified not only for each intervention, but also for the totality of the child's medical picture. An inability to achieve the goals of care necessitates consideration of withdrawing or withholding specific treatments. Informed, structured communication allows families to understand and to live better with the outcomes, and to appreciate the value of all they gave their child. Poor communication can interfere with a team approach and may hinder the ability of the team and the family to ensure the best quality of life for each child, based on each one's specific needs and circumstances.

A decision to withdraw or withhold treatments is only the first part of the process. Even if the child will die, aggressive treatments should continue. The goals of these treatments should be palliative, and should be focused on alleviating symptoms, maximizing quality of life, family interactions, and facilitating decision-making. This should continue throughout the child's life, whether it lasts minutes or years.

NOTE

1. These vignettes are based on experiences from the author's practice.

REFERENCES

Andresen, E. M., Seecharan, G. A., & Toce, S. S. (2004). Provider perceptions of child deaths. *Archives of Pediatrics and Adolescent Medicine, 158,* 430–435.

Beale, E. A., Baile, W. F., & Aaron, J. (2005). Silence is not golden: Communicating with children dying from cancer. *Journal of Clinical Oncology, 23,* 3629–3631.

Beauchamp, T. L., & Childress, J. F. (1994). *Principles of biomedical ethics* (4th ed.). New York: Oxford University Press.

Belasco, J. B. (2002). In memoriam 2001. *Journal of Palliative Medicine, 5,* 747–750.

Bluebond-Langner, M. (1978). *The private worlds of dying children.* Princeton, NJ: Princeton University Press.

Catlin, A. (2005). Thinking outside the box. Prenatal care and the call for a prenatal advance directive. *Journal of Perinatal and Neonatal Nursing, 19,* 169–176.

Center to Advance Palliative Care. (2007). *Pediatric palliative care: State of the art and science.* Retrieved October 31, 2007, from http://www.capc.org/support-from-capc/audio-conf/11–13–07-audio

Field, M. J., & Behrman, R. E. (Eds.). (2003). *When children die: Improving palliative and end-of-life care for children and their families.* Washington, DC: National Academy Press.

Hamilton, B. E., Miniño, A. M., Martin, J. A., Kochanek, K. D., Strobino, D. M., & Guyer, B. (2007). Annual summary of vital statistics: 2005. *Pediatrics, 119,* 345–360.

497

*Withdrawing
and Withholding
Life-Prolonging
Therapies in
Children*

Hammes, B. J., Klevan, J., Kempf, M., Williams, M. S. (2005). Pediatric advance care planning. *Journal of Palliative Medicine, 8,* 766–773.

Hilden, J. M., Emanuel, E. J., Fairclough, D. L., Link, M. P., Foley, K. M., Clarridge, B. C., et al. (2001). Attitudes and practices among pediatric oncologists regarding end-of-life care: Results of the 1998 American Society of Clinical Oncology survey. *Journal of Clinical Oncology, 19,* 205–212.

Hinds, P. S., Schum, L., Baker, J. N., Wolfe, J. (2005). Key factors affecting dying children and their families. *Journal of Palliative Medicine, 8*(Suppl. 1), S70–S78.

Hurwitz, C. A., Duncan, J., & Wolfe, J. (2004). Caring for the child with cancer at the close of life: "There are people who make it, and I'm hoping I'm one of them." *Journal of the American Medical Association, 292,* 2141–2149.

Kaempf, J. W. (2007, October 1). Periviability guidelines are helpful and rational. *Pediatrics.* Retrieved October 21, 2007, from pediatrics.aappublications.org/cgi/content/full/117/1/22

Kaempf, J. W., Tomlinson, M., Arduza, C., Anderson, S., Campbell, B., Ferguson, L. A., et al. (2006). Medical staff guidelines for periviability pregnancy counseling and medical treatment of extremely premature infants. *Pediatrics, 117,* 22–29.

Levetown, M. (2005). *Children and palliative care: It can be done!* From the 2005 Annual Assembly of the American Academy of Hospice and Palliative Medicine. Retrieved October 21, 2007, from http://www.medscape.com/viewarticle/499471

Mack, J. W., Hilden, J. M., Watterson, J., Moore, C., Turner, B., Grier, H. E., et al. (2005). Parent and physician perspectives on quality of care at the end of life in children with cancer. *Journal of Clinical Oncology, 23,* 9155–9161.

Mack, J. W., Wolfe, J., Grief, H. E., Cleary, P. D. & Weeks, J. C. (2006). Communication about prognosis between parents and physicians of children with cancer: Parent preferences and the impact of prognostic information. *Journal of Clinical Oncology, 24,* 5265–5270.

Mahon, M. M. (1990). The nurse's role in treatment decisionmaking for the child with disabilities. *Issues in Law & Medicine, 6,* 247–268.

Meyer, E. C., Ritholz, M. D., Burns, J. P. & Truog, R. D. (2006). Improving the quality of end-of-life care in the pediatric intensive care unit: Parents' priorities and recommendations. *Pediatrics, 117,* 649–656.

Miniño, A. M., Heron, M. P., Murphy, S. L., & Kochanek., K. D. (2007). Deaths: Final data for 2004. *National Vital Statistics Report, 55*(19), 1–120.

Nuffield Council on Bioethics. (2006). *Critical care decisions in fetal and neonatal medicine.* London: Author.

Nyquist, A. C., Gonzales, R., Steiner, J. F., & Sande, M. A. (1998). Antibiotic prescribing for children with colds, upper respiratory tract infections, and bronchitis. *Journal of the American Medical Association, 27,* 875–877.

Royal College of Paediatrics and Child Health. (2004). *Withholding or withdrawing life sustaining treatment in children. A framework for practice* (2nd ed.).

Retrieved October 23, 2007, from http://www.rcpch.ac.uk/doc.aspx?id_Resource=2002

Singh, J., Fanaroff, J., Andrews, B., Caldarelli, L., Lagatta, J., Plesha-Troyke, S., et al. (2007). Resuscitation in the "gray zone" of viability: Determining physician preferences and predicting infant outcomes. *Pediatrics, 120,* 519–526.

Spence, K. (2000). The best interest principle as a standard for decision making in the care of neonates. *Journal of Advanced Nursing, 31,* 1286–1292.

Steel, R. (2000). Trajectory of certain death at an unknown time: Children with neurodegenerative life-threatening illnesses. *Canadian Journal of Nursing Research, 32*(3), 49–67.

Tournay, A. E. (2000). Withdrawal of medical treatment in children. *Western Journal of Medicine, 173,* 407–411.

Wolfe, J, Klar, N., Grier, H. E., Duncan, J. Salem-Schatz, S., Emanuel, E. J., et al. (2000). Understanding of prognosis among parents of children who died of cancer. Impact on treatment goals and integration of palliative care. *Journal of the American Medical Association, 284,* 2469–2475.

Youngner, S. J. (1996). Medical futility. *Critical Care Clinics, 12,* 165–178.

43

Ethical Challenges in Pediatric Dialysis and Kidney Transplantation

BERNARD S. KAPLAN, CYNTHIA GREEN, H. JORGE BALUARTE, AND KEVIN E. C. MEYERS

DIALYSIS AND TRANSPLANTATION have prolonged the lives of large numbers of infants, children, and adolescents with permanent kidney failure (end-stage kidney failure) over the past 40 years. Yet these treatments, once extraordinary but now routine, can pose significant ethical challenges to medical professionals and patients' families.

From their inception, it was recognized that neither dialysis (the removal of waste products and fluid from the blood by machine) nor renal transplantation were cures for permanent kidney failure; despite decades of technological advances, this remains true today. Dialysis patients must spend many hours a week connected to an artificial kidney that is a poor substitute for one's natural organs; they must carefully limit what they eat and drink and take multiple medications that can have side effects. Transplant recipients, while free of the dialysis machine, still must take medications everyday and face the prospect that the replacement kidney will not last a lifetime, necessitating future dialysis or retransplantation. In addition, even successful transplant patients are always at risk for serious infections or cancers as complications of the powerful immunosuppressive agents. As early as 1970, Reinhart posed queries about dialysis and transplant in children that continue to trouble us: "What does the child gain from the prolongation of life and at what cost? What price does the child pay to postpone parents' grief? What is the price of the physician's reluctance to permit death? Who makes decisions about the child's management, and on what basis are these decisions made?" (Reinhart, 1970, p. 505). He concluded by stating that "programs of dialysis and renal transplant for children should be evaluated not in terms of gross survival but in parameters of meaningful growth and development-living" (Reinhart, 1970, pp. 505–507). Yet who should decide what constitutes a so-called meaningful quality of life?

The basic ethical principles of *nonmaleficence, beneficence,* and *distributive justice* are called into question for any patient with renal failure because of the intrusive, even painful nature of the treatments and the shortage of organs available for transplant. For children, these questions loom even larger as parents and caregivers take on the profound responsibility of *making decisions for them.* The principle of *autonomy* is a cornerstone of medical decision-making, but children do not have the decision-making capacity to necessarily act in their own best interests. Adolescents may or may not be equipped to make medical decisions, but there are legal constraints, and the stakes of an error in judgment are extremely high. Yet even with concerned adults acting as the minor's proxy, ethical problems can arise when there are differences of opinion among team members and the child's parents or guardians about how best to proceed.

PEDIATRIC DIALYSIS

PEDIATRIC DIALYSIS IN many ways runs counter to the principle of *nonmaleficence* because it is painful and often frightening to the child, fraught with complications, restrictive, and costly to families and to society. Dialysis is never curative and at best serves as a bridge to transplant. For the same reasons, dialysis may also conflict with the notion of *beneficence.* Whereas the maintenance of life is usually considered to be an ultimate good, it poses profoundly challenging ethical difficulties when a high degree of pain and suffering is involved.

Starting dialysis can raise many tensions among different caregivers and family members who need to balance the ethical principles of *nonmaleficence, beneficence,* and *autonomy.* This is especially true in some cases in the intensive care unit, when the child's grave condition

501

*Ethical Challenges
in Pediatric
Dialysis
and Kidney
Transplantation*

essentially makes the treatment at best palliative and at worst medically futile. Decisions about whether to dialyze a severely ill neonate whose parents insist on treatment despite long odds against survival, or whether to withhold dialysis from a potentially viable neonate whose parents refuse treatment because of these same odds, are emotionally traumatizing and ethically challenging for families and medical staff alike. The American Academy of Pediatrics Committee on Bioethics (1996) wisely advocated that individualized decisions should be made jointly by clinicians and parents in a partnership based on full communication of facts and feelings, because the conflicts, agony, and burdens are too great for either side to carry alone (Shooter & Watson, 2000).

Our renal service at The Children's Hospital of Philadelphia was asked to take care of a normal female baby born at 31 weeks gestational age. She weighed 1.5 kg with Apgar scores of 5 and 9. She had been diagnosed in utero by ultrasound with oligohydramnios secondary to bilateral renal dysplasia with nonfunctioning kidneys. Her parents were offered termination but opted for intervention with serial amniotic fluid infusions. Do not resuscitate orders were instituted in accord with the parents' wishes, but comfort care was provided with fluids and feeds. The serum creatinine increased to 10.6 mg/dl by day 18, but parents were unwilling to allow peritoneal dialysis and the nephrologist concurred and was reluctant to start dialysis. The baby was fed a combination of oral and nasogastric feeds and steadily gained weight. There was a great deal of disagreement among the parents, the nephrologists and the neonatologists taking care of this neonate. Several medical personnel could not understand why these Catholic parents chose not to abort the fetus and elected infusions of saline to *give the baby the best chance* but did not want to start peritoneal dialysis. When the baby was born, they decided initially to let nature take its course and agreed to allow all comfort measures to be given to the baby. However, they did not want to allow a nasogastric feeding tube to be inserted or to subject her to peritoneal dialysis. The parents were advised that peritoneal dialysis would be an option if she were bigger and that a renal transplantation could be done when she had reached a weight of 10 kg. The baby was managed without dialysis until she was several months of age. At a year of age she received a kidney from her father and is now an intelligent thriving 11-year-old.

Deciding whether or not to offer chronic dialysis can also become a religious issue, as in the case of an Orthodox Jewish child. The Orthodox teaching is that once a medical procedure has been started, it cannot be stopped. Some have argued that when a procedure is not *continuous,* it *can* be stopped (Ravitsky, 2005), and that dialysis falls into this category of procedures. But it is not always a simple decision for an ultra-Orthodox family. This is especially the case when the patient may initially require a type of dialysis called continuous hemodiafiltration for initially unknown and unspecified periods of time. The principle of *autonomy* is breached when a family does not allow any direct discussion with an adolescent patient, particularly if the patient is 18 years of age. This is based on the view that autonomous decisions that do not comply with required halachic moral standards are superseded by these higher moral values that derive from the divine law and value system that governs the life of each individual, whether patient or physician. It is therefore considered impossible, for the Orthodox person, to solve moral problems in medical practice on the basis of the patient's or the physician's proclivities or personal feelings.

Withholding dialysis from a profoundly delayed child or adolescent whose parents insist on this treatment raises other ethical problems. For example, a boy aged 5 years was blind, deaf, and profoundly delayed developmentally and physically. He was born at 26 weeks to an 18-year-old mother who was the legal guardian even though the child was in foster care. He was in end-stage renal failure, and the mother wanted everything to be done for her child including dialysis and renal transplantation from a deceased donor. The patient's nephrologist wanted to institute palliative care. The mother was angry with the nephrologist, but both agreed to meet with an ethics committee. The boy subsequently underwent a short period of dialysis during which he almost died several times. He then received a kidney from a deceased donor and has normal renal function 5 years later.

Respecting the wishes of an emotionally competent adolescent who does not want to continue with dialysis or who refuses a procedure can be emotionally devastating for the treating team. We described the case of a 19-year-old African American girl who presented with end-stage kidney failure and numerous medical and psychosocial problems at the age of 10 (Salerno et al. 2004). At 19 years of age, she asked us to stop dialysis and wrote a farewell letter. Although we had agreed to accept her wishes, we were unable to let her die. A visiting vascular surgeon suggested that a graft could be created from the subclavian artery to the right atrium of the heart. After being informed fully of the high risk of the procedure and the possibility of failure, she eagerly agreed to undergo the operation. She had severe septic shock postoperatively but recovered. She was discharged to a stable foster home, returned to high school, and was transferred to an adult hemodialysis unit where she received dialysis three times a week. She was alive 5 years later (see Table 43.1).

Even when dialysis is clearly feasible and the child's medical condition is relatively stable, there are ethical issues that must be tackled. For example, many children and families prefer home-based dialysis, which can be done at night and which allows patients to attend school during

503

*Ethical Challenges
in Pediatric
Dialysis
and Kidney
Transplantation*

TABLE 43.1   Situations in Which Withholding or Withdrawing Dialysis Might Be Considered

The brain-dead child	In the older child where two practitioners agree that brain-stem death criteria have been met, it may still be technically feasible to maintain the patient's life by providing basic cardio-respiratory support. It is agreed within the profession that dialysis in such circumstances is futile and withdrawal is appropriate.
The permanent vegetative state	The child who develops a permanent vegetative state following insults such as trauma or hypoxia is reliant on others for all care and does not react or relate with the outside world. It may be appropriate to withdraw/withhold dialysis.
The "no chance" situation	The child has such severe disease that life-sustaining treatment delays death without significant alleviation of suffering. Dialysis in this situation may thus be deemed inappropriate.
The "no purpose" situation	Although the patient may be able to survive with dialysis, the degree of physical or mental impairment will be so great that it is unreasonable to expect them to bear it. The child in this situation will never be capable of taking part in decisions regarding dialysis or its withdrawal.
The "unbearable" situation	The child and/or family feel that in the face of progressive and irreversible illness further dialysis is more than can be borne. They wish to have it withdrawn or to refuse further treatment, irrespective of the medical opinion on its potential benefit.

Note. Adapted from Shooter and Watson (2000).

the day and generally lead more normal lives. However, this may not always be possible, because of medical or anatomical issues or because of profound social and/or economic deprivation in the family, which can make home treatment unsafe or financially prohibitive. Deciding whether a family or patient is up to the task of dialyzing at home brings up issues of *autonomy,* when the desires of those who will undergo or carry out the home treatment are weighed against the expertise and experience of medical staff who have seen home treatment fail with serious, even deadly, consequences for the child (see Table 43.2).

PEDIATRIC RENAL TRANSPLANT

THEORETICALLY, ALL CHILDREN with end-stage renal disease are considered candidates for renal transplantation. Nevertheless, there are indications and contraindications for transplant that

TABLE 43.2   Ethical Decisions in Pediatric Dialysis and Transplant:
Practice Guidelines

Equal consideration for all children
The child's best interest comes first
Gather all available facts before making decisions
Allow all team members to contribute their opinions
Come to a consensus whenever possible
Discuss issues with the entire family
Appreciate the difficulties of the situation and the decision
Provide support for all involved, including the child, family, and health care team
Avoid or allay guilt for all involved
Remember that often there is no *one best solution* or correct answer

should always be kept in mind when renal replacement therapy is first being considered. Currently, absolute contraindications include incompatibility between the donor pool and recipient's blood or tissue (this usually occurs after the loss of the first graft); an active, progressive, or untreated malignancy; severe multiorgan failure; chronic active hepatitis or HIV; and irreversible severe brain injury. With technological advances, however, transplantation between incompatible blood types and for patients with HIV is being attempted in selected adults and may eventually become available for pediatric patients. Transplantation is currently withheld when a patient has active autoimmune disease or chronic infection with hepatitis C, until the disease can be brought under control. Other contraindications to transplant may include profound psychomotor retardation, psychiatric illness that requires custodial care, lack of family support or home supervision, and nonadherence with medical recommendations, although these factors are all relative and must be weighed in each individual case against the positive reasons for proceeding.

For the child or adolescent who receives a kidney transplant that is later lost because of failure to take necessary medications, questions of *distributive justice* arise in determining whether to offer a second transplant or subject the child to long-term maintenance dialysis. Many questions arise as to who is responsible for the loss of the graft. Was it the patient or the family? Should an individual receive a second kidney transplant from the finite and insufficient pool of available deceased organ donors when others are awaiting their first? What if a living relative is willing to donate—should that person be placed at even minimal risk when there is no guarantee that the patient will adhere to treatment? How long should the patient wait after losing the first transplant, and what measures need to be taken to improve adherence and increase the chances that retransplantation will be successful? We simply do not have the answers to these questions and must decide each case according to its unique circumstances. We have not been able to

505

*Ethical Challenges
in Pediatric
Dialysis
and Kidney
Transplantation*

arrive at a consensus in regard to these ethical issues. Therefore, every effort is made prior to and after transplant to educate the patient and family on the importance of adherence. Despite all our efforts, some patients stop taking the medications, and, unfortunately, it is often difficult to predict who they will be.

THE LIVING DONOR

A POTENTIAL LIVING DONOR risks physical and economic harm to self by giving up a kidney. While medical complications from donor surgery are rare, they can occur, and donors must take time off from paid work in order to recuperate. Although there may be psychological advantages to donating an organ, there may also be adverse psychological repercussions, including those of an unsuccessful transplant surgery or a transplant lost to nonadherence by the recipient. The safety and well-being of the living donor are important concerns, and therefore the evaluation of living related donors is extremely important, in order to screen out candidates who have physical, psychiatric, psychological, or social contraindications for donation (Sterner, Zelikovsky, Green, & Kaplan, 2006).

It is sometimes difficult to balance the interests of recipients and donors as they may not necessarily coincide, even when the donor is a patient's parent. A parent may try to or even insist on donating a kidney to a child at great risk to the parent's own health, in which case the donor may require protection from his or her own selflessness by the medical team refusing to proceed (*beneficence* balanced against *nonmaleficence*). At the other extreme, family members may be unwilling to donate but feel that others will think badly of them if they refuse. Candidate donors who feel pressured to donate and are unable to tell the recipient and the family of their decision are offered the opportunity to cover themselves by telling the recipient that a medical issue has ruled out the donor (*truth-telling* versus *nonmaleficence*).

THE ALTRUISTIC DONOR

A CCEPTING A KIDNEY donated by a nonrelative or a stranger (*altruistic donor*) is controversial and emotionally charged (Broyer & Affleck, 2000; Kaplan & Polise, 2000). One study asks whether such donors should be praised for their selflessness or evaluated for their sanity (Henderson et al., 2003). It may seem to some that organ acquisition for renal transplantation has been moving down a slippery slope from deceased donors to biologically or legally related living donors, to nonrelated but emotionally involved donors—and finally to strangers. However, when there are no living related donors within a family, the patient may face a difficult, complicated dialysis course of several years' duration while awaiting a cadaver kidney. Proposed altruistic donors have included persons with close emotional relationships to the family, such as longtime family friends; casual emotional ties, such as the parent of a young patient's former schoolmate or an older adolescent patient's college classmate of short duration; and total strangers who have come to know of the family's situation through information disseminated in a religious community, workplace, media exposure, Internet chat room, or family-initiated Web site.

Some medical institutions in the United States have performed transplants with kidneys from altruistic donors. However, there are several concerns that are unique to altruistic donation. An objection frequently raised against allowing altruistic donations is the possibility that recipients or their families may secretly offer money or otherwise unduly influence donors (buying/selling organs is illegal in most countries). In fact, this is an equally strong possibility within families, and already part of donor psychosocial screening is set up to ensure that no monetary or psychological inducement or coercion has affected the potential donor's decision. Another objection is that wanting to give up an organ of one's own free will to a stranger is prima facie evidence of a psychological problem (Henderson et al., 2003). But we allow, even encourage, donation of blood, plasma, and bone marrow; firefighters, police officers, and soldiers who give their lives for strangers are hailed as heroes. Whichever view one takes, there is the possibility that mental health concerns could rule out an otherwise physically healthy donor, and psychological screening is recommended for all potential donors.

MINORS AS LIVE KIDNEY DONORS

THE PARTICIPANTS OF the Consensus Conference on the Live Organ Donor concluded that the person who gives consent to be a living donor should be competent, willing to donate, free of coercion, medically and psychosocially suitable, fully informed of the risks and benefits as a donor, and fully informed of the risks, benefits, and alternative treatment available to the recipient (Live Donor Author Group, 2000). The Consensus Conference participants were generally opposed to live organ donation from a minor because it obviously strains the concept of voluntarism, the ethical underpinning of live donation. In instances when an infant recipient received a kidney from a teenage parent, the donor was emancipated to adulthood by virtue of being a parent. Although this may not be ethically objectionable, it

507

*Ethical Challenges
in Pediatric
Dialysis
and Kidney
Transplantation*

does open the door to other circumstances in which minors might be used as donors. There might be circumstances, however, such as in the case of identical twins, when it is justified to use a minor donor. Surprisingly, an analysis of the United Network for Organ Sharing (UNOS) database found that live minor kidney donors were used in clinical circumstances not endorsed by the recommendations of a Consensus Conference on Live Organ Donation. Minor donor kidneys were transplanted more frequently to adult than to pediatric recipients, only 12% of recipients were identical twins, and use of a minor donor provided no better outcome than that expected from an adult donor (Delmonico & Harmon, 2002). These data raise ethical concerns regarding the justification for allowing a minor to donate a kidney.

CONCLUSION

Sir Cyril Chantler, in 1992, summed up the advances and problems of pediatric transplantation as follows:

> Amazing advances have been achieved over the last 20 years in transplantation. As well as the problems of rejection and its control there are other difficulties which have to be confronted. There are shortages of donors, problems of selection for treatment and the problems of funding this expensive form of therapy. The need to make choices has to be considered and the criteria in determining choice have to be determined. Of particular concern in paediatrics are the problems that arise in relation to rehabilitation and the need to provide a multidisciplinary approach to care. Finally, we have to remember that our enthusiasm for the possibilities of saving life and new treatments must not interfere with the basic responsibility to prevent suffering; at times the preservation of life at all costs is not justified, but in such circumstances doctors and other health care professionals have a responsibility for providing support both to the patient and to the family. (Chantler, 1992, p. S81)

It is clear that in 1992 Chantler echoed Reinhart's concerns from 1970 (p. 505), and we continue to deal with similar issues 38 years later. We believe that the scientific and medical problems of pediatric dialysis and renal transplant will never be completely resolved because the goal posts will always shift. We will continue to deal with the ethical issues in a sensitive, collaborative, nonconfrontational manner that is in keeping not only with the zeitgeist but also the cultural, ethnic, and religious affiliations of the patient and the family.

REFERENCES

American Academy of Pediatrics Committee on Bioethics. (1996). Ethics and the care of critically ill infants and children [review]. *Pediatrics, 98,* 149–152.

Broyer, M., & Affleck, J. (2000). In defense of altruistic kidney donation by strangers: A commentary. *Pediatric Nephrology, 14,* 523–524.

Chantler, C. (1992). Transplantation—a new dimension for paediatrics. *European Journal of Pediatrics, 2,* S81–S84.

Delmonico, F. L., & Harmon, W. E. (2002). The use of a minor as a live kidney donor. *American Journal of Transplant, 2,* 333–336.

Henderson, A. J., Landolt, M. A., McDonald, M. F., Barrable W. M., Soos, J. G., Gourlay, W., et al. (2003). The living anonymous kidney donor: Lunatic or saint? *American Journal of Transplant, 3,* 203–213.

Kaplan, B. S., & Polise, K. M. (2000). In defense of altruistic kidney donation by strangers. *Pediatric Nephrology, 14,* 518–522.

Live Donor Author Group. (2000). Consensus statement on the live organ donor. *Journal of the American Medical Association, 284,* 2919–2926.

Ravitsky, V. (2005). Timers on ventilators. *British Medical Journal, 19,* 415–417.

Reinhart, J. B. (1970). The doctor's dilemma: Whether or not to recommend continuous renal dialysis or renal homotransplantation for the child with end-stage renal disease. *Journal of Pediatrics, 77,* 505–507.

Salerno, A. E., Green, C., Zelikovsky, N., Gruber, P. J., Lodge, A., Meyers, K. E., et al. (2004). Creation of a novel hemodialysis bridge graft to extend the life of an adolescent. *Pediatric Nephrology, 11,* 1297–1299.

Shooter, M., & Watson, A. (2000). The ethics of withholding and withdrawing dialysis therapy in infants. *Pediatric Nephrology, 14,* 347–351.

Sterner, K., Zelikovsky, N., Green, C., & Kaplan, B. S. (2006). Psychosocial evaluation of candidates for living related kidney donation. *Pediatric Nephrology, 21,* 1351–1363.

44

The Ethics of Perinatal Palliative Care

CHRIS FEUDTNER AND DAVID MUNSON

PERINATAL PALLIATIVE CARE is the emerging specialty devoted to providing health care to fetuses diagnosed prenatally with life-threatening conditions, as well as supportive care to the prospective parents and families (Leuthner, 2004; Leuthner & Jones, 2007; Munson & Leuthner, 2007). "Perinatal" implies that this care is provided during the time surrounding birth (but sometimes continues for a far longer period of time). The range of medical conditions that can affect these patients is vast, spanning from major congenital anomalies or genetic syndromes that are invariably lethal to imminent extreme premature birth occurring before the fetus is viable. Much of pediatric mortality occurs near the time of birth: of the approximately 53,000 persons under 20 years of age who die each year in the United States, just over half (52%) are less than 1 year of age; and for every 1,000 pregnancies that enter the last trimester, 6.2 end in the death of the fetus or newborn (Hamilton et al., 2007). With such a large proportion of deaths during childhood occurring during the perinatal period, the field of pediatric palliative care would be remiss if it did not endeavor to assure that these infants and their families have access to perinatal palliative care.

Compared to more routine neonatal or palliative care (Carter & Levetown, 2004; Goldman, Hain, & Liben, 2006; Kang et al., 2005; Kang, Munson, & Klick, 2007; Lantos & Meadow, 2006), this novel domain of clinical practice and medical ethics has both similarities and some singular differences. In this chapter, we will examine seven aspects of perinatal palliative care, highlighting certain details of medical care, as we believe that understanding these details helps us to formulate a more complete depiction of the challenges—medical and moral—that these grievously ill fetuses, newborns, and their families confront. Throughout, we will pay particular attention to how high-quality perinatal palliative care can enhance three ethically important outcomes, namely (a) empowering families to reflect broadly on the situation and to mold medical care to conform to their deepest values, (b) maximizing the benefit and minimizing the harms of medical care for the child (whose best interest is the primary concern) and family (who are also important, and whose interests sometimes need to be compared and contrasted with the interests of the fetus or newborn), and (c) assuring that all families and infants have equal access to this mode of care. Having laid this groundwork, in the final of the seven sections we will turn to questions regarding the status of the fetus and the problem of being born into suffering, questions that loom large in the minds of many and that we believe are best addressed after being suitably framed within a well-developed perspective of the context surrounding specific fetuses or newborns and their families.

BEYOND A FORCED DICHOTOMY

FOR MANY PARENTS, the beginning of the journey that leads to perinatal palliative care is receiving news about an abnormal test result during pregnancy. With advances in prenatal care, clinicians may have to deliver worrisome information more frequently, as the number of screening tests offered during pregnancy increases, heightening the public health importance of defining and improving best practices for discussing disease or medical condition risk information with parents. The problem is compounded by the fact that available interventions for affected fetuses are not keeping pace with the ability to diagnose in utero problems.

Once the diagnosis is confirmed with subsequently more definitive diagnostic tests, clinicians often frame the cardinal clinical decision as having only two options: either (a) carry the pregnancy to term and provide maximal life-extending care to the baby or (b) abort the pregnancy. Parents have reported, anecdotally, that they have felt pressured to terminate the pregnancy because the other option of subjecting the live-born but extremely ill infant to a series of life-extending interventions—invasive, painful, and ultimately futile—is portrayed as cruel and inappropriate, a portrayal with which the parents often concur but also feel trapped by because they also believe that abortion is not an appropriate act. Clinicians, on the other hand, usually perceive themselves as acting out of genuine benevolence if they believe they are protecting families from ongoing grief by suggesting an early end to a bad situation.

The prospect of perinatal palliative care fleshes out the true range of options by including a third possible course of action, namely (c) carry forward with the pregnancy, and after the delivery provide comfort-maximizing care to the baby. Such interventions certainly include drying, warming, and holding of the infant, and may include breast feeding, the provision of oxygen or comfort-promoting drugs, the performance of baptisms or other meaningful rites or rituals with family members and friends of the family, and a wide variety of acts that would foster comfort and enhance meaning and relationships. They may even include some aggressive interventions depending on the underlying diagnosis and goals of care.

In this capacity of expanding the number of available treatment options, perinatal palliative care serves the same ethical function as more routine palliative care, namely, empowering parents to avoid a forced dichotomous choice and instead to select a mode of care that most closely corresponds to their beliefs and values. Likewise, perinatal palliative care also can diminish the moral distress of clinicians who may likewise have felt trapped by the limited two-option framework, or who may have had abiding misgivings about feeling compelled to perform invasive procedures on an infant who they perceive as dying. At the same time, unlike other modes of palliative care, prenatal counseling of parents about the possibility of palliative care for their unborn infant directly touches on the highly contentious issue of abortion. How to create a context for these discussions, and then facilitate the myriad issues that the ensuing dialogue often raises, are the topics to which we turn next.

CREATION OF A SAFE HARBOR

SEVERAL ASPECTS OF perinatal palliative care require clinicians to be mindful of the psychosocial environment in which first the parents and then the infant reside, and to seek to make this environment as safe and supportive as possible (Feudtner, 2007; Levetown, 2008).

First, the parents are most likely still trying to comprehend the information that they have been given by the obstetrical clinicians, information that may be bewildering in terms of the rarity, complexity, and uncertainty of the medical conditions that can affect the fetuses or in terms of the esoteric nature of the treatment options that exist. Their questions need to be answered clearly and patiently, in a manner that is both compassionate and forthright.

Second, parents are often buffeted by powerful emotions, including feelings of sadness, anxiety, anger, guilt, as well as an overwhelming sense of love, devotion, and responsibility. Consequently, all dialogue and actions have to recognize, honor, and engage both negative and positive emotions.

Third, during the prenatal phase, as mentioned previously, perinatal palliative care often involves discussions about the option of terminating the pregnancy. Families are owed full and unbiased information regarding this course of action, as well as support from the clinical staff regarding their thoughts and feelings, and ultimately their decision, about pursuing or declining abortion.

How can clinicians work to create a safe (or at least, safer) harbor? Such an environment would not only be respectful, truthful, and free from coercive or threatening influences but also perceived by the parents as such, allowing them to digest and ponder the information provided to them, to ask questions or otherwise respond in an uninhibited manner, and to make decisions and plans. One means to promote such an environment is for clinicians to explicitly state that this is one of their goals—that they seek to work with the parents to create a safe space for them to decide the best way to care for their future child. Physicians and nurses can also communicate their empathy toward the parents and the fetus by expressing to the parents how they wish that things were very different, and that you did not have to deal with these problems (Quill, Arnold, & Platt, 2001). When parents express emotion, either in words or behaviors, clinicians can provide support for these emotions by simply saying words to the effect that "I hear what you are saying about feeling so sad." Health care providers can further lay the foundations for this sense of safety and respect by again saying how they will provide the parents with complete information about the various treatment options, including options that they may not want to consider or pursue, in order to assure that the parents were aware of the range of possibilities. Finally, the physicians, nurses, and medical office can further accommodate the psychosocial needs of the mother and father by offering office visit times before or after regular hours (so that the parents do not have to wait in a room full of happily expectant parents), or visits with members of the extended family present.

THE CERTAINTY OF UNCERTAINTY

IF A SENSE of safety pervades the conversations between parents and clinicians, their dialogue and relationship is better positioned to handle two cardinal factors that make the provision of perinatal palliative care such a dynamic endeavor: uncertainty and emotion. Here, let us consider uncertainty. Indeed, the only aspect of perinatal palliative care that is certain is that the future is uncertain—a cliché that bears repeating in order to avoid one of the major mistakes that can be made in counseling parents, namely, to prognosticate with certainty that a specific infant patient will die soon. While some clinicians feel that parents need to hear this reality, the problem is that the information that a child has an extremely high probability of dying in a short period of time is not definitive: the truth is that some infants live longer than expected. Take, for instance, live-born infants with trisomy 18: while many die shortly after birth, and most die within the first 10 days of life, approximately 10% are alive at 1 year of age (Rasmussen, Wong, Yang, May, & Friedman, 2003). The challenge then is to talk about this uncertainty without evading the worry that the child is likely going to die in the near future. We find that couching all predictions in terms of this worry is an effective means of communicating this information; when discussing what might happen, a clinician could say: "I wish I knew for sure, but I don't. What I do know, based on my knowledge of other infants who have the condition that your child has, is that I am very worried that the baby may die shortly after birth, so I think we need to plan what to do if that is what is happening. At the same time, the baby may be with us longer, so we need to plan for that possibility as well."

THE FRAY OF EMOTIONS

A CORE ASPECT OF all pediatric palliative care is the management of the range of emotions that affect both parents and clinicians (Feudtner, 2005a). A prospective mother normally develops a deep sense of attachment to her fetus; this process often occurs unabated even when the pregnancy is shrouded by an ominous diagnosis. A profound sense of grief and loss frequently occurs when the future parents learn of a life-threatening illness in their fetus. At the same time, the knowledge can seem surreal because it is only known through images and tests. The consequence of this battle between what is a physical experience of a pregnancy versus a far more abstract cognitive processing of the diagnostic and prognostic information usually results in an emotional roller coaster: the reflexive elation that accompanies the feeling of the fetus's movements transforms into sadness, anger, or despair with the growing awareness that all is not well, that something is dreadfully wrong. For the family that chooses to carry to term, the care provider can assist the prospective parents in coping with these extremes of emotion. Simply preparing them for the fact that day-to-day experiences can trigger a grief reaction can be a powerful anticipatory tool, validating their experience. Clinicians can also help prospective parents to generate a variety of stock responses for the well-intended stranger who congratulates them for their "good fortune," and for the parents to feel empowered to ask for help from family and friends to be the gatekeepers of information about the pregnancy and the fetus.

The clinician may also be wrestling with emotions that may stem from their own cultural, spiritual, or philosophical beliefs, or from their own intimate personal experience regarding childbearing, illness, or death. Working to bring these emotions into conscious awareness enables one to evaluate them in light of the clinician's sense of duty toward the prospective parents and the fetus or newborn, asking: are my emotions assisting or interfering with the clinical decisions at hand? Fostering within oneself a healthy skepticism for one's personal belief system and developing a broadly tolerant viewpoint promotes a sense of equipoise when helping a family navigate difficult decisions (Feudtner, 2005b). Compassion is one emotion that should not be held in check, but instead abundantly displayed, as families find solace and support if they sense the clinician genuinely cares.

MAKING DECISIONS REGARDING CARE DURING AND AFTER THE DELIVERY

GIVEN THE UNCERTAINTY and emotional challenges outlined previously, how—in practical terms—can the sometime hectic postpartum care of the baby be managed? While some individuals respond to these challenges by drafting ever more detailed care plans in an effort to maintain control, there is also need for clarification of some key guiding principles that steer care if and when events go in an unanticipated and thus uncharted direction. For example, it can be very helpful to talk about what will be the "True North" that will guide care: what is the most important goal? For many families with whom we have worked, this goal expresses a desire to make the baby as comfortable as possible, and to keep the child in the arms of the family. Some families also want a concurrent goal to provide all forms of care that would prolong life but not cause suffering. This common combination of goals can be captured by a credo "to neither overdue nor underdo."

Equipped with these overarching orienting goals, whatever they are, the clinician and parents can respond to potentially surprising circumstances, evaluating the situation and potential interventions, and creating an updated care plan. Suppose, for example, that the infant is born with such a small mandible (chin) that the baby labors to breathe; while the prebirth plan may have aimed to avoid inserting any tubes, the placement of a small nasopharyngeal airway (a tube through one of the nostrils can allow air to be inhaled more easily) may become a useful therapeutic option to consider, given that it may make the baby more comfortable and enable the family to more readily hold the infant.

ASSURING THE DELIVERY OF CARE

MAKING A CARE plan is like making a promise, a promise to provide a certain mode of care. If for whatever reason this plan cannot in fact be effectively enacted, the underlying promise—wittingly or unwittingly—is broken. Our point here is that the ethics of perinatal palliative care must address whether or not palliative care will in fact be provided to the babies whose parents have opted for this mode of care—a fact that hinges on the cooperation of potentially many individuals, ranging from the clinician who delivers the baby through to the nurses, physicians, respiratory therapists, and others who will attend to the baby after birth.

When planning the postpartum care of the infant, the default should be to assume that not all members of the clinical staff will be willing to provide palliative care. Consequently, one of the most important planning tasks is to identify which health care providers will be part of the care team for the baby, and to develop contingency plans if any of these individuals happen to be unavailable at the time that the child is born (as this timing is unpredictable). For instance, which neonatologist will be summoned to the delivery to supervise the early care of the baby, and who will be the backup neonatologist? A similar line of planning has to occur for all of the key personnel. Furthermore, the planning should include inquiry regarding whether the hospital (if the delivery occurs in a hospital) has formal policies or legal opinions, or informal but highly influential views, regarding the appropriateness of providing palliative care to babies. While the delivery of perinatal palliative care, as we are describing here, is in full accord with the guidance set forth by the so-called Baby Doe regulations promulgated in the 1980s, the time to clarify this point with all concerned parties is before the baby is born.

The question of who should be on the care team can influence the answer of where care should be provided. While ideally the delivery and care of the child is provided as close to the family's home residence as is possible (so as to minimize the burdens of being far from home and, if desired, maximize the ability of other family members to meet the baby and participate in meaningful events), this goal sometimes is of lesser priority than assuring that the mode of care is completely palliative, or more capable to responding to an unpredictable turn of events, goals that may be more readily accomplished at another site of care.

The promise of care may also extend beyond the infant to other family members, especially in the form of bereavement care offered to the mother, father, and any siblings. Here, too, plans should be made carefully to assure that these services are of high quality and are respectful of the difficult choices that the family made on behalf of the infant. In this regard, group therapy may not be as appropriate as individual therapy.

Careful planning, and then vigilance to assure that the plan unfolds properly, is paramount: a noble plan followed by undesired care is not ethically sound. Ultimately, however, acknowledging the irreducible uncertainty and the limited ability to control how events will unfold is a cornerstone to the honest and forthright dialogue that is essential to perinatal palliative care.

THE ETHICS OF RESPONDING TO MORAL INDETERMINACY

THE FINAL ASPECT of perinatal palliative care that we will consider is a combination of two questions that may have been uppermost in the minds of readers when first approaching this chapter: First, should a fetus be the object of a medical team's attention? And second, what should our response be when we learn that a fetus will be born into a life that will be short and may be marked by suffering? If asked without an adequately developed sense of an individualized context, both questions are mired by the reality that in the United States the fetus has ambiguous moral and legal status as an individual: at 23 weeks estimated gestational age, a fetus could be aborted, delivered and resuscitated, or evaluated for fetal surgery.

While perinatal palliative care need not resolve this society-level ambiguity, this domain of practice should seek to examine and manage any ambiguities at the level of individual fetuses and their families. To this end, we believe that clinicians can best support prospective parents who are grappling with a nearly incomprehensible situation using the tenets of palliative care, which ultimately derives its principles from a deep respect for persons. In this setting, respect must be shown to the parents as well as the fetus, with as open a dialogue as possible about how the perceived best interest for the fetus and the parents appear to overlap or diverge. The prospective parents may be weighing real concerns regarding the potential suffering that their baby might experience with their own philosophical, religious, and cultural beliefs that may either permit or prohibit abortion. Within the potential pull of these concerns, parents wonder: is the suffering associated with delivery and ultimately death from respiratory failure in an infant with renal agenesis (congenital absence of kidneys) too much to ask a baby to bear? At the same time as parents are grappling with this question, the parents may be wrestling with a rapidly progressing sense of attachment to the fetus on the one hand, and on the other a sense of being personally unable to cope with an overwhelming situation, emotionally, morally, or even financially. What is the best, most loving way to be a parent under these unimaginable circumstances?

Perinatal palliative care does not seek to address such questions with simple or definitive answers. Instead, by painting a picture of what the various therapeutic paths would look like, if chosen, a family can better visualize and evaluate what they believe is the most appropriate path. The ethically appropriate role of the clinician, then, is to acknowledge the prevailing moral indeterminacy of the questions regarding the status of fetuses and appropriate response to their potential future suffering, and to collaborate with the prospective parents in working out well-informed individualized answers to these questions.

CONCLUSION

OUR EXPLORATION OF the ethics of perinatal palliative care, a novel and demanding area of medical practice, encourages us to view the most important ethical challenges of this care as fully embodied in the care itself and in the persons giving and receiving this care. Within this framework, understanding and managing behaviors and emotions, relationships and self-awareness, are crucial to promoting the best interest of the fetus or newborn and the family, and thus to an effective medical ethic.

REFERENCES

Carter, B. S., & Levetown, M. (2004). *Palliative care for infants, children, and adolescents: A practical handbook*. Baltimore, MD: Johns Hopkins University Press.

Feudtner, C. (2005a). Hope and the prospects of healing at the end of life. *Journal of Alternative and Complementary Medicine, 11*(Suppl. 1), S23–S30.

Feudtner, C. (2005b). Tolerance and integrity. *Archives of Pediatriatrics and Adolescent Medicine, 159*(1), 8–9.

Feudtner, C. (2007). Collaborative communication in pediatric palliative care: A foundation for problem-solving and decision-making. *Pediatritric Clinics of North America, 54*(5), 583–607.

Goldman, A., Hain, R., & Liben, S. (2006). *Oxford textbook of palliative care for children*. Oxford, UK: Oxford University Press.

Hamilton, B. E., Minino, A. M., Martin, J. A., Kochanek, K. D., Strobino, D. M., & Guyer, B. (2007). Annual summary of vital statistics: 2005. *Pediatrics, 119*(2), 345–360.

Kang, T., Hoehn, K. S., Licht, D. J., Mayer, O. H., Santucci, G., Carroll, J. M., et al. (2005). Pediatric palliative, end-of-life, and bereavement care. *Pediatric Clinics of North America., 52*(4):1029–1046, viii.

Kang, T. I., Munson, D., & Klick, J. C. (Eds.). (2007). Pediatric palliative care. *Pediatric Clinics of North America, 54*(5), xv–xvii.

Lantos, J. D., & Meadow, W. (2006). *Neonatal bioethics: The moral challenges of medical innovation*. Baltimore, MD: Johns Hopkins University Press.

Leuthner, S. R. (2004). Fetal palliative care. *Clinics in Perinatology, 31*(3), 649–665.

Leuthner, S., & Jones, E. L. (2007). Fetal Concerns Program: A model for perinatal palliative care. *MCN: The American Journal of Maternal and Child Nursing, 32*(5), 272–278.

Levetown, M. (2008). Communicating with children and families: From everyday interactions to skill in conveying distressing information. *Pediatrics, 121*(5), e1441–e1460.

Munson, D., & Leuthner, S. R. (2007). Palliative care for the family carrying a fetus with a life-limiting diagnosis. *Pediatritric Clinics of North America, 54*(5), 787–798.

Quill, T. E., Arnold, R. M., & Platt, F. (2001). "I wish things were different": Expressing wishes in response to loss, futility, and unrealistic hopes. *Annals of Internal Medicine, 135*(7), 551–555.

Rasmussen, S. A., Wong, L. Y., Yang, Q., May, K. M., & Friedman, J. M. (2003). Population-based analyses of mortality in trisomy 13 and trisomy 18. *Pediatrics, 111*(4 Pt. 1), 777–784.

Part VIII

Access to Health Care

45

Health Care Access in the United States: American Exceptionalism Once More!

Stephen E. Lammers

THERE IS AN ever-growing literature in many different fields of study about what is identified as American exceptionalism, the sense that Americans have of themselves as not subject to the same vicissitudes and limitations as the rest of the world. Originally this applied to Americans' understanding of themselves vis-à-vis their forebears in Europe; today it might apply to their understanding of themselves vis-à-vis peoples anywhere in the world.

When it comes to health care, often the claim is put forward that the United States has the best health care in the world. As will become clear, this statement, if taken as an indication of outcomes, is false. When the comparative work is done, questions begin to emerge, not simply about the correctness of the claim, but about the attitude that gave rise to the claim in the first place. This chapter will address American exceptionalism in the area of access to health care and will explore related issues that are raised by the way bioethics is practiced in the United States.

BACKGROUND

THE UNITED STATES does not have a health care system that covers all citizens. Nor does it have in place public policies that have universal coverage as their goal. Almost all other industrialized countries do. The policy differences are well known; the outcome differentials between the United States and other countries are less well known. Those policy differences are only the beginning.

The United States spends more, relatively and absolutely, on health care, than any other nation in the world. According to a study released by the Organization for Economic Development (OECD), the United States spends 15.3% of its GDP on health care compared to 9.6% on average for other OECD countries. Ironically, this is done with fewer physicians and nurses on average in the United States than in comparison with other countries, and with shorter hospital stays in the United States. The increased expense does not lead to longer years of life when compared to the other OECD countries. The differences between the other OECD countries and the United States in life expectancy can be dramatic, up to 8 years longer life expectancy for Japanese women, for example (Organization for Economic Development, 2007).

For those without health insurance in the United States, the reality is that their lives will be shorter still. Those without insurance at some point in any given year constitute at least 15% of the population. This includes at least 9 million children. Most persons receive health care insurance through their employer, and there is no universal requirement for what those employer-based policies must cover, nor a requirement that employers provide any health insurance options whatsoever. There are other insurance programs in addition to employer-based insurance. Persons will be insured if they are veterans, suffer from certain disabilities, or are over 65. Depending upon the standards of individual states, children and families are eligible for Medicaid. Finally, health insurance is also available on the open market for those who would buy it as individuals.

The consequences of this nonsystematic approach to health care leads to results that are dramatic when the United States is compared to other industrialized countries. For example, if one uses the World Health Organization (WHO) databases, maternal and child mortality and morbidity statistics are higher in the United States when compared to other industrialized countries. Expected life span for men and women is also lower. At the beginning and the end of life, the United States does not perform as well as many countries to which it is often compared (World Health Organization, 2007).

And yet no one questions that Americans have the best medical technologies in the world. Indeed, those technologies are celebrated

523

*Health Care Access
in the United
States: American
Exceptionalism
Once More!*

in the popular culture. Major news networks routinely report on what they consider major medical findings, findings that are supposed to make a difference in the lives of Americans. As will become clear, this is only true for citizens who have some form of health care coverage or who are independently wealthy so that they can buy the latest medical technology, even if it is not covered by their health insurance.

According to the most recent data, the United States is not improving as quickly as the other countries with respect to so-called amenable mortality. Amenable mortality refers to those deaths that should not occur in the presence of effective health care. The United States has improved in this area, but the improvements have been less than those in other OECD countries to which the United States was compared (Nolte & McKee, 2008). Americans spend more money than others, yet their health outcomes are not as good. Health care access, health outcomes, the expense of the system and the consequences of that expense for other social goods are the outstanding issues when health care in the United States is examined comparatively. It is not simply access to the system but what the system provides and at what cost to the country that are important matters from this perspective. There is a fair amount of discussion of the issue of access to health care in the political arena in light of the upcoming presidential election of 2008. Thus far the public discussion has paid less attention either to the concomitant problem of the cost of health care in the United States in comparison with other industrialized countries or to the disparities in results between the health care systems of other countries and the health care system in the United States.

This comparative data is well known in health policy circles, but it does not elicit as much comment from the bioethics community as does the latest difficult case that engages the press. One would think that this comparative data would bring forth questions from the bioethics community. First, why are there such disparities in access to health care? Second, why are resources being used here that could be invested in other social goods? Although work is being done on access to health care and the allocation of resources to health care, these issues have generally not captured the attention of the bioethics community. This chapter will offer one interpretation for this phenomenon.

THE ORIGINS OF BIOETHICS IN THE UNITED STATES

WHEN CONSIDERING THE origins of bioethics in the United States, two elements stand out. First, bioethics in America began as a reaction to wrongs done by researchers to subjects who were not told that they were participants in research. Second, there was a reaction to what was considered the tendency of physicians to over-treat their patients when these patients desired to be cared for but not treated aggressively with therapeutics at the end of their lives. The answer to both of these concerns was found in protecting the patient's liberty to accept or refuse treatment and the participant's liberty to participate or not in research. All of this was cast in terms of patient autonomy versus physician beneficence (Jonsen, 1998).

Given this background, it is not surprising that a remarkable amount of attention was given to the clinical setting. One outcome was the establishment of ethics consultations, which presuppose that the patient is already a part of the health care system and something is amiss within the system. The stories of the clinical encounters were and are compelling; what was not noticed were the stories of those who were not part of the system. Likewise, the research participant was a person already within the health care system. Within that context, the consent of the participant was quite important. So too was the quality of the research design. What received little attention was the person who was not present either as a patient or as a research participant. Again, this should not be surprising. Many bioethicists found that part of their responsibilities had to do with ethics consultations or memberships on institutional review boards (IRBs). To put this directly, bioethicists were not being paid to think about persons who were not present in the health care systems that the same bioethicists were advising.

The third principle of bioethics, justice, understood as equal treatment, did not receive the attention that beneficence or respect for autonomy did. It is not that it was ignored, but justice, understood as equality in terms of access to treatment, simply did not capture the interest of the bioethics community in the United States in the way that conflicts between respect for autonomy and beneficence did. As developed by Beauchamp and Childress, justice was supposed to be considered equally alongside respect for autonomy and beneficence, but in practice, it was not (Beauchamp & Childress, 1979). The emphasis upon rights as they are typically articulated in this country contributes to this inattention to issues of justice.

RIGHTS AND SELVES

THE AMERICAN FOCUS on rights, and the arguments around a right to health care, is revealing. Colleagues in other countries are not as involved with such conversations. As a Dutch colleague made the point, "we see ourselves in solidarity with one another and

525

*Health Care Access
in the United
States: American
Exceptionalism
Once More!*

we begin the conversation there" (Theo Boer, Utrecht, Netherlands, personal communication, June 5, 2001). At least twice in Michael Moore's film *Sicko* the comment is made that the speakers thought they were in the (human) situation together with others and that those who were financially fortunate should be willing to pay for the health care of others. In both cases, the speakers were not Americans. These comments are a hermeneutical clue to the difficulties of speaking about a right to health care in the United States.

It is well known that there is contention about the idea of a human right. One way around some of this contentiousness is to focus on the Declaration of Human Rights and note that health care is considered to be a human right (United Nations General Assembly, 1948). This is too often not done.

There are at least two issues involved. The first is the American preference for negative rights, which are rights that protect individuals against interference by others, particularly government, unless harm is being done to someone. This means that there is less attention to positive rights, which are rights to assistance and services provided by the state, such as education or health care. In such a framework, access to health care is automatically assumed to be of secondary importance because it is a right that demands that some contribute to the upkeep of a health care system within which others may, should it be necessary, exercise their right of access to health care.

The second issue is the conception of the person who is claiming her rights. Here there appears to be a divide in American bioethics. On the one side are the bioethicists who, consciously or not, adopt a view of the person that is fundamentally consistent with that of economics. In that view, we are primarily invested in our own well-being, and we seek to maximize our self-interest. One can begin with this point of view and end with an argument for universal access to health care as the best way to protect one's self-interest, but the conception of the self remains fundamentally self-interested and, unlike the Dutch colleague mentioned previously, there is little attention at the beginning of the conversation to concepts of solidarity and what persons might owe others in this arena.

There are alternative ways of thinking about the self. For example, one competing conception begins with a self that is constituted by a body and thus is limited. The limits can be those of persons with bodies in general or the limits of my particular body, limits that include disease or disability (MacIntyre, 1999). If one sees human beings as sharing these possibilities of disease or disability, it is much more likely that attention will be given to access to health care as a way of addressing the inequalities of circumstance that grow out of being a body or in a body. Another conception of the self begins with the self in a community of persons. What leads to the good of that community becomes the focus of attention (Cahill, 2005).

LIBERTY, EQUALITY, AND DISABILITY

EVEN THOUGH A lot has been written about the tension between liberty and equality in American bioethics, in practice Americans prefer to give the nod to liberty. In that context, access to health care is not given priority. Further, the ways in which disability and illness limit a person are rarely addressed. If one is disabled because of illness, often one does not have the liberty to participate in the life of a society, large or small. The constraints to liberty caused by illness and disability, permanent or temporary, become ethically problematic when the illness is amenable to treatment and yet that treatment is not provided because there is no health care coverage. The consequence is that a nation that does not have a system of universal health care is a nation that is willing to live with a large number of inequities and with a large number of persons with significant constraints on their liberty.

These inequities are not simply moments in the lives of persons but rather have effects that persist across time. For example, children who are without access to health care when they are young do not flourish as much as those who do have this access. The effects of not having access to health care will persist over the life of the person. It is not accidental, in this context, to note that Article 25 of the Universal Declaration of Human Rights pays special attention to mothers and children. A system of universal access to health care increases the likelihood that persons will not be hindered in participation because of illnesses that, if left untreated or undertreated, will debilitate them.

From this perspective, discussions of justice and liberty must be kept combined and not separated. One cannot begin the discussion of liberty without a discussion of the real choices that individuals have. If in fact individuals cannot choose to have basic health care because of their circumstances, then they are constrained. As Jones (2007) has shown in his discussion of assisted suicide, even when liberties (physician-assisted suicide in Oregon) are offered, in the absence of access to high quality health care, real choices are in fact limited (Jones, 2007).

The medical technologies that fascinate us are developed for those persons who are already in the system, and little attention is given to those currently outside of it. Paul Farmer is unsparing in his critique of a health care system that is designed not simply *not* to serve the poor, but also to make sure they have no voice in how health care is delivered (Farmer, 2005). The focus of his comments most often is the international community, but the critique applies just as well to access to health care in the United States.

527

*Health Care Access
in the United
States: American
Exceptionalism
Once More!*

CONCLUSION

WHERE DOES THAT leave us? This chapter is not an argument for the claim that universal access to health care will solve all of the difficulties that face the health care system in the United States. Indeed, there is a very good chance that universal access will exacerbate the tendency of this country to spend far more on health care than other countries to which we compare ourselves. All that is being argued here is that comparative work is useful for understanding where in fact our health care system succeeds and where it might do better. Bioethicists need to become more familiar with the data generated by this work. In doing so, we better understand how our own history has influenced the way in which the discussion about universal health care is conducted. It may turn out that we need to worry less about being exceptional and more about being better.

REFERENCES

Beauchamp, T. L., & Childress, J. F. (1979). *Principles of biomedical ethics*. New York: Oxford University Press.

Cahill, L. (2005). *Theological bioethics: Participation, justice and change*. Washington, DC: Georgetown University Press.

Farmer, P. (2005). *Pathologies of power: Health, human rights and the new war on the poor*. Berkeley: University of California Press.

Jones, R. P. (2007). *Liberalism's troubled search for equality: Religion and cultural bias in the Oregon assisted suicide debates*. Notre Dame, IN: University of Notre Dame Press.

Jonsen, A. R. (1998). *The birth of bioethics*. New York: Oxford University Press.

MacIntyre, A. (1999). *Dependent rational animals: Why human beings need the virtues*. Chicago: Open Court.

Nolte, E., & McKee, C. M. (2008). Measuring the health of nations; updating an earlier analysis. *Health Affairs, 27*, 58–71.

Organization for Economic Development. (2007). *OECD health data 2007: How does the United States compare?* Retrieved January 11, 2008, from http://www.oecd.org/dataoecd/46/2/38980580.pdf

United Nations General Assembly. (1948). *Universal declaration of human rights* Retrieved February 1, 2008, from http://www.un.org/Overview/rights.html

World Health Organization. (2007). *WHOSIS*. Retrieved January 3, 2008, from http://www.who.int/whosis/en/index.html

46

Does the U.S. Constitution Protect a Right to Unapproved Drugs?

Theodore W. Ruger and Mahnu Davar

FEW LEGAL QUESTIONS implicate the poignant clash of competing constitutional and ethical values like a dying patient's claim of the right to use promising but not yet government-approved experimental drugs. Patients' arguments in this area resonate with the traditional legal and ethical values of individual autonomy, freedom over one's own body, and the long-standing proposition in American law that medical decisions are most appropriately made at the bedside by the patient and her treating physician. On the other side of the equation stands the venerable federal Food and Drug Administration (FDA) as an expert, scientific—and generally well-regarded—public

The views expressed in this chapter are those of the authors and not those of Mr. Davar's firm (Arnold & Porter LLP, Washington, DC) or its clients.

health agency with absolute gatekeeping authority over new medicines entering the U.S. market.

Despite these highly contested ethical and policy concerns, the formal constitutional doctrine on this question has for many decades been settled in favor of the FDA's absolute authority to restrict or prohibit use of new substances until it has completed its full regulatory review. In the 1979 case of *United States v. Rutherford,* the Supreme Court pointedly considered the question of whether the Food, Drug, and Cosmetic Act "makes special provision for drugs used to treat terminally ill patients" (*United States v. Rutherford,* 1979). (The case involved a group of cancer patients seeking preapproval access to Laeterile.) The Court answered that query in the negative, finding a clear congressional intent to give the FDA gatekeeping authority over *all* new medicines, and did not find any constitutional barrier to such jurisdiction.

Rutherford remains a good law as of 2008, but its durability was cast into question recently in a controversial and notable 2006 decision titled *Abigail Alliance for Better Access to Developmental Drugs v. Von Eschenbach* (2006). In that case, a three-judge panel of the federal District of Columbia Circuit did find a novel constitutional right grounded in the Due Process Clause of the Fourteenth Amendment for terminal patients to access potentially lifesaving drugs prior to FDA approval. In 2007, the full D.C. Circuit Court (a group of 10 federal judges sitting together) reversed the original three judges (*Abigail Alliance for Better Access to Developmental Drugs v. Von Eschenbach,* 2007)—returning the legal rule to its earlier regime of FDA exclusive control over new medicines. In January 2008 the U.S. Supreme Court declined to review or modify that decision (see *Abigail Alliance for Better Access to Developmental Drugs v. Von Eschenbach,* 2008, denial of certiorari). As a matter of formal constitutional doctrine, then, the law is once again settled: patients have no individual right of access to new therapies that the FDA has not yet approved.

But the *Abigail Alliance* case, and the contested issues it raises, continue to resonate both in ethical and legal discourse and in concrete debates about access to new drugs in other public policy venues such as Congress and the FDA itself. Several scholars have been sharply critical of the full D.C. Circuit's decision to deny an individual the right to use potentially lifesaving medications, arguing that it unduly transgresses principles of individual autonomy and self-preservation (e.g., Volokh, 2007). Others have argued strenuously in support of the ultimate affirmation of FDA control, maintaining that a contrary holding in favor of the terminally ill patient would have effectively been the end of the FDA's role as primary guarantor of drug safety (Jacobsen & Parmet, 2007). On a case-by-case basis some federal judges are employing more particularized legal doctrines to enable desperate patients to access potentially useful drugs (Goldstein, 2008). Moreover, though the constitutional law doctrine remains settled in favor of the FDA, the

531

*Does the U.S.
Constitution
Protect a Right
to Unapproved
Drugs?*

debate over earlier access to promising but unproven new medicines has not ended but has instead shifted to the political and regulatory settings and can be expected to continue for the foreseeable future.

This brief chapter will address these topics in turn. First, we provide a summary of existing constitutional law and the challenge, and ultimate resolution, provided by the sequential decisions in the *Abigail Alliance* case. Second, we describe some of the legislative and administrative reform initiatives that the *Abigail Alliance* case appears to have catalyzed. Finally, we conclude by assessing the decision and the issues it raises from a variety of legal and ethical perspectives, particularly focusing on conceptions of informed consent as they interact with the constitutional ruling in the case.

ACCESS TO UNAPPROVED THERAPIES AND THE U.S. CONSTITUTION

THE QUESTION OF whether patients might have judicially enforceable constitutional rights to choose the terms of their own therapy even against FDA policy is one that implicates long-standing disputes over the content of the vague language of the Constitution itself. There are two substantially different kinds of rights that individuals plausibly might advance in relation to accessing new medicines. The first is the most complete from the perspective of egalitarian moral theory: the state has an affirmative obligation not merely *to permit* the use of but also *to provide funding for,* and access to, essential medicines for all its citizens. This sort of claim for affirmative entitlement is what standard constitutional vocabulary labels a positive right, and is clearly *not* the sort of right that American courts have typically been willing to recognize in the health care context or virtually any other. Indeed, the Supreme Court has stated that even such near-universal political entitlements as Social Security and public education are creations of legislative design rather than fundamental constitutional rights (e.g., *Fleming v. Nestor,* 1960). Even while expressly constructing and reaffirming protection for basic negative rights, such as the right to choose an abortion in some circumstances (*Planned Parenthood of Pa. v. Casey,* 1992; *Roe v. Wade,* 1973), the Court has pointedly refused invitations to enshrine correlative rights to affirmative public funding for abortions (*Beal v. Doe,* 1977; *Maher v. Roe,* 1977). Under standard doctrines of American constitutional law, then, no individual can plausibly claim an affirmative entitlement to get the government to pay for a costly new drug therapy, no matter how essential to medical outcomes.

The plaintiff in *Abigail Alliance,* however, asserted a more straightforward negative liberty claim—the right to be free from government interference in using a drug that she was prepared to pay for herself, under the supervision of a private physician who recommended the therapy, and with a willing manufacturer ready to sell it to her. The sole barrier to her effectuation of this individual medical choice was the FDA's regulatory limitation on access. This sort of libertarian right is more consistent with the general path of constitutional jurisprudence in the United States, and so it presented a much closer and more divisive question for the federal courts. Most of the tremendous expansion of judicial protection of individual liberty in the second half of the 20th century has been in this realm of negative liberties—the rights of persons to be free of government intrusion in their most intimate and meaningful personal choices.

Although the U.S. Constitution's text only partially specifies the individual behaviors and choices that American courts have held to receive special protection from government interference, a number of cases in the past few decades lent some support for the *Abigail Alliance* patient's claim. In the past 40 years, the U.S. Supreme Court and other federal courts have gradually expanded individual rights under the implicit privacy or liberty guarantees of the Constitution's Due Process Clause.[1] Many of these fundamental interests involve rights of autonomy over medical procedures and bodily integrity (e.g., *Eisenstadt v. Baird*, 1972; *Griswold v. Connecticut*, 1965). So, for instance, the Court in a series of notable cases involving contraception and abortion has protected numerous features of reproductive autonomy from direct government interference. These cases expressly invoked rights of personal autonomy and self-determination over intimate choices regarding the body, a line of reasoning that provided support for the plaintiffs in the *Abigail Alliance* case. Perhaps even more pointedly, the Court has assumed that patients have a right to refuse lifesaving medication even against the objection of public health authorities (*Cruzan v. Director, Missouri Dept. of Health*, 1990; *Washington v. Glucksberg*, 1997), a concept that the *Abigail Alliance* plaintiff sought to extend to her decision to choose not-yet-approved medication. Finally, in the *Gonzales v. Oregon* decision in 2006, the Supreme Court rebuked Attorney General John Ashcroft's efforts to bar Oregon physicians from using federally controlled substances in accordance with that state's Death With Dignity Act, finding a strong presumption against federal regulation of the practice of medicine, an area traditionally left to the states. All of these precedents formed the basis for a solid, and at least temporarily persuasive, claim by the *Abigail Alliance* patient.

Arrayed against these conceptual analogs, however, was a fact that the plaintiff and the federal courts could not ignore: the decades-long presumption that the FDA had absolute regulatory authority over the initial approval of new medicines. This regulatory exclusivity had been upheld even when applied to desperate terminal patients in the

533

*Does the U.S.
Constitution
Protect a Right
to Unapproved
Drugs?*

Rutherford case and other lower-court litigation, and was a significant (and in the final analysis, determinative) barrier to the plaintiff's claim. How could she assert a "fundamental right" that was "deeply rooted in the nation's history and tradition" (*Abigail Alliance for Better Access to Developmental Drugs v. Von Eschenbach*, 2007) if the governmental practice for the second half of the 20th century appeared to repudiate just such a freedom? For the initial D.C. Circuit panel that ruled in her favor, the answer was found in a much longer view of history. The court examined drug regulatory and prescribing practices dating back to the colonial era and concluded that the FDA's absolute gatekeeping authority over both safety *and* efficacy was a relatively new phenomenon. For most of American history, according to the original three-judge panel, Americans were free to ingest any therapeutic substances they or their physician could get their hands on.

In this historical inquiry, it was important to the court that the drug that the *Abigail Alliance* plaintiff sought had already passed the FDA's Phase I regulatory approval hurdle. The FDA process has many steps, with Phase I directed at ascertaining an initial safety profile and Phases II and III entailing larger controlled studies to determine relative safety and efficacy. For the original *Abigail Alliance* court, the successful completion of Phase I testing meant that the drug has been proven safe—all that was left was for the FDA to complete its efficacy review. This was important for the court's historical claim: since the FDA only received authority to monitor medicines for effectiveness in 1962 (whereas the basic safety authority arose in 1938), the court was able to claim that for the vast majority of American history terminal patients were able to access drugs regardless of a government finding of effectiveness.

This original 2006 court opinion that *did* find a constitutional right of access was not the final chapter of the litigation. The federal Courts of Appeals (the penultimate level of the federal system, below only the U.S. Supreme Court) initially hear and decide cases in randomly chosen panels of three judges despite often having a dozen or more active judges in total. Before seeking Supreme Court review, parties who lose before the initial three-judge panel have the right to seek "en banc" review, meaning that all active judges on the court (in the case of the D.C. Circuit, 10 judges) will hear and decide the case. This is what the FDA sought and received in the *Abigail Alliance* litigation. And after reargument and new briefing, a year later in 2007 the full en banc court reversed the earlier decision, returning the law to the earlier settlement in favor of absolute FDA authority over new drugs. Though the en banc ruling differed from the original panel decision in multiple respects, its central distinction was in the role that history played; for the en banc majority, the decades-long history in the 20th century of a strong FDA authority outweighed any fainter lessons to be gleaned from the lack of direct regulation in a preindustrial past. Moreover, the full en banc court was clearly persuaded by the FDA's argument that to grant one exception here would necessarily create others, thus ultimately gutting the FDA's ability to monitor drug research and the clinical trial process. The en banc decision is the last judicial opinion in this particular case, given that in January of 2008 the U.S. Supreme Court declined to review or correct the decision.

The end of this chapter of judicial involvement produces the same constitutional doctrine as the beginning: the FDA has virtually absolute gatekeeping authority to control access to unproven new therapies, even over the medical and personal claims of individual patients. In this sense the law is stable and settled. But a broader conception of law and legal rules fairly embraces legal forms beyond court-made doctrine. And in these other venues for lawmaking—administrative law and practice and perhaps even statutory change—the law is far from static. Indeed, the controversy raised by the conflicting judicial opinions in *Abigail Alliance* has largely shifted outside the courts, where it continues to roil congressional debates, public discourse, and administrative practice at the FDA.

The FDA has long sought to mediate the tension between its role as guarantor of drug safety and the potentially objectionable barriers to access that its regulatory supremacy produces. In order to blunt the absolute effect of its absolute authority, the FDA provides various avenues whereby patients in need can access new therapies that have not yet undergone the full normal approval process. First, terminal patients may access promising but unapproved new therapies through participation in Phase III clinical trials of the drug. This route to access is incomplete and inadequate for some patients, given the fact that some may not meet criteria for inclusion in the clinical trials, and even those enrolled in controlled trials risk random assignment to the control, or placebo, group (see chapter 23 of this volume). Beyond participation in clinical trials, the FDA offers two other routes to early access to new drugs. First is the Treatment IND (Investigational New Drug) program, which permits some terminally ill patients to receive drugs that have completed Phase II but not yet Phase III approval. Such IND treatments require discretionary approval by the commissioner of the FDA, and as such are not available to all patients who might wish to access a given new therapy. Finally, the FDA also has instituted various expedited review programs, such as the Fast Track approval and the Accelerated Approval programs, both of which exist to speed ordinary approval times where "physicians and patients are generally willing to accept greater risks and side effects" in light of their life-threatening or debilitating illness.[2]

The *Abigail Alliance* litigation and the public controversy it generated provided an additional impetus for the FDA to further loosen restrictions on access for terminal patients in various circumstances. Just months after the original *Abigail Alliance* court had found in favor of the patient's constitutional right, the FDA announced that it had "proposed significant regulatory changes to make experimental drugs more widely and easily available to seriously ill patients" ("FDA Proposes Rules Overhaul," 2006). The main thrust of these regulatory reforms would be to expand access that individual patients had to unapproved drugs via the IND treatment programs, by removing various regulatory hurdles to participation in those programs. In proposing these changes the FDA stated that its revisions "will result in more patients with serious or immediately life-threatening diseases or conditions getting the earliest possible access to...therapies" ("Expanded Access to Investigational Drugs for Treatment Use," 2006).

The *Abigail Alliance* controversy not only spurred administrative reform, it also catalyzed proposals for new legislation in Congress. A bill currently pending in the Senate titled the ACCESS Act would amend the Food, Drug, and Cosmetic Act to allow more lenient access for terminal patients. The text of this proposed bill takes a sharply critical posture toward the FDA, declaring that "the current standards of the Food and Drug Administration for approval of drugs, biological products and devices deny the benefits of medical progress to seriously ill patients who face morbidity or death from their disease" (ACCESS Act, 2008). Whether or not this or a similar bill passes Congress, the legislative and public interest in this question has clearly provoked a more permissive attitude on the part of the FDA, as described previously. Through this dynamic, the *Abigail Alliance* litigation has produced through administrative means some measure of the increased access that it sought, and failed to receive, as a matter of formal constitutional doctrine.

REMAINING ETHICAL TENSIONS
AND PROBLEMATIC INCENTIVES

IN EVALUATING WHETHER the law should include a right to access experimental drugs not yet approved by the FDA, it is important to consider the effect of any proposal on existing protections of patient or consumer autonomy. As we discussed earlier, the complex FDA regulatory system was created to protect the public health. Implicit in this model is a shifting of rights; the consumer gives up an absolute right to have access to goods in favor of a conditioned right that limits the world of goods to only those that have been cleared by an agency. Normatively, this is for the consumer's own good—a consumer, who lacks the sophistication or access to information to independently verify whether a product is safe and effective, is asked to rely on the judgment of an agency to make this determination on his behalf. The drug approval process also protects consumers from falling prey to unscrupulous vendors of untested or sham medicines.[3] The FDA's public health role does not end when a drug is approved; the agency has continued oversight over the promotion, risk and safety information, and adverse event history of the drug. Acting alone or through health care professionals, the FDA endeavors to ensure that consumers have all of the relevant information to make informed decisions. This last section explores whether patients could ever be adequately informed about the risks and benefits of an experimental treatment, absent FDA review, such that access to that treatment would be ethical. In particular, if a desperate consumer was granted a limited right to purchase an unapproved treatment from a drug manufacturer, could informed consent to the treatment's potential risks be assured?

Informed consent in the health care context is essentially a test of the quality of information an individual has at the time he faces an important health care decision. In the law, informed consent developed out of medical battery tort cases, which turned on whether the treatment in question that caused harm had been consented to.[4] On the heels of the Nuremberg trials and the public outcry at the Tuskegee studies, informed consent became vested in the legal and ethical discourse in international documents such as the Nuremberg Code and the Declaration of Helsinki (Caplan, 1992; Weinberg, 2000). Informed consent was eventually codified, in the drug use context, with the advent of our modern FDA drug-approval process, where ethical and legal discourse overlap. FDA regulations require that clinical research subjects give informed consent and that the conditions of their consent and the subsequent treatment be monitored by an institutional review board (IRB).[5] A patient is deemed adequately informed about the risks and benefits of a treatment if he consents to the potential risks and benefits in writing. Consent can be abrogated by infancy, duress, and delusion but also by a misconception of risks and benefits or lack of relevant information (Faden & Beauchamp, 1986). The modern view of informed consent is that it is a process (Weinberg, 2000). A health care provider or researcher has a duty to work with a patient or subject to ensure that his autonomy is protected through an ongoing discussion about a treatment's benefits and risks.

Informed consent does not require the potential benefits of a potential treatment to outweigh its risks, but where the risk is extremely high, protections to autonomy must be heightened. A patient could consent to a life-threatening treatment that most of us would consider to be virtual suicide, and assuming the decision was voluntary and fully informed, the treatment could proceed. However, in such a situation, the voluntary nature of the consent and degree of information about the risks and benefits would have to be assured. When a patient

537

*Does the U.S.
Constitution
Protect a Right
to Unapproved
Drugs?*

does not fully understand the risks and benefits of a drug, or harbors misconceptions, he is not properly informed and meaningful consent is not possible.

Misconceptions about a course of treatment can arise from a variety of circumstances. In practice the information holders and information learners must maintain an open and well-informed dialogue. For approved drugs, the information available to the doctor and patient is generated by drug companies, the FDA, and academic research. To be fully informed, a patient must, in theory, process and understand this information, to the best of his ability, before consenting to a treatment regimen. However, scientific risk information can be very complex, and a very sick patient may be susceptible to desperation. It is generally the duty of the physician, as a learned intermediary between the drug consumer and the drug manufacturer, to provide accurate and realistic information. Although the system is not perfect, regulations and ethical norms mandate that physicians, the FDA, and drug companies all play a role in educating a consumer on a drug's risks and benefits.

The FDA regulations that currently govern so-called treatment use of an investigational new drug attempt to protect patients by codifying informed consent and assuring the flow of available risk and benefit information. A drug company that is in Phase II (or later) of the FDA-approval process for a new experimental drug can make that drug available to patients for "treatment use," if they have a "serious or life-threatening disease," and if "there is no comparable or satisfactory alternative drug or other therapy available to treat that stage of the disease in the intended patient population" (21 C.F.R. 312.34(b)(i)–(iii), 2008). Drug companies that have products eligible for treatment use must get informed consent from patients, assure IRB oversight, and only distribute the experimental drug through "qualified experts" (21 C.F.R. 312.34, 2008). If a treatment protocol is administered by a drug company directly, the informed consent process must be detailed, along with the other requirements, in a report to the FDA.[6] Alternately, if a health care provider is seeking an experimental treatment on a patient's behalf, the provider must not only comply with the same requirements of a drug company but must also certify his familiarity with the available safety and effectiveness information of the particular experimental drug (21 CFR 312.35(b), 2008).

Contrast the approved drug setting with that of the experimental or unapproved drug. In a true experimental use setting, very little may be understood about a drug. Informed consent to experimental use requires a patient to understand not only that an experimental drug could carry potentially deadly side effects, but that it may not work at all. Further, a desperate, severely ill patient may operate under the misconception that an experimental drug will actually work even when there is no data to support that belief. This so-called therapeutic misconception abrogates the requirements of informed consent. *Therapeutic misconception* is a term generally applied to placebo-controlled trials where a trial subject cannot give meaningful consent if he fails to recognize that he may not receive any therapeutic benefit by enrolling. The term may be applied to the *Abigail Alliance* context where the lines between consumer, patient, and research subject blur. Under the current drug approval laws, a drug must be both safe and effective to be approved for sale and use. The *Abigail Alliance* argued that during the foundational years, the standard was that drugs, including some cancer drugs, simply be "unadulterated" and that the new safe and effective threshold was too high for certain life-saving drugs (21 CFR 312.35(b), 705, 2008). The *Alliance* contended that if patients were required to wait for Phase II or later trials it would be "too late" for patients with critical life-threatening diseases (Volokh, 2007, p. 699). This argument suggests that safety, or Phase I, is a suitable point at which experimental use should be permitted. Leaving aside the effect this proposal would have on the decades of contrary legal and legislative history, we must evaluate the effect on consumer protections.

First, the language is important. To talk about an experimental drug as a *therapy* is to essentially fall into the therapeutic misconception trap. A drug which has been proven safe, has not automatically been proven effective. There is another whole phase of efficacy studies that a drug must undergo to actually show that it works. Thus, a drug that is simply safe cannot be considered a therapy. Consumers who then take these drugs under the Phase I, *Abigail Alliance* model could only give informed consent to the risks of such drugs if they were clear that those drugs not only had a low chance of actually working but that it was unknown if the drugs could work at all. Ensuring true consent would be difficult at this stage in light of the consumer's rationale for seeking experimental drugs. A consumer who requests experimental drugs generally does so after approved remedies have failed. The danger that a consumer in such a situation would pin his hopes on a highly risky, possibly inefficacious Phase I drug working, would be arguably higher than a Phase II drug that at least had efficacy data to support a conclusion that the drug could be a viable therapy. Finally, there would simply not be enough available safety and efficacy information to predict the potential risks and side effects of a Phase I drug, let alone any benefits, at such an early stage of usage.

Ultimately, requisite protections of autonomy in the experimental use context boil down into two key areas: voluntariness and quality of information. Informed consent is ideally a method of assuring both. When a patient is desperate and his emotions override logic, his consent

539

*Does the U.S.
Constitution
Protect a Right
to Unapproved
Drugs?*

is not meaningful because it is not truly voluntary. Where a patient is unable to comprehend risk information about a drug, or gather and access such information, his consent is not meaningfully informed. The ethical stakes are highest when a terminally ill patient is seeking an early-stage experimental drug, believing it to hold therapeutic benefit. Convincing proof that such a patient has given his informed consent to proceed with an unapproved use could only exist in a system with strong legal protections in place to prevent misconception or abuse.

We conclude this section with some reasons why it will be extremely difficult to protect consumers who seek expanded access to unapproved drugs, without working with the FDA. As our understanding of science and technology has grown, so too has the difficulty in striking a balance between protecting the autonomy of the individual on the one hand, while providing effective treatment on the other. While critics of the informed consent model question its practicality, it remains an effective measure for protecting consumers. As information grows complex, so too must the system of checks and balances that filter and break down that information for the consumer. Absent strong, codified protections of autonomy, the incentives to assure that patients have all the facts about the risks of a drug simply don't exist in the marketplace. Even with such a system in place, things can go wrong, as evidenced by the high-profile prescription drug scandals involving poorly understood or underreported side effect information for diet drugs, birth control, and antipsychotics. While this is a fair criticism of the success of the FDA oversight system, we must examine the consumer landscape without it.

Working outside the FDA system is not a practical solution. The incentives of drug manufacturers to over-inform are undercut by the need to prevent bad publicity and to sell products. The very scandals over adulterated or misbranded medical products that gave rise to the modern FDA show the dangers of entrusting an unregulated industry with consumer protection. Further, the incentives of doctors to truly act as learned intermediaries have changed with the rise in frequency of malpractice suits. Many physicians would rather give in to demands by patients to receive the newest therapies than to stand their ground on risk information and risk allegations of malpractice. In the absence of FDA or other oversight and policing, neither the drug company nor the doctor have adequate incentives or information to assure that the consumer is adequately informed of the risks of an experimental drug.

While some may argue that consumers have the freedom to contract to buy and use dangerous things everyday, without complex and time-consuming regulatory intervention, they miss the point. The permutations of risks of an experimental drug are millionfold when compared to, say, a butane torch or a chainsaw. It is impossible for a consumer, without help from a combination of doctor, drug company, and independent scientists, to educate himself in a fair and balanced way about the risks of a drug. Without a system of laws or an agency to assure that the incentives of doctors, drug companies, and others are aligned and centered on consumer interest, such a synergistic relationship would be impossible. Thus, if proponents of expanding access succeed and Congress expands access to experimental drugs, it would likely be wiser to do so by using FDA's oversight and resources and acknowledging the role the agency plays as a stakeholder in this public health debate. Absent agency oversight, protection of consumer autonomy and decision-making cannot be assured under the current legal landscape, and expansion of access to unapproved drugs could have potentially tragic consequences.

CONCLUSION

BECAUSE THE JUDICIARY in the United States is supreme over questions of doctrinal constitutional law, a court's decision to establish a new constitutional right carries with it significant institutional implications. When a right—such as access to unapproved drugs—is declared fundamental and thus constitutionally protected, individual decisions in that area are deemed by courts to be largely outside of government control. Viewed in this institutional perspective, the full D.C. Circuit's en banc decision to deny the *Abigail* plaintiffs strong-form constitutional protection in their choice of drugs reflects an allocational choice to situate the poignant debate over the competing values of drug safety and early access in the more calibrated, and perhaps more expert, venues of the FDA and Congress. The court's denial of complete constitutional freedom of choice hardly ends the debate, but to the extent that it continues, it will be, and should remain, under the traditional supervision of an expert agency and a well-established regulatory scheme.

NOTES

1. The guarantee of "due process of law" appears twice in the Constitution's text, in the Fifth Amendment (applicable to the federal government), and the Fourteenth Amendment (governing the States). In recent decades the Supreme Court has interpreted the substantive commands of the two clauses equivalently.

2. See 21 C.F.R. § 312.80 (2005), describing the purpose of expedited approval programs as being to "expedite the development, evaluation, and marketing of new therapies intended to treat persons with life-threatening…illnesses, especially where no satisfactory alternative therapy exists."

3. Articles in *Collier's Weekly* in 1905 and 1906 and Upton Sinclair's *Jungle* reflect public outcry against the practices of the food and drug industry at the turn of the 20th century and the need for more robust regulation. State regulation, which was initially thought to be the most constitutionally sound method of policing misbranded or adulterated foods and drugs, was inadequate for policing interstate trade in these products. See Regier (1933).

4. *Schloendorff v. Society of New York Hospitals* (1914), stating that "every human being of adult years and sound mind has a right to determine what shall be done with his own body; and a surgeon who performs an operation without his patient's consent commits an assault."

5. See 21 C.F.R. Part 312 (2008) for a discussion of IND requirements and 21 C.F.R. Part 56 (2008) for IRB regulations; 21 C.F.R. Part 50 (2008) (informed consent and human research protections); 21 C.F.R. Part 56 (2008) (IRB regulations); 21 C.F.R. Part 312 (2008) (requiring informed consent and IRB oversight of clinical trials, as requirements for a New Drug Application or "NDA").

6. 21 C.F.R. 312.35. In particular, the sponsor must evidence "a commitment…to assure compliance of all participating requirements of 21 C.F.R. Part 50," which codifies informed consent in the FDA regulations. 21 CFR 312.35(a)(3).

REFERENCES

21 C.F.R. Part 312 (2008).

21 C.F.R. § 312.34(b)(i)–(iii) (2008).

21 C.F.R. § 312.35(a)(3) (2008).

21 C.F.R. § 312.35(b) (2008).

21 C.F.R. § 312.80 (2005).

21 C.F.R. Part 56 (2008).

Abigail Alliance for Better Access to Developmental Drugs v. Von Eschenbach, 445 F.3d 470 (D.C. Circ. 2006).

Abigail Alliance for Better Access to Developmental Drugs v. Von Eschenbach, 495 F.3d 695 (D.C. Cir. 2007).

Abigail Alliance for Better Access to Developmental Drugs v. Von Eschenbach, 128 S. Ct. 1069 (2008) (denial of certiorari).

ACCESS Act, Bill No. S-1956, 109th Cong., 1st. Sess. (2008).

Beal v. Doe, 432 U.S. 438 (1977).

Caplan, A. L. (1992). Twenty years after: The legacy of the Tuskegee syphilis study—When evil intrudes. *Hastings Center Report, 22*, 29–32.

Cruzan v. Director, Missouri Dept. of Health, 497 U.S. 261 (1990).

Eisenstadt v. Baird, 405 U.S. 438 (1972).

Expanded access to investigational drugs for treatment use. (2006). *Federal Register, 71*, 75147, 75150.

Faden, R. R., & Beauchamp, T. L. (1986). *A history and theory of informed consent.* Oxford, UK: Oxford University Press.

FDA proposes rules overhaul to expand availability of experimental drugs. FDA news [Press release]. December 11, 2006.

Fleming v. Nestor, 363 U.S. 603 (1960).

Goldstein, J. (2008, August 21). Judge rules PTC therapeutics must give experimental drug to teen. *Wall Street Journal Health Blog*. Retrieved November 4, 2008, from http://blogs.wsj.com/health/2008/08/21/judge-rules-ptc-therapeutics-must-give-experimental-drug-to-teen/

Gonzales v. Oregon, 546 U.S. 243 (2006).

Griswold v. Connecticut, 381 U.S. 479 (1965).

Jacobsen, P., & Parmet, W. (2007). A new era of unapproved drugs. *Journal of the American Medical Association, 297*, 205–208.

Maher v. Roe, 432 U.S. 464 (1977).

Planned Parenthood of Pa. v. Casey, 505 U.S. 833 (1992).

Regier, C. C. (1933). The struggle for federal food and drug legislation. *Law & Contemporary Problems, 1*(3), 3.

Roe v. Wade, 410 U.S. 113 (1973).

Schloendorff v. Society of New York Hospitals, 211 N.Y. 125, 129–130 (New York, 1914).

United States v. Rutherford, 442 U.S. 544 (1979).

Volokh, E. (2007). Medical self-defense, prohibited experimental therapy and payment for organs. *Harvard Law Review, 120*, 1813.

Washington v. Glucksberg, 521 U.S. 702 (1997).

Weinberg, M. (Ed.). (2000). *Medical ethics: Applying theories and principles to the patient encounter*. New York: Prometheus Books.

47

Fair Pricing and Access to Medicines for the Poor

DONALD W. LIGHT

ACCORDING TO OXFAM (2002), 14 million people die every year from infectious diseases, and the great majority of them are poor. Chronic diseases cause about 35 million of all 58 million deaths a year and are rising rapidly toward more than 50 million by 2020 (Strong, Mathers, Leeder, & Beaglehole, 2005; Yach, Hawkes, Gould, & Hofman, 2004). Although there is much concern about diseases prevalent in poor regions and therefore neglected by the pharmaceutical industry, cardiovascular disease and cancer are the first and second in causes of death in developing countries. More than three-quarters of deaths and disease burden from noncommunicable diseases occur in low- and middle-income countries, where 84% of the world's population lives (Outterson, 2006b). This simple fact raises the possibility that advanced medicines for diseases shared by rich and poor alike could be made available to the poor for cost, while investments are recovered and profits made in affluent markets.

Infectious and chronic diseases limit people's capacities to take care of themselves or be productive so that the burden of disease impedes economic growth and return on investment. Among high-mortality developing countries, that burden amounts to 420 million disability life years (DALYs) a year, a calculation that estimates the burden of limited functioning across all diseases (World Health Organization [WHO], 2002). Many factors contribute to these conditions: malnutrition; lack of shelter, safe water, and basic sanitation; illiteracy and poor education; poor health care and lack of medicines or vaccines; dysfunctional and corrupt health or welfare services; and the multiplying effect of poverty itself. Here we will focus on just one factor, the accessibility to medicines and vaccines that can quickly increase the capacity of individuals and families to care for themselves, work, and even flourish.

Many newly effective vaccines and effective medicines, particularly for HIV/AIDS, cancers, and heart disease, are priced far above what poor countries or the individuals living in them can afford. Using an ingenious method for surveying all the elements that make up final prices, WHO and Health Action International have translated them into how many days an unskilled government worker has to work to pay for one month's supply of a given drug (Gelders, Ewen, Noguchi, & Laing, 2006). Although low-level government jobs are a prize in many countries, they barely pay for shelter, food, clothing, and transportation. Yet it takes on average 5.5 days' work to earn enough to pay for a month's supply of a patented medicine for asthma and 4.2 days' wages each month for a diabetic to pay for the patented medicine he needs. Field reports testify the obvious: an inhaler or bottle of pills can only be paid for by sacrificing meals or other essential needs. Many patients go without and suffer, as they also do in the United States (Safran et al., 2005). Prices vary widely, and the mark-ups by importers, wholesalers, and retail pharmacists each increase final costs substantially, as do import taxes and other fees. Still, a generic equivalent can cost the diabetic only 0.7 days of work for a month's supply, though often in developing countries they are in short supply because pharmacies often do not stock them.

The reason drugs cost so much, companies explain, is quite simple. While drugs and vaccines cost little to manufacture, the costs of research to discover, develop, and test them in human trials is immense, an average estimated in 2003 to be $800 million and now is declared to be $1.2 billion each (DiMasi, Hansen, & Grabowski, 2003; Tufts Center for the Study of Drug Development, 2006). This includes the costs of all the failures, and about half of these estimates consists of how much would have been made had the money been invested in stocks rather than sunk into research and development (R&D) project. Risks are also said to be high. Only one in every 5,000 candidate drugs makes it to market. Prices under patent protection must therefore be set high enough to recover all these costs and generate a reasonable profit before the patent expires (Pharmaceutical Research and Manufacturers of America, 1999). For these widely accepted reasons, prices have to be high. Even European and Canadian prices (an average of European prices) do not allow companies to recover R&D costs, so that

Americans have to make up the difference (United States Department of Commerce, 2004). These high costs and risks mean important medicines will be unaffordable to at least half the people in the world. Without high patent-protected prices, companies would have to cut back their research, causing future patients and generations to suffer even more (Aldonas, 2004).

In researching this moral dilemma, a pragmatic approach is most effective (McGee, 1999). First, one should investigate the realities of a situation in as much detail as possible and deconstruct what the claims and language really mean. This often clarifies the original dilemma in powerful ways. Second, one should look at how the situation arose and the roles of powerful actors in shaping it. One can then not only gauge the benefits and harms at stake but also have the information and perspective to suggest alternatives.

INVESTIGATING THE REALITIES BEHIND PATENT-PROTECTED PRICES

RESEARCH COSTS

BECAUSE THE MULTINATIONAL companies do not back their claims of huge R&D expenditures with verifiable figures, it is difficult to know the facts. However, the National Science Foundation has been tracking basic and applied research in all industries for over 50 years, and their latest figures show that pharmaceutical companies spent 12.4% of revenues on R&D (details in Light & Lexchin, 2005). Of that 12.4%, 18% went to basic research to discover new drugs. The rest is devoted to developing variations on existing molecules and testing. Thus, Glaxo-SmithKline's slogan that explains how high prices support breakthrough research—"Today's medicines pay for tomorrow's miracles"—is true only for 2.2% ($.18 \times .124$) of revenues, not 18% as the industry claims. Tax credits and savings reduce the net cost to the company to only 1.3% of revenues. A more detailed cost breakdown of R&D costs by the industry's trade association indicates that basic research accounted for only 9.3% of R&D, about half the NSF figure (summary in Light, 2006a), or 0.7% of revenues. This analysis indicates that the central claim made since the 1950s that high patented prices are essential to pay for huge R&D costs is not supported by even the industry's unverified facts.

The industry has devoted millions to supporting economists and their policy research centers to produce high estimates of R&D costs per new drug. What about the so-called fact that R&D costs $800 million, or $1.2 billion per new drug? These estimates are based on confidential numbers submitted by companies to the industry's leading policy research center. They are subject to several kinds of bias and variability that cannot be verified (Light & Warburton, 2005). Moreover, the sample used in the last two estimates was based on a small, nonrandom sample of firms and on the most costly subsample of new molecular entities (NMEs). The cost estimates were then claimed to be the estimate for all new drugs. Correcting that simple error alone drops the estimate in half and therefore suggests prices could be lower (overview in Light, 2007b).

There are indicators that company figures for R&D may include research-related costs such as legal expenses for crafting and defending patents, grants, and fees to doctors to participate in trials often larger than needed in order to sign them up as promoters of new products, companywide technical upgrades like a better computer or data-management system, smaller, unscientific trials used for marketing, medical writers to ghost-write favorable articles for publication, search costs for finding new R&D partners, and contract costs for signing them up. These are not actual costs of discovering new drugs and developing them but may be included in reporting high R&D costs. Moreover, companies do not reveal the actual cost of research to discover new molecules because it is so difficult to calculate. The industry-supported economists handle this problem by adding a large assumed amount that contributed 42% of the 2003 estimate of $800 million for R&D per new drug (DiMasi et al., 2003). Because of the way the analysis was done, the free contributions from basic research paid for by the National Institutes of Health (NIH) and large public research programs in the United Kingdom, Japan, Germany, France, Sweden, and elsewhere that often identify how a given pathogen and part of the body works were not counted as free research costs. Overall, about 84% of all funds for basic research to discover new medicines comes from public sources (Light, 2006a). If it were possible to correct for these sources of overstatement, the median costs of R&D would be still lower.

The industry's estimated costs of R&D are doubled by building in a high profit for all the years it takes to develop each drug and calling those estimated profits *cost of capital*. We normally think that cost of capital means the cost of borrowing, say, to buy a home. But this cost of capital is compounded at two to three times the cost of borrowing. The multiplier used by the pharmaceutical industry is more than twice the one recommended by government. If this exaggeration is corrected, the estimated cost of R&D becomes even smaller. One can even question whether cost of capital should be included at all. It is commonly calculated by companies to estimate whether a project is worth investing in, but should an estimate of profits forgone be claimed as several hundred million dollars that patients, governments, and society owe?

Other outside evidence indicates that the average costs of R&D are lower still. Previous investigations have found that the average size of trials used in the industry's high estimates are two to three times greater than reported independently by the FDA and about four times more costly than what is reported by the NIH (Love, 2003). The large trials we read about in the press are usually much larger than needed by the FDA for approval because they serve to sign up scores of leading specialists with handsome fees for recruiting and monitoring some patients in the trial, who then become the market launchers as they are paid lecture fees to talk up the new drug at professional meetings and clinical courses, most of which are also paid for by companies. Thus a sizable fraction of large trial costs are part of marketing, not R&D (Barton & Emanuel, 2005).

RISKS

RISKS ARE MUCH lower than claimed as well. As Angell (2004) and Goozner (2004) point out in two well-researched books, companies can say they screen 3,000, 5,000, or 10,000 drug candidates for each one that gets approved—it matters little because high-speed computerized screening methods are used (Angell, 2004; Goozner, 2004). By the time the best candidates begin phase-1 clinical trials, the risk is less than one in five (DiMasi et al., 2003). Phase-1 and phase-2 trials are relatively small. Two-thirds of costs occur in phase-3 trials when the risk is less than one in two. Thus, the high-risk investments at the beginning of a search for a new drug are relatively small. Further, companies spread these risks over many projects, each at different stages of rapidly declining risk in what is called portfolio management. Total corporate R&D risk is thus a fraction of the risk for any given project, and as major companies have combined into fewer, larger global corporations, their risk has declined even further.

MANUFACTURING COSTS

MANUFACTURING COSTS ARE equally secret, but from evidence that emerges from time to time, it appears that most pills cost $0.05–$0.10 each for the multinational companies to manufacture in bulk at a high standard of quality. Quality generic manufacturers, who are more focused on maximizing manufacturing efficiency, can produce pills for even less, $0.03–$0.05. Some AIDS drugs appear to cost only $100–$200 to manufacture a year's supply (evidence in Light, 2006b). Thus patent-protected prices are often 40–100 times manufacturing costs. Such large gross profit margins justify spending a great deal more on marketing, management, and development than other consumer products priced at 4–10 times costs, which result in companies reporting costs much higher than they would be if pharmaceutical companies were run to be efficient rather than to maximize profits from patent-protected prices by paying anything to sell more drugs.

GOOD PROFITS AT LOWER PRICES

ALTHOUGH A MAJOR pharmaceutical campaign claims that companies cannot earn back their R&D costs at European prices, industry and government reports show that companies earn back all costs, with good profits, at those prices (Light & Lexchin, 2005). Americans pay extra prices for extra profits. This fact reframes the extension of patent-protected prices built into the free trade agreements (FTAs) that the United States is requiring many poorer and smaller countries to sign (Light, 2007a). While most of the FTAs deal with lowering trade barriers for international companies in many other areas of trade, the section relevant to prescription drugs prohibits free trade and requires signees to extend market protections for several more years beyond patent expiration because the industry claims it is losing money everywhere except in the United States (Aldonas, 2004; United States Department of Commerce, 2004). This claim, however, is not supported by their own data.

FEW PROFITS OUTSIDE AFFLUENT COUNTRIES

NEARLY ALL PROFITS from medicines are made in the affluent sixth of the world (Outterson, 2006b). The seminal role of pharmaceutical companies in the World Trade Organization (WTO) movement to extend strong, long patents aims to extract more profits from less affluent countries that have weaker or no patent provisions. The claim is that stronger patent protections will foster investment and innovation in developing countries, but the reality is that "for diseases affecting millions of poor people in developing countries, patents are not a relevant factor or effective in stimulating R&D and bringing new products to the market" (Commission on Intellectual Property Rights, 2006, p. 34). In fact, leading experts in patent law and economics have concluded that patents have become more of an obstacle to innovation and a higher cost to society than a boon (Blonder, 2005; Clarkson & deKorte, 2006; Lessig, 2001). "Encouraging research through patents creates static distortions, underinvestment in research, and distortions of research toward duplicating existing innovations," concluded Michael Kremer (1998, p. 1140), the Gates Professor of Economics at Harvard. "Patents also distort the direction of research by creating too much incentive to develop substitutes for patented goods" (Kremer, 1998, p. 1140). Support comes from detailed evaluations that find that six out of every seven new drugs in the past 20 years offer no substantial benefit over existing drugs (Prescrire International, 2007).

In response to fierce criticism from Medecins sans Frontieres, Oxfam, and scores of advocacy groups for patients with HIV/AIDS that vital medicines are priced far above affordability, companies are offering lower prices to poorer countries. Although presented as a humanitarian response to make precious patented drugs available to poorer patients, tiered pricing is a well-known way to maximize profits, because one makes more money selling drugs at lower prices than if poorer people do not buy them at all.

Many people believe that low prices for the poorest countries, for example, $100–$150 for a year's supply of an AIDS drug, are a loss that is made up by affluent countries, a sort of charitable cross-subsidization built into their $10,000 price. But in a brilliant paper, Plahte (2005) shows that companies profit from sales even at the lowest tier. In fact, large-volume, low-price sales increase profits in the high-priced sixth of the world by lowering production costs. However, the lowest tiered prices may still have quite a bit of profit built into them and could be even lower, while the prices for so-called emerging markets of patients in countries with an average income of $3,000–$8,000 a year have a sizable profit. For example, in its analysis of tiers and prices for the new global vaccines for pneumococcal diseases, the GAVI Alliance calculates their price as averaging $55.07 a dose in affluent markets for 43 doses, $26.36 a dose in emerging markets for 131 million doses, and $7.54 in low-income markets for 178 million doses (GAVI pneumoADIP, 2006). Given that the vaccines cost $1–$2 to manufacture in bulk (Applied Strategies, 2006), the price for the huge poor markets is 3.7–7.5 times the cost, and for the large middle-income markets is 13–26 times the cost. If the goal is to eradicate diseases such as pneumococcal diseases, not only to end suffering and death but to help poor countries thrive, then vaccine prices for countries with a per capita budget of less than $100 a year to spend on all health care should be near cost or $1–$2 a dose, not $7 or $26. The same argument would hold for patented vaccines for other serious diseases of the poor that also have large affluent markets, like rotavirus and cervical cancer.

Even free samples and donated drugs generate profits, a point rarely recognized. As tax-deductible expenses, free samples and donation appear to save more in taxes than they cost. Consider Bayer's drug, Cipro, because we have quite good evidence that it costs about $0.10 to manufacture in volume (in Light, 2006b). If the average wholesale price of $4.67 is used to deduct it as a business expense, and if the marginal tax rate is 35%, then the tax savings are $1.67, or $1.57 in pure profit over cost. To sum up, globalizing long patents has more to do with extracting additional profits from poorer countries than with increasing innovation. Tiered prices as a concession are used by some companies in some markets, but set at levels still unaffordable to many.

MORAL PERSPECTIVES

IN 1972, SINGER wrote a seminal essay on our moral obligations to the distant poor and victims of tragedies, such as the millions destitute in East Bengal in 1971 (Singer, 1972). If we believe we should wade in and rescue a child drowning in a shallow pond, then, Singer maintained, "It makes no moral difference whether the person I can help is a neighbor's child ten yards from me or a Bengali whose name I shall never know, ten thousand miles away" (Singer, 1972, pp. 231–232). Our moral obligations are not distance-dependent. Secondly, Singer's principle "makes no distinction between cases in which I am the only person who could possibly do anything and cases in which I am just one among millions in the same position." The principle is that "if it is in our power to prevent something bad happening, without thereby sacrificing anything of comparable moral importance, we ought, morally, to do it." This principle "requires us only to prevent what is bad, and not promote what is good" (Singer, 1972, p. 231). If millions of others can help—donate to the victims of 9/11, or a tsunami, or a hurricane—so much the better. But it does not diminish one's own duty. Singer concludes that "The traditional distinction between duty and charity cannot be drawn" (Singer, 1972, p. 235). We may call what we give *charity* and the organizations that take it *charities,* but the term falsely implies there is nothing wrong with not giving. Singer maintains there is.

The research summarized here about the facts of R&D costs and risks, manufacturing costs, and pricing leaves no defensible reason for pharmaceutical companies not to make all patented and nonpatented medicines available to the world's poor, either free (and thus profiting from the tax deductions) or at very low cost.

In *Living High and Letting Die,* Unger (1996) extends and refines Singer's original work through a series of test cases, such as the man with a very nice car who sees a person lying by the road with a gash in his leg, waving for help as he bleeds profusely. Should you take the time and trouble to drive him to the hospital and have the inside of your nice car get soaked with blood? Even more dire is the case of Bob, who leaves his priceless vintage Bugatti on a railroad siding when he sees a runaway empty train barreling toward a child playing on the tracks. Bob could run and throw the switch so the train would avert the child but destroy his Bugatti. Should he? Most people think he should. Leaving aside fine points, responses indicate that people should be ready not only to help those in need but make material sacrifices. An implication of Singer's argument is that most people in affluent countries can give quite a bit of money—thousands of dollars—by just not spending it on clothes, accessories, and other things they really don't need to live a comfortable life. By analogy, if very low prices for the poor led pharmaceutical companies to earn a percent or two less return on capital, the bonuses and stock options of officers would be somewhat lower, but they would still be very well-off.

Unger takes readers through several kinds of moral distinctions, which include "fallacious futile thinking" (Unger, 1996, p. 63). Since my little gift or effort will make no difference anyway, the fallacy goes, there's no point of doing anything. Unger's book begins by urging readers to send $100 to the UNICEF oral rehydration therapy program, where $0.15 of salts will save a child's life. Saving one child, or several, matters.

Conservatives, however, are unconvinced. Responding to Singer, Narveson (2003) writes, "I have seen no plausible argument that we *owe* something, as a matter of general duty, to those to whom we have done nothing wrong" (p. 419). But an extensive historical literature documents the ways in which wealthy nations benefited from and exploited both the lands and the people they colonized. Many postcolonial forms of exploitation have developed, and Pogge (2002) argues that more compelling than the moral imperative to rescue those who are dying or seriously suffering is the imperative to help those one has harmed or exploited and also to stop those invidious legal, institutional, or economic practices. But Wade (2004), among others, has found that poor regions have suffered and inequality has worsened.

The reality of global poverty, ironically exacerbated by the globalization of so-called free trade and strong intellectual property (IP) protections from open competition, is ethically more like ambitious marathoners who knock weaker runners off the trail and down a precipice than it is like a passer-by seeing a child drowning in a shallow pond. If they stop to help those they have harmed, they will fall behind. Even more realistically, the marathoners are in a tight pack, and they knock others down but do not realize it until someone points it out. Do they say, "Oh really? Well, things happen in a tough race. That's too bad"? This is apparently how many corporate leaders respond in their global race for revenue growth, market share, and profits. Our first moral priority, Pogge contends, should be to address the harms that we as persons, corporations, and institutions inflict on others.

Making medicines unaffordable and less accessible to poor patients with HIV/AIDS and other serious disorders is an even more direct consequence of the WTO agreements concerning patents for pharmaceuticals. The small number of American-based global companies that crafted the Agreement on Trade Related Aspects of Intellectual Property Rights (TRIPS) required any nation that wanted to trade to end a long tradition in Europe and around the world of exempting medicines from patents as a social and humanitarian good and to extend patents from 7 or 10 or 13 years (depending on the country) to the global maximum of 20 years (Sell, 1998, 2003). Among the companies were Bristol-Meyer-Squibb, Johnson & Johnson, Merck, and Pfizer, the fierce promoter of government-protected pricing since the 1960s. The explicit goal was to *prohibit* free trade and low-priced generics from the emerging pharmaceutical industries in developing countries so that maximum, government-protected prices can be imposed on all nations that did not already have them. As the doctors and nurses of Medecins Sans Frontieres testify, needed drugs for patients with HIV/AIDS, cancer, and other life-threatening diseases are becoming unaffordable (Medecins Sans Frontieres, 2003; Medecins Sans Frontieres—Campaign for Access to Essential Medicines, 2007). Because generics shadow-price patented drugs, their prices are rising sharply too.

CONCLUSION

LONG, STRONG PATENTS and other IP rights for medicines in less affluent countries neither promote R&D, which largely takes place in a small number of affluent countries, nor generate much revenue. Relaxing or removing these rights qualifies as a moral duty under both Singer's and Pogge's concepts of justice. Outterson (2006a) has explored some of the options and legal issues. Unlike most property, patents are nonrivalrous, so allowing others to use them produces neither congestion nor exhaustion. Further, traditional property may be taken for public use and is subject to duties when others are harmed; so why should the intellectual property of patents on drugs needed to meet a public health need not be treated in similar ways? Compulsory licenses are analogous to eminent domain yet are less injurious to owners because they are partial and leave intact the owner's rights to profit in all other markets while they receive royalties for the licenses. Incentives for innovation are not weakened. It seems to be a win-win option. Since the mid-1980s, however, companies have vigorously advocated an expansion of their IP rights, like the marathoners, even if they harm others (Sell, 1998, 2003). At the behest of industry leaders, the United States Trade Representative's Office has vigorously opposed compulsory licensure and pressured poorer countries not to use TRIPS flexibilities in order to get affordable medicines to their patients (Abbott, 2004). Companies offer a variety of voluntary programs to provide vital medicines at little or no cost to poor patients. Thus the issue of how the rights of property owners should be balanced against the needs of poor patients with serious illnesses remains controversial.

REFERENCES

Abbott, F. M. (2004). *The DOHA declaration on the TRIPS agreement and public health: Contradictory trend in bilateral and regional free trade agreements.* Geneva: Friends World Committee for Consultation.

Aldonas, G. D. (2004). *International trade and pharmaceuticals.* Washington, DC: U.S. Senate Finance Committee, Subcommittees on Health and Trade

Angell, M. (2004). *The truth about the drug companies: How they deceive us and what to do about it.* New York: Random House.

Applied Strategies. (2006). *Advance market commitments: Financial implications and risk model.* London: Author.

Barton, J., & Emanuel, E. (2005). The patent-based pharmaceutical development process: Rationale, problems, and potential reforms. *Journal of American Medical Association, 294,* 2075–2082.

Blonder, G. (2005, December 20). Cutting through the patent thicket. *Business Week.* Retrieved August 21, 2008, from http://www.morgenthaler.com/content/Ventures/Articles/Articles%20documents/BusinessWeek%2012-20-05.pdf

Clarkson, G., & deKorte, D. (2006). The problem of patent thickets in convergent technologies. *Annals of the New York Academy of Sciences, 1093,* 180–200.

Commission on Intellectual Property Rights. (2006). *Public health innovation and intellectual property rights.* Geneva: Author.

DiMasi, J. A., Hansen, R. W., & Grabowski, H. (2003). The price of innovation: New estimates of drug development costs. *Journal Of Health Economics, 22,* 151–185.

GAVI pneumoADIP. (2006). *GAVI alliance investment case: Accelerating the introduction of pneumococcal vaccines into GAVI-eligible countries.* Baltimore, MD: Johns Hopkins Bloomberg School of Public Health.

Gelders, S., Ewen, M., Noguchi, N., & Laing, R. (2006). *Price, availability and affordability: An international comparison of chronic disease medicines.* Geneva: WHO and Health Action International.

Goozner, M. (2004). *The $800 million pill: The truth behind the cost of new drugs.* Berkeley: University of California Press.

Kremer, M. (1998). Patent buyouts: A mechanism for encouraging innovation. *The Quarterly Journal of Economics, 113,* 1137–1167.

Lessig, L. (2001). *The future of ideas: The fate of the commons in a connected world.* New York: Random House.

Light, D. W. (2006a). Basic research funds to discover important new drugs: Who contributes how much? In M. A. Burke (Ed.), *Monitoring the financial flows for health research 2005: Behind the global numbers* (pp. 27–43). Geneva: Global Forum for Health Research.

Light, D. W. (2006b). Pricing pharmaceuticals in the USA. In N. J. Temple & A. Thompson (Eds.), *Excessive medical spending: Facing the challenge* (pp. 63–79). Oxford, UK: Radcliffe Publishing.

Light, D. W. (2007a, March). Globalizing restricted and segmented markets: Challenges to theory and values in economic sociology. *The ANNALS,* 232–245.

Light, D. W. (2007b). Misleading Congress about drug development. *Journal of Health Politics, Policy and Law, 32,* 895–913.

Light, D. W., & Lexchin, J. (2005). Foreign free riders and the high price of US medicines. *BMJ, 331,* 958–960.

Light, D. W., & Warburton, R. N. (2005). Extraordinary claims require extraordinary evidence. *Journal of Health Economics, 24,* 1030–1033.

Love, J. (2003). *Evidence regarding research and development investments in innovative and non-innovative medicines.* Washington, DC: Consumer Project on Technology.

McGee, G. (1999). Pragmatic methods and bioethics. In G. McGee (Ed.), *Pragmatic bioethics* (pp. 18–29). Nashville, TN: Vanderbilt University Press.

Medecins Sans Frontieres. (2003). *Trading away health: Intellectual property and access to medicines in the Free Trade Area of the Americas (FTAA) agreement.* Paris: Author.

Medecins Sans Frontieres—Campaign for Access to Essential Medicines. (2007). *Submission to second public hearing on public health, innovation and intellectual property.* Retrieved August 21, 2008, from http://www.who.int/phi/public_hearings/second/contributions_section1/Section1_tHoen Ellen-MSF.pdf

Narveson, J. (2003). We don't owe them a thing! *The Monist, 86,* 419–433.

Outterson, K. (2006a). Fair followers: Expanding access to generic pharmaceuticals for low- and middle-income populations. In J. Cohen, P. Illingworth, & U. Schuklenk (Eds.), *The power of pills: Social, ethical and legal issues in drug development, marketing, and pricing* (pp. 164–178). London: Pluto.

Outterson, K. (2006b). Patent buy-outs for global disease innovations for low and middle income countries. *American Journal of Law and Medicine, 32,* 159–173.

Oxfam. (2002). Fatal side effects: Medicine patents under the microscope. In B. Granville (Ed.), *The economics of essential medicines* (pp. 81–99). London: Royal Institute of International Affairs

Pharmaceutical Research and Manufacturers of America. (1999). *Why do prescription drugs cost so much…and other questions about your medicine.* Washington, DC: Author.

Plahte, J. (2005). Tiered pricing of vaccines: A win-win-win situation, not a subsidy. *The Lancet Infectious Diseases, 5*(1), 58–63.

Pogge, T. W. (2002). *World poverty and human rights.* Malden, MA: Polity Press.

Prescrire International. (2007). A look back at pharmaceuticals in 2006: Aggressive advertising cannot hide the absence of therapeutic advances. *Prescrire International, 16*(88), 80–86.

Safran, D. G., Neuman, P., Schoen, C., Kitman, M., Wilson, I., Cooper, B., et al. (2005). Prescription drug coverage and seniors. *Health Affairs—Web Exclusive, W5*, 152–166.

Sell, S. K. (1998). *Power and ideas: North-south politics of intellectual property*. Albany: State University of New York Press.

Sell, S. K. (2003). *Private power, public law*. New York: Cambridge University Press.

Singer, P. (1972). Famine, affluence, and morality. *Philosophy and Public Affairs, 1*(3), 229–243.

Strong, K., Mathers, C., Leeder, S., & Beaglehole, R. (2005). Preventing chronic diseases: How many lives can we save? *Lancet, 336*, 1667–1671.

Tufts Center for the Study of Drug Development. (2006). *Average cost to develop a new biotechnology product is $1.2 billion, according to the Tufts Center for the Study of Drug Development*. Retrieved August 21, 2008, from http://csdd.tufts.edu/NewsEvents/NewsArticle.asp?newsid=69

Unger, P. (1996). *Living high and letting die: Our illusion of innocence*. New York: Oxford University Press.

United States Department of Commerce. (2004). *Pharmaceutical price controls in OECD countries: Implications for U.S. consumers, pricing, research and development and innovation*. Washington, DC: Author.

Wade, R. H. (2004). Is globalization reducing poverty and inequality? *World Development, 32*(4), 567–589.

World Health Organization. (2002). *Global chronic disease burden: 1990–2020*. Retrieved November 8, 2007, from http://www.who.int/dietphysical activity/media/en/gsdoc_principles_charts.pdf

Yach, D. Y., Hawkes, C., Gould, C. L., & Hofman, K. J. (2004). The global burden of chronic diseases. *Journal of American Medical Association, 291*, 2616–2622.

Part IX

Community and Public Health

Public Health Ethics: An Update on an Emerging Field

Michael Yudell

WRITING SHORTLY BEFORE his untimely death in 1998, the doctor and scholar Jonathan Mann called attention to a "crisis of identity about the nature, roles, and responsibilities of public health" and issued a clarion call for the field's "rebirth" (Mann, 1998, p. 118). Mann maintained that the source of this crisis was public health's "reluctance and inability to work directly on the societal roots of health problems" (Mann, 1998, p. 118). A rebirth of public health, Mann insisted, could begin only once the field developed a unifying ethos and language, and an ethics to govern it (Mann, 1997, 1998). These elements would give the field focus, unity, and direction, and would consequently give public health the moral authority to address its myriad research and clinical challenges. One does not have to agree with Mann's provocative admonition, now 10 years old, to find value in it. Indeed, a burgeoning literature exploring matters of public health ethics points to a growing interest in addressing what Mann articulated so plainly: that public health is in need of both an ethos and ethics to unify its disparate traditions and help advance its primary goal of making the public healthy.

WHAT IS PUBLIC HEALTH?

IT HAS BEEN challenging for a field that encompasses so many disparate disciplines and methodologies to define itself and articulate a common mission. The often-cited 1988 Institute of Medicine (IOM) report on public health defines the field as "what we, as a society, do collectively to assure the conditions in which people can be healthy" (IOM, 1988). This definition emphasizes public health's collective focus on improving the health of populations, thereby distinguishing it from clinical medicine, a field concerned primarily with improving the health of individual patients. The difference between medicine and public health, however, cannot simply be considered one of degree, nor should it be used as the sole basis for defining the field. It must not be overlooked that significant overlap exists between medicine and public health, that many medical doctors have training in public health and medicine, and that several subspecialties in medicine—including infectious disease and occupational and environmental medicine—are concerned with population health. Indeed, what sets public health apart is more than just its collective focus on the health of populations; it is that it strives to coordinate multiple disciplines, literatures, and methodologies into a coherent approach to making both the public as a whole and its subpopulations healthier.

In a sense, what makes public health so difficult to define is that ultimately the field itself is an ideal; a noble, multidisciplinary ambition whose sole goal is to improve the public's health. Under its umbrella epidemiologists, sociomedical scientists, biostatisticians, environmental health scientists, community and health policy experts, municipal workers, health care workers, and ethicists, among others, work in academia, private enterprise, the nonprofit sector, and government to fulfill the field's shared goals. And because of this disciplinary and bureaucratic diversity, the IOM's definition for the field inevitably falls short—it provides a common goal but lacks a shared vision and spirit for how public health is supposed to accomplish its tasks. Mann hoped to overcome this by calling for a public health ethic.

BEYOND AN IDEAL: AN ETHOS FOR A NEW PUBLIC HEALTH

THE FUNCTION OF a public health ethos would be to shape the field's core values, goals, boundaries, and duties, providing the discipline with purpose and intent and a framework to motivate both the ideals and intellects of its practitioners. Excepting its collective focus on population health, no dominant framework has yet unified public health practitioners.

THE HUMAN RIGHTS FRAMEWORK

MANN BELIEVED THAT a human rights framework was best suited to contribute to, if not shape, the core values of a renewed public health. "Modern human rights is an effort to identify, promote, and protect the societal pre-conditions for human well-being," Mann wrote in 1998, arguing that such an effort provided "public health with a more useful framework, vocabulary, and guidance for analysis and direct response to the societal determinants of health than any framework inherited from the past biomedical or public health tradition" (Mann, 1998, p. 120). A human rights framework would also create standards for the "societal foundation of individual and collective well-being" (p. 118). The foundation for human rights is the Universal Declaration of Human Rights, adopted by the United Nations in 1948. The declaration states that certain rights and freedoms should be held to a "common standard," including the right to life, liberty, and security of person. Article 25 of the declaration specifically names health as a right, acknowledging that a person has "the right to a standard of living adequate for the health and well-being of himself and his family" (United Nations, 1948).

Human rights can be understood in a legalistic sense (human rights as outlined and guaranteed by participation in international treaties) or in an aspirational sense (human rights as an ambition to which governments and peoples should strive; Gostin, 2001). A legalistic approach is hindered in the United States because it is neither a signatory to several of the legally binding international human rights treaties, nor are its legal precedents necessarily amenable to human rights interpretations. Nations that have seen success in the application of human rights principles to health seem to either have existing laws codifying a right to health or a judiciary eager to involve themselves in health reforms (Singh, Govender, & Mills, 2007). The concepts of health and human rights may therefore be most valuable in nations without such a legal framework when used to shape thinking and encourage action in public health practice.

An aspirational human rights framework also has its limits. According to Lawrence Gostin, the idea of human rights as applied to public health remains too broadly defined. Gostin also questions whether the individualistic focus of human rights is "consistent with public health's focus on collective well-being" (Gostin, 2001, p. 129). A significant challenge to integrating a human rights framework into an American context is that the language of human rights does not necessarily comport with the traditions of American political and legal culture. In the United States, rights "generally refers to individual civil rights based on non-interference rather than the more expansive rights articulated in the human rights framework" (Knowles, 2001, p. 256). Finally, in asserting claims that a human rights framework would address public health's failure to address the social origins of health problems, Mann and others ignore a long tradition of social justice in public health practice (Oppenheimer, Bayer, & Colgrove, 2002).

THE SOCIAL JUSTICE FRAMEWORK

THE APPLICATION OF social justice to public health—a framework that understands disparities in health as caused by social inequalities and seeks to identify and redress these problems—dates back more than 150 years (Daniels, Kennedy, & Kawachi, 1999). Some of the earliest work identifying social determinants of health was done in nineteenth-century France and England. In France, René Villermé's work exposed the relationship between poverty rates and morbidity and mortality rates. Despite the fact that Villermé opposed attempts to remedy these disparities (the conditions he exposed reflected "the nature of things"), his work established the sociomedical nature of the relationship between health and social status (Oppenheimer et al., 2002, p. 525). Edwin Chadwick's work in England was undertaken in order to understand origins of disease among the working class. Chadwick's report maintained that the environment (filth, excrement, and decaying organic matter) caused disease, and that sanitary measures were necessary for its prevention. By reducing the causes of illness to sanitation, Chadwick's work and advocacy removed "poverty, wretched housing, overwork, and hunger from the debate over social class and disease," and "gave aid and comfort" to those who supported the harsh labor policies of industrial England (Oppenheimer et al., 2002, p. 526). While these early examples linking social inequalities to health status may seem primitive by today's standards, they did initiate debates over the social determinants of health.

Contemporary social justice approaches to public health try to incorporate both an analysis of the social determinants of health and a means by which to address their impact. Social determinants of health include socioeconomic status, race, ethnicity, gender, sexual orientation, age, culture, social organization, and political participation (Daniels et al., 1999). Ideally, a social justice framework seeks to control hazards to health, prevent death and disability through collective action, and create a system whereby burdens of health are "shared equally by all except where unequal burden results in increased protection of everyone's health and especially potential victims of death and disability" (Beauchamp, 1999, p. 107). The social justice paradigm has been faulted because there is no universal agreement on determining "which inequalities in health outcomes are unjust," nor is there consensus on how to address these inequalities (Peter, 2004, p. 94).

Ultimately, a social justice framework can provide public health with the motivation and awareness that the social determinants of health must be studied, but it does not necessarily tell us what to do about them (other than eliminate or mollify them). Therefore, unlike human rights, which legislates or proposes minimum standards for health, a social justice framework "only points in the right direction," leaving "open how we should go about making judgments of unfairness and injustice" (Peter, 2004, p. 94).

THE COMMUNITARIAN FRAMEWORK

A THIRD FRAMEWORK offered by the ethicist Dan Beauchamp proposes a communitarian language of public health that elucidates the field's focus on populations and provides a community-based justification for public health interventions. Beauchamp draws on the literature of American political history to explore the intellectual precedents for a communitarian ethos for public health, noting that democracy in the United States can sustain two complementary ideologies: a traditionally liberal one that emphasizes "private interests and private rights" and the protection of these rights, and a communitarian one that emphasizes that "individuals are members of a political community—a body politic" (Beauchamp, 1985, p. 29; Gerstle, 1994; Gibson, 2000). A communitarian ethos, Beauchamp maintains, provides a language of public health that is an alternative to "the dominant discourse of political individuals" that relies "on the harm principle or a narrow paternalism justified on the grounds of self-protection alone" (Beauchamp, 1985, p. 34). Instead, the protection of the public's health is regarded as a community interest. This ethos provides the intellectual foundation for "encouraging citizens to share in reasonable and practical group schemes to promote a wider welfare," for community based participatory research, and for the unity of the public health community itself (Beauchamp, 1985, p. 35). While this framework offers important foundational thinking and justifications for public health practice, its general definition of community may not always serve public health well, especially in a republic where minority communities may not always factor into definitions of community interest.

THE JURIDICAL FRAMEWORK

FINALLY, THE BIOETHICIST and legal scholar Mark Rothstein is critical of recent attempts to expand the definition of public health, arguing that it is "incongruous to embrace the broadest meaning of public health at the same time that our legal system and public health infrastructure are based on a narrow definition of public health juris-diction, authority, and remedies" (Rothstein, 2002, p. 148). Rothstein instead advocates for a "government intervention as public health" framework, described as "public officials taking appropriate measures pursuant to specific legal authority, after balancing private rights and public interests, to protect the health of the public" (Rothstein, 2002, p. 146). This narrow, juridical approach to public health reduces the field's practice to one that "involves government action, coercive powers, and societal interests taking precedence over individual rights" (Rothstein, 2002, p. 147). In this framework, public health is a reactionary force, paternalistic at its core, wielded in limited circumstances to protect population health when threatened or when government expertise is unique or most efficient. And while this framework certainly accounts for some of contemporary public health practice, it fails to acknowledge the breadth of the field.

A PROPOSAL FOR SYNTHESIS

A S STAND-ALONE FRAMEWORKS, these four models do not offer a comprehensive ethos for public health. Separately, I do not believe they can address Mann's concern that public health lacks "a conceptual framework for identifying and analyzing" the social factors that influence health (Mann, 1997, p. 8). However, a synthesis of the aforementioned frameworks would address Mann's concerns about our field's shortcomings and capitalize on public health's traditions to shape its future. The four models contain the fundamentals of a new public health ethos: minimum standards for the public's health (human rights), methods by which to identify and address the social determinants of health (social justice), an explanation of and a rationale for why communities and populations are the focus of public health practice (a communitarian ethos), and the understanding that paternalistic interventions that sacrifice individual liberties can be justified in the interest of the public's health (government intervention as public health). From these basic tenets we can work toward shaping a new public health ethos, an aspirational framework and values system for public health practitioners. Integrating a value system into public health cannot simply be about the shared skills and competencies of public health. Instead, we can instill these values into public health professionals by incorporating human rights and social justice courses into public health curricula and by teaching students about the history of public health, a history that acknowledges the contradictory strains of community and liberalism in our democratic beliefs.

IN SEARCH OF A PUBLIC HEALTH ETHICS

IN 2002, THE American Public Health Association (APHA) published its first code of ethics for public health practitioners. The code's authors hoped that their work would "make clear to populations and communities the ideals of public health institutions that serve them, ideals for which the institutions can be held accountable" (Thomas, Sage, Dillenberg, & Guillory, 2002, p. 1057). Titled *Principles of Ethical Practice of Public Health*, the code lists 12 principles written to establish acceptable behaviors and values for public health practitioners. The principles stress social justice, human rights, community, and the protection of research subjects. Its authors hope that its "adoption by key national agencies and organizations will imbue the code with a degree of moral authority that will increase both its utility and the likelihood that it will be adopted and used by national, state, and local institutions" (Thomas et al., 2002, p. 1058).

The code is written in a tentative language of what public health institutions and practitioners should do in terms of ethical conduct. The bioethicist Robert Olick points out that the code "does not offer a comprehensive moral system of ethics, nor is it an ethics prescription for practitioners seeking specific action-guides for concrete decisions" (Olick, 2004, p. 89). The code does seek to balance the interests of populations and individuals (Principle 2: "Public health should achieve community health in a way that respects the rights of individuals in the community"), "but it does not tell us how to balance these commitments when they are in conflict; it does not tell us what we ought to do in particular cases" (Thomas et al., 2002, p. 1058; see also Olick, 2004, p. 89). This question of how to balance the interests of populations and individuals is the central question of formulating a public health ethics. These limitations to the code reflect a failure to engage both specific ethical principles and the legal underpinnings of public health practice. In essence, the APHA issued an ethos for the field but failed to produce a code that could govern behavior in public health and hold public health institutions and practitioners accountable.

Public health ethics still lacks the theoretical foundations and the synergy between theory and practice that is exploited, for example, in a field like bioethics. The ethicist Nancy Kass notes that public health practitioners are often forced to turn to medical ethics and research codes "for professional moral direction" (Kass, 2001, p. 1777). Bioethical theory and principles are well documented and, in the United States, are integrated into the protection of human subjects in biomedical research. The "Belmont Report," published in the *Federal Register* in 1979, outlines the general principles of bioethics (respect for person, beneficence, and justice) and mandates requirements for research practice (informed consent, risk/benefit assessment, and just selection of the subjects for research; Jonsen, 1998). Public health research has no comparable underlying theory or *Belmont Report*–like protections specific to public health practice and research (National Commission for the Protection of Human Subjects of Biomedical and Behavioral Research, 1979).

There are competing emerging theoretical frameworks for a public health ethics that seek to address both of these concerns. James Childress and colleagues have outlined, for example, five "justificatory conditions...intended to help determine whether promoting public health warrants overriding such values as individual liberty or justice." These conditions are *effectiveness* (will the intervention protect public health?); *proportionality* (will "benefits outweigh the infringed general moral considerations?"); *necessity* ("is there a supportable, good faith belief that justifies a coercive approach?"); *least infringement* (does the intervention "seek to minimize the infringement of general moral considerations?"); and *public justification* (does the action "explain and justify" itself to effected parties?) (Childress et al., 2002, p. 172).

An alternative approach has been proposed by Ronald Bayer and Amy Fairchild. Bayer and Fairchild believe that public health ethics requires "a population-based analysis and a willingness to recognize that the ethics of collective health may require far more extensive limitations on privacy...and on liberty," unlike the autonomy-based focus of bioethics (Bayer & Fairchild, 2004, p. 490). In other words, the theoretical bases for a public health ethics concern "paternalism and subordination of the individual for the good of the commonwealth" (Bayer & Fairchild, 2004, p. 488). Bayer and Fairchild do not offer the kind of "justificatory conditions" that Childress and colleagues propose. They instead call on ethicists "to define those moments when public health paternalism is justified and to articulate a set of principles that would preserve a commitment to the realm of free choice" (Bayer and Fairchild, 2004, p. 492).

The theoretical approaches outlined here do little, however, to address questions specific to the ethics of public health research. This is an area that has received far less attention in the nascent public health ethics literature, in part, because current institutional review boards already review public health-related research and because of the more traditional focus of ethicists on questions of balancing individual rights with population health. David Buchanan and Franklin Miller argue that the moral obligations of protecting population health affect the "ethical norms to guide research ethics" (Buchanan & Miller, 2006, p. 729). They would amend research ethics to include the following considerations: "the duty to protect the population as a whole; a fiduciary obligation to realize the social value of research; and the moral responsibility to distribute the benefits and burdens of research fairly across society" (Buchanan & Miller, 2006, p. 732). Ethicists have also drawn attention to the idea of community consent and review as a part of population research ethics. Richard Sharp and Morris Foster have shown, for example, that in public health genomics research "all members of a socially identifiable group may be affected by genetic information obtained from just a few individual members of that group." To protect these groups they advocate "the need for members of study populations to be directly involved in the review process" (Sharp & Foster, 2000, p. 41). Sandra Crouse Quinn proposes that one way to protect populations in public health research would be to involve, when possible, community advisory boards that can help protect communities and foster meaningful research. Quinn advocates the adoption of the principle of "respect for communities" to complement the principles of the "Belmont Report" (Quinn, 2004, p. 922).

Finally, one area of public health ethics that is already well formed can be found in public health law. Public health law has the "explicitly moral purpose…of promoting and protecting the lives of citizens" (Callahan & Jennings, 2002, p. 173). Existing legal mechanisms can be used, as ethicists Daniel Callahan and Bruce Jennings write, in order to "coerce citizens into behaving in some approved, healthy way." Examples of public health laws include the compulsory vaccination of children, antismoking laws, and the use of quarantine to limit the spread of disease (Callahan & Jennings, 2002, p. 173).

CONCLUSION

THE FRAMEWORKS AND concerns outlined above regarding public health ethics are only part of the ongoing discussions and debates that are shaping this new field. While there have been various proposals for an ethos that would shape public health, it does not yet seem possible to articulate a definitive ethics for the entire field. This may be because public health still remains a poorly integrated profession, made up of disparate disciplines with different methodologies and already existing ethical standards for their work. Indeed, creating a public health ethics will be a challenge for this field. But if bioethics serves as an example, a consensus will eventually emerge on this matter, driven by the needs of an ever-evolving field and by threats, both social and biological in nature.

Jonathan Mann will long be remembered for his visionary work in HIV/AIDS care and policy and for his creative insight into the needs of the rapidly changing field of public health. It is a terrible loss that his death prevented him from engaging in what has become a fertile discussion about the nature of public health and how the field should define its values and its ethics. But Mann's imprint remains unmistakable in the evolving literature of public health ethics. The debates about public health ethics will continue to shape our field, and, like bioethics before us, will, over time, become integrated into public health practice. Until that day comes, we owe it to the public we serve to define our values and to articulate a governing ethics that can hold us all accountable for our actions.

REFERENCES

Bayer, R., & Fairchild, A. L. (2004). The genesis of public health ethics. *Bioethics, 18*, 473–492.

Beauchamp, D. E. (1985). Community: The neglected tradition in public health. *Hastings Center Report, 15*, 32–38.

Beauchamp, D. E. (1999). Public health as social justice. In D. E. Beauchamp & B. Steinbock (Eds.), *New ethics for the public's health* (pp. 101–109). New York: Oxford University Press.

Buchanan, D. R., & Miller, F. G. (2006). A public health perspective on research ethics. *Journal of Medical Ethics, 32*, 729–733.

Callahan, D., & Jennings, B. (2002). Ethics and public health: Forging a strong relationship. *American Journal of Public Health, 92*, 169–176.

Childress, J. F., Faden, R. R. Gaare, R. D., Gostin, L. O., Kahn, J., Bonnie, R. J., et al. (2002). Public health ethics: Mapping the terrain. *Journal of Law, Medicine, and Ethics, 30*, 170–178.

Daniels, N., Kennedy, B. P., & Kawachi, I. (1999). Why justice is good for our health: The social determinants of health inequalities. *Daedalus, 128*, 215–251.

Gerstle, G. (1994). The protean character of American liberalism. *American Historical Review, 99*, 1043–1073.

Gibson, A. (2000). Ancients, moderns, and Americans: The republicanism-liberalism debate revisited. *History of Political Thought, 21*, 261–307.

Gostin, L. O. (2001). Public health, ethics, and human rights: A tribute to the late Jonathan Mann. *Journal of Law, Medicine, and Ethics, 29*, 121–130.

Institute of Medicine. (1988). *The future of public health*. Washington, DC: National Academy Press.

Jonsen, A. R. (1998). *The birth of bioethics*. New York: Oxford University Press.

Kass, N. E. (2001). An ethics framework for public health. *American Journal of Public Health, 91*, 1776–1782.

Knowles, L. P. (2001). The lingua franca of human rights and the rise of a global bioethic. *Cambridge Quarterly of Healthcare Ethics, 10*, 253–263.

Mann, J. M. (1997). Medicine and public health, ethics and human rights. *The Hastings Center Report, 27*, 6–13.

Mann, J. M. (1998). Society and public health: Crisis and rebirth. *Western Journal of Medicine, 169,* 118–121.

National Commission for the Protection of Human Subjects of Biomedical and Behavioral Research. (1979). *The Belmont Report.* Retrieved October 31, 2007, from http://www.hhs.gov/ohrp/humansubjects/guidance/belmont.htm

Olick, R. S. (2004). Codes, principles, laws, and other sources of authority in public health. *Journal of Public Health Management and Practice, 10,* 88–89.

Oppenheimer, G. M., Bayer, R., & Colgrove, J. (2002). Health and human rights: Old wine in new bottles? *Journal of Law, Medicine, and Ethics, 30,* 522–535.

Peter, F. (2004). Health equity and social justice. In S. Anand, F. Peter, & A. Sen (Eds.), *Public health, ethics, and equity* (pp. 93–106). New York: Oxford University Press.

Quinn, S. C. (2004). Protecting human subjects: The role of community advisory boards. *American Journal of Public Health, 94,* 918–922.

Rothstein, M. A. (2002). Rethinking the meaning of public health. *Journal of Law, Medicine, and Ethics, 30,* 144–149.

Sharp, R. R., & Foster, M. W. (2000). Involving study populations in the review of genetic research. *Journal of Law, Medicine, and Ethics, 28,* 41–51.

Singh, J. A., Govender, M., & Mills, E. J. (2007). Do human rights matter to health? *The Lancet, 370,* 521–527.

Thomas, J. C., Sage, M., Dillenberg, J., & Guillory, V. J. (2002). A code of ethics for public health. *American Journal of Public Health, 92,* 1057–1059.

United Nations. (1948). *Universal declaration of human rights.* Retrieved October 31, 2007, from http://www.un.org/Overview/rights.html

49

Bioethics "On the Ground": Public Health Matters

JOANNE GODLEY

PUBLIC HEALTH PRACTITIONERS regularly encounter ethical challenges (Kass, 2004). For instance, an environmental health services sanitarian who is offered money to overlook violations assessed during a restaurant inspection may be aware that there is an ethical matter at hand because she has been specifically trained to be vigilant about possible bribes (and trained to refuse them!). However, some ethical issues may not always be so apparent. For example, flu vaccine was in scarce supply during a recent flu season. The decision to distribute a limited quantity of vaccine that is insufficient to immunize an at-risk population is an ethical issue (Melnick, Kaplowitz, Lopez, & Murphy, 2005). The decision to allow patients to queue up at a public health clinic at 6 A.M. in inclement weather (because the medical care is free and the number of persons who can be seen daily is limited) has ethical implications. One could question whether it is ethical to channel federal money earmarked in the local health department's budget for bioterrorism activities to fund more critically needed public health services. These are examples of ethical dilemmas that can arise in the public health arena. There are several reasons why a public health practitioner may fail to frame them as ethical quandaries: (a) the decision-maker may be unaware that they are ethical issues, (b) the decision-maker may be aware and choose not to be transparent about her ethical decision-making process, or (c) the decision-maker may be aware that these are ethical dilemmas and not know how to address them.

A public health code of ethics was created in 2002 in order to provide public health practitioners with a moral framework that would serve as the basis for all public health activities (Public Health Leadership Society, 2002) (see Exhibit 49.1). The code expresses a common value system (Thomas, Sage, Dillenberg, & Guillory, 2002). Public health practitioners can employ the code practically, as a template, in order to recognize and understand the underlying ethical elements of a situation. And it can be used as a guide for an appropriate professional response. This chapter describes specific on the ground experiences in a local health department to demonstrate the practical utility of the ethics code and the associated principles.

EXHIBIT 49.1

Principles of the Ethical Practice of Public Health

1. Public health should address principally the fundamental causes of disease and requirements for health, aiming to prevent adverse health outcomes.
2. Public health should achieve community health in a way that respects the rights of individuals in the community.
3. Public health policies, programs, and priorities should be developed and evaluated through processes that ensure an opportunity for input from community members.
4. Public health should advocate for, or work for the empowerment of, disenfranchised community members, ensuring that the basic resources and conditions necessary for health are accessible to all people in the community.
5. Public health should seek the information needed to implement effective policies and programs that protect and promote health.
6. Public health institutions should provide communities with the information they have that is needed for decisions on policies or programs and should obtain the community's consent for their implementation.
7. Public health institutions should act in a timely manner on the information they have within the resources and the mandate given to them by the public.
8. Public health programs and policies should incorporate a variety of approaches that anticipate and respect diverse values, beliefs, and cultures in the community.

9. Public health programs and policies should be implemented in a manner that most enhances the physical and social environment.

10. Public health institutions should protect the confidentiality of information that can bring harm to an individual or community if made public. Exceptions must be justified on the basis of the high likelihood of significant harm to the individual or others.

11. Public health institutions should ensure the professional competence of their employees.

12. Public health institutions and their employees should engage in collaborations and affiliations in ways that build the public's trust and the institution's effectiveness.

HIV PREVENTION IN JAIL

WHILE REVIEWING THE medical policies and records at the local jail (at the request of the city's jail commissioner), a physician from the local health department noted the following deficiencies.

There were no health education programs or screening policies in place for inmates or prison staff for HIV or for hepatitis C; there were no HIV prevention policies in place. The treatment protocols for sexually transmitted infections (STIs, e.g., chlamydia and gonorrhea) were outdated. There had been a recent tuberculosis (TB) outbreak involving a few inmates and a staff member. When she raised the issue of HIV prevention policies for the inmates, the jail commissioner showed her the results of a recent survey among the correction officers—the majority of whom were against the distribution of condoms. He informed her that the consensus among the staff was that the distribution of condoms would encourage sexual activity and that sex was illegal in the jail system. The jail commissioner indicated that the issue was closed.

Consider the following hypothetical scenario: In a town of well-meaning people, at the end of Main Street, there is a large black hole in the middle of the street that no one talks about. Each week, two or three different people, inadvertently, fall into the hole. They eventually reappear covered with a gross rash that is itchy and very contagious. The rash quickly spreads throughout the town. Health authorities are summoned from an outside town to control the dissemination of the rash. However, no one mentions the hole.

DISCUSSION

THE LATE JONATHAN Mann championed the idea that medicine, public health, ethics, and human rights are intimately related. He maintained that protecting the public's health meant promoting and protecting human rights. He was one of the original supporters of the concept that public health should have its own code of ethics. The code reflects his strong bias for a human rights–oriented framework and incorporates human rights language (Mann, 1997). The first sentence of the 12 values underlying the code belies its human rights–based conceptual foundation, "Humans have a right to the resources necessary for health" (Public Health Leadership Society, 2002). This principle also applies to incarcerated humans.

Because the public health ethics code is human rights–based, public health practitioners who advocate for quality medical and preventive health care for prisoners and for educating the public about the importance of this issue to the public's health are following the code's basic tenets. Prisons and jails are known to be huge reservoirs of infectious diseases, such as STIs, TB, methicillin-resistant Staphylococcus aureus (MRSA), hepatitis C, HIV, and AIDS. HIV infection is three times more prevalent in prison than in the general community (Kantor, 2006). Prison inmates are members of our society. They return from prison and, if they have acquired an infectious disease, they risk transmitting it throughout the community. If, as was described in the earlier thought experiment, prisons are regarded as black holes and ignored, it will be impossible to ever gain control of these important public health diseases.

In addition to human rights, the other key values upon which the public health code of ethics is based are human interdependence, prevention, and social justice. Interdependence is a key value in public health just as respect for autonomy is a key value in medical ethics (Thomas, 2005). Interdependence speaks to the fact that there is fluidity between prisons and the larger society. People from the community staff the prisons, and family and friends of inmates visit and go home. The high prevalence of infectious diseases in the prisons poses risks to the staff and visitors as well as to the inmates. There are few hand-washing facilities in prisons, there is limited personal protective equipment for staff usage, and staff are subject to encountering blood-borne pathogens while carrying out routine duties in the laundry, during interactions with inmates (body searches, potentially being gassed by inmates with body fluids), and while working in the clinical area of the prison (Bick, 2007).

In the aforementioned case, condoms served as an example of a prevention measure for HIV/AIDS and STIs for which public health practitioners should advocate. Another prevention measure is a policy that would allow inmates to receive nonoccupational postexposure prophylaxis for HIV on demand—following potential exposure to blood-borne pathogens (Bick, 2007). The Centers for Disease Control and Prevention (CDC) have recently recommended that HIV screening be performed routinely and without informed consent in all health care settings (including prisons) and that patients only be able to opt out. Those at high risk (i.e., prisons) should be screened annually (CDC, 2006).

The public's health is inextricably tied to the manner in which the most vulnerable members are treated. Traditionally, the indicator of a society's level of health or quality of life has been the infant mortality rate. Another index of societal well-being ought to be the degree of morbidity within a society's inmate population. These are issues about which public health practitioners should be educating policy makers and the public. "The challenges for public health officials in balancing the goals of promoting and protecting public health and ensuring that human rights and dignity are not violated call urgently for ethical analysis. The official nature of much public health work places public health practitioners in a complex environment, in which work to promote rights inevitably challenges the state system within which the official is employed" (Mann, 1997, p. 9). As suggested by the late Jonathan Mann, the *failure* of public health practitioners to consistently call into question the health policies of their own institutions raises ethical concerns.

REDUCING FETAL LOSS

A LOCAL HEALTH department was asked to provide birth data for a multicenter study designed to reduce fetal loss in women at high risk for repeat preterm births. The proposed study was a randomized controlled trial targeting minority and economically disadvantaged women who had just experienced a preterm birth. The treatment arm of participants would be evaluated and known risk factors for preterm birth would be addressed, including: identification and treatment of vaginal infections and identification and treatment of gingival infections. Housing and job assistance would be given to women identified as being in need of those social supports, they would be screened and treated for depression, routine medical care would be administered, nutritional status would be assessed and addressed, literacy would be tested, educational assistance given, and they would be counseled about delaying a repeat pregnancy. The women in the control arm of the study would be screened for all of the parameters listed above and simply followed on a monthly basis. If any of the parameters screened were found positive, the women in the control group would be advised to follow up with their usual source of care. The institutional review board for the local health department approved the study. However, the health department's chief ethics officer did not.

DISCUSSION

THE PUBLIC HEALTH ethics code is composed of a series of statements. If one changes the statements in the public health code of ethics to questions, they can be used as a template that one can apply to ethical problems. The first four questions developed from the ethics code are useful in the evaluation of the proposed study to reduce fetal loss.

1. Are public health providers addressing the basic causes of disease, assessing what is needed for health and trying to prevent adverse health outcomes?

The answer to the first question is no. In the study design of the experiment described above, the control group of women would not have been not be treated. If any one of them were diagnosed with an infection, they would be told to seek care as per usual. The problem with this scenario is that economically disadvantaged women typically do not have a usual source of care or have poor quality care. The study design exploits the fact that a majority of the women in the control group would have ended up having most of their medical problems untreated. If any of these women were to become pregnant, she would, then, be at increased risk for preterm birth.

2. Are public health providers approaching community health in a manner respectful of the individuals in the community? Would the provider feel comfortable implementing the same program/policy in his community?

This second question speaks to the concept of transparency, one of the underlying values framing the code of public health ethics. Transparency means that public health professionals have been entrusted to act on behalf of the common welfare and that honesty and truth telling are part of the implicit pact. Being transparent in this study would require the researcher to divulge the fact that an untreated vaginal or gum infection would put a woman at risk for preterm birth, among other things (Goldenberg & Culhane, 2006; Wadhwa et al., 2001). It would require the researcher to divulge the fact that high blood pressure might be discovered and nothing would be done about it and a stroke or heart attack might be one of the outcomes. If one were unlucky enough to be assigned to the control group, one would simply be tested and followed but not treated.

3. Were the public health policies/programs/priorities developed and evaluated with the community?

The answer to this question is no. There were institutional review boards (IRBs) that approved the study in question, but it was not presented to a community board. Community consultation or presentation of research proposals to communities representative of those for whom the studies are targeted has been recommended as a means of aligning research ideas with local community interests (Parker, Alvarez, & Thomas, n.d.).

4. Are public health providers advocating to achieve the conditions necessary for health for the most disenfranchised community members?

Even if this study were to answer a critical question about preterm birth, it would do so at the expense of the lives of a group of vulnerable women and their potential birth outcomes. This study would violate the public health code of ethics by exploiting (rather than helping) vulnerable women who do not have good medical care, literacy training, or money.

SCREENING IN HIGH SCHOOL

IN RESPONSE TO statistics indicating that gonorrhea and chlamydia infections were at epidemic levels among urban teenagers, a local health department partnered with the city's education board and instituted a citywide STI screening and treatment program in all public high schools. There are state laws and city statutes that support the screening and treatment of minors. Meetings were held with parents and school boards. All students were informed that their decision to participate in this program was voluntary. The feasibility of the program was based on the fact that the infections could be tested from a urine sample. After listening to a peer-based presentation on STIs, all students were given paper bags with a urine container inside and all students were required to go to the bathroom and turn in the bag. Each student could then decide whether or not to submit a urine sample for STD testing when they turned in their bag. Those teens testing positive were notified and treated and given partner notification cards. Rescreening was done in 3–4 months.

At the onset of the screening program, the decision was made to *not* give out condoms or test for HIV. An FDA-approved rapid test for HIV was commercially available at the time that the high school screening program was instituted.

DISCUSSION

THIS PROGRAM TARGETED youth attending public high schools in a large urban city, the majority of whom were Black and Hispanic. The major failing of this program is that it focused on only one facet of the epidemic of sexually transmitted diseases in that age group (i.e., gonorrhea and chlamydia infections). It failed to test for and offer specific prevention methods for the most serious of all STIs, HIV. CDC data confirms that HIV prevalence among teenagers, particularly African American young women, is on the rise. Having an STI like gonorrhea or chlamydia greatly increases a person's risk of acquiring or transmitting HIV. HIV/AIDS is now epidemic among African Americans of all ages (CDC, 2006). If one applies the public health ethics code as a template, the failure to test for HIV among this population can be viewed as a social justice issue. It is a missed opportunity to address a significant racial health disparity, namely, the burgeoning epidemic of HIV among African Americans. Screening for and treating STIs without addressing HIV/AIDS in an at-risk population is like using a water pistol on a raging fire. Simply put, it is unjust. Jonathan Mann alluded to such practices as potentially stemming from bias. He stated,

> Public health practice is heavily burdened by the problem of inadvertent discrimination. For example, outreach activities may "assume" that all populations are reached equally by a single, dominant-language message on television; or analysis "forgets" to include health problems uniquely relevant to certain groups, like breast cancer or sickle cell disease; or a program "ignores" the actual response capability of different population groups, as when lead poisoning warnings are given without concern for financial ability to ensure lead abatement. Indeed, inadvertent discrimination is so prevalent that all public health policies and programs should be considered discriminatory until proven otherwise, placing the burden on public health to affirm and ensure its respect for human rights. (Mann, 1997, p. 5)

Public health policies and public health institutional practices need to better reflect the social justice and human rights principles espoused in the ethics codes. Gostin terms this the "justice perspective": vigorously challenging policies and practices that maintain poor health among the already disadvantaged, and promoting programs and policies that address the social determinants of poor health (Gostin & Powers, 2006).

BANNING TRANS-FATS

IN RESPONSE TO an alarming rise in obesity rates in a major urban area, several local board of health members suggested that the city health department follow the lead of another urban health department and ban the citywide use of trans-fats in restaurant food.

DISCUSSION

THE RISK OF developing heart disease or becoming obese is an individual risk that is frequently tied to an individual behavior (i.e., a trans-fat-laden diet). Banning the use of trans-fats in restaurant food could be considered paternalistic and construed as potentially restricting an individual's autonomy or right to choose (Bayer, 2004). The commitment to the importance of health is delineated in the first principle of the public health ethics code: "Humans have a right to the resources necessary for health." In other words, everyone should have the opportunity to make the healthiest possible choices. And that may not happen if all of the foods have been prepared using trans-fats. The role of public health is to facilitate the public's ability to make healthier individual lifestyle choices.

The commitment to prevention, another central value in public health ethics, often requires the adoption of a paternalistic stance. Robert Goodin is a philosopher who supports public policy development based on utilitarian principles. He notes that critical issues of public safety and health are not left to individual determination (e.g., whether or not to drink polluted water or eat contaminated food). One of the basic tenets of public health is the protection of the public. This is an inherently paternalistic principle. Public health measures that could be interpreted as imposing on an individual's rights (e.g., community water fluoridation) are defended by governmental agencies on the basis of the calculated benefit afforded to the larger majority (Goodin, 2006). Public health has taken up a similar prevention mantle in the past in advocating for seat belts in cars or advocating against the marketing of alcohol and certain fast foods to youth. Public health is a practical and action-oriented discipline. Public health policies are often developed based on imprecise evidence. While trans-fats do not definitely cause disease, the precautionary principle would dictate that the best action is to avoid them.

THE BIKER AND THE MONKEY

THE MOTORCYCLE SLOWED and stopped as the traffic light turned red. A tiny furred head peeped out from the inner confines of the biker's leather jacket. Within seconds, the monkey leaped down from the motorcycle and hopped over to the little girl who stood on the street corner next to her mother. The girl shrieked when she saw the monkey, who promptly bit her on the leg. The girl was taken to a hospital where the wound was attended. The local health department was contacted. Later that afternoon, the monkey was seized and placed into quarantine at the city's animal control division. The owner was fined for keeping a nondomestic animal as a pet. The following day, the health department's communicable disease director appeared before a judge (in an emergency judicial hearing) to request permission to euthanize the animal and examine its brain for evidence of rabies. The events were leaked to the press and the health commissioner's office was inundated with calls from animal rights groups protesting the monkey's treatment.

DISCUSSION

IN THEIR MANDATES to promote and protect the public's health, federal, state, and local health agencies maintain a list of reportable diseases. These diseases are considered to be of great significance to public health, and physicians and laboratories are required to submit a report to the local public health agency when they diagnose any of these conditions. Rabies is a reportable disease. Any animal suspected of being infected with rabies (i.e., exhibiting bizarre or unusually aggressive behavior) is quarantined and observed for signs of rabies for a specific period of time. The animal control division frequently handles animals that are considered a menace or a threat to the public's health. There are city statutes that give the health department the power to seize such animals. The animal control division had not had experience with rabid monkeys (nor had the primate experts that the health department consulted), and it was determined that the most precise diagnostic method for the detection of rabies in this monkey would be direct examination of the brain.

Several ethical issues are depicted in this scenario: (a) wild animals are considered by many to be inappropriate pets (i.e., respect for animals can be interpreted as allowing wild animals to remain in the wild), (b) the biker's claim of autonomous ownership of a wild animal violates the city's public health statues, and (c) the health department's plan involves killing an experiencing being (the monkey). The health department acted in accordance with the code of public health ethics by seeking to maintain the health of the little girl and prevent her (and, possibly, others) from developing rabies. If the monkey were found to have rabies, the girl would require a series of postexposure vaccinations to eradicate the virus. Keeping the monkey in quarantine while a diagnosis was being established protected others from potentially being bitten by the monkey. The critical issue was to determine whether the monkey was rabid.

Prevention is a core value of public health and also represents an underlying principle for the public health code of ethics. Public health actions are fundamentally anticipatory and employ preventive steps to reduce harm in the face of limited scientific evidence. This is the precautionary principle (Weed, 2004). In this example, public health law was used to seize an animal and, ultimately, euthanize it with limited objective information. However, the underlying motive was to protect the health of the little girl and protect the health of the public at large.

This situation also raises the question of the individual worth of an animal relative to that of a human being. Presenting the case to the court and asking the court to decide the monkey's fate was a direct acknowledgment of the monkey's right to life. The judicial hearing was valuable because it showed respect for the animal's welfare (Aaltola, 2005). This case illustrated the measured use of public health powers in protecting the health of the public (Martin, 2006).

CONCLUSION

T HE FOREGOING SCENARIOS demonstrate the fact that ethical dilemmas are common occurrences in everyday public health practice and impact everything from public health prevention programs, to public health research, to public heath advocacy issues, to the allocation of limited health resources, to public health law. Recognizing and addressing the ethical issues requires an understanding of public health and how it operates within Western society. There is a conceptual demarcation between the values of Western medical ethics and those underlying the field of public health. The public health code of ethics is an articulation of these distinctive values that form the basis of the field. Public health seeks to assure the health of an interdependent community of individuals. The good of the individual is largely subordinated to the good of the group. The language of the public health ethics code is human rights–driven and emphasizes principles of collaboration, prevention, and social justice. The public health ethics code serves as a roadmap of principles for the public health practitioner.

APPENDIX: TEMPLATE FOR PUBLIC HEALTH ETHICAL ANALYSIS (BASED ON THE PUBLIC HEALTH CODE OF ETHICS)

1. Are public health providers addressing the basic causes of disease, assessing what is needed for health and trying to prevent adverse health outcomes?
2. Are public health providers approaching community health in a manner respectful of the individuals in the community? Would

the provider feel comfortable implementing the same program/policy in his/her community?

3. Were the public health policies/programs/priorities developed and evaluated with the community?

4. Are public health providers advocating to achieve the conditions necessary for health for the most disenfranchised community members?

5. Are public health providers seeking the information needed to implement effective policies and programs that protect and promote health?

6. Are public health institutions providing communities with the information they have that is needed for decisions on policies or programs? Did these institutions obtain the community's consent for their implementation?

7. Are public health institutions acting in a timely manner on the information they have within the resources and the mandate given to them by the public?

8. Do the public health programs and policies incorporate a variety of approaches that anticipate and respect diverse values, beliefs, and cultures in the community?

9. Are public health programs and policies implemented in a manner that most enhances the physical and social environment?

10. Do public health institutions protect the confidentiality of information that can bring harm to an individual or community if made public? (Exceptions must be justified on the basis of the high likelihood of significant harm to the individual or others).

11. Do public health institutions ensure the professional competence of their employees?

12. Do public health institutions and their employees engage in collaborations and affiliations in ways that build the public's trust and the institution's effectiveness?

REFERENCES

Aaltola, E. (2005). Animal ethics and animal interest conflicts. *Ethics and the Environment, 10*, 19–48.

Bayer, R., & Fairchild, A. L. (2004). The genesis of public health ethics. *Bioethics, 18*, 473–492.

Bick, J. A. (2007). Infection control in jails and prisons. *Clinical Infectious Diseases, 45*, 1047–1055.

Centers for Disease Control and Prevention. (2006). Revised recommendations for HIV testing of adults, adolescents, and pregnant women in health-care settings. *Morbidity and Mortality Weekly Report, 55*, 1–17.

Goldenberg, R. L., & Culhane, J. F. (2006). Preterm birth and periodontal disease. *New England Journal of Medicine, 355,* 1925–1927.

Goodin, R. (2007). No smoking: The ethical issues. In R. Bayer, L. O. Gostin, B. Jennings, & B. Steinbock (Eds.). *Public health ethics.* New York: Oxford University Press.

Gostin, L., & Powers, M. (2006). What does social justice require for the public's health? *Health Affairs, 25,* 1053–1060.

Kantor, E. (2006). HIV transmission and prevention in prison. *HIV InSite.* UCSF Center for HIV Information. Retrieved August 20, 2008, from http:// hivinsite.ucsf.edu/InSite?page=kb-07-04-13

Kass, N. E. (2004). Public health ethics: From foundations and frameworks to justice and global public health. *Journal of Law, Medicine and Ethics, 32,* 232–242.

Mann, J. (1997). Medicine and public health, ethics and human rights. *Hastings Center Report, 27,* 6–13.

Martin, R. (2006). The limits of law in prioritization of public health and the role of public health ethics. *Public Health, 120,* 71–77.

Melnick, A., Kaplowitz, L., Lopez, W., & Murphy, A. (2005). Public health ethics in action: Flu vaccine and drug allocation strategies. *Journal of Law, Medicine & Ethics, 33,* 102–105.

Parker, L., Alvarez, H., & Thomas, S. (n.d.). Module 2: The legacy of the Tuskegee syphilis study. In Association of Schools of Public Health (Ed.), *Ethics and public health: Model curriculum* (pp. 37–73). Retrieved November 16, 2007, from http://www.asph.org/document.cfm?page=782

Public Health Leadership Society. (2002). *Principles of the ethical practice of public health.* Retrieved November 16, 2007, from http://www.apha. org/NR/rdonlyres/1CED3CEA-287E-4185-9CBD-BD405FC60856/0/ethics brochure.pdf

Thomas, J. (2005). Skills for the ethical practice of public health. *Journal of Public Health Management and Practice, 11,* 260–261.

Thomas, J., Sage, M., Dillenberg, J., & Guillory, V. J. (2002). A code of ethics for public health. *American Journal of Public Health, 92,* 1057–1059.

Wadhwa, P. D., Culhane, J. F., Rauh, V., Barve, S. S., Hogan, V., & Sandman, C. A. (2001). Stress, infection and preterm birth: a biobehavioural perspective. *Paediatric and Perinatal Epidemiology, 15,* 17–29.

Weed, D. (2004). Precaution, prevention, and public health ethics. *Journal of Medicine and Philosophy, 29,* 313–332.

50

Disease Control Policy: Individual Rights Versus the Common Good

JASON L. SCHWARTZ

O N MAY 30, 2007, media outlets throughout the United States reported on the federal government's compelled isolation of an American traveler infected with a highly dangerous, drug-resistant form of tuberculosis. The previous afternoon, a press conference by the Centers for Disease Control and Prevention (CDC) outlined the circumstances surrounding the patient's diagnosis and his subsequent travel itinerary, which involved multiple flights in North America and Europe. The assistance of the media was requested in asking those who took the same flights to seek tuberculosis testing and possible prophylactic treatment. Notably, the press conference was led personally by the director of CDC—a quite rare occurrence reflecting the apparent gravity of the medical threat.

In the weeks that followed, the traveler, 31-year-old lawyer and newlywed Andrew Speaker, became the star of a media frenzy. Numerous questions emerged as to the actions of public health officials as well as those of Speaker himself. A particular focus was his decision to proceed with a planned European honeymoon after being instructed not to fly due to the possibility of exposing others to tuberculosis in the close quarters of an airplane. Observers asked whether the government could or should have actively prevented Speaker from traveling. By the time the CDC press conference was held, Speaker was under government care as a result of a federal isolation order, the first issued in over 40 years (CDC, 2007).

Several weeks later, physicians determined that Speaker did not actually have the highly dangerous extensively drug resistant tuberculosis (XDR TB) but, rather, a less severe type of tuberculosis that responds better to treatment. Nevertheless, the very public nature of the Speaker case brought national and international attention to perhaps the core challenge of public health efforts, namely, balancing a respect for individual liberty while protecting the health and well-being of society as a whole.

While this tension is present throughout many aspects of public health programs, it becomes particularly challenging in matters of infectious disease control and prevention. Here, uncertainties abound, as the specific risks of exposure, infection, and transmission as well as the severity of a disease threat are rarely known with any precision. Moreover, the very nature of infectious disease control means that prompt actions by public health officials are essential to addressing emerging outbreaks. While attempts may be made to understand risks, possible benefits, and other variables as well as possible, decisions invariably must be made based on incomplete information. As the case of Andrew Speaker demonstrated, subsequent investigation after the immediate threat subsides may amend those facts.

The spectrum of infectious disease control activities by public health officials is broad, including mandatory reporting of diseases to central health departments, epidemiological investigations of outbreaks and their sources, and required treatment for transmissible diseases (such as directly observed therapy for tuberculosis patients). While the tension between individual rights and the common good is present in varying degrees in all of these initiatives, this discussion will focus on perhaps the two most ethically complex tools available to public health officials, isolation and quarantine. In both cases, decisions are made to limit some of the basic tenets of individual liberty—the freedom to move freely and to interact with others of one's choosing—in order to protect the health of others and the community as a whole. The ethics of isolation and quarantine pose challenges for traditional principles of bioethics, yet these principles remain highly relevant to the articulation of the ethics of public health.

THEMES IN THE HISTORY OF ISOLATION AND QUARANTINE

ISOLATION, THE VOLUNTARY or compelled separation of a contagious person from others, and quarantine, the temporary segregation of people, animals, or products that may have been exposed to an infectious disease, have long been used by public health authorities. (Not included in this context is the routine, noncontroversial isolation of hospitalized patients to protect against the spread of disease within the hospital.) While descriptions of separating the ill and those at risk of sickness from the healthy appear in the Old Testament and the literatures of ancient Greece and Rome, the practices became more systematically applied during the Renaissance. *Quarantine,* from the Italian word for *forty,* referred initially to the 40-day period when all traffic entering the Port of Venice in the 14th and 15th centuries was to remain onboard their ships prior to disembarking (Markel, 1997, p. 3).

The use of isolation and quarantine became an increasing interest of public health officials in the closing decades of the 19th century as the germ theory of disease gained wider acceptance. Over time, the concept of disease being transmitted through specific microbes gradually supplanted less concrete explanations of outbreaks linked to miasmas, general filth, or other causes. Concurrent with these developments in bacteriology, the turn of the 20th century saw the establishment of permanent departments of health in many American cities and states (Leavitt, 1982; Rosenkrantz, 1972). No longer assembled following the onset of a specific outbreak and dissolved upon its conclusion, standing health departments now developed extensive programs in disease prevention, surveillance, and response, utilizing the "scientific" knowledge provided by germ theory and the often-expansive authority delegated by state and municipal governments.

The New York City Health Department was at the forefront of robust public health activities that sought to apply advances in scientific knowledge to its policies and practices. The combination of massive immigration around the turn of the century, overcrowding as a result of often substandard living conditions, and an infrastructure straining to meet the growing demands of the city meant that New York was particularly susceptible to disease outbreaks. Accordingly, city health officials acted quickly upon finding evidence of a possible emerging outbreak. During a typhus epidemic in 1892, nearly 1,200 people, nearly all Eastern European Jewish immigrants, were quarantined for 2 months. The vast majority never became ill, despite being sequestered alongside the very infected patients who were being isolated from the rest of the community (Markel, 1997, p. 59). Here and elsewhere, restrictive policies made in the name of protecting public health were often difficult to distinguish from anti-immigrant sentiments present in American society at the time.

Perhaps the most well known example of an aggressive strategy of protecting public health by means of isolation occurred in the case of Mary Mallon, better known as Typhoid Mary. Despite showing no signs of typhoid herself, Mallon, a typhoid carrier who worked as a cook, was detained for 26 years on an island in the East River in New York City. The decades of isolation of Mallon, an unmarried Irish immigrant, came even as other known carriers of typhoid were not subject to the same restrictions (Leavitt, 1996, p. 55).

Other accounts of isolation and quarantine by public health authorities in the 20th century raise similar questions about the just application of these restrictive policies ostensibly implemented in order to protect public health. Following the death of a Chinese man in San Francisco in 1900 by bubonic plague, health officials ordered a quarantine of the entire Chinatown District and its residents, to begin only after all whites had been removed from the area (Shah, 2001, p. 120). During World War I, 18,000 women—many, but not all of whom were prostitutes diagnosed with a sexually transmitted disease—were placed under quarantine by the federal government. In facilities with barbed wire and armed guards, the women were confined as part of a program to reduce the spread of syphilis and other diseases, particularly among the military (Brandt, 1987, p. 89). Decades later, tuberculosis patients in Washington in the 1940s and 1950s were subject to quarantine and detention in state hospitals, a policy that largely targeted alcoholic, itinerant laborers in the Skid Road area of Seattle (Lerner, 1998, p. 118).

Each of these historical case studies of the use of isolation and quarantine suggests that the decisions made by public health officials failed to show respect for justice or other rights of the individuals subject to these requirements. The involuntary restriction of liberty by the state in order to protect other members of the community is a very significant decision. The use of such practices can only be ethically justified when consistently applied to all affected members of a community based on well-founded facts and conclusions about the nature of the disease threat, the necessity of such measures, and the absence of less intrusive alternatives. Similar requirements have been articulated by courts reviewing challenges to isolation and quarantine (Parmet, 2007, p. 434). The seemingly arbitrary use of isolation and quarantine in these examples, coupled with motives that seem to be linked more closely to biases and anti-immigrant attitudes rather than a compelling public health necessity, raise questions about the place of these practices in public health efforts during the period in American history when they were relied upon most heavily.

ISOLATION AND QUARANTINE IN CONTEMPORARY PUBLIC HEALTH

IN THE YEARS following World War II, antibiotics, vaccines, and general improvements in standards of living, particularly in cities, led to a decrease in infectious disease outbreaks for which isolation and quarantine would be a worthwhile large-scale tool for public health officials. As noted previously, the last federal isolation order prior to the case of Andrew Speaker was issued in 1963. Likewise, neither measure has been a major tool of state and local public health efforts in recent years (Bayer & Fairchild, 2004, p. 482).

While their use has become less widespread, compulsory isolation and quarantine have not disappeared entirely. One study of isolation orders in New York City during the 1990s revealed that non-White and homeless individuals constituted a large majority of those targeted (Gasner, Maw, Feldman, Fujiwara, & Frieden, 1999). Whether simply a reflection of disease trends and compliance challenges or the result of less justifiable policies, this trend underscores the need for ongoing discussions and scrutiny regarding the use of isolation and quarantine in public health programs.

Recent infectious disease threats for which pharmaceutical interventions are not available have refocused attention on broad isolation and quarantine programs. As noted previously, months after the height of public attention surrounding Andrew Speaker, it was determined that he actually had a less serious, more easily treatable form of tuberculosis. The handling of the Speaker case by officials at the CDC represented a departure from the agency's previous and subsequent handling of travelers with similar diagnoses, particularly with respect to the federal isolation order and press conference. The actions have led some tuberculosis experts to wonder publicly whether the CDC was motivated by a desire to generate attention toward the more-serious XDR TB in hopes of generating increased research funding (Young, 2007). Government officials have rejected these claims.

The Speaker case involved the compelled isolation of a single individual, but the 2002–2003 outbreak of severe acute respiratory syndrome (SARS), a previously unknown viral infection, brought much attention to the use of large-scale restrictive measures to limit the impact of an epidemic. Initially observed in China in November 2002, SARS was subsequently identified in countries throughout the Americas, Europe, and Asia, with a particularly large number of cases in Canada. By the time the outbreak concluded in July 2003, over 8,000 cases and 750 deaths were attributed to the disease (CDC, 2005).

With essentially no effective treatment available for SARS and much of its rapid worldwide spread attributable to international air and sea travel, the isolation of confirmed, hospitalized patients was a particularly effective tool for public health officials. Given the condition of those infected, this practice was generally noncontroversial. China, the country most affected by the epidemic, also quarantined tens of thousands of citizens thought to have been exposed to the virus. A CDC analysis after the epidemic concluded that, while effective in reducing the transmission of SARS, the quarantine could have been far more efficient by employing stricter criteria regarding candidates for the action (CDC, 2003). Also during this period, Canada implemented a voluntary, home-based quarantine program, with very little need for legal orders to achieve compliance.

PANDEMIC INFLUENZA PLANNING AND THE ROLE OF QUARANTINE

THE EXPERIENCE OF quarantine—both voluntary and compulsory—during the SARS epidemic provided valuable, contemporary evidence that has informed ongoing planning efforts concerning the global threat of pandemic influenza. Upon the arrival of a pandemic, health officials will be facing a disease for which pharmaceuticals are of limited use and effective vaccines will be unavailable for several months. As a result, planning efforts have given substantial attention to nonpharmaceutical interventions (NPIs), actions including isolation and quarantine in addition to the temporary closing of schools and public gathering places. Researchers studying the 1918–1919 influenza pandemic have found that cities that used isolation and quarantine, usually as part of comprehensive NPI programs, successfully reduced the impact of the pandemic in their areas (Markel et al., 2007).

While considerable public attention has been directed toward efforts to stockpile antiviral medications and develop vaccines, isolation and quarantine are significant components of the pandemic response strategies of federal, state, and local public health officials. The extensive planning document released in late 2005 by the U.S. Department of Health and Human Services (DHHS) examines at length the important role of these measures as part of a comprehensive response program (DHHS, 2005). The discussion of quarantine here reflects a clear awareness of the public concerns surrounding the practice, many of which have been influenced by the abuse of quarantine powers in past epidemics. The extensive content outlining the design and implementation of quarantine in pandemic planning and response acknowledges the importance of public acceptance of its use and trust for the public health officials shaping the response.

While the DHHS plan expresses optimism about public support for quarantine policies, if needed, the potential use of quarantine provides an opportunity for a national dialogue about the ethical questions and challenges it raises. It must be noted that while quarantine and isolation receive considerable attention in the planning document, material included within a 400-page government document is far from constituting a national conversation on these complex topics. While senior government officials have spoken at length about the status of planning with respect to antiviral and vaccine stockpiles, quarantine has received extraordinarily limited attention in the public arena, even though it will be central to pandemic response efforts. In the planning report, distinctions between voluntary and compulsory quarantine are ambiguous, if not absent entirely, even though the latter involves radically different circumstances and challenges.

Despite talk of the police powers of the state, forced confinement, and other accounts of the legal authority of public health agencies, it would be incredibly difficult to enforce a large-scale isolation or quarantine program in the face of widespread public opposition, even with assistance from other government or military agencies. Particularly during the confusion that would follow a public health emergency severe enough to require such actions, significant public support will be essential to the success of any response program.

In one area of pandemic planning, the prioritization of limited vaccine supplies, the government has been extraordinarily proactive in publicizing the development of allocation strategies, soliciting public feedback through various channels, and offering detailed explanations for the decisions being made. A parallel effort aimed at preemptively building public understanding of the circumstances when isolation and quarantine would be warranted seems similarly worthwhile.

Also important is a frank discussion regarding the presumably limited circumstances when involuntary quarantine may be required. Even though the abuses of past instances of isolation and quarantine are unlikely to be repeated, we know from other areas of bioethics— particularly human subjects research—that the legacies of past transgressions endure in the public consciousness. Provided that early public engagement regarding these measures is done in a way so as not to raise unnecessary alarm, an explicit discussion of the tension between individual rights and public health in a pandemic or other health emergency can only be advantageous to subsequent disease control efforts.

AMBIGUITY AND ETHICS IN THE LANGUAGE OF PUBLIC HEALTH POLICY

Mᴏʀᴇ ɢᴇɴᴇʀᴀʟʟʏ, ᴀᴛᴛᴇɴᴛɪᴏɴ toward the use of compulsory isolation and quarantine could shine light on the largely unarticulated continuum of the strategies available to public health leaders to prevent and respond to disease outbreaks, each with unique ethical considerations. There are important differences between public health activities based upon education, persuasion, coercion, or compulsion, respectively. These differences merit closer study. While no consensus exists on the definition of each term in the context of public health, one could define *education* as strictly informative efforts by public health officials, *persuasion* as activities in which public health leaders generally endorse and recommend a specific health-related behavior, *coercion* as efforts that link acceptance of such recommendations to a specific benefit or penalty (such as a cash bonus or access to certain facilities), and *compulsion* as action forced by the state that either severely limits civil liberties or occurs under threat thereof (such as involuntary isolation or forced treatment).

These distinctions in public health programs are neither trivial nor simply a matter of semantics. For example, one term often used in discussions of public health, *mandatory,* can refer to as many as three of the four categories noted above, as in the case of "mandatory" vaccination requirements that most often can be better described as opt-out programs. Similarly, the practice of quarantine discussed in this chapter can similarly refer to a spectrum of activities, ranging from involuntary confinement by the state to a voluntary recommendation to remain inside one's own home during a disease outbreak.

This ambiguity in terms is problematic in fostering public understanding and support for public health initiatives. Similarly, it complicates efforts to identify and examine the embedded ethical questions raised by specific subsets of these hydralike terms. Even if not explicitly perceived or described as such by public health officials, the decision to pursue a particular set of actions represents the resolution of an ethical debate over the rights of the infected, the rights of the exposed, the rights of the uninfected, and the responsibility of government and public health authorities. These often-implicit ethical analyses that inform public health policies are frequently hidden from public view.

The relatively recent emergence of scholarly attention to a population-centered public health ethics (Bayer & Fairchild, 2004; Buchanan, 2008; Childress et al., 2002), often framed in contrast to the individual-focused bioethics, has provided valuable insights on the relationship and tension between individual liberty and the societal aims of public health programs. For example, Childress and colleagues (2002, p. 173) propose five conditions that must be met to justify overriding personal liberty or other values, as would occur in cases of compulsory isolation or quarantine. Those conditions require the proposed policy to be *effective, proportionate* with respect to its benefits compared to the rights infringed, *necessary,* the *least infringement* of the relevant values compared to alternative actions, and *publicly justified* in order to preserve accountability and public trust. Once again, the importance of public understanding of disease control programs is seen as inseparable from the epidemiological goals of health officials.

CONCLUSION

THE SOCIETAL FOCUS of public health makes it extremely well suited to consequentialist analyses that discount the interests of any specific person in favor of community benefits. Admittedly, this is the justification for any instance of involuntary isolation or quarantine. Nevertheless, it must be remembered that population-wide policies ultimately affect individuals with rights deserving respect. The history of isolation and quarantine practices reveals that these rights have been too often and too easily trumped by prejudices or seemingly arbitrary decisions couched in the language of public health. These past abuses should serve as both a reminder and a caution to policy makers considering isolation and quarantine as part of present-day disease control efforts.

Isolation and quarantine present a seemingly intractable tension between competing and compelling values—individual rights and the common good. These tensions reflect the significance of these measures and underscore that they should be used rarely and only after considerable reflection. Essential to the just use of isolation and quarantine is an ongoing, preemptive dialogue among the bioethics and public health ethics communities, public health officials, and the general public. From such sustained attention to the ethics of these measures, the important objectives of local, national, and global disease control efforts are best positioned to succeed while striving to respect personal liberty and other individual rights.

REFERENCES

Bayer, R., & Fairchild, A. L. (2004). The genesis of public health ethics. *Bioethics, 18,* 473–492.

Brandt, A. M. (1987). *No magic bullet: A social history of venereal disease in the United States since 1880* (expanded ed.). New York: Oxford University Press.

Buchanan, D. R. (2008). Autonomy, paternalism, and justice: Ethical priorities in public health. *American Journal of Public Health, 98,* 15–21.

Centers for Disease Control and Prevention. (2003). Efficiency of quarantine during an epidemic of severe acute respiratory syndrome—Beijing, China, 2003. *Morbidity and Mortality Weekly Report, 52,* 1037–1040.

Centers for Disease Control and Prevention. (2005). *Fact sheet: Basic information about SARS.* Retrieved June 2, 2008, from http://www.cdc.gov/ncidod/ sars/factsheet.htm

Centers for Disease Control and Prevention. (2007). *Public health investigation seeks people who may have been exposed to extensively drug resistant tuberculosis (XDR TB) infected person.* Retrieved June 3, 2008, from http://www. cdc.gov/media/transcripts/2007/t070529.htm

Childress, J. F., Faden, R. R., Gaare, R. D., Gostin, L. O., Kahn, J., Bonnie, R. J., et al. (2002). Public health ethics: Mapping the terrain. *Journal of Law, Medicine and Ethics, 30,* 170–178.

Department of Health and Human Services. (2005). *HHS pandemic influenza plan.* Retrieved June 3, 2008, from http://www.hhs.gov/pandemicflu/ plan/pdf/HHSPandemicInfluenzaPlan.pdf

Gasner, M. R., Maw, K. L., Feldman, G. E., Fujiwara, P. I., & Frieden, T. R. (1999). The use of legal action in New York City to ensure treatment of tuberculosis. *New England Journal of Medicine, 340,* 359–366.

Leavitt, J. W. (1982). *The healthiest city: Milwaukee and the politics of health reform.* Princeton, NJ: Princeton University Press.

Leavitt, J. W. (1996). *Typhoid Mary: Captive to the public's health.* Boston, MA: Beacon Press.

Lerner, B. H. (1998). *Contagion and confinement: Controlling tuberculosis along the Skid Road.* Baltimore, MD: Johns Hopkins University Press.

Markel, H. (1997). *Quarantine! East European Jewish immigrants and the New York City epidemics of 1892.* Baltimore, MD: Johns Hopkins University Press.

Markel, H., Lipman, H. B., Navarro, J. A., Sloan, A., Michalsen, J. R., Stern, A. M., et al. (2007). Nonpharmaceutical interventions implemented by U.S. cities during the 1918–1919 influenza pandemic. *Journal of the American Medical Association, 298,* 644–654.

Parmet W. E. (2007). Legal power and legal rights—isolation and quarantine in the case of drug-resistant tuberculosis. *New England Journal of Medicine, 357,* 433–435.

Rosenkrantz, B. G. (1972). *Public health and the state: Changing views in Massachusetts, 1842–1936.* Cambridge, MA: Harvard University Press.

Shah, N. (2001). *Contagious divides: Epidemics and race in San Francisco's Chinatown.* Berkeley: University of California Press.

Young, A. (2008, March 13). Did CDC hype TB case as a fund-raising ploy? *The Atlanta Journal-Constitution.* Retrieved August 25, 2008, from http://www. ajc.com/search/content/health/stories/2008/03/13/tbpublicity_0113.html

51

Bioethics and National Security

Jonathan D. Moreno and
Michael S. Peroski

T**HE APPLICATION OF** bioethics in the area of national security often focuses on the tension between individual rights and the public interest of ensuring national security. For example, the development of ethics protocols for the approval of experiments with human subjects required balancing the protection of individuals from harm against the public interest of conducting experiments that may produce significant benefits for the United States. Post-9/11, bioethics has traveled far from these origins to address new relevant issues in national security such as bioterrorism preparedness and response, triage in mass casualty medicine, and the role of doctors in interrogations. Emerging technologies with potential implications for national security, such as the use of genetically modified bacteria by sophisticated terrorists, further complicate issues and intensify the tension between individual rights and national security.

HUMAN SUBJECTS RESEARCH AND NATIONAL SECURITY

T**HE CONNECTION BETWEEN** bioethics and national security begins with Walter Reed's dispatch in 1900 to quell a yellow fever pandemic affecting American soldiers in Havana, Cuba. Through human experimentation, Reed confirmed that the vector of yellow fever was the female silver-backed mosquito. By using primitive consent forms that informed subjects of the risks and benefits of his study, Reed showed that medicine, particularly military medicine, was compatible with medical ethics. These experiments largely inoculated both medical experimentation and military medicine from association with scandal.

This adequate condition lasted about 50 years, until the horrendous World War II experiments conducted by doctors in Nazi concentration camps were revealed. Many German officials were charged, tried, and convicted at the Nuremberg war crimes tribunal for their abuses of humans. A 10-point statement known as the Nuremberg Code resulted from these trials and calls for voluntary consent of research subjects, prior animal experimentation, the elimination of undue risk, the right of the subject to terminate involvement in an experiment at any time, and medical scientists' responsibility for the well-being of subjects.

At around the same time, the Atomic Energy Commission (AEC) discovered that scientists in the United States had been conducting experiments since 1945 that involved the administration of plutonium injections without consent. The fact that judges from the United States played a significant role in the formation of the Nuremberg Code made this situation particularly challenging. To avoid the embarrassment of exposing these experiments and potential lawsuits from subjects, the AEC decided in 1947 to keep the experiments secret (Moreno, 2001, pp. 119–155). After this episode, the AEC developed a policy to prevent future misuse of radio nuclides by requiring informed consent. The requirement of informed consent and the first official use of the term *informed consent* in this policy indicate that special attention was given to the Nuremberg Code (Moreno, 2001, p. 141). This policy proved inadequate, because it offered neither a systematic articulation nor a mechanism for implementation. The AEC's role in the human experiments issue extended to its relationship with other national security agencies. For example, between 1948 and 1951, an intense discussion on the risks of radiation to the crew of a nuclear-powered aircraft occurred in an interagency committee between the AEC and the Department of Defense (DoD).

During its complex postwar reorganization, the DoD discovered that the Pentagon lacked a policy for human experimentation. Thus, from 1950 to 1953, several internal advisory panels deliberated on how to proceed. Both the military and medical members of these panels largely preferred to rely on an unwritten code of ethics and the virtues of those in charge rather than a formal ethics code that would invite legal scrutiny. As this debate progressed, rampant offenses implicating the government occurred, such as the death of tennis professional

Harold Blaur in a mescaline-derivative study sponsored by the Army Chemical Corps. Efforts made by New York State and the Army Chemical Corps to cover up this experiment underscored the need for a formal policy on human experimentation (Moreno, 2001, pp. 195–199).

It was President Eisenhower's defense secretary Charles E. Wilson who finally signed off on the top-secret, so-called Wilson memorandum in 1953, adopting the Nuremberg Code verbatim as the Pentagon's policy. Although the policy included a written consent requirement, its secrecy made implementation just as difficult as the earlier AEC policy. The disappointing story of the actual effect of this policy seems attributable to numerous cultural factors that characterized both the military establishment and the medical profession in the 1950s. In the late 1950s, the Nuremberg Code–based policy withered as it was variously interpreted and sporadically applied. The fact that defense officials wanted to introduce a clear policy to protect the government from human experiment scandals may surprise those who suppose that expanded governmental power leads to practices that are antithetical to the high ethical principles of the Nuremberg Code, like the Central Intelligence Agency's (CIA's) experiments with hallucinogenic substances.

In these experiments, soldiers were exposed to lysergic acid diethylamide (LSD) and seem to have known they were going to be given a hallucinogen but were not aware of other details, such as the time of exposure, the quantity of LSD administered, or the goals of the study. On the other hand, the infamous case of Dr. Frank Olson, an army doctor to whom LSD was administered by the CIA in 1953 and who later appeared to have killed himself, indicates that LSD trials were sometimes applied to unsuspecting persons who were clearly unable to give consent (Moreno, 2001, pp. 191–192).

At the same time, the uniformed services created written policies on human experiments, beginning with the Army's Regulation 70–25, which contained vestiges of the Nuremberg Code's language. Ironically, these regulations received few objections. A set of exemptions to the written consent requirement stated, among other things, that the written consent requirement did not apply if the study was a "training exercise" (United States Army, 1962). Even activities that involved medical monitoring were often called training exercises. And for roughly 20 years after the Wilson memorandum, the more the activities in question were considered training exercises, and the less they resembled a clinical intervention, the less likely it was that consent would be sought.

Despite these struggles, a highly publicized and apparently successful human experiment program, called Project Whitecoat, took place at Fort Detrick from 1953 to 1974. Part of President Nixon's directive to shut down the biological weapons program at Fort Detrick terminated this program, eliminating a primary source of human subjects. As a result, the Medical Research Volunteer Subjects (MRVS) program was born, with participants recruited from groups of medics assigned to Fort Detrick's infectious disease lab. It is fascinating and ironic that, following a mixed history of human subjects' protections, the Army MRVS is one of the most admirably ethical human research programs in the world.

Although the military's discourse on issues of human experimentation was far in advance of any in the civilian world, human experimentation was largely unencumbered by the resulting rules of ethics until 1975, when revelations of the CIA experiments, army experiments, and media converge of the Tuskegee syphilis study compelled both congressional and intra-agency investigations. In the wake of these scandals, as well as Watergate and the national reaction to the chaotic conclusion to the Vietnam War, public mistrust in government reached historic proportions. Human research protections, both in the civilian and military sectors, became far more restrictive and accountable. Accordingly, human experiments for national security purposes appear to have been severely limited for the past 30 years, with the exception of defensively oriented studies.[1]

The fact that, historically, the rules that governed human subject protections could be so easily ignored in the context of military- and government-run human experiments is instructive. In today's national security environment, regulations governing human research conducted or sponsored by the U.S. military are at least as stringent as those that apply to civilian research. Exemptions to ethics codes still exist but do not apply to clinically oriented research that involves interventions with discrete individuals (United States Army, 1990). Therefore, informed consent and prior institutional review board (IRB) approval (known in the U.S. Army as a Human Use Committee) would be required under these rules for this nonexempt research.

Classified research necessitates expanded guidelines. For example, to satisfy the standard criteria of valid informed consent, protocols require security clearances for all parties, including the IRB members and human subjects. Such experiments lack public scrutiny; therefore at least one member of the classified IRB should not be a federal employee. There should also be a method of appealing an IRB decision to a superior authority. A letter signed by President Clinton in 1996, still technically applying to all 17 federal agencies that conduct or sponsor human experiments, including those with classification authority, incorporated these elements. Currently, the federal government reports that no classified human research is taking place, but it is not difficult to imagine circumstances in which such activities would be thought important so that terrorist groups would be denied information about American capabilities.

BIOETHICS AND BIOTERRORISM

UNTIL THE TERRORIST attacks of September 11, 2001, and the subsequent anthrax scare, modern bioethics paid little attention to preparation for and response to bioterrorism (Moreno, 2002). The term *bioterrorism* has become shorthand for terror through the use of unconventional weapons, especially chemical, nuclear, and radiological weapons, or so-called dirty bombs. Although the tactical notion of using biological or chemical agents to spread terror among enemy forces reaches back to World War I, the novelty of 21st-century bioterrorism lies in its combination of political radicalism and techniques that were once largely the province of military establishments.

The 2001 anthrax scare highlighted what many in the United States regarded as weaknesses in preparedness and in the legal framework empowering public health workers. To address these issues and provide comprehensive legal standards for responding to a catastrophe while respecting civil liberties, a group of public health law scholars developed the Model State Emergency Health Powers Act (MSEHPA). Critics charged that it was based on post-9/11 hysteria and represented unjustifiable infringements on freedoms in the name of bioterrorism preparedness (Annas, 2003).

For successful bioterrorism preparedness and response, government approval of vaccines and therapies for bioweapons agents that cannot be ethically tested in humans needs to be addressed. Because of the bioweapons potential of smallpox, the U.S. government undertook vaccine trials, demonstrating a general public enthusiasm about volunteering for clinical trials when faced with widespread fears of bioterrorism. As these fears become greater, protections for human subjects can seem less important. Despite the fact that the initial phase of clinical research took place before September 11, 2001, the public took little interest until after the anthrax scare (Frey et al., 2002). To overcome the challenge of testing smallpox *in vivo* in humans, the FDA adopted the so-called animal rule, allowing the approval of therapies for potential bioweapons agents based on animal rather than human efficacy testing. This alternative to human testing became law in the Bioterrorism Act of 2002 (Moreno, 2003).

To support the development of new vaccines and antibiotics for the War on Terror, President Bush secured funding for Project BioShield in 2004. This combination of regulation and funding promises to propel a great deal of science in the coming years; whether it will distort research priorities or complement new approaches to naturally occurring diseases remains to be seen. This highlights the general issue of investing resources in bioterrorism preparedness rather than in more familiar sources of morbidity and mortality (e.g., current infectious diseases, food-borne illness, and drug and alcohol abuse) for which prevention or treatment is available but underutilized. The rationality of this critique runs afoul of the powerful symbolism of national security as somehow transformative of what might otherwise be a straightforward allocation question.

There is also the issue of already overburdened emergency workers dedicating time to bioterrorism preparedness. In the event of a terrorist attack, they are often better prepared to introduce methods to save lives as a result of their training. For example, emergency physicians sometimes find themselves implicitly in the position of agents of law enforcement, as when they care for individuals whose injuries may have been incurred in the course of a crime, which may prepare them to work with security agencies in catastrophic events.

After determining how to act, emergency workers must assess the nature of the threat. Having ties to national security would be useful for threat assessment because, in this context, security agencies in particular are in a position to support or hinder the flow of information necessary to threat assessment. Their decision-making must take into account not only the public health implications of withholding sensitive information but also social implications. Thus the broader implications of decisions by national security agencies can compromise not only threat assessment but also the public cooperation that makes emergency intervention more effective (Eckenwiler, 2003). Advanced preparation with these agencies proves problematic, however, because systematic ties to national security agencies in preparation for a terrorist attack may be viewed by some as likely to compromise the ideals of independence of medical practice and transparency of public health practice. Following threat assessment, emergency response should follow from advance planning, with the broadest possible public participation, transparency, and accountability, relieving health care workers of any unfair burden of determining allocation criteria on their own.

Considerations of national security assume unique relevance in communicating information that has public health consequences when the source of the threat is thought to be a terrorist attack. Justifiable expectations about the privacy of health information records honor the ethical principle of respect for persons and give individuals confidence that presenting themselves for medical care will not expose them to stigmatization or other social risks. However, when the implications of personal health information are relevant to actions that can preserve public health, these expectations may be overridden.

Arguably, considerations of national security may also justify the release of personal health information as needed, to help identify the source of an outbreak, for example. Conversely, national security authorities may determine that the health status of certain groups that would normally be available to health officials should be especially safeguarded (Eckenwiler, 2003). For example, releasing health information about operatives needing cover that were exposed to a dangerous bioweapon might tip off adversaries.

When faced with these extreme conditions, it is likely that emergency workers will require privately held resources, like pharmaceuticals, for the public good (Mills & Werhane, 2003). In this context, advanced planning of industry is essential. Drug manufacturers, for example, should plan for special pricing strategies in the event of a widespread public health threat, a prudent step in any case as they risk losing control over a product if the government chooses to assert its prerogatives for the greater good and withdraw patent protection. Some corporations, engaged in the production and distribution of substances that could be turned to terrorist advantage, also have an obligation to develop adequate security measures and provide educational programs for their employees. Cooperation with local, regional, and, depending on the nature of the business, even national authorities may be required, especially if the company's facilities could be directly exploited and toxic substances released (DeRenzo, 2003).

With the advancement of technology, these practical concerns may be coupled with other, atypical issues. In the late 1990s several government advisory groups warned that the conclusion of the Human Genome Project and subsequent advances in genetics created risks for the United States concerning genetically modified bioterror organisms. Possible efforts to modify viruses so that they will elude currently available vaccines, or perhaps agents that could act on agriculture, are of particular concern (Meslin, 2003). Just as terrorists may employ genetic technologies, they may attempt to develop and use nerve agents. Fortunately, most of these concerns are highly speculative, but in the era of bioterrorism, even a scientific event that would normally cause unalloyed celebration, the publication of the map of the human genome on the World Wide Web, raises concerns about the openness of science and the role of government in both utilizing and constraining scientific activity (Meslin, 2003).

This problem illustrates how far bioethics has traveled from its original concerns with the rights of patients and research subjects, the allocation of life-saving technology, and the implications of genetics for the future of humanity. Yet the bioethical issues stimulated by bioterrorism also revive each of these topics in a new light while creating new ones, challenging the creativity and resourcefulness of those interested in the life sciences and human values. One such challenge in bioterrorism preparedness guidelines is how to develop a framework for effective use of triage in mass casualty medicine.

TRIAGE

THE NAPOLEONIC ARMIES first practiced a system of sorting casualties of war in order to maximize the good for the greatest number of injured combatants. This utilitarian approach is also thought to satisfy the formal requirement of justice: equity or the treatment of similar cases similarly. Equitable treatment varies in its detail but should be guided by the greater likelihood that some benefit from treatment more than others, both in quality and duration, and in the urgency of treatment.

Both medical utility and social utility operate in civilian and military disasters. Social utility refers to the value for the entire fighting force of returning wounded soldiers to duty. It may also apply to a larger sense of common good that could justify an expanded form of triage in which egalitarian principles are modified to take into account the exceptional value of certain individuals to society, such as political leaders or those with rare technical expertise. A broad version of social utility provides little guidance for specific judgments in the event of a terrorist attack or similar catastrophic event. A narrower version that provides more guidance combined with medical utility, namely the multiplier effect of salvaging medical personnel so that they can provide medical care to others, is much more useful (Childress, 2003). Although triage may justifiably compromise human equality, egalitarian approaches could be applied within sorted groups. In this way the principle of equal human worth is honored while social utility is recognized. Today, successful triage efforts involve assessing patients as they enter hospitals, monitoring patients for whom treatment is delayed, caring for patients most in need, sufficient staffing at all times, freeing of hospital infrastructure, and cooperation of patients and patient families (Moreno, 2007).

Individual physicians and other health care professionals should not be the only ones to bear the burden of developing triage criteria for these complex necessities. Shared accountability that accompanies decisions that may result in the death or suffering of some rather than others is essential, for example, when justifying instances in which care may have to be provided in homes and civic institutions.

In catastrophic events, if victims are collected near those not exposed, medical care will have to be provided outside of hospitals. Planning for this sort of emergency must be far-sighted as it entails decentralizing health resources in various community settings rather than in hospitals. Community acceptability of triage arrangements will, as indicated, be especially important if an incident is of such magnitude that the infrastructure of health care institutions themselves is compromised by the scale of the attack and the subsequent number of injured, by the infliction of massive casualties upon health care workers themselves, or by the nature of the attack that causes some patients to be a danger to many others.

In the event of a catastrophic bioterrorism attack, it is not far fetched to imagine a case in which the military has more resources to address a given circumstance than do civilians. In this circumstance, significant cooperation between civilian medical forces, military medical forces, and national security organizations must occur. The infrastructure under which such a distribution of resources would now occur is in need of reform to respond to potential threats (RAND Corporation, 2004). The cooperation between medical professionals and military officials extends to interrogation methods in some cases outside of civilian issues.

THE ROLE OF DOCTORS IN INTERROGATIONS

ASSISTANCE FROM DOCTORS in interrogations and the administration of torture has occurred since the 15th century (Miles, 2006, p. 24). The early 20th century, however, marked the beginning of U.S. doctors' involvement, when they developed methods of capital punishment and interrogation (Miles, 2006, pp. 28–29; Reynolds & Bernstein, 1989). Throughout the 1940s and 1950s, doctors conducted research, informing future interrogation techniques, often funded inconspicuously by national security agencies. These studies were used to develop the CIA's KUBARK manual on counterintelligence interrogation in 1963 and "The Human Resource Exploitation Training Manual," in 1983, both of which specifically call for physician and psychologist involvement (CIA, 1963, 1983). The latter of these manuals precipitated congressional interest after reports of its encouragement of coercive methods surfaced.

Although congressional interest in interrogations peaked, in this instance in the 1990s, it wasn't until after the events of 9/11 that significant public concern regarding doctors' involvement in interrogations arose. After 9/11, national security organizations needed to extract information quickly from suspects to gauge further threats. One of the first actions of the Secretary of Defense, Donald Rumsfeld, in these efforts, was to call for the involvement of military doctors in monitoring interrogations (Sullivan, 2006).

Images of detainees, declassified reports of interrogation programs, and the release of a transcript of the interrogation of a suspect in the 9/11 plot all contributed to a renewed public interest in interrogations. With each of these stories also came the revelation that trained medical professionals were involved in these interrogations. Given the previously mentioned history, this involvement is not surprising. However, medical ethics has come a long way since the early 20th century, making the involvement problematic for the profession and difficult to excuse simply on "we didn't know any better" grounds.

Doctors fill one or more central roles in interrogations, classified as certification, medical supervision, and participation (Gross, 2006). Certification might involve examining detainees and qualifying them to receive certain forms of interrogation, signing medical documents verifying the condition of a prisoner after an interrogation, designing specific interrogation methods, and signing death certificates. When doctors provide supervision, they give medical care to detainees suffering from illness or injury, for rehabilitation, or to allow them to continue interrogation. Although infrequent, there are accounts of direct participation of doctors in some detention facilities (Gross, 2006, p. 231). In this role doctors may act as passive agents, through actions such as withholding pain-relieving medication until a detainee cooperates, or may participate actively as fellow interrogators.

The involvement of doctors in interrogations raises ethical flags for some who argue that regulations, such as the third Geneva Convention and national laws, prohibit them from acting in interrogations (Gross, 2006, p. 232). In spite of these objections, some military physicians and national security officials argue in favor of continued doctor involvement, contesting that when doctors assist in interrogations they act as combatants, not medical practitioners. This claim is only validated if the doctors involved maintain only one of two potential roles, which are caregiver and expert consultant. On this front, difficulty arises when the opinions of equally qualified professionals differ with regard to the appropriate course of action.

In attempting to address these issues, the American Psychological Association prohibits psychologists from participating in interrogations that rely on coercion, permits so-called indirect but not direct involvement, requires psychologists to report ethical violations to the chain of command, and distinguishes the health care provider from the consultant. This code of ethics is derived from a dual consideration of nonmaleficence and social responsibility. However, the American Psychological Association recently approved changes to its policy that will take effect in August 2009. These changes prohibit psychologists from working in any facility that violates international law or the U.S. Constitution unless they are working for the persons detained or as part of a human rights effort. By contrast, the American Psychiatric

Association maintains that nonmaleficence is the chief concern and affirms that psychiatrists should not be involved in interrogations; however, this is not an ethical rule. Much to do with the alignment of psychologists with the mission of national security, DoD officials indicated their desire to use psychologists as "behavioral consultations" and physicians to administer treatment (Hausman, 2006). Some suggest that harmonizing these and other codes of ethics might solve dilemmas that arise in the context of interrogations (Miles, 2007).

The sophistication of interrogation technologies promises to create new ethical dilemmas. Evidence suggests that certain chemicals are present in the brain when people trust others. It is not hard to imagine the value of chemically inducing feelings of trust and the necessity for doctors in using this possible regimen in interrogations (Moreno, 2006, p. 74). National security funding also supports efforts to develop and refine functional magnetic resonance imaging (fMRI) technologies for lie detection. In fact, researchers are already successful at detecting simple lies using fMRI, such as whether or not a subject recognizes a certain face or language (Moreno, 2006, p. 100). Doctors involved in other studies are refining technologies to find loci of brain activity during lying (Moreno, 2006, pp. 103–105). Despite the current technical limitations of using fMRI for lie detection, at least one former intelligence officer reports that it has been used in the War on Terror (Peroski, 2008). If developing these technologies provides some potential advantages, it would be foolhardy and perhaps immoral not to explore them, under carefully constructed constraints (Moreno, 2006, p. 165).

CONCLUSION

BIOETHICS HAS COME far from its original focus on the protection of human subjects in experiments for national security purposes. Although human subjects' protections are challenging and the development of protocols to protect human subjects was complicated, the current issues faced by the field are even more difficult. In a post-9/11 United States, bioethics not only continues to face the challenges posed by human subjects' research, but also faces issues related to bioterrorism, triage in mass casualty medicine, and the involvement of physicians in interrogations. Whereas analysis of many of these issues might be straightforward in a strictly civilian context, the tension between civil rights and national security makes decision-making inextricably complicated. Surely, the unique challenges presented by a combination of advancing technology, potential threats, and the national security enterprise promise to continue pushing bioethics into novel territory.

NOTE

1. Although this impression is hard to quantify, it is a conclusion reached based on Dr. Moreno's work for the Advisory Committee on Human Radiation Experiments and his many conversations with agency officials.

REFERENCES

Annas, G. E. (2003). Terrorism and human rights. In J. D. Moreno (Ed.), *In the wake of terror: Medicine and morality in a time of crisis* (pp. 33–50). Cambridge: MIT Press.

Central Intelligence Agency (CIA). (1963). KUBARK counterintelligence interrogation. Retrieved January 10, 2008, from www.gwu.edu/~nsarchiv/NSAEBB/NSAEBB27/01-01.htm

Central Intelligence Agency (CIA). (1983). The human resource exploitation training manual. Retrieved August 10, 2008, from http://www.gwu.edu/~nsarchiv/NSAEBB/NSAEBB27/02-01.htm

Childress, J. F. (2003). Triage in response to a bioterrorist attack. In J. D. Moreno (Ed.), *In the wake of terror: Medicine and morality in a time of crisis* (pp. 77–94). Cambridge: MIT Press.

DeRenzo, E. G. (2003). The rightful goals of a corporation and the obligations of the pharmaceutical industry in a world with bioterrorism. In J. D. Moreno (Ed.), *In the wake of terror: Medicine and morality in a time of crisis* (pp. 149–166). Cambridge: MIT Press.

Eckenwiler, L. A. (2003). Emergency health professionals and the ethics of crisis. In J. D. Moreno (Ed.), *In the wake of terror: Medicine and morality in a time of crisis* (pp. 111–132). Cambridge: MIT Press.

Frey, S. E., Newman, F. K., Cruz, J., Shelton, W. B., Tennant, J. M., Polach, T., et al. (2002). Dose-related effects of smallpox vaccine. *New England Journal of Medicine, 346*(17), 1275–1280.

Gross, M. L. (2006). *Bioethics and armed conflict: Moral dilemmas of medicine and war* (pp. 230–232). Cambridge: MIT Press.

Hausman, K. (2006). Military looks to psychologists for advice on interrogations. *Psychiatric News, 41,* 4.

Meslin, E. M., (2003). Genetics and bioterrorism: Challenges for science, society, and bioethics. In J. D. Moreno (Ed.), *In the wake of terror: Medicine and morality in a time of crisis* (pp. 199–218). Cambridge: MIT Press.

Miles, S. H. (2006). *Oath betrayed: Torture, medical complicity, and the war on terror*. New York: Random House.

Miles, S. H. (2007). Medical ethics and the interrogation of Guantanamo 063. *The American Journal of Bioethics, 7*(4), 5–11.

Mills, A. F., & Werhane P. H. (2003). After the terror: Health care organizations, the health care system, and the future of organization ethics. In

J. D. Moreno (Ed.), *In the wake of terror: Medicine and morality in a time of crisis* (pp. 167–182). Cambridge: MIT Press.

Moreno. J. D. (2001). *Undue risk*. New York: Routledge Press.

Moreno, J. D. (2002). Bioethics after terror. *The American Journal of Bioethics, 2*(1), 60–64.

Moreno, J. D. (2003). The BioShield bonanza and human experimentation. *Research USA, 1*(2), 29.

Moreno, J. D. (2006). *Mind wars: Brain research and national defense*. Washington, DC: Dana Foundation Press.

Moreno, J. D. (2007). Bioethics and bioterrorism. In B. Stenbock (Ed.), *The Oxford handbook of bioethics* (pp. 721–734). Oxford, UK: Oxford University Press.

Peroski, M. S. (2008). They (might) know what you're thinking. *Science Progress*. Retrieved on August 10, 2008, from http://www.scienceprogress.org/2008/04/they-might-know-what-youre-thinking/

RAND Corporation. (2004). *Triage for civil support: Using military medical assets to respond to terrorist attacks*. Retrieved February 11, 2008, from http://www.rand.org/pubs/mon ographs/MG217/

Reynolds, T. S., & Bernstein, T. (1989). Edison and "the chair." *Technology and Society Magazine, 8*(1), 19–28.

Sullivan, A., (2006, June 26). *How doctors got into the torture business*. Retrieved January 9, 2008, from http://www.time.com/time/nation/article/0,8599,1207633,00.html

United States Army. (1962). *Army regulation 70–25: Use of volunteers as subjects of research:* Retrieved January 12, 2008, from http://ethics.iit.edu/codes/coe/us.gov. army.research.1962.html

United States Army. (1990). *Regulation 70–25*. Retrieved March 9, 2004, from http://www.apd.army.mil/pdffiles/r70_25.pdf

52

Bringing the Public to the Private: Increasing the Accountability of Nonprofit Health Organizations

ROBERTA M. SNOW

WHEN WE TALK about the health care system on a global, national, or local level, we are actually talking about networks of organizations. Within these networks, nonprofit organizations—private enterprises serving the public good—play major and diverse roles. And in the public health arena, nonprofits are the major organizational vehicle used to put government policies into practice. They develop, promote, and deliver the goods and services that fight disease and enhance community well-being.

Health-focused nonprofits differ widely in the work they do. A nonprofit might be an advocacy, policy, or educational group, a scientific research institution, an organization delivering health services directly to the public, a professional society or accrediting body, or a charitable foundation that provides funding to sustain and further develop the network. Health-focused nonprofits also vary greatly in size. Some are large international bureaucracies like the World Health Organization, while others are small, informal, local collaboratives like patient and caregiver support groups.

NONPROFIT STRUCTURE AND ORGANIZATIONAL ACCOUNTABILITY

WHATEVER THEIR SIZE or scope, as a group, health-related nonprofits differ from public agencies and commercial businesses in terms of their legal status and formal structure. One facet of their structure, accountability, poses practical ethical challenges for everyday management. While government agencies are ultimately accountable to the voters and for-profit enterprises are accountable to their shareholders, nonprofits are for the most part accountable to no one.

As a private entity, a nonprofit determines internally what it is going to do and how it is going to do it. A nonprofit sets its mission and develops specific strategies for pursuing it. For example, when the Bill and Melinda Gates Foundation was established, the founders made innovation in global health a major focus; therefore much of its programming supports breakthrough science.

A nonprofit's formal external accountability—that is, accountability to the public whom the nonprofit serves—is limited to standardized filings required by government authorities. In the United States, which has the most stringent oversight of the sector, a nonprofit is required to file standard forms with the Internal Revenue Service (IRS). This documentation provides a limited view of the nonprofit's activities, primarily through financial statements. The organization complies in order to maintain its tax-exempt status. Beyond that, there is negligible regulation and enforcement.

Until relatively recently, there has been little interest or investment in developing additional oversight procedures and infrastructure, largely because the importance of nonprofits' work and assumptions about their efficiency has created a general attitude of good will and support.

A SHIFT IN ATTITUDE TOWARD THE NONPROFIT SECTOR

THESE LONG-STANDING VIEWS, however, are beginning to change. In recent years, nonprofits have come under increased scrutiny as the result of two driving forces: significant sector growth and a general erosion of public trust in corporate entities.

INCREASED SECTOR GROWTH

FIRST, ACCORDING TO Salamon (2002), the size and composition of the nonprofit health sector has changed significantly. The number of international nonprofits addressing health issues across national borders (commonly called nongovernmental organizations or NGOs) has increased by 50% between 1990 and 2000. In the United States, the number of health-related nonprofits has remained relatively stable, but the nonprofit sector as a whole has grown enormously in the past decade. The number of nonprofit organizations registered with the IRS has shown a 30% increase in the past 10 years, and the rate of sector growth is accelerating (Independent Sector & Urban Institute, 2002).

Moreover, Savas (2000) explained how commercial organizations are increasingly doing the work once done by government and non-profits. Over the past quarter-century, governments have experimented with privatization, contracting with for-profit companies to supply basic services. The argument for privatization is that businesses, driven by market and profit incentives (that is, accountability to the consumer and the bottom line), can carry out the work more effectively and efficiently. This assumption has led to the increased commercialization of a number of nonprofit health care services in the United States. Roughly two-thirds of dialysis centers, rehabilitation hospitals, home health agencies, and HMOs are now for-profit, and one-third are nonprofit. In the 1980s the percentages were the reverse—two-thirds were nonprofit and one-third was for-profit.

Dramatic sector growth coupled with increased for-profit involvement has led international and domestic policy makers to begin asking basic accountability questions. Are all these organizations legitimate? Are they all necessary? Do sufficient resources exist to support them all? Would the available private and public funding be better spent elsewhere? (Light, 2004).

EROSION OF TRUST IN CORPORATE ENTITIES

SECOND, THE PUBLIC is less trusting of corporate entities. This is in large measure the result of a series of scandals that began in the late 1990s involving prominent businesses: Enron and MCI WorldCom in the United States and Vivendi and Parmalat in Europe. Fraud and corrupt practices in large, publicly traded companies have had significant economic impact and have eroded the confidence of investors and the general public.

The past decade has also been marked by a large number of cases of improper practices in the health sector, some affecting local communities and others having international impact. For example, a significant number of U.S. hospitals and home health care agencies—both non-profit and commercial—were involved in highly publicized cases of Medicare and Medicaid fraud (*Medicaid Fraud and Abuse,* n.d.). Cases of so-called patient dumping resulted in legislation protecting patients' access to treatment (*Examinations and Treatment for Emergency Medical Conditions,* 2007). Conflicts of interest between commercial sponsors and professional organizations—such as the partnership between the American Academy of Pediatric Dentistry and Coca-Cola (American Academy of Pediatric Dentistry Founation, 2003)—have been criticized by their members as well as by public interest groups (Miller, 2006). The Red Cross's highly publicized mismanagement of funds and blood supply in the wake of the September 11 terrorist attacks raised issues of donor accountability. Finally, the issue of so-called phantom aid has been the focus of increased scrutiny internationally as a significant amount of funding intended to build health infrastructure in poor countries has gone instead to consultants and intermediary organizations (Carey, 2005).

These commercial and health-related examples plainly illustrate why public confidence in institutions is waning. As a result, there is greater demand for organizational accountability at the board and executive levels, for more accurate and open reporting, for greater internal checks and balances, and for more government oversight.

INCREASED ACCOUNTABILITY THROUGH REGULATION

THE UNITED STATES has accordingly developed a first generation of regulatory strategies that are currently being explored and modified for adoption in other countries. The American Corporate Accountability Act of 2002, commonly known by the name of its authors, Sarbanes-Oxley, has set the regulatory framework for improved governance, management accountability, and accuracy in financial reporting. While the primary targets of the regulations are publicly traded commercial entities, portions of the law apply to all corporations, including nonprofits. Many health-related nonprofits are adopting the broader Sarbanes-Oxley guidelines as a set of best practices to demonstrate a commitment to careful and responsible management practices (ABA Coordinating Committee on Nonprofit Governance, 2006).

In addition, the IRS has supported the development of GuideStar, a national database of nonprofit organizations. The GuideStar Web site publicly posts the Form 990s that nonprofits have filed with the IRS. It includes an overview of financials, a list of board members, and a breakdown of executive compensation. In effect, it opens up any nonprofit filing with the IRS to the scrutiny of funders, regulators, competing organizations, and concerned citizens. Anyone with a link to the Internet has access to this information.

TOWARD A COMPREHENSIVE APPROACH TO NONPROFIT ACCOUNTABILITY

Cᴸᴇᴀʀᴸʏ, ᴛʜᴇʀᴇ ɪꜱ increasing external pressure for more systematic accountability. Transparency in financial reporting is a start. The question then becomes, what else should a nonprofit do to become fully accountable to its public?

UNDERSTANDING THE ROLE OF STAKEHOLDERS

Tᴏ ʙᴇɢɪɴ, ᴡᴇ first have to understand what *public* means in practical terms for the health sector as a whole and for individual nonprofits. It is useful to borrow a concept from corporate ethics and view a nonprofit's public as all of its stakeholders taken together (Friedman & Miles, 2006). *Stakeholder* in this context means any individual or group that gives something of value to the organization or gets something of value from it. So stakeholders have a direct interest, involvement, or investment. While the specific stakeholders for any health care nonprofit will differ, several general categories apply to most organizations:

Government. As we have seen, government assures the legal and tax status of health-related nonprofits. It also provides regulatory oversight and enforcement through public health authorities, and it is a source of funding through grants and contracts. For instance, the U.S. Food and Drug Administration regulates health products to assure their safety and efficacy, and the National Institutes of Health provide research and training grants.

Consumers. Institutions and individuals constitute the market for what the nonprofits produce. For example, pharmaceutical companies constitute a market for research universities. Businesses as well as individuals buy HMO and other forms of health coverage from nonprofit insurers. Patients are the consumers in hospital and clinic settings.

Employees. Employees include those who work in nonprofit health organizations: doctors, nurses, scientists, administrators, and so on. This category can be expanded to include the groups that support and represent employees, such as the American Medical Association and various trade unions.

Competing organizations. Both nonprofits and for-profit businesses can fall into this category, since it includes organizations that have the same consumers and the same products or services. For instance, hospitals with similar specialties compete for patients. Research institutions working on similar problems compete for limited sources of funding.

Complementary organizations. As with competing groups, this category can include both nonprofits and commercial entities. Complementary organizations are those that can increase each other's effectiveness. For instance, local mental health clinics usually work with nonprofit human service organizations as well as commercial home health care companies to meet the needs of their clients.

Suppliers of goods and services. Nonprofit health organizations usually have a range of contractual relationships for goods and services. In these relationships, the nonprofit becomes the customer. Goods can range from highly specialized laboratory equipment to office supplies. Services can range from waste removal to outsourced payroll, from investment management to highly specialized scientific consultants.

Private funders. Charitable dollars, including foundation and corporate donations as well as individual gifts, significantly subsidize the nonprofit health sector. Grants and gifts support a wide range of projects: constructing new buildings, funding basic research, supporting education and advocacy, and underwriting direct patient care. There are numerous well-known examples. After his death in 1873, Baltimore merchant Johns Hopkins left $7 million to establish a university and hospital in his name (Fleishman, 2007). The large pharmaceutical corporation GlaxoSmithKline supports numerous global health programs addressing specific diseases such as HIV and AIDS, malaria, and lymphatic filariasis. And the Robert Wood Johnson foundation provides support to address current pressing national health care issues such as childhood obesity and insurance coverage.

Accrediting and credentialing groups. These are the independent nonprofits that set professional standards and monitor health-sector institutions and individuals for compliance. For example, the Joint Commission provides health care accreditation and related services to hospitals, assisted-living facilities, and behavioral health care groups.

Once a nonprofit has defined its public by identifying its stakeholders, it can develop a system of accountability. The next step is to determine how to engage the stakeholders most effectively.

PROCEDURAL ETHICS AND STAKEHOLDER ENGAGEMENT

P*ROCEDURAL ETHICS PROVIDE* an approach for engaging stakeholders and increasing nonprofit accountability. This is a practical form of ethics particularly appropriate for addressing questions of how complex and dynamic organizations should behave. Right and wrong actions are not determined by rules set out in advance but result from ongoing and structured dialogue and deliberation among the stakeholders. Procedural ethics balance the perspectives and interests of stakeholder groups so they can be integrated with existing management and decision-making routines.

In a number of cases within the health sector, procedural ethics have been applied to create decision-making processes that are open, transparent, and have broad stakeholder involvement. Clinical ethics committees are widely used in U.S. hospitals and include nurses, social workers, clergy, and academic ethicists. This approach has also been used to frame health policy discussion of contentious topics like stem cell research and pandemic flu preparedness. The application of procedural ethics to routine management decisions is by no means new, but most health-related nonprofits nonetheless find it a novel idea (Eiser, Goold, & Suchman, 1999).

In this approach, stakeholders should be involved in the decision-making process at both the strategic and programmatic levels. On the strategic level, stakeholder dialogue will inform the decisions that shape the future direction of the organization as a whole. On the programmatic level, stakeholder input will guide the development of the goods and services that the nonprofit provides.

PROCEDURAL ETHICS IN NONPROFIT STRATEGY

O*RGANIZATIONAL STRATEGY IS* the responsibility of the board and senior staff of the organization. Several core management activities at this level can be enriched by broader stakeholder involvement. These include the following:

> **Board composition.** Nonprofit boards should be representative of the public served by the nonprofit. By recruiting board members who represent its stakeholder groups, an organization builds

accountability into its structure. Boards with stakeholder involvement are more likely to develop plans, set policies, establish budgets, and make decisions that accurately reflect public need and opinion.

Strategic planning. Strategic planning is the process by which a nonprofit's leadership sets the organization's future course, usually for a 3- to 5-year period. Normative and participative methods of planning involve stakeholders throughout the process. The broader the stakeholder involvement, the more accurate the plans will be, and the greater the broader community's commitment to the plans' success. The nonprofit is thereby accountable to its stakeholders from the outset of planning, even before any action is taken (Allison & Kaye, 2003).

Values statements. Clear and nuanced values statements set the standard for behavior across an organization. These statements should include how the organization relates to its stakeholder groups. Values statements capture explicitly what the organization identifies as its most important core beliefs and activities—the right things to do. For example, a nonprofit providing direct care might embrace a certain therapy, limiting its clients' options. A research center might focus on certain problems to the exclusion of others, determining which funding streams it can and will pursue. An advocacy group might position itself to serve a certain geographical area and form competing and complementary relationships with other organizations in the area. The greater the stakeholder input when formulating the organization's values, the more easily these values can be communicated to and understood by the nonprofit's public.

Ethics policies. Stakeholder input is particularly important in developing the nonprofit's ethics policies because those policies establish guidelines for responsible behavior. Going beyond legal requirements, ethics policies help align internal performance with external expectations. They spell out in detail what constitutes a conflict of interest, confidentiality, and intended environmental impact. For example, an increasing number of academic medical centers have introduced policies that prohibit physicians from accepting gifts from pharmaceutical and other biomedical companies in an attempt to limit their potential influence.

By involving stakeholders in a formal leadership role at the board level or through advisory roles in designing strategic plans, articulating values, or developing ethics policies, the nonprofit develops a system of what we might call *accountability assurance*. That is, accountability is not an afterthought but is built into the organization's governance and senior management practices.

PROCEDURAL ETHICS IN NONPROFIT OPERATIONS

LIKEWISE, STAKEHOLDERS CAN play structured roles in a nonprofit's daily operations to assure accountability on a programmatic level. Formal management processes can include and encourage stakeholder participation, using the nonprofit's specific health programs, services, or goods as a focus. The extent of stakeholder involvement and the roles they play will depend on the decisions facing managers at the moment. With certain routine issues, stakeholders might have limited involvement. In more dynamic situations, they might be closely engaged on an ongoing basis. In this way, the organization becomes accountable to stakeholders through its everyday activities. Formal stakeholder involvement will have impact in the following areas:

Monitoring external conditions. The world of health care is increasingly dynamic and complex. For any nonprofit to operate effectively in the changing environment, it must develop ways to monitor external conditions. Representatives of stakeholder groups provide a way to maintain contact with the environment. For example, talking with human service groups can help clinics better understand social trends affecting the health of their clients. Discussions with foundation officers can help research and educational institutions understand emerging priorities in institutional giving and project support.

Design, review, and evaluation processes. Once a nonprofit has determined that a set of activities is in keeping with the needs of its public, stakeholders can play an active role in its further development. They can participate in the design, review, and evaluation processes of new and existing projects and programs. This approach can utilize common techniques for gathering input such as convening focus groups or surveying opinion leaders. Involvement before implementation assures that management will not miss important details, and it promotes transparency and buy-in.

Reconciling divergent points of view. Sometimes an organization is faced with multiple options, and divergent points of view arise within the organization about which one to choose. Stakeholder input can be beneficial in determining the optimum choice. Stakeholders might for example contribute important external information indicating the better choice from the public's point of view. The dialogue should be organized using an established method that results in open and focused discussion. Such methods include focus groups, structured interviews, and surveys.

At the program level, stakeholder involvement treats accountability as an emergent process developing alongside the organization's core activities. When stakeholder groups have well-defined roles in the discussion, they are in a position to inform decisions, and they are in a position to become better informed about programs and their impact. Participation creates a deeper understanding of the work a nonprofit does. The ultimate result is greater transparency and buy-in as programs evolve.

CONCLUSION

NONPROFIT HEALTH ORGANIZATIONS, no matter their size or scope, can effectively respond to increasing demands for accountability. By identifying their critical stakeholder groups and actively engaging them in management dialogue at both the strategic and program levels in a deliberate way, they put ethics into practice. Accountability is integrated into organizational structures and processes and becomes routine.

REFERENCES

ABA Coordinating Committee on Nonprofit Governance. (2006). *Guide to nonprofit corporate governance in the wake of Sarbanes-Oxley*. Chicago: American Bar Association.

Allison, M., & Kaye, J. (2003) *Strategic planning for nonprofit organizations* (2nd ed.). Hoboken, NJ: John Wiley & Sons.

American Academy of Pediatric Dentistry Foundation. (2003). *Campaign quarterly*. Chicago: Author.

Carey, R. (2005). *Real or phantom aid?* Retrieved August 13, 2007, from http://www.oecd.org/document/29/0,2340,en_2649_33721_34990749_1_1_1_1,00.html

Eiser, A., Goold, S., & Suchman, A. (1999). The role of bioethics and business ethics. *Journal of General Internal Medicine, 14*(Suppl. 1), S58–S62.

Examinations and treatment for emergency medical conditions and women in labor. (2007). Retrieved November 16, 2007, from http://www.ssa.gov/OP_ Home/ssact/title18/1867.htm

Fleishman, J. (2007). The foundation: A great American secret; how private wealth is changing the world. Cambridge, MA: Public Affairs.

Friedman, A., & Miles, S. (2006). *Stakeholders: Theory and practice.* Oxford, UK: Oxford University Press.

Independent Sector & Urban Institute. (2002). *The new nonprofit almanac and desk reference: The essential figures for managers, researchers, and volunteers.* San Francisco: Jossey-Bass.

Light, P. (2004). *Sustaining nonprofit performance.* Washington, DC: Brookings Institution Press.

Medicaid fraud and abuse. (n.d.). Retrieved September 8, 2007, from http://www.cms.hhs.gov/MDFraudAbuseGenInfo/

Miller, J. D. (2006). Conflict-of-interest spurs new rules, not consensus. *Journal of the National Cancer Institute, 98*(3), 1678–1679.

Salamon, L. (2002). *The state of nonprofit America.* Washington, DC: Brookings Institution Press.

Savas, E. (2000). *Privatization and public-private partnerships.* New York: Seven Bridges Press.

53

The Bioethics of Tobacco

ERIC A. FELDMAN

T OBACCO HAS BEEN the focus of countless lawsuits, the center
of bitter political conflict, the subject of careful historical analysis, and the engine of dramatic corporate and personal wealth. In
the literature on ethics, however, its impact has been modest. The only
serious, book-length treatment published over the past several decades
was Goodin's *No Smoking: The Ethical Issues* (1989), which did a fine job
of exploring the philosophical justifications for government regulation of smoking but has long been out of print. Academic publications
are rife with articles on the relationship between tobacco advertising
and smoking initiation, the addictive properties of nicotine, and the
intended and unintended consequences of FDA regulation of the tobacco industry, but they rarely make the ethical dimensions of such issues their primary concern (e.g., Gately, 2001; Glantz & Balbuch, 2000;
Kessler, 2001). Not even the mainstream bioethics journals show much
interest in tobacco; a search of the archives of the *American Journal of
Bioethics* leads to not a single article about either tobacco or smoking
(see http://www.bioethics.net/search/).

On the other hand, the contentious nature of the debate over smoking means that almost everything written about tobacco is, to some
extent, about ethics. Studies of the impact of advertising restrictions

I am grateful to Alison Stein for her excellent research assistance on this
chapter.

and bans, for example, frequently argue that they are justified if they can be shown to limit the number of people who smoke. The fight over zoning restrictions that separate smokers from nonsmokers, or prohibit smoking in certain places, is fundamentally about when it is appropriate to prohibit individuals from harming themselves, and what degree of harm to others is needed to justify placing limits on individual liberty. Analyses of the marketing of U.S. tobacco products overseas cannot avoid questions about the ethics of trade and to what extent, if at all, economic policy and health policy should be coupled. And many book-length treatments of tobacco, including Kluger's comprehensive *Ashes to Ashes* (Kluger, 1997), Sullum's cranky libertarian tract *For Your Own Good* (Sullum, 1998), and Brandt's magisterial *The Cigarette Century* (Brandt, 2007), take a strong ethical position, even if they are not explicitly engaged in ethical analysis.

Rather than rehash the most visible and politically volatile issues of tobacco control, this chapter examines several areas that have attracted only modest scholarly attention but raise pointed ethical concerns. First, it will examine smoking bans in light of the changing demographics of tobacco consumption, and it will raise questions about the ethics of policies that further marginalize particular social groups. Second, it will analyze the ethics of cigarette pricing; charging increasingly high prices has come to be seen as a legitimate public health strategy, even though one unintended consequence of higher prices is that low-income families may spend so much on tobacco that they have insufficient funds left for essential foods. Third, it will discuss the effort to require that the home institutions of American Legacy Foundation research grantees pledge to forgo receiving research money from any tobacco-related concern, thereby raising difficult questions about academic freedom.

SMOKING BANS AND SOCIAL MARGINALIZATION

O F THE MANY approaches to reducing the impact of smoking on health, perhaps the most widely used, both in the United States and internationally, is the zoning of social space.[1] In contrast to the default assumption of peaceful coexistence between smokers and nonsmokers, who for many years sat on adjacent barstools and dined at neighboring tables, those who smoke have found themselves increasingly relegated to designated smoking areas or exiled entirely. Not only have public areas like municipal buildings and train stations gone smoke-free, but privately owned restaurants, bars, stores, offices, and clubs have been deemed public spaces subject to laws that prohibit smoking. The medical justification for excluding smokers from a wide range of establishments rests on the harms caused by environmental tobacco smoke; not only are smokers making themselves sick, but their smoke is damaging the health of nonsmokers. As the data on such harms have strengthened and been amplified by academic studies and U.S. government reports (see *The Health Consequences of Involuntary Exposure to Tobacco Smoke. A Report of the Surgeon General, 2006*), states and localities have been emboldened to pass increasingly far-reaching smoking bans.

It is easy to appreciate the benefits of bans—the clinging stench of stale tobacco will no longer be ubiquitous, nonsmokers will not continue to be placed at risk by smokers, some smokers will smoke less or quit because smoking will be less convenient, and they may be spared the misery of tobacco-related disease—but one should also take account of the consequences. Increasing the restrictions on where people can smoke has made those who continue to smoke into social pariahs, pushed further and further into the geographic and conceptual margins of society. And while there are almost always ethical concerns with marginalization, they are dramatically amplified by the demographic reality of tobacco consumption.

Over the past several decades the percentage of adult smokers in the United States has steadily declined, from a high of 46% of adults in 1950 to 20.8% in 2006 (23.9% of men, 18% of women; Brandt, 2007, p. 499; Cigarette Smoking Among Adults, 2007). Crucial to that decline is the fact that well-educated, relatively affluent individuals increasingly have given up their smoking habits while among those with lower income and fewer resources, smoking continues to be widespread. Those below the poverty line smoke significantly more, at 29.1%, than those above the poverty line, at 20.6% (Brandt, 2007, p. 499; Cigarette Smoking Among Adults, 2007). More starkly, of those who have earned a graduate degree—including a masters, a doctorate, or a professional degree—only 8% are smokers, whereas those whose schooling terminated with a GED (a degree awarded to those who did not finish high school but passed a series of exams) smoke at a rate of 39.6% (Brandt, 2007, p. 499; Cigarette Smoking Among Adults, 2007).

Such patterns are neither new nor distinctive; highly educated individuals have smoked at a lower rate than those without a high school diploma for decades (Feldman & Bayer, 2004).[2] As smoking bans have reordered social space and pushed smokers to the margins, however, the implications of the education/income gap have become more pronounced. The physical expulsion of smokers from restaurants, bars, and other establishments has been accompanied by their symbolic rejection, with smoking recast as an activity that emits an unpleasant odor, pollutes the air, and signals a personal failing. Smokers, seen as too weak to overcome their shortcomings, increasingly have been treated as suffering from an illness that must be treated with medical interventions like nicotine replacement therapies and smoking cessation programs. As participants in an activity considered socially irresponsible and costly, smokers—disproportionately people who are relatively poor and poorly educated—have been pressed to either stop smoking or pay the price for continuing, which includes increasingly expensive cigarettes and social opprobrium (see the following section).

The unambiguous public health benefits of bans may justify the burdens placed on lower income/education smokers. Unquestionably, limiting the places where smoking is permitted has increased the likelihood that smokers will throw up their arms in despair and quit smoking (or will smoke less). Still, for those interested in social equity, the education/income gap in smoking rates is deeply disturbing, particularly when compounded by the way in which those who smoke increasingly are treated like social pariahs. If there is to be an ethics of smoking, it must carefully address the competing values at stake in a society that allows individuals to engage in a broad range of dangerous activities while reserving its scorn for only a few.

SMOKING, NOT EATING: THE IMPACT OF TOBACCO TAXES ON THE POOR

FOR CENTURIES, GOVERNMENTS have imposed taxes on tobacco in order to capture a portion of the revenues generated by the public's embrace of smoking. But only in the past decade or two has the state taken a different approach to the tobacco tax. Throughout the industrialized world, public health advocates have successfully argued that taxing tobacco is a legitimate way of inducing people to give up their smoking habits. By making a pack of cigarettes more expensive, the argument goes, some people will decide that smoking is no longer worth the money. The widely reported data for the developed world is that a 10% increase in the price of cigarettes will lead to a decrease in tobacco consumption of approximately 4% (Becker, Grossman, & Murphy, 1994, p. 407). By raising the price of a pack of cigarettes from $3.00 to $3.30, for example, tobacco consumption in a jurisdiction in which 1,000,000 cigarettes/day are consumed would decrease by 40,000 cigarettes/day. Unfortunately, raising the price of cigarettes does more than induce some people to quit; it also results in higher prices for those who continue to smoke. Given the population of current smokers, the consequence is a profoundly regressive tax.

The cost of smoking in many areas in the United States has risen dramatically. Indeed, prices are "eclipsing $8.00 a pack."[3] The 1998 Master Settlement Agreement (MSA) is one crucial factor in the price increase.[4] Payments made under the MSA go to state governments and are functionally identical to a tax; rather than tax cigarette smokers directly, however, the government gets paid by the tobacco companies, which have raised the price of cigarettes to enable them to amass the large sum of money they owe to the states (Melnick, 1999). Direct tax increases also were a major factor in the escalation of the cost of smoking. In 2002, New York City began implementing a comprehensive, five-component tobacco control strategy. The first component, an increase in the city's cigarette tax (from $0.08 to $1.50 per pack), became effective on July 2, 2002. New York State had already increased its tax from $1.11 to $1.50 per pack on April 1, 2002. Together, the state and city tax increases raised the cost of a pack of cigarettes by approximately 32%, to a retail price of approximately $6.85 (Frieden et al., 2005). This also results from the combined city and state cigarette tax of $3.00 per pack on all cigarettes possessed for sale or use in New York City ($1.50 is New York State tax; $1.50 is New York City tax; see http://www.nyc.gov/html/dof/html/services/services_fraud_cigarettes.shtml). In California, state taxes account for the $0.87 of the average $4.34 that people pay for a pack of cigarettes, or 20% of the cost of a pack ("State Cigarette Tax Ranks and Rate, Campaign for Tobacco Free Kids," 2007).

Viewed strictly from the perspective of limiting the negative health consequences of smoking—lung cancer, heart disease, and more— reducing the number of smokers is clearly desirable. Indeed, some public health scholars are so focused on the link between increased costs and smoking cessation that they do not view the tobacco tax as regressive, since it has a positive impact (individuals are less likely to be afflicted by a tobacco-related disease) on those lower-income people who quit rather than pay (e.g., Brandt, 2007). Unfortunately, there are relatively few such individuals; as discussed above, data on smoking rates makes clear that the overall drop in smoking rates is primarily the result of smoking cessation among people of higher income and education, not those in the lower brackets. Rather than focusing on the benefits accruing to a relatively distinct group of smokers, therefore, the tax should be evaluated with reference to its impact on all smokers, and particularly lower-income smokers. And there, the data is deeply discouraging.

In 1969, a senior executive at Philip Morris declared, "The cigarette will preempt even food in times of scarcity on the smoker's priority list" (Wakeham, 1969, p. 240). It appears that his prediction was accurate. A recent study confirms that smokers at the lowest end of the economic spectrum will buy cigarettes even when they do not have sufficient funds to cover the cost of essential groceries (Armour, Pitts, & Lee, 2008). More specifically, low-income families with earnings at or below 200% of the federal poverty level are 6% more likely to be "food insecure"—unable to purchase enough food for a healthy and active lifestyle—if there is a smoker in the family (Armour et al., 2008). Such families spend a significant amount of money on cigarettes, on average $33.70 per week, and as a result too frequently come up short when it comes to buying food (Armour et al., 2008). The study did not examine other purchases that may be forgone as a result of the money being spent on tobacco. But one can easily imagine the possibility that as cigarettes get increasingly expensive, families may buy fewer books, less clothing, attend fewer cultural events, and more.

Dropping the price of cigarettes, or subsidizing their cost for low-income families, would be a cynical solution to the problem of high tobacco taxes. The state has an interest in reducing unnecessary morbidity and mortality, and the health harms of smoking are an appropriate target. But we should not ignore the disparate impact of high tobacco taxes, and it is disingenuous to contend that increasing the price of a pack of cigarettes is a successful public health strategy when one consequence of that strategy is that it increases the likelihood that some families will end up with plenty of butts in the ashtray but not enough food in the pantry.

UNHOLY ALLIANCES AND TOBACCO RESEARCH FUNDING

IN 1998, AFTER a series of lawsuits over the costs of treating individuals with tobacco-related diseases had reached the courts, the defendant tobacco companies and plaintiff state attorneys general (AG) settled their dispute.[5] The settlement involved a huge sum of money—approximately $250 billion—and included a number of less orthodox terms. Among the most unusual was the creation of the American Legacy Foundation, which was charged with developing national programs to counter the health effects of smoking through "grants, technical training and assistance, youth activism, strategic partnerships, counter-marketing and grass roots marketing campaigns, public relations, research and community outreach" (http://www.amer icanlegacy.org/12.htm). Established in 1999, the foundation has been an important sponsor of academic research, giving away over $150 million to individuals and organizations involved in tobacco control research (http://www.americanlegacy.org/46.htm).

While the foundation quickly took its place as a crucial source of funding for academic public health researchers interested in tobacco, there was a catch. One of the conditions for receiving a grant, according to what is known as Clause 12 of the foundation's grant conditions, is that the researcher's institution must pledge in writing that no member of that institution is currently accepting, or will in the future accept, money or its equivalent from any tobacco manufacturer, distributor, or other tobacco-related entity.[6] For a faculty member to be funded by the American Legacy Foundation, in other words, one's dean must guarantee to the foundation that neither the school nor any individual faculty member is currently funded by a tobacco manufacturer or one of its affiliates, and will continue not to be for the entire duration of the foundation's grant.

There are obvious reasons why an academic researcher at a school of public health should be wary of accepting funding from a tobacco company. Indeed, concerns about undue influence are so pervasive in the tobacco control area, and in medicine generally, that many publishers now require authors of tobacco-related books and articles to reveal conflicts of interest on the first page of their publications. Moreover, skepticism should greet the claims of tobacco researchers whose work is funded by the tobacco industry, just as one would be skeptical of data on obesity generated by a researcher funded by McDonalds or any public health research sponsored by the industry under investigation. Nevertheless, the American Legacy Foundation's Clause 12 requires more than individual prudence and restraint. It denies potentially important funding to individuals based upon the decisions of their colleagues, decisions that however distasteful to the foundation are legal and, at least in certain circumstances, may be appropriate.[7]

Lorillard Inc., for example, which manufactures and sells Newport, Kent, and other cigarettes, is wholly owned by the Loews Corporation. Loews is controlled by the Tisch family, which has donated generously to educational institutions like Tufts and NYU. Indeed, Lawrence Tisch, who built Loews into a corporate powerhouse, was chairman of NYU's Board of Trustees for 20 years, a period during which the school raised $1.8 billion and endowed more than 140 professorships (http://www.nyu.edu/nyutoday/archives/17/06/PageOneStories/tisch-obit.html). Without any apparent sense of irony, NYU's 700-plus bed hospital, which houses the NYU Cancer Institute, bears his name. Are public health and medical researchers at that hospital, or working for NYU, tainted by the fact that they have directly profited from Tisch's largesse? Should the American Legacy Foundation refuse to provide funding to NYU tobacco researchers? Or would the foundation make a (dubious) distinction between funds given to universities and/or researchers by individuals, rather than by the companies controlled by those individuals? The value of academic freedom can be protected by leaving funding decisions to individual researchers, requiring them to be transparent about their support, and letting consumers/readers decide whether the quality of their research has been diminished by suspect funding. The foundation's willingness to impose funding rules on all faculty members at particular schools, and the willingness of many (but not all) schools to acquiesce to such a condition, opens the door to other groups who want to influence the academic research agenda—foundations that require a pledge that no faculty member is studying evolution, for example, or has taken money from the pharmaceutical industry, or is writing about needle exchange or teenage sexual behavior. The funding of tobacco-related research has long been contentious; unfortunately, the foundation's Clause 12 further polarizes the debate, and has created a rift between those public health researchers who prioritize the value of academic freedom (and thus bristle at Clause 12) and those who are willing to limit academic freedom in the interest of tobacco control.

CONCLUSION

THERE ARE, OF course, many areas in which tobacco and ethics cross paths. One could, for example, examine the U.S. government's trade policies, and its willingness to pressure foreign governments to eliminate trade barriers that limit their importation of American tobacco products, even when doing so is likely to increase tobacco-related morbidity and mortality. Punitive damages in tobacco tort litigation also raise ethical concerns—is it fair for a small number of successful plaintiffs to receive multimillion-dollar punitive damage awards when so many others receive neither compensatory nor punitive damages? And the hundreds of millions of dollars in legal fees awarded to certain attorneys who were involved in the MSA, viewed in light of the funds received by sick smokers—none—also deserves ethical scrutiny. This brief chapter cannot begin to examine the full range of issues at the intersection of bioethics and smoking. If it stimulates at least some consideration of that intersection, it will have satisfied its goal.

NOTES

1. See, for example, "City of Philadelphia Clean Indoor Air Worker Protection Law" (2006), which protects Philadelphians from the harmful effects of second-hand smoke by making virtually all workplaces in the city smoke-free.

2. See also Menvielle, Leclerc, Chastang, Melchior, and Luce (2007), who conclude that despite the overall decrease in cancer mortality rates, smoking has contributed to the continued existence of remaining substantial socioeconomic inequalities in cancer mortality among men.

3. Feuer and Sweeny (2006) describe the rising cost of cigarettes.

4. "Under the Master Settlement Agreement, seven tobacco companies agreed to change the way tobacco products are marketed and pay the states an estimated $206 billion. The tobacco companies also agreed to finance a $1.5 billion anti-smoking campaign, open previously secret industry documents, and disband industry trade groups which Attorneys General maintain conspired to conceal damaging research from the public" (http://ag.ca.gov/tobacco/msa.php).

5. For an explanation of the Master Settlement Agreement, see Becker et al. (1994).

6. The letter of intent guidelines for the American Legacy Foundation's Small Innovative Grants Program describes the policy in its section on special requirements and restrictions. "To avoid any real, potential, or perceived conflict of interest between Legacy's grant recipients and tobacco-related entities, Legacy will not award a grant to any applicant that is in current receipt of any grant monies or in-kind contribution from any tobacco manufacturer, distributor, or other tobacco-related entity. In addition, Legacy expects that a grantee will not accept any grant monies or in-kind contribution from any tobacco manufacturer, distributor, or other tobacco-related entity over the duration of the grant" (http://www.americanlegacy.org/Files/SIG_Letter_of_Intent_Guide lines_October_2007.pdf). See also Balas, Ramiah, and Martin (2004).

7. For a lively debate on Clause 12, see "Why Universities Should Not Accept Money From the American Legacy Foundation" (2006).

REFERENCES

Armour, B. S., Pitts, M. M., & Lee, C. (2008). Cigarette smoking and food insecurity among low-income families in the United States, 2001. *American Journal of Health Promotion, 22*(6), 386.

Balas, A. E., Ramiah, K., & Martin, K. (2004). ASPH/American Legal Foundation Step Up Program: An innovative partnership for tobacco studies in the schools of public health. *Public Health Reports, 119*(3), 380–385.

Becker, G., Grossman, M., & Murphy, K. M. (1994). An empirical analysis of cigarette addiction. *The American Economic Review, 84*(3), 396–418.

Brandt, A. M. (2007). *The cigarette century: The rise, fall and deadly persistence of the product that defines America.* New York: Basic Books.

Cigarette smoking among adults—United States, 2006. (2007). *Morbidity and Mortality Weekly Report, 54,* 1157–1161.

"City of Philadelphia Clean Indoor Air Worker Protection Law," June 15, 2006, Bill No. 050063-A.

Feldman, E. A. & Bayer, R. (2004). Conclusion to *Unfiltered: Conflicts over tobacco policy and public health* (pp. 303–306). Cambridge, MA: Harvard University Press.

Feuer, A. & Sweeny, M. (2006, January 25). Smoking, and venting about prices eclipsing $8 a pack. *New York Times,* sec. B, col. 3, p. 3.

Frieden, T. R., Mostashari, F., Kerker, B. D., Miller, N., Hajat, A. & Frankel, M. (2005). Adult tobacco use levels after intensive tobacco control measures: New York City, 2002–2003. *American Journal of Public Health, 95,* 1016–1023. Retrieved December 15, 2007, from http://www.pubmedcentral.nih.gov/articlerender.fcgi?&artinstid=1449302

Gately, I. (2001). *Tobacco: A cultural history of how an exotic plant seduced civilization.* New York: Grove Press.

Glantz, S. A., & Balbuch, E. D. (2000). *Tobacco war: Inside the California battles.* Berkeley: University of California Press.

Goodin, R. E. (1989). *No smoking: The ethical issues.* Chicago: University of Chicago Press.

The health consequences of involuntary exposure to tobacco smoke: A report of the Surgeon General. (2006). U.S. Department of Health and Human Services, Centers for Disease Control and Prevention, Coordinating Center for Health Promotion, National Center for Chronic Disease Prevention and Health Promotion, Office on Smoking and Health. Retrieved October 21, 2008, from http://www.surgeongeneral.gov/library/secondhandsmoke

Kessler, D. (2001). *A question of intent: A great American battle with a deadly industry.* New York: Public Affairs.

Kluger, R. (1997). *Ashes to ashes: America's hundred-year cigarette war, the public health, and the unabashed triumph of Philip Morris.* New York: Vintage Books.

Melnick, R. S. (1999). Tobacco litigation: Good for the body but not the body politic. *Journal of Health Politics, Policy and Law, 24*(4), 805–810.

Menvielle, G., Leclerc, A., Chastang, J-F., Melchior, M., & Luce, D. (2007). Changes in socioeconomic inequalities in cancer mortality rates among French men between 1968 and 1996. *American Journal of Public Health, 97*(11), 2082–2087.

"State cigarette tax ranks and rate, Campaign for Tobacco Free Kids." (2007). Retrieved December 15, 2007, from http://tobaccofreekids.org/research/factsheets/pdf/0099.pdf

Sullum, J. (1998). *For your own good: The anti-smoking campaign and the tyranny of public health.* New York: Free Press.

Wakeham, H. (1969). *Smoker psychology research.* Presentation to the Philip Morris board of directors, November 26, 1969. Richmond, VA: Philip Morris.

"Why universities should not accept money from the American Legacy Foundation. (2006, September 25). Retrieved December 15, 2007, from *http://tobaccoanalysis.blogspot.com/2006/09/in-my-view-why-universities-should-not.html*

54

HIV Exceptionalism and the Mutability of Ethical Boundaries

Marlene Eisenberg, Michael B. Blank,
and Ronald Bayer

We reach a new level of awareness when we approach the other as a Thou—as a relational being...I-Thou is a relationship of openness, directness, mutuality, and presence. I-It, in contrast, is the typical subject-object relationship in which one knows and uses other people and things without allowing them to exist for oneself in their uniqueness...Through the Thou a person becomes I.

—*Martin Buber (1923)*

N JUNE 1981, the first case of AIDS was diagnosed in the United States. Before effective treatments were available, diagnosis invariably carried with it the stigma of behaviors such as homosexuality and drug use, along with the expectation of death. Four years later, in 1985, the HIV antibody test became widely available. However, with the information provided by the test came the accompanying fear of forced testing, compulsory treatment, and isolation, which were the traditional public health approaches to infectious diseases (Colgrove & Bayer, 2005). There was also the pervasive questioning about the utility of testing, in the absence of effective treatment. In response to these concerns, in 1987, the Centers for Disease Control (CDC) developed guidelines to promote voluntary counseling and testing (VCT) to hemophiliacs, those who received blood transfusions, men who have sex with men (MSM), and injection drug users (IDUs), as they were considered to be in the highest risk groups for the transmission of HIV/AIDS. As an additional complement, routine testing was recommended for anyone seeking treatment for STDs regardless of health care setting. These guidelines resulted in the handling of HIV testing and diagnoses separate and apart from most other medical procedures to ensure that individuals undergoing the test did not suffer from discrimination or stigma associated with the behaviors that led to testing or with a potential positive diagnosis.

The resulting protections were three-pronged. First, informed consents were designed to focus solely on HIV/AIDS with the intent of expressing, in real terms, the ethical principal of individual autonomy within clinical practice. This provided the individual with an opportunity to be the ultimate decision-maker regarding whether or not to be tested (Appelbaum, Lidz, & Meisel, 1987), and it was a process that empowered individuals. It encouraged active participation in the promotion of an individual's own health care, as well as an opportunity to disseminate positive health care messages to others within their risk group. Second, there was concern that testing opportunities would be lost especially for those who needed them the most (Stall et al., 1996), so testing anonymity became de rigueur, particularly for those at highest risk for HIV (Fehrs et al., 1988).

Third, pre- and posttest counseling targeted both medical and psychological issues related to the testing process, testing outcomes, education, and the potential for positive behavior change. In the event of a positive finding, counseling and referral to appropriate treatment was provided to counter the variety of responses to a positive diagnosis, which often included suicidal ideation, depression, and severe anxiety (Coates, Moore, & McKusick, 1987; Ostrow et al., 1989). The timing of the delivery of the counseling component was also important. It was most relevant if it occurred immediately following notification, as that was when the most intense reactions to diagnosis were observed (Ironson et al., 1990; Perry et al., 1990). High-risk individuals often experienced anxiety associated with testing because, in the absence of viable treatment options, a positive diagnosis was a certain death sentence. Even after HAART (highly active antiretroviral therapy) treatment became available in 1995, and HIV/AIDS became a chronic illness, stigma associated with a positive test result lingered in the form of anxiety over disclosure to significant others. There was fear, legitimate

633

*HIV
Exceptionalism
and the Mutability
of Ethical
Boundaries*

for some, that even their health care providers would avoid contact and discontinue their care (Brimlow, Cook, & Seaton, 2003) because of fears about contagion and death (Weinberger, Conover, Samsa, & Greenberg, 1992). Perhaps less crippling, but creating no less of a barrier to treatment, health care providers expressed concerns about "courtesy stigma" (Goffman, 1963) or the stigma that comes from other providers knowing that they delivered HIV-related treatment services (Snyder, Omoto, & Crain, 1999).

WHAT IS HIV EXCEPTIONALISM?

HIV EXCEPTIONALISM DESCRIBES these extra provisions of informed consent, anonymous testing, and pre- and posttest counseling, which were targeted to high-risk groups (Bayer, 1989, 1991, 1999). During the 1990s, the CDC expanded the recommendations to include individuals receiving health care either in an inpatient or out-patient facility. In 2001, routine testing of pregnant women was initiated and prior recommendations for pretest counseling were relaxed. The 2001 recommendations were remarkable not necessarily for their content, which was consistent with older recommendations, but for the additional freedom with which they allowed providers to interpret implementation of HIV testing services. Later recommendations (CDC, 2003) continued this trend with specifications that encouraged providers to consider HIV testing within the traditional battery of diagnostic and screening tests, and to include universal testing of women either during labor and delivery, or postpartum. The most recently proposed recommendations (CDC, 2006a) continue to expand HIV testing into routine health care by encouraging voluntary HIV screening across health care settings for all individuals age 13 to 64, using an opt-out approach where an HIV test is performed unless an individual specifically refuses participation. The new guidelines additionally specify that high-risk individuals receive annual HIV tests, along with the recommendation that separate written consent for HIV testing and pretest counseling be eliminated.

The most recent recommendations are a response to a long-standing debate regarding the effectiveness of so-called HIV exceptionalism to reduce rates of HIV transmission, and its associated risk behaviors. Discussions regarding modifications to the special HIV protocol were formally initiated more than 17 years ago (Bayer, 1991), because the special circumstances present in the early 1980s that had initially justified separation of HIV from most other medical treatments no longer existed. More recently, it has been argued that the special public health considerations so thoughtfully crafted early in the epidemic may now be hindering public health efforts to fight the disease (Frieden, Das-Douglas, Kellerman, & Henning, 2005; Manavi, 2005).

VOLUNTARY COUNSELING AND TESTING (VCT): RISKS AND BENEFITS

FROM A PUBLIC health perspective, VCT has not been associated with a demonstrable increase in the number of individuals getting tested (Braithwaite, Hammett, & Mayberry, 1996), with approximately 25% of people infected with HIV unaware of their status (CDC, 2005). Those who remain unaware of their status are estimated to be more than three times more likely to transmit the disease to others (CDC, 2006b). The original testing protocol emphasized a focus on targeted risk groups, but according to Paltiel and colleagues (2005), up to 20% of HIV-infected individuals do not fall within a targeted risk group. The disease has already bridged from high-risk groups such as injection drug users and men who have sex with men into the general heterosexual population. Unfortunately, interventions found to be effective with these groups may not translate into similar success for newly identified risk groups such as Blacks and Latinos, who are actually less likely to engage in traditional high-risk behaviors but paradoxically have been observed with the highest rates of infection (Metzger, 2006).

Early diagnosis and initiation of therapy, especially while those infected are asymptomatic, are potent public health mechanisms that delay disease progression and limit opportunistic infections (Paltiel et al., 2005). But compliance with testing follow-up has been observed to be notoriously low, with follow-up rates of 10% for individuals referred from emergency rooms (Coil, Haucoos, Witt, Wallace, & Lewis, 2004). And onset of treatment for low-risk, nontargeted individuals may occur later in the life span of infection resulting in treatment that is initiated only when the disease has progressed into AIDS-related infections. This not only shortens the life span for the infected person but lengthens the time-frame available for disease transmission to others (Frieden et al., 2005). Anonymous testing precludes active surveillance and routine public health practices such as partner notification and testing used for other STIs (sexually transmitted infections), and reliance on those who do know of their HIV-positive status to share their status with current partners has not been reliable or widespread. For example, Landis and colleagues (1992) found that only 14% of a sample of HIV positives agreed to partner notification, and that tracing was only successful in 7% of these cases. These studies underscore the vulnerability inherent in a testing paradigm that relies solely on voluntary

635

*HIV
Exceptionalism
and the Mutability
of Ethical
Boundaries*

HIV counseling and testing protocols, with the possibility that VCT may actually inhibit partner testing and thereby facilitate another mechanism by which disease transmission can continue unabated.

The underlying goal of the CDC's 2006 recommendations was to expand HIV testing to identify individuals who are infected unknowingly and to direct them to needed health care services. In addition, it was hoped that by expanding HIV testing, it would be normalized and its associated stigma reduced. A final purpose of expanded testing was to identify infection earlier and more often.

ISSUES OF IMPLEMENTATION

THERE IS A great deal of support for the latest CDC recommendations. The American Medical Association and HIV Medical Association support routine testing, as does the American College of Nurse Midwives and the American Academy of Family Physicians (American College of Nurse-Midwives, 2003). For many AIDS advocates, however, the 2006 CDC recommendations to expand routine HIV testing into the sphere of low-risk populations has engendered considerable controversy, as the advocates perceive the changes to be a relaxation of protections they originally fought so hard to establish. Consequently, adoption of the new recommendations has been sporadic and inconsistent. In a practical sense, this slow diffusion may be due to conflict between these recommendations and state regulations that must undergo lengthy policy review in order to be updated (*Kaiser Daily HIV/AIDS Report,* 2007). In particular, 24 states still require pretest counseling, and 32 states continue to require separate informed consent prior to HIV testing, both items that were dropped from the 2006 CDC updates. But these changes have also elicited concern from HIV advocates who are wary of HIV testing without the prior protections. They charge that implementation of the CDC recommendations cannot occur in the current vacuum of treatment options (Gerber, 2007), when only one-third of infected individuals are actually receiving care (Fleming et al., 2002). Lack of insurance coverage for HIV treatment may be driving this finding, for it is estimated that 45% of HIV positives have no health insurance, with hospital emergency departments often being the sole provider of health care for many (Kaiser Family Foundation, 2004). Advocates note that HIV is "the only reportable disease that is not explicitly tied to care" (Chase, 2006).

Second, AIDS advocates are skeptical about the removal of pretest and posttest counseling, as its absence may increase the risk of infection for individuals engaging in high-risk behavior without the benefit of risk-reduction information (Valdiserri, 2007).

While one of the intents of expanded HIV testing is to normalize it for the larger population, the opt-out provision and the mandatory testing recommended by the CDC have provoked an enormous amount of comment from AIDS advocates due to continued concern about HIV stigma and discrimination. While the argument has been made that tuberculosis and cancer are similarly associated with stigma, high treatment costs, and employment discrimination (Bayer, 2007), advocates argue that the effect of a positive HIV test is fundamentally different than outcomes from these other diagnoses (Lambda Legal, 2007a). Employment-related HIV discrimination claims have remained fairly consistent since 1994 (Lambda Legal, 2007b), and stigma persists in the health care industry as well (Sears & Ho, 2006), with almost 50% of obstetricians and 56% of staff in skilled nursing care facilities reporting that they would refuse to treat an individual with HIV. This data is used by advocates to argue against elimination of counseling and education. While such data certainly reflects the need for professional education, it does not directly address the effect that elimination of pretest counseling might have on the behavior of at-risk individuals or the behavior of the general population that undergoes the testing using an opt-out approach.

The cost-effectiveness of the opt-out provision to increase the number of new infections being identified has been questioned by some, such as Holtgrave (2007), who found that targeted testing was much more efficient than universal testing. However, some empirical support for the opt-out provision was reported by Zetola (2007), who found an increase in HIV testing rates both before and after opt-out and pretesting were removed from the standard HIV testing protocol. Perhaps more importantly, the number of positive tests significantly increased as well. While there was an upwards trend in testing before the policy change, these data support the argument that relaxation of the special provisions inherent in HIV exceptionalism may not act to suppress testing.

THE ASCENDANCY OF ADVOCATES TO IMPACT PUBLIC HEALTH POLICY

THE PERCEIVED EVISCERATION of HIV exceptionalism has generated discussion and debate about the relevance of the original protections as well as the ethics associated with their alteration. Simply stated, advocates believe that the ethical and moral rights of people with AIDS are threatened when a shift from the exacting standards of opt-in are replaced by an opt-out approach with its assumptions of consent (Wynia, 2006). Both groups have effectively used empirical data

637

*HIV
Exceptionalism
and the Mutability
of Ethical
Boundaries*

to support divergent points of view. At what point does public health trump an individual's right to privacy? The narrative of HIV exceptionalism represents a potent example of how boundaries between vulnerable populations and health care providers, as well as among and between vulnerable populations themselves, must receive careful consideration before, during, and after implementation of health policy changes.

In reflecting on the tension associated with balancing individual rights with public health needs, the interests represented by this dichotomy have shifted from limited to expansive, as represented by HIV exceptionalism. During much of the 20th century, public health authorities often regulated behavior considered to be in the best interests of the public, but they rarely, if ever, sought the counsel of those most likely to be affected by their decisions. For example, the landmark Supreme Court decision of 1905, *Jacobson v. Massachusetts*, compelled Henning Jacobson to be vaccinated for smallpox (Colgrove & Bayer, 2005) in spite of his considerable reservations about the effect the vaccine might have on his health. The forced sterilization of Carrie Buck is another example of extreme coercion being exercised for the potential benefit of public health. While the *Jacobson v. Massachusetts* decision was prompted by the potential for an epidemic of smallpox, in the case of *Buck v. Bell*, and her forced sterilization, the threat of infection was much more distal to public health interests. Even so, Justice Oliver Wendell Holmes, Jr. argued that "It is better for all the world, if instead of waiting to execute degenerate offspring for crime, or to let them starve for their imbecility, society can prevent those who are manifestly unfit from continuing their kind. The principle that sustains compulsory vaccination is broad enough to cover cutting the Fallopian tubes.... Three generations of imbeciles are enough" (Lombardo, 1985, p. 30).

Buck v. Bell is commonly considered to be an embarrassment by ethicists today. In contrast to the complete disregard for individual choice that it typified, the provisions that created HIV exceptionalism were meant to be sensitive to the needs of vulnerable individuals at a time when there was significant misunderstanding and stigma concerning the disease, its methods of transmission, and the identity of those at highest risk for infection. The fear and panic evoked during the first few years of the epidemic resulted in a meaningful dialogue between AIDS advocates and public health officials that ultimately engaged a wide network of individuals in the planning and implementation of public health policy, a network that was not considered a key public health player during the early part of the 20th century.

Issues of respect and personal autonomy were brought to the forefront of a serious public health discourse by a group who refused to be silenced and quickly changed the complexion of HIV testing and treatment delivery. Their success in advocating for protections for those at greatest risk of discrimination and stigma is a potent story about the power of marginalized groups to alter the landscape of public health (Shilts, 1987). These early AIDS advocates prepared the groundwork for current consumers of public health policy who have been empowered and emboldened to expect a standard of care that is sensitive to their needs (Siplon, 2002) by expanding access to new drugs and shedding light on pharmaceutical pricing practices (Casarett & Lantos, 1998). As noted by Bayer (2007), health care policy makers will be hard pressed to ignore the impact of individual rights to privacy and civil liberties on the implementation of policy.

INDIVIDUAL RIGHTS AND PUBLIC HEALTH: TENSION OR SYNERGY?

INTERPRETATIONS REGARDING THE balance between individual and public health needs have evolved in unexpected directions. For example, in an effort to further promote targeted guidelines for HIV testing and treatment, AIDS advocates challenged the popular assumption that individual rights must necessarily be pitted against the public's health. A mutual synergy was advanced that proposed the benefit to public health in the presence of enhanced individual rights, and it was this argument that was used to create the original HIV exceptionalism protocols. While this paradigm shift was initially persuasive, and certainly appealing to all involved, under more careful reflection it is a relationship that is illusory at best, and disingenuous at worst, because it does not recognize the trade-offs that must necessarily be considered in order to implement effective public health policy (Gerber, 2007). In addition, it masks the more fundamental nature of the debate concerning state paternalism. As argued by Bayer (2007), "It would be more honest—and in the long term more protective of public health—to acknowledge that intervention is sometimes necessary to protect individuals from their own foolish or dangerous behavior because such efforts can have a broad and enormous impact at a population level" (p. 1102).

If the dichotomy between individual rights and societal collectivism should then be better considered as a tension instead of a synergy, perhaps the most intimate articulation of it is expressed via perinatal HIV testing, which inextricably rests the interests of one vulnerable group on another. Maternal privacy, stigmatization, and informed consent must be considered contemporaneously with the potential for vertical transmission to the child, and all corresponding negative effects that might then ensue. One-quarter to one-third of all infants born to

639

*HIV
Exceptionalism
and the Mutability
of Ethical
Boundaries*

HIV-positive mothers were infected either during pregnancy, parturition, or breastfeeding. In 1994, the percentages were dramatically reduced with the prophylactic use of zidovudine during pregnancy, the use of elective caesarian sections, and the avoidance of breastfeeding for women at high risk for HIV. The result was the almost immediate reduction of perinatal transmission rates to less than 2% (Cooper, Charurat, & Mofenson, 2002).

However, in spite of this evidence suggesting enormous public health benefits to mandatory testing for pregnant women, and in spite of evidence that opt-out prenatal testing is acceptable by a large majority of pregnant women (Yudin, Moravac, & Shah, 2007), challenges to routine testing for pregnant women have been made. In particular, the arguments of maternal rights to privacy guaranteed by the First, Third, and Ninth amendments to the constitution have been invoked (Zank, 2007), and AIDS advocates continue to argue that only in the presence of "legitimate and compelling state interest" can these rights be abridged or infringed upon (Zank, 2007, p. 626). Unfortunately, depending on the perspective being taken, the definition of a legitimate and compelling state interest has itself provoked avid debate and discussion that has resulted in wide variation in the implementation of policy and regulation. Two states, New York and Indiana, have implemented mandatory HIV screening for newborns; Indiana has incorporated the caveat that HIV screening may take place without maternal consent but only if the attending physician finds it medically necessary based on his or her evaluation of maternal risk factors. Other states, such as Massachusetts, continue to support and require written consent laws that are specifically in conflict with the most recent CDC recommendations and with the prior knowledge that federal dollars may potentially be jeopardized by such a policy (Smith, 2007).

RECOMMENDATIONS

IN RECOGNITION OF the subtle ways in which the "I-Thou" relationship may be considered, and in light of the vicissitudes of public health decision-making that are affected by the troika of cultural context, perceptions driven by fear and stigma, and the need to consider the potential for negative outcomes, we offer the following guidance to facilitate the implementation of policy and HIV treatment as the debate continues.

First, take care to identify the "thou" in public health policy making. At the beginning of the epidemic, vulnerable groups were easily identified as IDUs and MSM, and targeted interventions were designed to address issues specific to them. These interventions successfully led to reductions in risk behavior and, consequently, reduced infections and mortality. Unfortunately, bridges to a larger and more heterogeneous group of at-risk individuals require a different set of interventions as well as the need for a broader implementation of HIV testing and treatment options.

Second, while shared goals between individuals and the community may be a noble aspiration, it is a specious argument to posit synergy between the two without full appreciation of the tensions that exist between them. An ethical resolution of conflict requires that choices be made that involve balancing a variety of threats with the ultimate question of whose vulnerability takes precedence when specific policies are created and implemented.

Third, the process of policy making must identify key stakeholders, and they should be included in all relevant discussions. AIDS advocates were essential to the creation and design of special, exceptionalism protocols designed with the intent to respect the privacy and autonomy of vulnerable populations while improving prospects for wider testing and diagnosis with a voluntary counseling and testing program. In addition, the emphasis on autonomy and justice so important to an ethical perspective can be attributed to the persistence of AIDS advocates. The resulting policies, at least initially, were more effective for their efforts.

Fourth, immersion in the process should not obscure or eliminate the most important discussion of final endpoints: who lives and for how long, and who dies and how soon. While continuous and careful thought should be given to the slippery slope often associated with consequentialism in health care ethics (Crichton, 2007; Hinks, 2007), it has the potential to provide guidance to practitioners who are placed in situations with no obvious ethical resolution and who require clarity to deal with difficult ethical and moral dilemmas (Frith, 2005; Sokol, 2007).

Fifth, the individual versus public dichotomy is most often taken into account within the policy debate. However, the cultural context within which that debate occurs must also be considered. Power to make and implement policy was initially in the hands of physicians, then shifted to a negotiated partnership with advocates. Currently, the trend seems to be shifting back to public health professionals. In order to maintain equipoise, attention must be given to what we study and how we attempt to change communities, and this effort should be careful to reflect individual value systems as well as the collective values that we hold (Heller, 1989).

Last, while ethical principles can provide increased clarity to the issues surrounding HIV testing and treatment, there is bound to be conflict regarding determination of the most parsimonious strategies

641

HIV
Exceptionalism
and the Mutability
of Ethical
Boundaries

to implement. Respectful discourse should be encouraged, even when conflicts arise. Sontag (2007) cautions against being persuaded by easy solutions, and in an even more dispirited tone, Clauser (1993) poignantly observes that *"There is no refuge; there is one quagmire after another"* (p. S10, emphasis added). While these viewpoints may be considered by many to be pessimistic, public health advocates may also be encouraged by the progress demonstrated by the history and advances associated with HIV exceptionalism. The trajectory of HIV policy has displayed sensitivity to justice while promoting public health endpoints.

CONCLUSION

HIV EXCEPTIONALISM HAS become an ingrained element of health care delivery for groups at high risk for HIV, so much so that even as treatment alternatives have become available, and negative perceptions of HIV have softened, change has been vociferously challenged and delayed. Ultimately, discourse regarding changes to VCT and implementation of more rigorous public health standards has resulted in deliberations about ethics and morals that have served to better articulate the tensions and balances inherent in the discussion.

REFERENCES

American College of Nurse-Midwives. (2003). Position statement: Human Immunodeficiency Virus (HIV) and Acquired Immunodeficiency Syndrome (AIDS). Retrieved October 3, 2008, from www.midwife.org/prof/display.cfm?id=403

Appelbaum, P. S., Lidz, C. W., & Meisel, A. (1987). *Informed consent: Legal theory and clinical practice*. Fair Lawn, NJ: Oxford University Press.

Bayer, R. (1989). *Private acts, social consequences: AIDS and the politics of public health*. New York: Free Press.

Bayer, R. (1991). Public health policy and the AIDS epidemic: An end to HIV exceptionalism? *New England Journal of Medicine, 324*, 1500–1504.

Bayer, R. (1999). Clinical progress and the future of HIV exceptionalism. *Archives of Internal Medicine, 159*, 1042–1048.

Bayer, R. (2007). The continuing tensions between individual rights and public health. *EMBO Reports, 8*(12), 1099–1103.

Braithwaite, R., Hammett, T., & Mayberry, R. (1996). *Prisons and AIDS: A public health challenge*. San Francisco, CA: Jossey-Bass.

Brimlow, D., Cook, J., & Seaton, R. (2003). *Stigma and HIV/AIDS: A review of literature*. Retrieved October 3, 2008, from http://hab.hrsa.gov/publications/stigma

Buber, M. (1923). *Ich und Du*. Leipzig, Germany: Charles Scribners Sons.

Casarett, D., & Lantos, J. (1998). Have we treated AIDS too well? Rationing and the future of AIDS exceptionalism. *Annals of Internal Medicine, 128,* 756–759.

Centers for Disease Control. (2002). Voluntary HIV testing as part of routine medical care—Massachusetts. *Morbidity and Mortality Weekly Report, 53,* 523–526.

Centers for Disease Control. (2003). Advancing HIV prevention: New strategies for a changing epidemic—United States. *Morbidity and Mortality Weekly Report, 52,* 329–332.

Centers for Disease Control. (2005). *HIV/AIDS surveillance report 2004* (Vol. 16). Atlanta, GA: U.S. Department of Health and Human Services.

Centers for Disease Control. (2006a). Revised recommendations for HIV testing of adults, adolescents, and pregnant women in healthcare settings. *Morbidity and Mortality Weekly Report, 55,* 1–17.

Centers for Disease Control. (2006b). Epidemiology of HIV/AIDS—United States, 1981–2005. *Morbidity and Mortality Weekly Report, 55,* 589–592.

Chase, M. (2006, July 5). Plans to expand AIDS testing alarm activists. *Post-Gazette Now.* Retrieved December 4, 2008, from http://www.ph.ucla.edu/epi/seaids/plansexpandtesting.html

Clauser, K. D. (1993). Bioethics and philosophy. *Hastings Center Report, 23*(6), S10.

Coates, T. J., Moore, S. F., & McKusick, L. (1987). Behavioral consequences of AIDS antibody testing among gay men. *Journal of the American Medical Association, 258,* 1889.

Coil, C., Haucoos, J., Witt, M., Wallace, R., & Lewis, R. (2004). Evaluation of an emergency department referral system for outpatient HIV testing. *Journal of Acquired Immune Deficiency Syndromes, 35*(1), 52–55.

Colgrove, J., & Bayer, R. (2005). Manifold restraints: Liberty, public health, and the legacy of Jacobson v. Massachusetts. *American Journal of Public Health, 95,* 571–576.

Cooper, E. R., Charurat, M., & Mofenson, L. (2002). Women and infants' transmission study group. Combination antiretroviral strategies for the treatment of pregnant HIV-1-infected women and prevention of perinatal HIV-1 transmission. *Journal of Acquired Immune Deficiency Syndrome, 29*(5), 484–494.

Crichton, P. (2007). Too much on consequences and not enough on what is right. *British Medical Journal, 334,* 986.

Fehrs, L. J., Fleming, D., Foster, L. R., McAlister, R. O., Fox, V., Modesitt, S., et al. (1988). Trial of anonymous versus confidential human immunodeficiency virus testing. *Lancet, 2*(8607), 379–382.

Fleming, P., Byers, R., Sweeney, P., Daniels, D., Karon, J., & Janssen, R. (2002). HIV prevalence in the United States, 2000. Atlanta, GA: Centers for Disease Control.

Frieden, T. R., Das-Douglas, M., Kellerman, S. E., Henning, K. J. (2005). Applying public health principles to the HIV epidemic. *New England Journal of Medicine, 353,* 2397–2402.

Frith, L. (2005). HIV testing and informed consent. *Journal of Medical Ethics, 31,* 699–700.

643

*HIV
Exceptionalism
and the Mutability
of Ethical
Boundaries*

Gerber, E. (2007). California limits egg donor compensation in privately-funded research. *Journal of Law, Medicine, and Ethics, 35*(1), 220–227.

Goffman, E. (1963). *Stigma: Notes on the management of spoiled identity.* Englewood Cliffs, NJ: Prentice Hall.

Heller, K. (1989). The return to community. *American Journal of Community Psychology, 17,* 1–15.

Hinks, T. S. (2007). Ends never justify the means. *British Medical Journal, 334,* 985.

Holtgrave, D. (2007). Costs and consequences of the U.S. Centers for Disease Control and Prevention's recommendations for opt-out HIV testing. *PLoS Medicine, 4,* 1–8.

Ironson, G., LaPerriere, A., Antoni, M., O'Hearn, P., Schneiderman, N., & Klimas, N., et al. (1990). Changes in immune and psychological measures as a function of anticipation and reaction to news of HIV-1 antibody status. *Psychosomatic Medicine, 52,* 247–270.

Kaiser Daily HIV/AIDS Report. (2007, 13 June). Targeting HIV testing at high-risk groups might be more effective than routine testing, research article says. Retrieved December 4, 2008, from http://www.thebodypro.com/content/news/art41358.html

Kaiser Family Foundation. (2004). *Financing HIV/AIDS care: A quilt with many holes.* HIV Policy Issue Brief no. 1607-02.

Lambda Legal. (2007a). Increasing access to voluntary HIV testing: A summary of evidence of the importance of specific written consent and pre-test counseling in HIV testing. *ACLU AIDS Project.* Retrieved October 10, 2008, from http://www.aclu.org/hiv/testing/30249res20070308.html#attach

Lambda Legal. (2007b). *Quick facts about workplace discrimination.* Retrieved October 10, 2008, from www.lambdalegal.org/our-work/publications/facts-backgrounds/quick-facts-about-workplace.html

Landis, S. E., Schoenbach, V. J., Weber, D. J., Mittal, M., Krishan, B., & Lewis, K., et al. (1992). Results of a randomized trial of partner notification in cases of HIV infection in North Carolina. *New England Journal of Medicine, 326,* 101–106.

Lombardo, P. A. (1985). Three generations, no imbeciles: New light on Buck v. Bell. *New York University Law Review, 60,* 30–62.

Manavi, K. (2005). HIV testing should no longer be accorded any special status. *British Medical Journal, 330,* 492–493.

Metzger, D. S. (2006). *New perspectives on racial disparities in HIV infections.* Presentation to HIV Prevention Research Division, University of Pennsylvania, October 25, 2006.

Ostrow, D. G., Monjan, A., Joseph, J., VanRaden, M., Fox, R., & Kingsley, L., et al. (1989). HIV-related symptoms and psychological functioning in a cohort of homosexual men. *American Journal of Psychiatry, 146,* 737–742.

Paltiel, A. D., Weinstein, M. C., Kimmel, A. D., Seage, G. R., Losina, E., Zhang, H., et al. (2005). Expanded screening for HIV in the United States—an analysis of cost-effectiveness. *New England Journal of Medicine, 352*(6), 586–595.

Perry, S., Jacobsberg, L. B., Fishman, B., Weiler, P., Gold, J. W. M., & Frances, A. (1990). Psychological responses to serological testing for HIV. *AIDS, 4,* 145–152.

Sears, B., & Ho, D. (2006). *HIV discrimination in health care services in Los Angeles County: The results of three testing studies.* The Williams Institute, UCLA School of Law, Los Angeles, CA.

Shilts, R. (1987). *And the band played on: Politics, people, and the AIDS epidemic.* New York: St. Martins Press.

Siplon, P. D. (2002). *AIDS and the policy struggle in the United States.* Washington, DC: Georgetown University Press.

Smith, S. (2007, September 1). AIDS test consent at issue in Mass. *The Boston Globe,* Retrieved October 10, 2008, from http://www.boston.com/news/local/massachusetts/articles/2007/09/01/aids_test_consent_at_issue_in_mass/

Snyder, M., Omoto, A. M., & Crain, A. L. (1999). Punished for their good deeds: Stigmatization for AIDS volunteers. *American Behavioral Scientist, 42*(7), 1175–1192.

Sokol, D. K. (2007). Commentary on ethics of HIV testing in general practice without informed consent: A case series. *British Medical Journal, 334*(7601), 984–986.

Sontag, D. (2007). What is wrong with "ethics for sale"? An analysis of the many issues that complicate the debate about conflicts of interests in bioethics. *Journal of Law, Medicine, and Ethics, 35*(1), 175–186.

Stall, R., Hoff, C., Coates, T. J., Paul, J., Phillips, K. A., & Ekstrand, M., et al. (1996). Decisions to get HIV tested and to accept antiretroviral therapies among gay/bisexual men: Implications for secondary prevention efforts. *Journal of Acquired Immune Deficiency Syndromes and Human Retrovirology, 11,* 151–160.

Valdiserri, R. (2007). Late HIV diagnosis: Bad medicine and worse public health. *PLoS Medicine, 4,* 1–2.

Weinberger, M., Conover, C. J., Samsa, G. P., & Greenberg, S. M. (1992). Physicians' attitudes and practices regarding treatment of HIV-infected patients. *The Southern Medical Journal, 85,* 683–686.

Wynia, M. (2006). Routine screening: Informed consent, stigma and the waning of HIV exceptionalism. *The American Journal of Bioethics, 6*(4), 5–8.

Yudin, M. H., Moravac, C., & Shah, R. R. (2007). Influence of an "opt-out" test strategy and patient factors on human immunodeficiency virus screening in pregnancy. *Obstetrics and Gynecology, 110,* 81–86.

Zank, D. (2007). Is it time to revisit prenatal HIV testing laws? *Virtual Mentor, 9*(9), 625–629.

Zetola, N. (2007). Association between rates of HIV testing and elimination of written consents in San Francisco. *Journal of the American Medical Association, 297*(10), 1061.

Part X

Vaccines

55

The Ethics of Vaccination

James Colgrove

V**ACCINES ARE AMONG** the most valuable and cost-effective medical interventions. They have been responsible for dramatic reductions in morbidity and mortality from infectious diseases and for corresponding decreases in human suffering and health care expenditures. The Centers for Disease Control (CDC) recommends that children be vaccinated against 15 diseases before age 6. Vaccines are also recommended for populations such as health care workers, the elderly, and travelers to some disease-endemic areas, who are at heightened risk of contracting certain infections.

Vaccines raise unique ethical issues. Vaccination confers a dual benefit: on the individual who undergoes it and on the surrounding community via herd immunity, the phenomenon in which all members of a group will be protected against a contagion if a sufficiently large percentage of the group is immune. Like all medical procedures, vaccination carries the small risk of adverse reactions, but unlike other interventions, vaccines are generally given to healthy people rather than sick, and therefore the standard for their safety is higher and the acceptability of side effects lower (Clements, Evans, Dittman, & Reeler, 1999).

Ethical debates about vaccination have a long history. The first vaccine, against smallpox, was developed more than 200 years ago, and both its safety and efficacy were matters of intense dispute. Many of these conflicts were mediated in the legal system. In the 19th century, compulsory vaccination laws provoked dozens of court challenges from people who considered them an unacceptable intrusion on individual liberty. After decades of conflicting lower court rulings, the U.S. Supreme Court took up the question of whether compulsory vaccination contravened the Constitution in the 1905 case of *Jacobson v. Massachusetts*. In a seven–two ruling, the justices declared that such laws were a legitimate exercise of state governments' police powers to guard the health, welfare, and safety of citizens (Colgrove, 2006).

In the 1960s and 1970s, court cases drew new attention to the risks of vaccines. Individuals who claimed to have been harmed by vaccines brought suit against pharmaceutical companies, medical societies, and public health departments, claiming these entities had a legal duty to warn recipients of risks. Repeated verdicts in favor of plaintiffs ultimately led to the creation of government-run systems to compensate victims and indemnify manufacturers from damages for nonnegligent vaccine injuries. In the past two decades, a growing grassroots movement has alleged that vaccines are much riskier than medical professionals claim. Although public support for vaccination remains high, ethical debates around vaccines have grown more visible (Colgrove, 2006).

INDIVIDUAL AND COLLECTIVE RIGHTS AND RESPONSIBILITIES

THE OPTIMAL SITUATION for the community occurs when each member assumes the small risk of undergoing vaccination in order to protect both himself and the group as a whole. But an individual's most self-interested strategy would be to allow everyone else to assume the small risk of vaccination but avoid vaccination himself and get a free ride on the resulting herd immunity (Dare, 1998; Fine & Clarkson, 1986; Menzel, 1995). Herd immunity is susceptible to a version of the so-called tragedy of the commons: the decision of any one individual to refuse vaccination will not affect the group's protection, but if too many people make that choice, those decisions in the aggregate will undermine the protection (Diekema & Marcuse, 1998).

An issue closely related to individual choice about vaccine use is whether it is ethically acceptable for governments to mandate vaccines. The starting point for thinking about the ethics of compulsory vaccination is the political philosophy of John Stuart Mill, the 19th-century utilitarian whose *On Liberty* laid out a guideline known as the harm principle for evaluating the use of state coercion. Mill contended that the only justification for coercive action against an individual was the presence of imminent harm to other members of society; a person's own good, Mill wrote, is insufficient reason (Mill, 1956 [1849]).

While *being* vaccinated clearly *benefits* others, does the *failure* to be vaccinated *harm* others? Some vaccine opponents argue that the individual who declines a vaccine places only himself at risk; anyone wishing to be protected from a disease can choose to take the vaccine and therefore has neither a logical reason nor a moral basis for demanding that others receive it. This reasoning is flawed, however. No vaccine is 100% effective; a small number of people who receive a vaccine will fail to develop the intended immunity, and it is not practically possible to identify these individuals. Further, some people cannot receive vaccines because of medical contraindications. These two categories of people may be placed in danger by infectious diseases that unvaccinated members of the community may spread. Thus declining to be vaccinated (or declining to have one's child vaccinated) does have, to use Mill's term, "other-regarding" consequences. Nevertheless, ethicists disagree about whether refusing vaccination constitutes sufficiently severe or proximal harm to others to warrant state intervention (for contrasting views on this point, see, e.g., Dare, 1998; Silverman & May, 2001).

Because most vaccines today are given to infants and children, the issue of parental control over their children's well-being is overlaid on the potential conflict between individual and collective interests. Should the wishes of parents who oppose vaccination prevail over society's interest in protecting children from preventable illness and building herd immunity? All states in the United States require that children receive most of the routinely recommended vaccines as a condition of attending school; many states also have such requirements for enrollment in day care. Proponents of these laws characterize them as helpful prompts to action rather than tools of coercion. In their view, the laws are essentially persuasive and hortatory, and they cite data showing that the great majority of parents would have their children vaccinated even if there were no legal requirement. Nevertheless, there remains a subset of parents who oppose vaccines and for whom the laws are coercive.

Is such coercion ethically justified? Mill argued that children were fit subjects for paternalistic action, and the principle that the state may intervene to protect minors from the harmful acts of their parents is well-accepted in both ethics and law. Nevertheless, the circumstances under which society has a right or a duty to override parental choice are often ambiguous. This issue has sparked debate in both medical and nonmedical contexts, with controversies involving groups such as Christian Scientists, Jehovah's Witnesses, and the Amish, and issues such as compliance with mandatory education laws, prohibitions on child labor, and consent for life-saving blood transfusions (Merrick, 2003; Swan, 1999).

Almost all mandatory vaccination laws in the United States contain exemptions for parents who have religious objections to vaccination, and many laws also allow parents who have secular philosophical concerns to opt out as well. Legislators and health officials have included these provisions both to respect the conscientious choices of parents and to provide a kind of political safety valve to forestall grassroots resistance from vaccination opponents. Very small numbers of children are exempted by their parents, which suggest that the exemptions are an acceptable compromise that honors the decisions of parents without endangering the safety of their children or the community. However, research has shown that schools with exemption rates as low as 2%–4% are at heightened risk of disease outbreaks and that children who have been exempted from vaccine requirements have a much greater risk of acquiring infectious diseases than their vaccinated peers (Salmon et al., 2006). Therefore, health officials are justified in denying exemptions when herd immunity may be compromised.

The scope of exemptions has also been challenged on constitutional grounds. In some states exemptions are available only to adherents of so-called recognized or established religions. Some courts have found that such provisions represent an unacceptable establishment of religion by the state, unfairly favoring adherents of some faiths over others (Salmon et al., 2005). Conversely, others have argued that the very existence of exemptions violates the equal protection of the nonexempt majority (Silverman, 2003). In a 1944 case involving child labor, the Supreme Court noted in dicta that parents do not have the constitutional right to withhold vaccines from children for religious reasons. "Parents may be free to become martyrs themselves," the justices declared. "But it does not follow they are free, in identical circumstances, to make martyrs of their children" (*Prince v. Massachusetts*, 1944, p. 170). While states may choose to offer religious exemptions, they are under no obligation to do so (Hodge & Gostin, 2001).

Parents who refuse vaccines for their children present a challenge to health care providers, who may feel frustration or anger toward individuals they perceive to be acting against a child's best interests. A survey found that more than one-third of pediatricians would dismiss from their practice a family that refused all vaccines, and more than one-quarter would do so to a family declining selected vaccines (Flanagan-Klygis, Sharp, & Frader, 2005). Because of the trusting relationships they develop with patients, clinicians are in a position to assess reasons for vaccine refusal and educate and counsel parents so that they might reconsider their decision. As a last step, providers would be justified in contacting child welfare authorities if refusal of vaccines places the child in imminent danger, as would be the case, for example, if an outbreak of a severe vaccine-preventable disease were occurring locally (Diekema, 2005).

VACCINE SAFETY AND RISKS

VACCINES TODAY ARE generally very safe; the vast majority of side effects are transient and superficial, such as fever or pain and swelling at the injection site. But rare severe events do occur. For example, the measles vaccine can cause life-threatening encephalopathy in about 1 in 1,000,000 doses. The risk of encephalopathy from measles itself, however, is about 1 in 1,000 cases. As incidence of a vaccine-preventable disease declines, so does the ethical acceptability of adverse events associated with the vaccine. A vaccine that is known to carry the risk of harmful side effects might be acceptable when the disease is both highly prevalent and severe, but such side effects in a vaccine for a rare or mild disease would be neither ethically nor politically acceptable (Chen, 1999).

One of the most vivid illustrations of a changing risk-benefit calculation of vaccination occurred as the incidence of polio declined in the United States. The Sabin oral polio vaccine, introduced in 1961, was very effective in controlling the disease, but it carried a small risk of causing paralytic polio (estimated at approximately 1 case of the disease for every 11,000,000 people vaccinated). By the 1970s, one-third of the annual cases of the disease in the United States were caused by the vaccine itself (Nightingale, 1977). In 1995, after polio had been eliminated from the western hemisphere, the United States changed to exclusive use of the Salk vaccine, which is less effective but does not carry the risk of vaccine-induced paralysis. In developing nations, however, where polio remains endemic, the Sabin vaccine continues to be used because of its superior control properties.

Because people undergo vaccination or have their children vaccinated at least in part to benefit society, and often do so in compliance with laws, governments have recognized they have a moral obligation to provide compensation for the small number of people who are harmed by vaccines. Several European nations enacted vaccine-injury compensation programs in the 1960s and 1970s; the United States did so in 1986 (Mariner, 1987).

CASE STUDY: THE VACCINE AGAINST HPV

HUMAN PAPILLOMAVIRUS (HPV) is the most common sexually transmitted disease in the United States. Approximately 6.2 million people become infected each year; among girls and women, overall prevalence is about 27%, with prevalence increasing each year for ages 14 to 24 years. Although most HPV infections are cleared from the body without complication, HPV is the causal agent of cancer in several sites, including cervix, vulva, and anus (Dunne et al., 2007). In

June 2006, the Food and Drug Administration licensed Merck's vaccine Gardasil, which protects against four strains of the virus, including the two that are responsible for the majority of cases of cervical cancer. Because the vaccine is most effective when given before the onset of sexual activity, the CDC recommended that it be routinely administered to girls at age 11–12. (The vaccine is currently not licensed for use in boys, although Merck is reviewing data on the product's efficacy in males.) In addition to the issues described above, three characteristics of this vaccine have sparked especially vigorous ethical debates: it protects against an infection that is sexually rather than casually transmitted; it is given to adolescents rather than infants; and it is the most expensive vaccine recommended for routine administration.

Some religious conservatives express concern that the availability of a vaccine against a sexually transmitted disease will increase the likelihood that teens receiving it will engage in sex. (No empirical data support this conjecture.) Although these groups support availability of the vaccine, they remain opposed to mandating it. In their view, such a requirement constitutes an attempt by the state to force a child to undergo an intervention that is irreconcilable with her family's religious values and beliefs.

Requiring HPV vaccination by law will almost certainly achieve more widespread protection against the disease than policies that rely exclusively on persuasion and education. A utilitarian analysis might therefore conclude that compulsory HPV vaccination outweighs the intrusion on parental decision-making. But the evidence in support of such a conclusion is equivocal. Several important aspects of the vaccine remain unknown, including its ultimate effect on the incidence of cervical and other cancers, the duration of its protection, and its potential effects on the prevalence and severity of other HPV strains (Sawaya & Smith-McCune, 2007). If the level of protection provided is lower than initial data suggest, then both the population-level and individual-level benefits will be fewer and the argument for the use of government compulsion will become concomitantly weaker.

Bioethicists, who generally hold the values of patient autonomy and informed consent to be preeminent, tend to be skeptical toward the utilitarian justifications that underpin compulsory vaccination. It is thus not surprising that some have expressed wariness about or opposition to making the HPV vaccine mandatory (Gostin & DeAngelis, 2007; Lo, 2006; Zimmerman, 2006). Further, Mill's harm principle might lead one to conclude that mandates are unwarranted because HPV is not casually transmissible; in the absence of imminent harm to a third party, such laws may be considered unacceptably paternalistic, in contrast to laws requiring vaccines for measles or pertussis, for instance. There is precedent, however, for mandating vaccines against diseases that are not casually transmissible. Most states require that students be protected against hepatitis B, which is primarily transmitted through sexual contact and injection drug use, and tetanus, which is not communicable. Such mandates express the principle that the government has a justifiably paternalistic concern for the welfare of minor children.

Because the HPV vaccine is given to adolescents rather than infants, questions of consent/assent may be complicated. For most medical procedures, standard ethical guidelines declare that both the youth and the parent or guardian must give consent (American Academy of Pediatrics Committee on Bioethics, 1995). In an ideal situation, both the youth and her parents will agree to the youth's receiving the HPV vaccine. However, wishes of parents and youth may be discordant, with a youth either seeking or rejecting the vaccine against the parent's wishes. Because adolescents have developed a level of autonomous functioning that differentiates them from younger children, their right to receive or refuse the HPV vaccine should be respected (Lo, 2005).

The price of Gardasil, approximately $360 for a full course of three shots, raises ethical concerns. This price is much higher than for other routinely given childhood and adolescent vaccines. Criticism of the price became more vocal after it was revealed that Merck had lobbied aggressively to convince state legislators to enact compulsory vaccination laws and had channeled money through a private advocacy group, Women in Government, to lobby on behalf of the vaccine, a strategy that was seen as a conflict of interest (Gostin & DeAngelis, 2007).

As of June 2008, legislation related to HPV vaccination had been introduced in 41 states (National Conference of State Legislatures, 2008). The bills under consideration include measures to educate the public about the vaccine, fund its provision, or make it mandatory for middle school students. The vigorous, sometimes acrimonious, debates that have surrounded this legislation vividly illustrate the extent to which ethical issues of vaccination continue to command public attention.

CONCLUSION

BECAUSE OF THEIR communitywide implications, ethical decisions about vaccination extend beyond the doctor–patient relationship to the realm of public policy. The dualities described above—self and society, risk and benefit—lead to a set of rights and duties on the part of the government and individuals. Because people undergo vaccination at least partly to benefit their fellow citizens, governments have an obligation to compensate the few who are harmed by vaccine side effects. They also have a duty to provide vaccines to those who are unable to afford them. The danger that severe infectious diseases may pose to vulnerable third parties provides an ethical imperative for people to receive recommended vaccines and to have their children vaccinated. Governments are justified on grounds of beneficence and justice in compelling people to be vaccinated in situations where their failure to do so could lead to severe and imminent harm to others. Whether such a situation exists—whether a vaccine-preventable disease is sufficiently dangerous and/or prevalent to warrant state intervention—is an empirical question that should be answered by people with expertise in medicine and epidemiology with input from representatives of the public. As new vaccines are licensed against diseases that are rarer or less life-threatening than the infectious killers of past eras, such deliberations will grow more complex. As is true in all areas of public health law, this decision-making must be transparent, and laws must be written in ways that are least restrictive and most respectful of individual autonomy.

REFERENCES

American Academy of Pediatrics Committee on Bioethics. (1995). Informed consent, parental permission, and assent in pediatric practice. *Pediatrics, 95,* 314–317.

Chen, R. (1999). Vaccine risks: Real, perceived and unknown. *Vaccine, 17,* S41–S46.

Clements, C. J., Evans, G., Dittman, S., & Reeler, A. V. (1999). Vaccine safety concerns everyone. *Vaccine, 17,* S90–S94.

Colgrove, J. (2006). *State of immunity: The politics of vaccination in twentieth-century America.* Berkeley: University of California Press.

Dare, T. (1998). Mass immunisation programmes: Some philosophical issues. *Bioethics, 12,* 125–149.

Diekema, D. S. (2005). Responding to parental refusals of immunization of children. *Pediatrics, 115,* 1428–1431.

Diekema, D. S., & Marcuse, E. K. (1998). Ethical issues in the vaccination of children. In G. R. Burgios and J. D. Lantos (Eds.), *Primum non nocere today* (pp. 37–47). Amsterdam, The Netherlands: Elsevier.

Dunne, E. F., Unger, E. R., Sternberg, M., McQuillan, G., Swan, D. C., Patel, S. S., et al. (2007). Prevalence of HPV infection among females in the United States. *Journal of the American Medical Association, 297,* 813–819.

Fine, P. E. M., & Clarkson, J. A. (1986). Individual versus public priorities in the determination of optimal vaccination policies. *American Journal of Epidemiology, 124,* 1012–1020.

Flanagan-Klygis, E. A., Sharp, L., & Frader, J. E. (2005). Dismissing the family who refuses vaccines: A study of pediatrician attitudes. *Archives of Pediatrics and Adolescent Medicine, 159,* 929–934.

Gostin, L. O., & DeAngelis, C. D. (2007). Mandatory HPV vaccination: Public health versus private wealth. *Journal of the American Medical Association, 297,* 1921–1923.

Hodge, J. G., & Gostin, L. O. (2001). School vaccination requirements: Historical, social, and legal perspectives. *Kentucky Law Journal, 90,* 831–890.

Lo, B. (2005). *Resolving ethical dilemmas: A guide for clinicians* (3rd ed.). Philadelphia: Lippincott Williams and Wilkins.

Lo, B. (2006). HPV vaccine and adolescents' sexual activity. *BMJ, 332,* 1106–1107.

Mariner, W. K. (1987). Compensation programs for vaccine-related injury abroad: A comparative analysis. *Saint Louis University Law Journal, 31,* 599–654.

Menzel, P. (1995). Non-compliance: Fair or free-riding. *Health Care Analysis, 3,* 113–115.

Merrick, J. (2003). Spiritual healing, sick kids, and the law: Inequities in the American health care system. *American Journal of Law and Medicine, 29,* 269–299.

Mill, J. S. (1956 [1849]). *On liberty.* Indianapolis, IN: Bobbs Merrill.

National Conference of State Legislatures. (2008). *HPV vaccine.* Retrieved October 19, 2007, from http://www.ncsl.org/programs/health/HPVvaccine.htm

Nightingale, E. O. (1977). Recommendation for a national policy on poliomyelitis vaccination. *New England Journal of Medicine, 297,* 249–253.

Prince v. Massachusetts. (1944). 321 U.S. 158.

Salmon, D. A., Sapsin, J. W., Teret, S., Jacobs, R. F., Thompson, J. W., Ryan, K., et al. (2005). Public health and the politics of school immunization requirements. *American Journal of Public Health, 95,* 778–783.

Salmon, D. A, Teret, S. P., MacIntyre, R. C., Salisbury, D., Burgess, M. A., Halsey, N. A. (2006). Compulsory vaccination and conscientious or philosophical exemptions: Past, present, and future. *Lancet, 367,* 436–442.

Sawaya, G. F., & Smith-McCune, K. (2007). HPV vaccine—more answers, more questions. *New England Journal of Medicine, 356,* 1991–1993.

Silverman, R. (2003). No more kidding around: Restructuring non-medical childhood immunization exemptions to ensure public health protection. *Annals of Health Law, 12,* 277–294.

Silverman, R. D., & May, T. (2001). Private choice versus public health: Religion, morality, and childhood vaccination law. *Margins, 1,* 505–521.

Swan, R. (1999). On statutes depriving a class of children to rights to medical care: Can this discrimination be litigated? *Quinnipiac Health Law Journal, 2,* 73–95.

Zimmerman, R. K. (2006). Ethical analysis of HPV vaccine policy options. *Vaccine, 24,* 4812–4820.

56

The Ethics of Allocating Vaccines

Robert I. Field

For lethal, rapidly spreading diseases, public health officials anticipate demand for vaccines that may far outstrip supply. This is a special concern in the early stages of an epidemic, before sufficient time has elapsed for vaccine production to reach full capacity. There are conflicting views on how best to prioritize potential vaccine recipients in such a situation.

Recent disease threats have heightened public health concerns that an epidemic of worldwide proportions, a pandemic, could emerge in the next several years. In 2002, smallpox was identified by some experts as a potential tool of biological warfare almost 30 years after its eradication as a naturally occurring peril, amid concerns that virus stockpiles safeguarded by the former Soviet Union were no longer secure (Breman & Henderson, 2002). In 2004, severe acute respiratory syndrome (SARS) killed hundreds in China and threatened to spread worldwide before vigorous government interventions successfully contained it (Riley et al., 2003). Since 2003, avian influenza (avian flu) has killed millions of birds across much of Asia and a few hundred humans, who have come into contact with infected birds (World Health Organization, 2008). Scientists have warned of its potential to become a virulent pandemic should it mutate into a form that could be transmitted directly between people (Purdue & Swayne, 2005). As globalization increasingly encourages and facilitates travel between nations, similar threats are likely to arise over coming decades.

AVIAN FLU AND SIMILAR PANDEMICS

As of 2008, avian flu represented the most pressing pandemic disease risk. A 2005 estimate by the U.S. Department of Health Human Services (DHHS) predicted that a pandemic in America would result in 90 million cases of illness, 10 million hospitalizations, 1.5 million intensive care unit patents, and 1.9 million deaths (DHHS, 2005). The last influenza pandemic of similar scope, which arose in 1918, is estimated to have caused as many as 50 million deaths worldwide (Morens & Fauci, 2007) and 500,000 in the United States (Noymer & Garenne, 2000). Considerable attention, both in the United States and globally, has focused on containment strategies, all of which emphasize vaccination as a central component.

Public health officials anticipate that an effective vaccine can be developed against avian flu, as has been the case for less virulent seasonal strains (Stohr & Esveld, 2004). However, logistical challenges abound (Wynia, 2007). The virus that causes the disease has been isolated by researchers and classified as H5N1, and vaccines against it are in development. However, it is not possible to verify that a vaccine will be effective against a strain that is communicable between humans until such a strain actually emerges. Uptake by the population of vaccines that are in development while a pandemic is still speculative is likely to be limited because of concerns over possible vaccine risks (McNeil, 2008). Therefore, full-scale manufacture and distribution of a vaccine with known effectiveness must await the start of an actual outbreak (Stohr & Esveld, 2004). The time lag between isolation of a pandemic strain and the start of widespread vaccine production is estimated to be at least 4 months (DHHS, 2005).

Once an outbreak begins, an estimated 6.7 billion doses would be needed for global protection, which is more than current manufacturing capacity (World Health Organization, 2007). The vaccine must be distributed worldwide, including delivery to remote locations in the developing world. Perhaps most challenging of all from an ethical perspective, initial supplies would have to be allocated among potential recipients until sufficient quantities became available.

The ethical challenges involved in distributing a scarce medical resource are not new. For example, the American health care system regularly faces allocation dilemmas with regard to organs for transplantation. Patients requiring transplants are placed on waiting lists administered by the United Network for Organ Sharing (UNOS), a private nonprofit organization funded by the federal government (UNOS, 2008). They are prioritized according to various criteria, most importantly medical need. Ethicists have grappled with the complexities of such allocation criteria since the first heart transplants were performed in the early 1960s, and they continue to do so today (Halpern, Ubel, & Caplan, 2002).

Vaccination allocation, however, presents distinct challenges that create the need to plan for a pandemic in advance. Decisions must be made rapidly, as a pandemic could spread nationwide in a matter of weeks. There would be no time to ponder the circumstances of potential recipients on waiting lists. A pandemic, unlike most other kinds of medical threats, presents not only health risks but also significant economic and strategic threats to the entire country because of its scope. Widespread absenteeism could jeopardize economic productivity, loss of essential personnel could impair key services and industries, and contagion within the military could impair national defense. The need for medical intervention would apply to everyone in the country, not just to a relatively small number of patients with advanced conditions.

BIOETHICAL CONSIDERATIONS

THE TASK FOR bioethics is to weigh competing approaches to the prioritization of vaccine distribution when supply is limited and everyone is potentially in need (Gostin, 2006). The assessment of these approaches from an ethical perspective depends on the underlying value to be promoted (Zimmerman, 2007). While there is no consensus as to the relative importance of each value in an absolute sense, a structured ethical analysis can help in evaluating the various options. This is an essential step in devising an advance plan that can be put into effect when a pandemic strikes.

RELEVANT ETHICAL PRINCIPLES

FOUR ETHICAL PRINCIPLES bear on decisions relating to vaccine allocation priorities. Beneficence is the imperative to do good for others (Weed & McKeown, 2001). In the context of vaccine allocation policy, it is the directive to protect those most at risk. Nonmaleficence is the dictate to avoid causing harm. It is the first teaching of the Hippocratic oath that is taken by physicians, and it instructs that medical interventions should, at the very least, not make patients worse. With regard to vaccine allocation, inappropriate apportionment decisions could divert supplies from their optimal uses. Justice calls for the equitable allocation of scarce resources. It requires fairness and reasoned decision-making in determining who will receive and who will be denied a benefit, such as vaccination. Finally, utilitarianism is the principle of doing the greatest good for the greatest number of people. Utilitarian distribution of vaccines would favor actions that protect society overall without regard for individual need.

VACCINE ALLOCATION STRATEGIES

Grant Priority to the Most Vulnerable

A COMMON STARTING point in allocating medical resources is to target those most at risk, based on the principle of beneficence. They represent the greatest medical need, because they are most likely to become ill or to die without an intervention. For seasonal influenza and many other infectious conditions, this category includes the elderly, very young children and infants, those with preexisting respiratory ailments, and those who are immunocompromised because of illness or medication use (Cox & Subbarao, 2000). The rest of the population is more likely to resist or recover from this disease without medical assistance.

Despite the obvious intuitive appeal, this approach raises practical questions. It is difficult to determine in advance who will face the greatest peril from a newly emerging disease. The influenza pandemic of 1918 presented the highest risk for those between the ages of 20 and 40 (Simonsen et al., 2004). Those in greatest danger from the disease may also be those who face the greatest danger from adverse reactions to the vaccine itself. Furthermore, the oldest, youngest, and frailest members of society are not likely to be among the most productive or among those most likely to spread the disease, so their survival presents the smallest relative benefit to the population overall (Dushoff et al., 2007).

Grant Priority to Those Most Essential to Protecting Public Health

FROM A UTILITARIAN perspective, the greatest good is achieved if limited vaccine supplies can be used to halt or retard the spread of disease in the general population. Some individuals are more likely than others to contract pandemic flu and to pass it along to others. These would include, for example, airline personnel, who come into close contact with travelers from around the world, and health care workers, who treat contagious patients. If these people are immunized first, likely vectors for infection can be contained until larger supplies of vaccines can be manufactured. This approach may save the most lives in the long run but at the expense of those in high-risk groups who nevertheless become ill.

A similar strategy would grant priority to essential workers in the public health and national defense infrastructures. This is the basis for guidance on government vaccine allocation policy developed by a task force of the DHHS (DHHS, 2007). This approach calls for vaccine supplies to be targeted to maintain security, health care, and essential services according to four tiers. Those protected first would be workers in homeland and national security, including intelligence gathering, boarder protection, and service as members of the active military. Next are those whose work involves critical infrastructure, such as emergency medical services, law enforcement, energy and communications personnel, and in key industries, including transportation, pharmaceuticals, and oil. The next tier includes those who provide health care and community support services. The final tier includes members of the general public.

This approach relies heavily on utilitarian considerations. The focus is solely on considerations of national needs to the exclusion of other factors, such as therapeutic benefit or disease vulnerability. To implement a utilitarian system, numerous judgments must be made regarding the relative indispensability to societal functioning of members of each category of the population. The emphasis is on the governmental role of protecting overall national interests, rather than on the role of assisting those members of society who are most in need.

The strategy of emphasizing utilitarian protection of essential workers raises questions about the boundaries of national concern. Noncitizens may work in essential jobs, and would certainly be members of the general public. Is a distinction based on citizenship appropriate? Allocation of vaccines to foreign countries where a disease first emerges may more effectively halt its spread than immunizing Americans who will not be exposed until later; however, such a preemptive use could divert supplies from potential American recipients. Key industries that are international in scope may have access to their own vaccines from abroad, so American supplies that are allocated to them may be wasted. Overall, it may be difficult as a practical matter to isolate national interests in the face of a global threat.

GRANT PRIORITY TO THOSE MOST LIKELY TO BENEFIT

VACCINES ARE WASTED on recipients whose immune systems are too impaired to develop sufficient disease resistance or who are particularly vulnerable to adverse effects. The principle of nonmaleficence would be violated if precious supplies were squandered on those least likely to benefit. However, those most likely to benefit from vaccination may be the healthiest, who could fight the disease most effectively without medical assistance. Granting priority to them may also violate the principle of beneficence, because it would disregard many in the greatest need, and of justice, because it would allocate resources to those who deserve them the least.

A similar strategy would grant priority to those with the most years of life ahead based on the premise that the value of saving a life may differ between individuals according to the extent of life that the beneficiary can be expected to gain as a result. Someone who is elderly would likely realize fewer additional years of life from avoiding a lethal disease than would a child. Justice can be seen to favor those who have not yet had the opportunity to experience a full life. One proposed framework refines this notion further based on a life-cycle principle that delineates gradations within a life span (Emanuel & Wertheimer, 2006). It would grant priority to those between early adolescence and middle age, because they have invested the most in developing life interests, hopes, and plans in relation to the amount of time that they are likely to have to realize them.

GRANT PRIORITY TO THE MOST PRODUCTIVE

FROM THE PERSPECTIVE of society overall, not all people contribute equally to the common good. Some contribute to the economy through gainful employment, provision of essential services such as health care or security, or achievement of artistic or scientific advances. At the other extreme, some commit crimes that degrade the general quality of life. Utilitarianism would protect those who contribute the most and who are likely to continue to do so. However, this result would contradict the principle of beneficence, since the greatest contributors may be those who need help the least. They are likely to enjoy the greatest economic advantages and hence the greatest access to medical care were they to become ill.

RESPECT THE NEEDS OF THE MOST DISADVANTAGED

SOCIETIES TEND TO favor those who are most economically prosperous, and vaccine allocations could follow the same path. This result would clearly violate the principle of justice. The Bellagio Group, an international collection of experts in public health, medicine, bioethics, law, and related fields, issued a *Statement of Principles* in 2006 that called for vaccine access policies that pay particular attention to traditionally disadvantaged groups and that are fair and nondiscriminatory (Bellagio Meeting on Social Justice and Influenza, 2006). This strategy does not resolve the larger issue of where priorities should lie, but it emphasizes a paramount need to ensure that justice is respected with regard to society overall.

GLOBAL CONCERNS: RESPECT FOR GENETIC PROPERTY RIGHTS AND CONTRIBUTIONS TO VACCINE INNOVATION

IN 2006, THE government of Indonesia declared a moratorium on shipment of avian flu virus isolates to the World Health Organization (McKenna, 2007). It, along with several other Southeast Asian counties, is a breeding ground for the organism that causes avian flu (Hien, De Jong, & Farrar, 2004). These countries seek a vaccine distribution system that equitably allocates supplies to the developing world. They fear that without one, they may see limited benefits from vaccines produced with their indigenous virus strains by industrialized nations.

Intellectual property rights to vaccines and vaccine technologies raise broader concerns. Naturally occurring substances, such as viruses, are generally not patentable, but modified organisms that serve as seed strains for vaccine production along with the processes for manufacturing them can be (Doll, 1998). Royalties charged by patent-holders, including nations, for these products could raise prices and slow production to the disadvantage of all potential vaccine recipients (Caplan & Curry, 2007).

Recognition of intellectual property rights creates incentives that can spur innovation. Countries that breed virus strains and companies that develop vaccine technologies can rely on the principle of justice to advocate for fair compensation for use of their property. However, the principle of beneficence is violated if a life-saving product is delayed or withheld because of national or economic self-interest. The global nature of an avian flu pandemic presents special challenges in balancing these principles.

CONCLUSION

VACCINES ARE CENTRAL to strategies for responding to pandemic diseases. Avian flu lurks as such a threat, but other lethal diseases with the ability to spread rapidly worldwide may also arise in the decades ahead. Large-scale production cannot begin on a vaccine that is known to be effective against such a condition until a microorganism that actually causes it emerges, and until large quantities have been manufactured and distributed, supplies will be limited. The bioethical principles of beneficence, nonmaleficence, and justice, combined with utilitarian considerations, underlie debates over how best to allocate this scarce resource, but they lead to conflicting allocation strategies.

The apportionment of vaccines against pandemic diseases raises various logistical challenges that are distinct from those related to the allocation of other scarce medical resources. Distribution must be rapid, because pandemics spread quickly. Economic and security interests must be considered, because large portions of the population could be incapacitated. Response strategies must be global in nature, because the microorganism involved could move quickly around the world. As a result, should a global pandemic arise, debates will play out with tremendous urgency, so advance planning is crucial. Conflicts between underlying ethical principles will have a central role in shaping this process.

REFERENCES

Bellagio Meeting on Social Justice and Influenza. (2006). *Bellagio statement of principles*. Retrieved January 22, 2008, from http://www.unicef.org/avianflu/files/Bellagio_Statement.pdf

Breman J. G., & Henderson, D. A. (2002). Diagnosis and management of smallpox. *New England Journal of Medicine, 346*(17), 1300–1308.

Caplan, A. L., & Curry, D. R. (2007). Leveraging genetic resources or moral blackmail? Indonesia and avian flu virus sample sharing. *The American Journal of Bioethics, 7*(11), 1–2.

Cox, N. J., & Subbarao, K. (2000). Global epidemiology of influenza: Past and present. *Annual Review of Medicine, 51*, 407–421.

Doll, J. J. (1998). The patenting of DNA. *Science, 280*(5364), 689–690.

Dushoff, J., Plotkin, J. B., Viboud, C., Simonsen, L., Miller, M., Loeb, M., et al. (2007). Vaccinating to protect a vulnerable subpopulation. *Public Library of Science Medicine, 4*(5), e174, 921–927.

Emanuel, E. J., & Wertheimer, A. (2006). Who should get influenza vaccine when not all can? *Science, 312*(5775), 854–855.

Gostin, L. O. (2006). Medical countermeasures for pandemic influenza: Ethics and the law. *Journal of the American Medical Association, 295*(5), 554–556.

Halpern, S. D., Ubel, P. A., & Caplan, A. L. (2002). Solid-organ transplantation in HIV-infected patients. *New England Journal of Medicine, 347*(4), 284–287.

Hien, T. T., de Jong, F. R. C. P., & Farrar, J. (2004). Avian influenza—a global challenge to global health care structures. *New England Journal of Medicine, 351*(23), 2363–2365.

McKenna, M. (2007, February 6). System for global pandemic vaccine development challenged. *Center for Infectious Disease Research and Policy News*. Retrieved January 19, 2008, from http://www.cidrap.umn.edu/cidrap/content/influenza/panflu/news/feb0607who.html

McNeil, D. G. (2008, January 22). A pandemic that wasn't but might be. *The New York Times*, C1.

Morens, D. M., & Fauci, A. S. (2007). The 1918 influenza pandemic: Insights for the 21st century. *The Journal of Infectious Diseases, 195,* 1018–1028.

Noymer, A., & Garenne, M. (2000). The 1918 influenza epidemic's effects on sex differentials in mortality in the United States. *Population and Development Review, 26*(3), 565–581.

Purdue, M. L., & Swayne, D. E. (2005). Public health risk from avian influenza viruses. *Avian Diseases, 49*(3), 317–327.

Riley, S., Fraser, C., Donnelly, C. A., Ghani, A. C., Abu-Raddad, L. J., Hedley, A. J., et al. (2003). Transmission dynamics of the etiological agent of SARS in Hong Kong: Impact of public health interventions. *Science, 300*(5627), 961–1966.

Simonsen, L., Olson, D. R., Viboud, C., Heiman, E., Taylor, R. J., Miller, M. A., et al. (2004). Pandemic influenza and mortality: Past evidence and projections for the future. In S. L. Knobler, A. Mack, A. Mahmoud, & S. M. Lemon (Eds.), *The threat of pandemic influenza: Are we ready?* (pp. 89–114). Washington, DC: National Academy Press.

Stohr, K., & Esveld, M. (2004). Will vaccines be available for the next influenza pandemic? *Science, 306*(5703), 2195–2196.

United Network for Organ Sharing. (2008). "What we do: Organ center." Retrieved January 18, 2008, from http://www.unos.org/whatwedo/organ center.asp

U.S. Department of Health and Human Services (2005). *HHS pandemic influenza plan.* Washington, DC: U.S. Government Printing Office.

U.S. Department of Health and Human Services (2007). *Draft guidance on allocating and targeting pandemic influenza vaccine.* Retrieved January 22, 2008, from http://www.pandemicflu.gov/vaccine/prioritization.html

Weed, D. L., & McKeown, R. E. (2001). Ethics in epidemiology and public health I. Technical terms. *Journal of Epidemiology and Community Health, 55*(12), 855–857.

World Health Organization. (2007). *Reports by the director-general, Intergovernmenal Meeting on Pandemic Influenza Preparedness: Sharing of influenza viruses and access to vaccines and other benefits. A/PIP/IGM/2 Rev. 1.* Retrieved January 22, 2008, from http://www.who.int/gb/pip/pdf_files/PIP_IGM_2Rev1-en.pdf

World Health Organization. (2008). *Cumulative number of confirmed human cases of avian influenza A/(H5N1) reported to WHO.* Retrieved January 18, 2008, from http://www.who.int/csr/disease/avian_influenza/country/cases_table_2008_01_18/en/index.html

Wynia, M. K. (2007). Ethics and public health emergencies: Rationing vaccines. *The American Journal of Bioethics, 6*(6), 4–7.

Zimmerman, R. K. (2007). Rationing of influenza vaccine during a pandemic: Ethical analyses. *Vaccine, 25*(11), 2019–2026.

57

Influenza Vaccination of Health Care Workers

Michael J. Smith

NFLUENZA IS RESPONSIBLE for nearly 200,000 hospitalizations and 36,000 deaths in the United States each year, with the highest mortality rates in young children and the elderly. Immunocompromised patients and those with chronic respiratory and neuromuscular medical conditions are also at increased risk of severe infection. Influenza vaccine, which is safe and effective in healthy adults, is not as effective in these high-risk patients. Because they are frequently hospitalized during influenza season and may acquire influenza during hospitalization, one effective method to protect them is to vaccinate health care workers against influenza. With this goal, the Advisory Committee on Immunization Practices has recommended for nearly 20 years that all health care workers (HCWs) should be vaccinated against influenza each winter. While some centers have achieved adequate levels of vaccination, overall rates of health care worker influenza vaccination remain dismally low; the latest nationally representative data show that only 36% of health care workers are vaccinated against influenza each year (Walker, Singleton, Lu, Wooten, & Strikas, 2006). This includes physicians and nurses in the hospital setting as well as employees of nursing homes, long-term care, and assisted living facilities.

Is there a moral obligation for health care workers to vaccinate themselves to protect the patients under their care? If vaccination rates remain low despite educational campaigns and freely available vaccine, should a hospital or local or state government have the authority to mandate vaccination as a condition of employment? In this chapter we discuss the ethical principles of beneficence and nonmaleficence as they relate to patient care and explore how health care workers decide whether or not to be vaccinated against influenza. We also discuss the role of autonomy of the individual health care worker to make decisions about his or her own medical care when patient safety is at stake.

IS INFLUENZA VACCINE EFFECTIVE?

BEFORE ADDRESSING THE ethical implications of HCW vaccination, we must review the efficacy and safety of influenza vaccination, both for the individual HCW and the patient. In a randomized controlled trial of healthy 18- to 64-year-old adults, Nichol (1995) found that influenza vaccine was highly effective. Specifically, there was a 25% decrease in episodes of acute respiratory illness, a 43% decrease in days of sick leave due to respiratory illness, and a 44% decrease in visits to a physician due to a respiratory illness. Additionally, the vaccine was found to be safe. Only arm soreness was reported more frequently in vaccine recipients as compared to placebo. There was no difference in the likelihood of fever, tiredness, headache, or muscle ache after receipt of the vaccine versus the placebo. Effectiveness studies focusing specifically on HCWs have demonstrated that they receive personal protection from the influenza vaccine through decreased absenteeism during influenza season, and shorter duration of influenza symptoms (Saxen & Virtanen, 1999; Wilde et al., 1999).

It is clear that influenza vaccine works and that it is safe. But does effectiveness among HCWs translate to protection for patients? Two randomized controlled trials of HCW vaccination in long-term care facilities demonstrated that vaccination of HCWs decreases mortality during influenza season, whether or not the residents are vaccinated (Carman et al., 2000; Potter et al., 1997). In addition, high levels of influenza vaccination among nursing homes residents do not prevent outbreaks if the staff is inadequately vaccinated (van den Hoven & Verweij, 2003). There is also evidence that higher rates of HCW vaccination in acute care hospitals are associated with decreased incidence of hospital-acquired influenza infections in both patients and HCWs. At one center, the number of patients with hospital-acquired infection dropped to zero in the same year that staff immunization rates reached 67% (Salgado, Giannetta, Hayden, & Farr, 2004).

ETHICAL AND PROFESSIONAL RESPONSIBILITY

THERE IS STRONG epidemiologic evidence that influenza vaccine is safe and effective in healthy adults, and that vaccination of HCWs also protects patients. Why then are so few HCWs vaccinated? While influenza vaccine does offer the HCW certain personal benefits, most HCWs are young, healthy individuals who are not at high-risk for severe disease or death. Because of this, HCW vaccination affords greater protection to patients than it does to the HCWs themselves. This is in contrast to other occupational health practices such as tuberculosis screening and hepatitis B vaccination, which offer significant protection to both HCWs and the patients under their care. While HCWs would ideally be motivated by their patients' well-being, the low rates for HCW vaccination suggest that this is not always the case. Not surprisingly, a sense of professional responsibility is highly correlated with HCW vaccination. In a study by Cowan, Winston, Davis, Wortley, and Clark (2006), the greatest predictor of influenza vaccination status was the belief that health care workers have a professional responsibility to be vaccinated. HCWs who claimed vaccination was a professional duty were four times as likely to receive influenza vaccine as those who did not. However, only half of the interviewed HCWs felt this responsibility.

Do all HCWs have a moral responsibility to be vaccinated against influenza? Absolutely. HCWs have been implicated in the spread of influenza in long-term care facilities, oncology units, intensive care units, and general medical and pediatric floors, resulting in patient death. There is a safe and effective intervention that can significantly reduce this transmission. The principle of beneficence states that individuals should engage in actions that benefit others, especially when the action carries little risk (Beauchamp & Childress, 2001). This is precisely the case for influenza vaccination. However, there are even more compelling reasons for HCWs to be vaccinated. The related concept of nonmaleficence, the obligation not to inflict harm on others, also needs to be considered (Beauchamp & Childress, 2001). This theme is ingrained in medical ethics and dates back to the days of the Greek physicians and Hippocrates' *The Epidemics:* "As to diseases, make a habit of two things—to help, or at least do no harm" (quoted in Herwaldt, 1993, p. 15). Given the prevalence of influenza in the United States, there is little doubt that any HCW employed during the winter months will be exposed to influenza and may therefore transmit disease to his or her patients. While nonmaleficence usually refers to the avoidance of actions that result in harm, it can be argued that inaction—not receiving influenza vaccination—results in direct harm to patients given the certainty of influenza exposure. Additionally, HCWs have special professional relationships with their patients that exceed those of mere beneficence; they are expected to act in their patients' best interest even if that means accepting some risk.

This role of ethical and professional responsibility has not been specifically studied in other analyses of HCW vaccination, but the importance of patient protection as a motivating force has been well documented. For instance, Nichol and Hauge (1997) found that those who felt that annual influenza vaccinations were very important for the protection of patients were more likely to be vaccinated. However, most HCWs get vaccinated to protect themselves. In a recent review of 25 studies of HCW attitudes concerning influenza vaccination, self-protection was the strongest motivation (33%–93% of all HCWs) to get vaccinated overall, whereas patient protection was less frequently mentioned. Only two identified studies found that patient protection was the main motivator (Hofmann, Ferracin, Marsh, & Dumas, 2006).

A recent analysis of HCW immunization practices at 16 hospitals caring for high-risk pediatric patients reached a different conclusion (Bryant et al., 2004). In these institutions, which reported data from pediatric and neonatal intensive care units as well as oncology units, a desire to protect patients was the most commonly reported reason for vaccination. Within these high-risk units, HCWs working on the oncology unit were significantly more likely than those on other units to report patient protection as their primary motivation for being vaccinated. The causal direction in this relationship is unclear. Certainly, oncology patients in general, and particularly bone marrow transplant patients, are at risk for life-threatening influenza infections. HCWs on the oncology unit may be motivated by personal experience with these complications. However, it is equally plausible that an innate concern for the well-being of others is what attracts HCWs to work with pediatric cancer patients. This distinction is crucial because the two explanations require different interventions. In the first case, simply educating HCWs about the consequences of influenza in high-risk patients might be effective. In the second, instilling concern for the welfare of others in individuals who do not already possess this trait is much more challenging, if possible at all. In this case, a mandatory policy might be needed to maximize HCW vaccination.

KNOWLEDGE ABOUT INFLUENZA AND INFLUENZA VACCINE

IDEALLY, EDUCATIONAL CAMPAIGNS would be able to maximize voluntary compliance with immunization. In this ideal scenario, there would be no moral dilemma, as HCWs would be vaccinated under their own free will without need of coercion. However, the evidence that knowledge about influenza is associated with vaccination status is mixed. One study assessed HCW knowledge about influenza vaccination using five questions about influenza, the vaccine, and HCW risk for acquiring influenza and transmitting it to their patients (Martinello, Jones, & Topal, 2003). The study revealed that 84% of vaccinated but only 66% of unvaccinated HCWs answered all five questions correctly, suggesting that knowledge may increase acceptance of vaccination. Watanakunakorn, Ellis, and Gemmel (1993) studied the effect of an influenza education session on HCW vaccination rates. While a higher proportion of vaccinated as compared to unvaccinated workers attended this session, most attendees had received the vaccine in prior years, and this was the only factor significantly associated with current immunization status. Heimberger and colleagues (1995) found that only one belief—that influenza vaccine does not cause influenza—was associated with vaccination. Other influenza-related knowledge was not associated with vaccination status. Specifically, awareness that HCWs can transmit influenza to their patients (held by 98% of physicians and nurses) and awareness that patients can die of influenza (held by 93% of physicians and nurses) did not translate into vaccination. These findings are cause for concern and suggest that education is not enough to optimize HCW vaccination rates. What are the obligations of the health care institution in this situation?

MOVING TOWARD MANDATORY VACCINATION

BOTH **HCW**s **AND** institutions have responsibility for patient safety. At the institutional level, influenza vaccine should be made readily available for all employees. One way to do this is by making the vaccine free for all HCWs. Other strategies include using mobile carts and offering extended hours at employee health so that hospital workers on overnight shifts are able to receive the vaccine. However, while increasing access to influenza vaccine is an essential part of any vaccination campaign, it is not sufficient to maximize uptake. For instance, the use of mobile vaccination carts that move from unit to unit resulted in a fivefold increase in staff immunization rates, but this was only from 7% to 35% (Sartor et al., 2004). These results are encouraging, but still quite far from both the rates needed to adequately protect patients and the 60% goal set forth by the CDC as part of the Healthy People 2010 goals (U.S. Department of Health and Human Services, n.d.). It is equally important to promote attitudes and beliefs that are associated with vaccination while addressing those that are associated with declination. As discussed previously, HCW vaccination is different from many other health behaviors in that the majority of benefit is derived by the patients, not the HCWs themselves. It has been suggested that framing HCW vaccination as a patient safety issue may encourage more personnel to become vaccinated (Hoffmann & Perl, 2005). Nevertheless, the previously cited data demonstrate that even HCWs who are aware that influenza vaccination protects patients remain unvaccinated.

Because of unacceptably low rates of HCW vaccination, several national organizations have suggested more aggressive tactics to improve vaccination rates. The Society for Healthcare Epidemiology of America now recommends mandatory declination—that is, all employees must either be immunized against influenza or sign a declination form stating that they understand the risks that remaining unvaccinated poses to themselves, their patients, and their families (Talbot et al., 2005). As of January 2007 the Joint Commission on Accreditation of Healthcare Organizations requires that all hospitals implement programs to increase HCW vaccination and monitor uptake. Finally, the Infectious Diseases Society of America (IDSA) also recommends a comprehensive vaccination program including "mandatory annual influenza vaccination among health care workers (with an allowance for a written declination to permit health care workers to object for religious or philosophical reasons, or if medically contraindicated)" (IDSA, 2007, p. 6).

Many institutions now use declination forms, though there is little evidence that they increase vaccination rates. Other institutions are moving toward mandatory vaccination of all hospital personnel as a condition of employment. In the fall of 2004, Virginia Mason Hospital in Seattle implemented a mandatory vaccination policy, claiming that influenza vaccination should be part of the employee fitness for duty requirement. In response, the Washington State Nurses Association argued that the requirement violated their nursing union contract. The union was not against vaccination per se but argued that coercion was neither necessary nor appropriate. A local arbitrator and U.S. District Court agreed that the hospital violated the union contract. While Virginia Mason may have violated the specific union contract, the question remains, does a health care institution have the ethical responsibility to infringe on the autonomy of its employees when patient safety is at stake?

Clearly, the same rules of beneficence and nonmaleficence that apply to the individual HCW apply to the larger medical community as well. That is, hospitals have an ethical obligation to promote actions, including influenza vaccination, that benefit their patients. Making the vaccine available and educating HCWs about influenza and influenza vaccine are necessary steps toward fulfilling this obligation. However, when comprehensive educational campaigns and increased vaccine accessibility are unable to maximize vaccine acceptance, it is the responsibility of the health care institution to ensure that all patients are protected against influenza. Therefore, a mandatory policy is justified. While such a policy may infringe on the autonomy of some HCWs, the net benefit to patients far outweighs this loss of HCW autonomy, especially given the favorable safety profile of the influenza vaccine.

This conflict between the greater good and individual rights is a recurring theme in public health and infection control ethics (Bryan, Call, & Elliott, 2007). Quarantines and isolation procedures in the hospital protect healthy patients but infringe on the personal liberties of the source patient. Similarly, policies that restrict use of antibiotics contribute to the greater good by preventing the emergence of multi-drug resistant bacteria, but limit the options for individual physicians caring for individual patients. None of these policies are questioned. In addition to being ethically justifiable, mandatory vaccination policies are effective. Rates of childhood vaccination in the United States exceeded 90% only after the introduction of school-entry requirements (Poland, Tosh, & Jacobson, 2005). At Virginia Mason Hospital, HCW vaccination rates have reached 98.5% each of the past 2 years, the highest reported rate in the country.

CONCLUSION

INFLUENZA IS RESPONSIBLE for 200,000 hospitalizations in the United States each year, and is a leading cause of health care–associated infection and death. There is a safe and effective vaccine that has been shown to protect HCWs and the patients under their care. Nevertheless, influenza rates among HCWs in the United States remain low. HCWs have a moral obligation to be vaccinated based on the principles of beneficence, nonmaleficence, and professional responsibility. Likewise, health care institutions have the obligation to ensure that their patients are protected against influenza. While every effort should be made to increase voluntary compliance with influenza vaccination, mandatory vaccination policies are justifiable and effective, and may be required in certain settings.

REFERENCES

Beauchamp, T. L., & Childress J. F. (2001). *Principles of biomedical ethics* (5th ed.). New York: Oxford University Press.

Bryan, C. S., Call, T. J., & Elliott, K. C. (2007). The ethics of infection control: Philosophical frameworks. *Infection Control and Hospital Epidemiology, 28*(9), 1077–1084.

Bryant, K. A., Stover, B., Cain, L., Levine, G. L., Siegel, J., & Jarvis, W. R. (2004). Improving influenza immunization rates among healthcare workers caring for high-risk pediatric patients. *Infection Control and Hospital Epidemiology, 25*(11), 912–917.

Carman, W. F., Elder, A. G., Wallace, L. A., McAulay, K., Walker, A., Murray, G. D., et al. (2000). Effects of influenza vaccination of health-care workers on mortality of elderly people in long-term care: A randomised controlled trial. *Lancet, 355*(9198), 93–97.

Cowan, A. E., Winston, C. A., Davis, M. M., Wortley, P. M., & Clark, S. J. (2006). Influenza vaccination status and influenza-related perspectives and practices among US physicians. *American Journal of Infection Control, 34*(4), 164–169.

Heimberger, T., Chang, H. G., Shaikh, M., Crotty, L., Morse, D., & Birkhead, G. (1995). Knowledge and attitudes of health-care workers about influenza— why are they not getting vaccinated. *Infection Control and Hospital Epidemiology, 16*(7), 412–415.

Herwaldt, L. A. (1993). Greek philosophy, medical ethics, and the influenza vaccine. *Infection Control and Hospital Epidemiology, 14*(1), 15–16.

Hoffmann, C. J., & Perl, T. M. (2005). The next battleground for patient safety: Influenza immunization of healthcare workers. *Infection Control and Hospital Epidemiology, 26*(11), 850–851.

Hofmann, F., Ferracin, C., Marsh, G., & Dumas, R. (2006). Influenza vaccination of healthcare workers: A literature review of attitudes and beliefs. *Infection, 34*(3), 142–147.

Infectious Diseases Society of America. (2007). *Pandemic and seasonal influenza principles for U.S. action.* Retrieved November 30, 2007, from http://www.idsociety.org/WorkArea/showcontent.aspx?id=5728

Martinello, R. A., Jones, L., & Topal, J. E. (2003). Correlation between healthcare workers' knowledge of influenza vaccine and vaccine receipt. *Infection Control and Hospital Epidemiology, 24*(11), 845–847.

Nichol, K. L., & Hauge, M. (1997). Influenza vaccination of healthcare workers. *Infection Control and Hospital Epidemiology, 18*(3), 189–194.

Nichol, K. L., Lind, A., Margolis, K. L., Murdoch, M., McFadden, R., Hauge, M., et al. (1995). The effectiveness of vaccination against influenza in healthy, working adults. *New England Journal of Medicine, 333*(14), 889–893.

Poland, G. A., Tosh, P., & Jacobson, R. M. (2005). Requiring influenza vaccination for health care workers: Seven truths we must accept. *Vaccine, 23*(17–18), 2251–2255.

Potter, J., Stott, D. J., Roberts, M. A., Elder, A. G., O'Donnell, B., Knight, P. V., et al. (1997). Influenza vaccination of health care workers in long-term-care hospitals reduces the mortality of elderly patients. *Journal of Infectious Diseases, 175*(1), 1–6.

Salgado, C. D., Giannetta, E. T., Hayden, F. G., & Farr, B. M. (2004). Preventing nosocomial influenza by improving the vaccine acceptance rate of clinicians. *Infection Control and Hospital Epidemiology, 25*(11), 923–928.

Sartor, C., Tissot-Dupont, H., Zandotti, C., Martin, F., Roques, P., & Drancourt, M. (2004). Use of a mobile cart influenza program for vaccination of hospital employees. *Infection Control and Hospital Epidemiology, 25*(11), 918–922.

Saxen, H., & Virtanen, M. (1999). Randomized, placebo-controlled double blind study on the efficacy of influenza immunization on absenteeism of health care workers. *Pediatric Infectious Disease Journal, 18*(9), 779–783.

Talbot, T. R., Bradley, S. F., Cosgrove, S. E., Ruef, C., Siegel, J. D., & Weber, D. J. (2005). Influenza vaccination of healthcare workers and vaccine allocation for healthcare workers during vaccine shortages. *Infection Control and Hospital Epidemiology, 26*(11), 882–890.

U.S. Department of Health and Human Services. (n.d). *Healthy People 2010 midcourse review.* Retrieved April 29, 2007, from http://www.healthypeople.gov/data/midcourse/comments/faobjective.aps?id=14

van den Hoven, M. A., & Verweij, M. F. (2003). Should we promote influenza vaccination of health care workers in nursing homes? Some ethical arguments in favour of immunization. *Age and Ageing, 32*(5), 487–489.

Walker, F. J., Singleton, J. A., Lu, P., Wooten, K. G., & Strikas, R. A. (2006). Influenza vaccination of healthcare workers in the United States, 1989–2002. *Infection Control and Hospital Epidemiology, 27*(3), 257–265.

Watanakunakorn, C., Ellis, G., & Gemmel, D. (1993). Attitude of healthcare personnel regarding influenza immunization. *Infection Control and Hospital Epidemiology, 14*(1), 17–20.

Wilde, J. A., McMillan, J. A., Serwint, J., Butta, J., O'Riordan, M. A., & Steinhoff, M. C. (1999). Effectiveness of influenza vaccine in health care professionals: A randomized trial. *Journal of the American Medical Association, 281*(10), 908–913.

Part XI

Organ Transplantation

58

Organ Transplantation: The Challenge of Scarcity

Arthur L. Caplan

EVERY DAY ABOUT a dozen people in the United States die waiting for organ transplants. One of these is a child or a baby. These deaths are especially tragic because many of them could be prevented if there were more organs available (Tan, Marcos, & Shapiro, 2008). Because organs are scarce, hard choices have to be made about who will live and who will die. With close to 100,000 people on waiting lists at American transplant centers for kidneys, hearts, livers, lungs, and intestines, the pressure to distribute the organs fairly and to find ways to increase their supply is enormous.

Every year waiting lists grow faster than the supply of organs, first because the capacity to perform transplants increases every year as new programs open and second because transplant teams are willing to accept patients far sicker than those who were put on waiting lists 10 or 20 years earlier. And if transplant centers were to relax their standards to include those who lack insurance, have severe intellectual disabilities, very old persons, prisoners, illegal aliens, drug addicts, and foreigners who cannot get transplants in their own countries, then the waiting lists would explode, easily tripling or quadrupling.

To deal with this gap, a number of options are currently being debated for inducing people to donate organs and for expanding the pool of people who could be potential donors. These steps need to be carefully considered because public support for organ donation is somewhat fragile, with many in the United States and elsewhere hesitant to indicate a willingness to be an organ donor for fear they might not receive aggressive treatment or will not be able to have the kind of funeral they or their family might wish (Caplan, 1984). Mainstream religions also support organ donation but only within a framework that treats the body as something to be cared for and stewarded, not commodified and sold.

Even if ways are found to expand the donor pool, there is not, despite what many who advocate change suggest, any quick fix for the supply problem. Scarcity cannot be eliminated any time in the near future. The hidden demand for transplants of those currently not listed would in all likelihood swamp any gains made by changing public policy or procurement practices. New forms of transplantation will also put pressure on the supply of organs and tissues (Caplan, 2004a; Caplan, Perry, Salome, Plante, & Batzer, 2007). Hard choices are going to have to be made for the foreseeable future, until medicine learns how to grow tissues and cells from adult, embryonic, cloned, or induced pluripotent cells or finds durable mechanical substitutes. Still, because it is obviously important to try and save more lives, it is ethically incumbent on American policy makers and those in other societies to consider options that might increase the supply of transplantable organs without risking the willingness of those now involved to donate.

INCREASING THE SUPPLY—SHOULD WE ABANDON ALTRUISM?

SOLID ORGAN PROCUREMENT in the United States, Canada, Sweden, Germany, the United Kingdom, and many other nations has rested on a very distinct moral foundation. Voluntary altruism has been the moral norm that has shaped how organs are obtained (Caplan, 1984; Caplan & Coelho, 1999; Veatch, 2002). This framework is intended both to protect individual autonomy about the disposition of one's body and to protect against nonconsensual taking of organs from dead or living bodies. It is also intended to help protect the quality of the obtained organs by removing money as an incentive, because historically, paid sellers of organs and tissues have not told the truth about their health, leading to problems in transmitting diseases to recipients.

Procurement from cadaver sources has always relied on the so-called dead donor rule (Truog & Miller, 2008). Under this principle, no one may serve as the source of a vital organ until they are pronounced dead. And those diagnosing death must have no interest or stake in whether organs can be procured or not from the deceased's body. In this way, the public can be assured that no one is killed in order to obtain organs.

A number of steps have been taken in the United States over the years to try and increase the supply of organs while respecting voluntary altruism and the dead donor rule. These range from state laws permitting the use of organ donor cards or giving families the authority to consent to donate a deceased relative's organs in the absence of any known objection, to an idea of my own—requiring doctors to ask families about organ donation, or a required request (Caplan & Coelho, 1999). States began requiring hospitals to make requests to potential donor families in the 1980s in the United States. More recently, state laws requiring hospitals to honor a patient's donor card even when the family opposes donation have been enacted in some states such as Texas and Wyoming, while others are requiring those seeking a driver's license to state their preference as to organ donation in order to obtain one (Petechuk, 2006).

While useful, none of these newer policies has dramatically increased the supply of organs. Therefore, some now argue for a shift away from a reliance on voluntary altruism in organ donation toward either a paid market or a framework of presumed consent. Others suggest abandoning the dead donor rule to expand the pool of those who can be considered organ donors (Truog & Miller, 2008). I am not sure that these changes make ethical sense even though lives hang in the balance everyday because of the scarcity of organs for transplant.

Organ Markets

Two basic strategies have been proposed to provide incentives for people to sell their organs when they die. One strategy is simply to permit organ sale by changing the National Organ Transplant Act (NOTA), the 1984 federal law that bans organ sales (National Organ Tranplant Act, 1984). Then, individuals would be free to broker contracts with persons interested in selling at prices mutually agreed on by both parties (Caplan, 2004b). The other strategy is a regulated market in which the government would act as the purchaser of organs— setting a fixed price and enforcing conditions of sale. Both proposals have drawn heated ethical criticism (Tan et al., 2008).

But would markets really work in the United States or other economically advanced nations? It is hard to imagine many people in wealthy countries eager to sell their organs upon their death who do not now donate them. In fact, even if compensation is relatively high, few will agree to sell. Polls show that the disincentive to cadaver donation has more to do with aesthetic, emotional, or religious concerns than a lack of payment. That has been the experience with markets in human eggs for research purposes and paid surrogacy in the United States, with prices escalating through the roof and still relatively few sellers.

Perhaps living persons can be induced to sell nonvital organs. In fact the United States now obtains more kidneys for transplant from those who donate a kidney to a friend or a family member than from cadaver sources. However, markets that incentivize living persons have their own ethical problems.

One criticism is that only the poor and very desperate will want to sell their body parts. If you need money, you might sell your kidney to try and feed your family or to pay back a debt. This may be a rational decision, but that does not make it a matter of free choice. Watching your child go hungry while you lack a job and a wealthy person waives a wad of bills in your face is not exactly a scenario that inspires confidence in the fairness of a market for body parts. Talk of individual rights and autonomy is hollow if those with no options must choose to sell their organs to purchase life's necessities. Choice requires options as well as information and some degree of freedom. A man naked in a barren desert is free to do what he wants but he has relatively little choice.

Another very important ethical challenge to proposals to permit markets is that selling organs, even in a tightly regulated market, violates the ethics of medicine. The core ethical norm of the medical profession is the principle of nonmaleficence. The only morally defensible way to remove an organ from someone is if the donor chooses to undergo the harm of surgery solely to help another and if there is sufficient medical benefit to the recipient.

The creation of a market puts medicine and nursing in the position of removing body parts from people solely to abet those people's interest in securing compensation. Is this a role that the health professions can ethically countenance? In a market, even a regulated one, doctors and nurses still would be using their skills to help people harm themselves for money—solely for the money. The resulting distrust and loss of professional standing may be too high a price to pay for a gamble that a market in living sellers may secure more organs for those in need (Caplan, 2004b).

Presumed Consent

There is another option for increasing the organ supply that has not been tried in the United States but is practiced abroad. Spain, Italy, Austria, Belgium, and some other European countries have enacted laws that create presumed consent, or what I prefer to call *default to donation*. In such a system, the presumption is that you want to be an organ donor upon your death—the default to donation. People who don't want to be organ donors have to say so by registering this wish on a computer, carrying a card, or telling their loved ones. With default to donation, no one's rights are taken away—voluntary altruism remains the moral foundation for making organs available, and, therefore, procuring organs is consistent with medical ethics.

Based on the European experience, there is a good chance America could get a significant jump in the supply of organs by shifting to a default-to-donation policy. Rates in presumed consent countries in Europe are about 25% higher than for non–presumed consent countries (Abadie & Gay, 2006). Default-to-donation proposals have been submitted in several states. Great Britain is also considering implementing presumed consent, and if it does—and if the policy is successful—that may provide more momentum for trying it in the United States.

CHANGING THE SOURCE OF ORGANS: DEATH BE NOT PROUD

PRESSURE TO CHANGE the existing norms governing organ donation has led to proposals to give more weight to the desire to donate organs than to following the requests of those who are dying as to how they want their medical care managed.

A number of states have passed laws over the past 2 years allowing organ donation requests to trump what patients have said about discontinuing life-support and the use of pain medication in their living wills or advance directives (DeVita & Caplan, 2007). The proposed revisions would make it impossible to discontinue life support if organ donation were deemed a possibility until donation had been accomplished so that organs are not damaged even if there were explicit instructions to the contrary from the patient. These laws make it more important to obtain organs than follow explicit patient wishes.

While it makes sense to ask persons if they want their desire to donate organs to trump their wishes about their care at the end of their lives, it is especially dangerous to public trust to simply create laws that make this supposition. Fortunately, in my view, the effort to enact such laws has encountered vigorous criticism and has thus slowed somewhat in the United States.

Other proposals involve modifying or abandoning the dead donor rule. Some advocate allowing persons to serve as organ donors when they are in a permanent vegetative state if they have previously signed a donor card or directive (Veatch, 2002). Some advocate putting dying persons who would not otherwise be put on life support on this technology solely to make it possible for them to serve as donors. New York City has considered equipping a special ambulance that would carry this type of equipment so that a person who died outside the hospital could be maintained on life support long enough to return to the hospital where questions of donation could be raised with family, partners, or friends.

One idea to expand the donor pool that has made real headway in American hospitals is considering persons as donors for whom a determination of brain death cannot be made either because of a lack of technology and expertise or because of terrible trauma to the brain itself. Many hospitals have instituted policies for obtaining organs from persons who do not meet brain death standards but who are deemed dead by traditional cardiac and pulmonary standards (see chapter 61 in this volume). The problem is, however, that there is no national standard for determining cardiac death as there is for brain death. Some hospitals wait 3 minutes for the heart to not function on its own before pronouncing death, whereas others wait as long as 5. In the case of infants some hospitals, eager to procure hearts for a lengthy waiting list of children born with failing hearts, may wait as little as 75 seconds before declaring death and removing the heart and other organs (Truog & Miller, 2008).

DISTRIBUTING ORGANS: WHAT IS JUST AND FAIR?

RATIONING IS A fact of life with organ transplantation, but the system for allocating organs must be just and fair. Justice requires some rule or policy that ensures that the supply of donated organs is used wisely and that allocation is consistent with what donors and their families would wish—for example, giving priority to saving children's lives or giving priority of access to American citizens. Fairness demands that like cases be treated alike and that the allocation system be transparent so that all who wait know why some are selected and some are not.

There are valid questions about the justice and fairness of the current system in the United States (Caplan & Coelho, 1999; Petuchek, 2006; Veatch, 2002). Transplant centers are the gatekeepers who decide whom they will and will not admit as transplant candidates. Their policies vary. Many nonmedical values shape their decisions, and it can be argued that some centers invoke these values in ways that are not truly just. Among these considerations are:

- Many transplant centers will not accept people without insurance. A so-called wallet biopsy is routinely performed on those seeking to be listed for heart, lung, or liver transplants because these are very costly.

- Transplant teams rarely consider anyone over 75 years of age.
- Some centers exclude patients with moderate mental retardation, HIV, a history of addiction, or a criminal record.
- Though American transplant centers can list foreigners, they can make up no more than 5% of any center's list. Most listed non-U.S. citizens have substantial financial resources and pay in cash. Cases have occurred where known criminals have been admitted into U.S. transplant programs from Japan and other countries simply because they could pay the full cost of a transplant in cash.
- Some transplant programs will admit illegal aliens, but most are children. Some transplant centers have caused controversy by refusing to retransplant illegal aliens whose initial organs, received at the same hospital during childhood, have failed.
- Many centers will retransplant Americans even though survival rates for second and third transplants are well below those of persons getting organs for the first time (see chapter 67 in this volume).

Value judgments may also influence the process of matching cadaver organs with patients on the waiting lists. The United Network for Organ Sharing (UNOS), a national network based in Richmond, Virginia, bears this responsibility (Veatch, 2002). At present, its driving considerations are matching a donor and a recipient by blood type, tissue type, and the size of the organ. Some weight is also given to the urgency or need for a transplant as reflected by time on the waiting list and the person's physical condition. There has been some push in recent years to steer organs toward those who are not seriously ill so as to maximize the chances for successful transplantation. UNOS used to have to allocate organs locally, but recently it has moved to a more regional distribution, as organ preservation techniques have improved.

Debates are growing louder about the criteria that should be used to dominate UNOS's distribution process—should it be the urgency of a patient's medical need? Or should it be efficacy (Petuchek, 2006)? In recent years, there has been a shift toward efficacy. UNOS policies are made available in the federal record, so it is possible to offer comments and criticism of them in an effort to improve the fairness of the allocation process.

Furthermore, patients can increase their chances of getting a transplant by enrolling at more than one transplant center, a practice known as multiple listing. About 10% of the current waiting list consists of persons who are listed at more than one center. Critics of multiple listing say that it is unjust because it gives an advantage to people with the resources to pay for more than one evaluation and listing, which can cost tens of thousands of dollars for each evaluation (Veatch, 2002).

Distribution of the organs that are available is very different depending on whether they come from cadaver or living sources. Living persons may direct their donation to particular recipients presuming there is a sufficient biological and size match. Cadaver organs enter into the UNOS system and are distributed to those most in need with an eye toward efficacy as well. To date the system has been seen as relatively just and fair, but as scarcity mounts, the system will have to closely examine practices such as multiple listing, disclosing risk to potential recipients and allowing foreigners with money to access American organs (Halpern, Shaked, Hasz, & Caplan, 2008).

CONCLUSION

INCREASING THE SUPPLY of organs is, in the short run, the strongest ethical obligation we have toward those dying for want of a transplant. But it is very important not to violate donor rights and interests in pursuit of these organs. Nor can we risk losing public confidence and trust in the commendable effort to try and save more lives by radically changing existing public policy or the source of organs. The best way forward in order to cement continuing public participation in making organs available would seem to require preserving the ongoing and long-standing commitment to free choice and altruism. The policy most consistent with those values is one of presumed consent. Similarly, to maintain public confidence and support for donation it is dangerous to break with the dead donor principle. Efforts that require doing so ought to be viewed with extreme skepticism. And equally important to public support and confidence in the ethics of organ transplantation is the demonstration that the system is just and fair. Practices such as multiple listing or giving entrée to wealthy criminals from other nations—which call both justice and fairness into question—need to be reigned in to prevent a backlash against these practices that would undercut the willingness of the public to altruistically donate organs either when alive or after their deaths.

REFERENCES

Abadie, A., & Gay, S. (2006). The impact of presumed consent legislation on cadaveric organ donation: A cross-country study. *Journal of Health Economics, 25,* 599–620.

Caplan, A. L. (1984). Organ procurement: It's not in the cards. *Hastings Center Report, 14,* 6–9.

Caplan, A. L. (2004a). Facing ourselves: Ethical issues in face transplantation. *American Journal of Bioethics, 4*(3), 18–20.

Caplan, A. L. (2004b). Transplantation at any price? *American Journal of Transplantation, 4*(12), 1933–1934.

Caplan, A. L., & Coelho, D. (Eds.). (1999). *The ethics of organ transplants: The current debate.* Buffalo, NY: Prometheus.

Caplan, A. L., Perry, C., Salome, J., Plante, L. A., & Batzer, F. (2007). Moving the womb: The ethics of uterine transplants. *Hastings Center Report, 37*(3), 18–20.

DeVita, M., & Caplan, A. L. (2007). Caring for organs or for patients? Ethical concerns about the Uniform Anatomical Gift Act. *Annals of Internal Medicine, 147,* 876–879.

Halpern, S. D., Shaked, A., Hasz, R. D., & Caplan, A. L. (2008). Informing solid-organ transplant candidates of donor risk factors. *New England Journal of Medicine, 358,* 2832–2837.

National Organ Transplant Act Public Law 98-507 (1984).

Petechuk, D. (2006). *Organ transplantation.* Westport, CT: Greenwood Press.

Tan, H. P., Marcos, A., & Shapiro, R. (Eds.). (2008). *Living donor organ transplantation.* New York: McGraw Hill.

Truog, R. D., & Miller, F. G. (2008). The dead donor rule and organ transplantation. *New England Journal of Medicine, 359,* 674–675.

Veatch, R. (2002). *Transplantation ethics.* Washington, DC: Georgetown University Press.

59

The Importance of Embodiment in Transplant Ethics

NORA L. JONES

THOSE OF US in a current state of health (in that there is nothing happening to give us complaint) are probably not thinking about our bodies. True, we may get distracted by a rumbling stomach, a numb leg from sitting poorly at our desks, or a dry eye from wearing too old contact lenses. But we eat, shift position, or use eye drops, and move on. An organ donor or a transplant recipient, however, can never not think about his or her body.

In saying this, I mean more than the simple recognition that the transplant recipient is able to sit and read this because of the replacement of one or more body parts (organ, tissue, blood, or even an entire face, although I will limit my discussion to solid organs). And I mean more than the acknowledgment that living organ donors sit with a bit less of themselves and a permanent scar to remind them of the experience. Bodies themselves are at the core of organ donation and transplant. They underlie moral, ethical, legal, and medical debate and decision-making: how to increase the supply of bodies for donation; how to expand the parameters of clinical compatibility between bodies; and how to decide where to send the body parts that are regularly flown across the country to be moved from one body to another. Where bodies often get less attention is in the influence that the physical body itself has in the lived experiences of donors and recipients.

So in noting that a donor or recipient can never not think about his or her body, I mean to say something about the relationship between physical bodies, identity, and worldview in general.

A worldview is essentially that, the particular view of the world we hold that gives coherence to experience. A worldview encompasses our beliefs, attitudes, and the motivations underlying our behaviors. It affects both how we make sense of the things and people we observe and how we present ourselves to those around us. On a very fundamental level, our worldview is determined by the particular body we inhabit. I don't mean this in a literal sense, that you are your body. Numerous authors have noted the difficulty here, by asking us to consider what happens when we apply this equation to an amputee or a blind person, for example. A leg or functioning eyes do not make you "you." What is you is how you understand yourself as you move through the world without a leg or without eyesight. If we are not our bodies, then perhaps it is better to say that we have bodies. However, this too is insufficient. Take our fictional amputee. She had lived some portion of her life in the world with two legs, and now with only one (she *has* a changed body). But also changed is she herself (she *is* her body, sans leg). She is aware of the way the physical environment is established for the conventionally mobile. She is aware that certain jobs are now off-limits for her. And she comes to learn that her one-legged status is different enough from the so-called norm to elicit stares from anonymous passersby. Her worldview has changed, because her body has changed. And so neither side of the equation wins outright; we must be content with the ambiguity that we both have and are bodies.

If we are comfortable with this ambiguity, we can see that our worldview is in fact an *embodied* worldview. Consider a child of color growing up in the segregated South or a little girl being told she is pretty and that her appearance gives her self-worth and definition. As an adult, this African American sees and experiences himself in his Black and White world in ways fundamentally different from an African American child born today in southern California. And our young girl has grown into a woman whose extreme dedication to her appearance is integral to her identity and who doesn't understand young emo girls today with their unbrushed hair and simple jeans and t-shirts.

As these examples show, embodiment is subject to pressures from one's surrounding moral and legal systems, political power relations, and sociocultural norms. As these sources of pressure or influence are not static, embodiment too becomes a process, open to revision at any time, given a change in either a moral or legal system (e.g., when we experience desegregation), political power relations (e.g., when women break the glass ceiling), or sociocultural norms (e.g., the different options for self-expression open to young people in different generations).

I've used these more straightforward, nonbioethical examples to illustrate the general process of embodiment. More complex is that embodiment may also be influenced by more immediate changes in one's
own body. How taking note of embodiment helps us understand the
amazing process of organ transplantation is the focus of this chapter.
My primary concern is with the question of what the transplant of
a bodily organ does to the embodiment, worldview, and identity of a
transplant recipient. And, complementing that, what is the relationship between embodiment and the decision to donate a part of one's
own or a loved one's body?

THE TRANSPLANTED SELF

T HE INFLUENCE OF the body on worldview and identity in times
of sickness, illness, or disease that alters the body is profound. It is
through our senses that we move through and know our social worlds.
When there are changes to those senses (ability to eat normally, ability
to move without aid, for example), we have a change in embodiment
itself and a change in the capacity to see that our identities and worldviews are embodied in the first place. It is when we are sick that we
can no longer take our bodies for granted. We are forced to notice our
bodies, and in the case of kidney disease or other organ failure, the important aspects of even the smallest portions of those bodies.

When someone has been deemed sick enough to be placed on a
transplant waiting list, her life's orientation faces forward, toward an
unspecified time in the future when her so-called broken part will be
replaced with a new one and she can return to her presickness stage.
She is literally awaiting the gift of life. The life she is anticipating (that
she has in fact been led to expect) is one that is full, vital, productive,
and independent (Crowley-Matoka, 2005; Sharp, 1995).

There are two problems with this transplant ideology. The first is
biological. Recipients, having lived with the expectation (enhanced by
length of time on the waiting list) that transplant would return them
to a normal state, find that instead of being returned to a state of normalcy they have simply been converted into another type of patient
(Crowley-Matoka, 2005). The broken-part metaphor doesn't hold up,
as even with a new part you aren't working as well as you used to. Recipients are chained to immunosuppressants, susceptible to illnesses
that people with suppressed immune systems get, and can be seen by
family and employers as disabled and uninsurable.

The second problem with the ideology that the gift of life returns
you to the person you were prior to transplant is that there is no prior
self to return to (Kierans, 2005). The prior self has been irrevocably

altered through the process of listing and transplant. A transplant recipient has come to view her body differently, as something with breakable parts, as something still living only because of a combination of altruism and technology. This is a special worldview related to a very particular process of embodiment that is not shared by many and not wholly understood by outsiders.

The majority of studies of life posttransplant are clinically oriented toward organ functionality, life expectancy, and posttransplant health complications. The few studies focused on psychological indicators of quality of life were published early in this organ transplant age, and generally paint a rosy picture of life posttransplant. Some claim that these early studies are biased, arguing that this positive picture emerges based on a variety of methodological problems: lacking a standard instrument to measure quality of life; being conducted by the same team responsible for the transplant and in charge of the life-saving experience; and being done immediately after transplant (Joralemon & Fujinaga, 1996).

As more social scientists contribute to the literature, the rosy picture begins to fade. In qualitative, interview-based studies, recipients talk about the social pressure to be a noble receiver and not to complain about posttransplant side effects and social difficulties. There are reports of constant worry over losing the organ. Recipients talk about the isolation of recipiency, the feeling that one has to diminish the negative aspects of living posttransplant in order to protect the people around them. Others report health professionals disregarding their current health complaints (Crowley-Matoka, 2005; Kierans, 2005; Sharp, 1995). It may be that recipients need the intimacy and trust of qualitative research to share these stories. For example, one organ transplant recipient spoke in a series of researcher interviews about posttransplant depression, isolation, and the loneliness he felt without the dialysis support. But on a public radio program discussing quality of life in organ transplantation, recorded after his interviews with the anthropologist, he mentioned none of this and instead extolled the virtues of this life-saving technology (Kierans, 2005).

The majority of these qualitative studies of transplant, embodiment, and identity have been conducted and published in Europe. U.S. researchers and publishers may be more hesitant to validate such questions because they run counter to the dominance of the biomedical model and establishment, in that these questions don't center on clearly defined outcomes. They ask us instead to consider more amorphous and nonquantifiable issues such as people's understandings of the relationship between organs, bodies, and human identity. For recipients of cadaveric organs, for example, the characteristics of the unknown donor-body become important. Recipients, with no *real* data to draw on, conjure their own *imagined* portraits of the donors (Sharp, 1995). These portraits often draw on the fear of contamination. An example of this, made all the more noteworthy because of the source, is the transplant surgeon who reported to anthropologist Margaret Lock that he was uncomfortable letting death-row prisoners donate organs because he personally wouldn't want to have within him the heart of a murderer (Lock, 2007). Similarly, there is also the fear when the donor is unknown that the residual spirit of the donor that resides in the organ will cause the organ to reject the *recipient,* as seen in the case of a Black kidney transplant recipient who feared that the White donor woman's kidney would reject him (Sharp, 1995).

The stress stemming from the fact that organ transplantation is not solely or merely a biomechanical process can be seen in the comments of a young woman who had received an initial kidney transplant that ultimately failed, followed by a liver-kidney transplant: "I still think of it as a different person inside me—yes I do, still. It's not all of me, and it's not all this person either. In a way I wish I could have a pig's liver or kidney—it would be much simpler then" (Lock, 2007, p. 228). What this quote reflects is the idea that there is something that is *us* that in some way *owns* and *is* our bodily parts, and that this level of consciousness of ourselves is either unique or infinitely more complex in humans than in other animals.

I explore this question further by turning from the transplanted self to its complement: the sources of transplantable body parts and the influence of notions of embodiment in the decisions by families and individuals to donate organs.

CADAVERIC BODIES

THE FIRST INDICATION that a body is a potential donor is the declaration of brain death. Many have talked at length about revisions in the clinical definition of brain death and the difficulty in explaining this concept to families. A family is faced with a heart beating, respiring, color-in-the-face body, and are being told that life cannot be sustained because of damage to the brain. While this disconnect may be a factor in some families' reluctance to donate organs, there have been enough popular cases (Terri Schiavo) and public representations of brain death (episodes of the TV show *ER,* for example) that the brain death concept may be more common and admissible than many presume. In fact, one 2005 study of donor families found that no participants were confused about brain death (Haddow, 2005). One family member even explicitly illustrated his understanding by making a cutting action at the back of the neck demonstrating severance of the spinal cord and thus, "there was nothing else I needed to know" (Haddow, 2005, p. 100).

If we stipulate that the hesitancy of families to donate loved ones' organs does not always center around an intellectual understanding of a clinical definition of death, then the debate over the decision may involve larger questions of embodiment and identity. The root of these questions lies in the distinction between biological death and social death. Social death refers to the fact that we as individuals live lives embedded in social networks. We are children, parents, spouses, relatives, and loved ones. Social death involves the reworking of the social webs we have woven over our lifetimes after we are no longer present.

Assuming that something of significance, whether it be a soul or a vessel to the afterlife, remains after biological death is seen in the behavior of every culture of man since the time of our evolution as a species. Over 2.5 million years ago, Paleolithic men were buried with bear skulls and marine shells, strongly implying to archeologists that death was not considered an absolute end but that the dead were being sent to live on in other ways. Bringing our gaze closer to today, capital punishment for murderers in 18th-century Britain was designed explicitly to harm the person left in the body after hanging through dissection and further terror through assault to the body and soul (Richardson, 2006). Closer to home was the desperate search to find and identify even the smallest bit of bodily remains in the World Trade Center rubble (Joralemon & Cox, 2003). These examples are not meant to imply that we as humans are superstitious or hold primitive beliefs; they illustrate the fact that we are social beings embedded in a web of social relationships in which bodies play an important part (Joralemon & Cox, 2003).

The period between death and burial (in circumstances in which transplant is not being considered) allows time for our death rituals—Irish wakes, Islamic ritual washing of the body, or the Zuni bathing of the corpse in yucca seeds—to take place. These rituals allow time for the web of social relations to begin to be reconfigured in light of the recent loss. If it is true that many people say they don't want to donate their loved ones' organs because they don't want the person to suffer any more (Richardson, 2006), a reason for this, given the discontinuity between this belief and the growing understanding of brain death, may lie in the fact that in our highly mobile individualistic U.S. (Western) culture, we have a rather limited circle of others we are connected to and perhaps we don't have enough rites of passage (death rituals) to make us or our loved ones comfortable with organ donation. In other words, there is not enough time or ritual to give ourselves the distance needed to make this decision. Let us consider again how our worldview is formed. It is formed through the external objects and personal possessions we hold and through each of our particular collections of persons and places we have experienced. In other words, the identity our worldview reflects is due to our "extended selves" (Belk, 1988), or ourselves in the world, our social selves. If this is the case, then agreeing to donate a loved one's organ means a personal loss to our extended self.

It may be that it is this sense of loss that propels the practice of embodying organs with the donor body's identity. Families talk of how organ donation allowed their loved one to live on, and some families actively seek out recipients, creating new bonds of kinship with the bodies holding their loved one's organs. Such actions are highly discouraged by the transplant industry for a variety of reasons. Anonymity is considered paramount in the first stages of transplant when donors are approached so as to avoid any problems with donors attempting to make donation contingent on certain types of recipients. And after the transplant, donor/kin knowledge would make difficult the mitigation of conflicts in cases of rejection. Knowledge of a recipient also makes it more difficult to maintain the organ transplant ethos that donating an organ is a freely given gift of life. The industry strives to maintain this ethos as it prevents other more commercial (i.e., the organ trade) interpretations or interests from taking hold. The key problem here, and the reason donor-families may fight anonymity, is that the transplant industry is failing to take into account the key element of gift-giving—the notion of reciprocity (Mauss, 1954/2002). Donor families want something in return, whether it is costs covered or a reweaving of the social webs that were ruptured by the death of a loved one. For recipients, however, knowledge of the giver heightens the burden of being unable to reciprocate. How does one repay the ultimate gift of life that stems from death? This paradox is the reason some commentators refer not to the gift of life but rather to the tyranny of the gift (Fox & Swazey, 1978).

LIVING DONOR BODIES

T HE EMBODIMENT OF donated cadaveric organs has similarities and differences to donation from living donors. In contrast to families of nonliving donors, a living donor is more likely to consider the donated liver lobe or kidney as a spare part. After all, they can continue to function more or less normally postdonation. This makes perfect sense if we consider the social function of embodying organs. A living donor can maintain social relations with the recipient—his organ doesn't have to do that work for him in absentia. And the notion that a liver lobe or kidney is a spare part is reinforced by the actions of the medical members of the transplant team. Living donors often complain of lack of follow-up and attention to their needs, both medical and emotional, after the organ's removal.

On the other hand, despite the pragmatism just expressed, live donors do stay attached to their donated organs. A donor may seek to protect the organ, monitoring those aspects of the recipient's behavior that may affect the health of the organ, such as drinking, smoking, or bungee jumping. The behavior of other family members may also reinforce the belief in embodied organs. A recipient living with a transplanted kidney may refer to the kidney as his, while the donor and rest of the family continue to reference "Uncle John's" kidney. Uncle John has given a part of himself, but that part carries with it no essence of Uncle John. Niece Jane doesn't take on the traits of John (as we saw claimed above for recipients of cadaveric organs). The dialogue resembles what may be imagined if Uncle John had loaned Niece Jane his classic Mustang.

CONCLUSION

WHILE QUESTIONS OF allocation and compatibility are important to patients on transplant waiting lists, embodiment may be closer to the daily concerns and preoccupations of recipients and donors as they struggle with the lived realities of organ donation. Taking embodiment into consideration in transplant ethics teaches us about the complexities resulting from this amazing technology and carries implications for questions of identity, worldview, and selfhood. Yes, organ transplant is a gift of life, but the life in question is more nuanced than a purely biologically functioning system.

REFERENCES

Belk, R. W. (1988). Possessions and the extended self. *Journal of Consumer Research, 15,* 139–168.

Crowley-Matoka, M. (2005). Desperately seeking "normal": The promise and perils of living with kidney transplantation. *Social Science and Medicine, 61*(4), 821–831.

Fox, R. C., & Swazey, J. P. (1978). *The courage to fail: A social view of organ transplantation and dialysis.* Chicago: University of Chicago Press.

Haddow, G. (2005). The phenomenology of death, embodiment and organ transplantation. *Sociology of Health and Illness, 27*(1), 92–113.

Joralemon, D., & Cox, P. (2003). Body values: The case against compensating for transplant organs. *Hastings Center Report, 33*(1), 27–33.

Joralemon, D., & Fujinaga, K. M. (1996). Studying the quality of life after organ transplantation: Research problems and solutions. *Social Science and Medicine, 44*(9), 1259–1269.

Kierans, C. (2005). Narrating kidney disease: The significance of sensation and time in the emplotment of patient experience. *Culture Medicine and Psychiatry, 29*(3), 341–359.

Lock, M. (2007). Human body parts as therapeutic tools: Contradictory discourses and transformed subjectivities. In M. Lock & J. Farquhar (Eds.), *Beyond the body proper: Reading the anthropology of material life* (pp. 224–231). Durham, NC: Duke University Press.

Mauss, M. (1954/2002). *The gift: Form and reason for exchange in archaic societies.* London: Routledge Classics.

Richardson, R. (2006). Human dissection and organ donation: A historical and social background. *Mortality, 11*(2), 151–165.

Sharp, L. A. (1995). Organ transplantation as a transformative experience: Anthropological insights into the restructuring of the self. *Medical Anthropology Quarterly, 9*(3), 357–389.

60

Organ Trafficking and Transplant Tourism

Debra A. Budiani-Saberi

STRIDES IN MEDICAL advancements of organ transplantation have designated transplants as the preferred therapy for
many organ-failure patients, particularly for failure of the kidneys, liver, heart, lungs, and pancreas. These advancements have also
resulted in a global search for organ supplies, especially for kidneys and
partial livers, to meet patients' overwhelming demand for this scarce
human resource. The buying and selling of organs in global markets has
become widely practiced and an ethical issue for clinicians, brokers, patients, and donors. Donors in these circumstances, commercial living
donors (CLDs), mainly consist of poor and vulnerable individuals who
are exploited by—and bear the heaviest burden of—the organ trade.[1]

Transplant specialists have largely expressed a recipient-centered
focus in their work to enhance transplant technology in measurable
outcomes of patient and graft survival rates. This general disregard for
the organ donor, particularly the living donor, has led to considerable
criticism from those concerned with medical ethics, human trafficking, and human rights and increasingly also by a few leading voices
within the transplant profession. This situation has produced satu-
rated debates about what constitutes ethical incentives for organ donation, including altruism, required response, presumed consent, organ
conscription (i.e., via executed prisoners), paid donation, or other forms

of compensated donation (i.e., free social services). Developing ethical and socially just systems for organ donation that do not target the poor is now imperative for assuring social trust in transplant practices.

BACKGROUND AND TERMS

TRANSPLANT PROCEDURES BEGAN within technically specialized medical settings and between genetically very similar individuals as with the first successful live donor kidney transplant between identical twins in 1954. They have since evolved to being practiced throughout developed and many developing countries in diverse clinical institutions and between recipients and donors (living and deceased) who are often strangers. Despite efforts in many countries to promote deceased donation as the principle supply source for therapeutic products of human origin (including organs, tissues, and cells), most transplants globally rely on living donors. The World Health Organization (WHO) reports that although the percentage of living to deceased kidney donors is relatively low in certain regions (Europe, 0.2; the western Pacific, 0.41; and the Americas, 0.67), the percentage is quite high in other regions such as Africa (3.93), the eastern Mediterranean region (14.96), and Southeast Asia (32.62; WHO, n.d., *GKT1 Activity and Practices*). The absence or ineffectiveness of a legal framework, infrastructure, or social acceptance for deceased donation are key factors that explain these figures.

Concerns that transplant science could become a victim of its own success and create a desperate demand far exceeding supply were imagined early in the development of this medical technology (Fox & Swazey, 1992). Various international and institutional declarations have been established to condemn organ trafficking as a way to increase organ supplies, including resolutions of the World Health Organization (*WHO Guiding Principles on Human Cell, Tissue, and Organ Transplantation*, 2008), the United Nations (United Nations Office on Drugs and Crime, 2000), the World Medical Association (World Medical Association, 2006), and the Transplantation Society (2008a).

Despite these efforts, demand has nevertheless created a global trade in human organs as well as tissues and cells. International research documents exploitative and unsafe practices of individuals who have been solicited, recruited, and/or trafficked to serve as CLDs (Abouna, 1993, 2003; Budiani, 2006, 2007; Scheper-Hughes, 2000; Zargooshi, 2001). CLDs have been reported to suffer significant health, economic, social and psychological consequences as a result of the organ procurement (Budiani, 2006; Goyal, Mehta, Schneiderman, & Sehgal, 2002; Naqvi, 2007; Scheper-Hughes, 2000; Shimazono, 2006; Zargooshi, 2001).

The *United Nations Protocol to Prevent, Suppress, and Punish Trafficking* describes "organ trafficking" as involving cases "where a third party recruits, transports, transfers, harbors or receives a person, using threats (or use) of force, coercion, abduction, fraud, deception, or abuse of authority or a position of vulnerability for the purpose of removing that persons organ/s" (United Nations Office on Drugs and Crime, 2000). This definition of organ trafficking captures the various exploitative measures used in the processes of soliciting a living organ donor in a commercial transplant. Exploitation has also been considered as circumstances in which the commercial transaction is given greater importance than the welfare of the living organ donor or recipient.

The term *transplant tourism* has been used as a connotation of organ trafficking. The United Network for Organ Sharing (UNOS) recently defined transplant tourism as "the purchase of a transplant organ abroad that includes access to an organ while bypassing laws, rules, or processes of any or all countries involved" (UNOS, 2007). However, not all medical tourism that entails the travel of transplant recipients or donors across national borders is organ trafficking. Tourism for a transplant may be legal and appropriate where travel of a related donor and recipient pair is from countries without transplant services to countries where organ transplantation is performed.

Illicit transplants may be coordinated in a variety of ways between recipients, CLDs, and transplant centers including transplants that occur: (a) in a transplant center within the same country of residence of the CLD and recipient, (b) when a recipient travels to a second country where the CLD and transplant center are located, (c) when a CLD travels to a second country where the recipient and transplant center are located, (d) when a CLD and recipient travel from the same country to a second country where a transplant center is located, and (e) a donor and recipient in different countries travel to a third country where a transplant center is located.

SCOPE AND COUNTRIES OF CONCERN

BECAUSE OF ITS clandestine nature, the scope of organ trafficking is difficult to assess. Countries that have facilitated organ trafficking do not often record or release precise data on the numbers of foreign patients that arrive for transplants. Nevertheless, the extent of organ trafficking has become evident.

At the Second Global Consultation on Human Transplantation of the WHO in March 2007, it was estimated that organ trafficking accounts for 5%–10% of the kidney transplants performed annually throughout the world. Shimazono (2007) assembled a sampling of the trafficking by an analysis of databases such as Lexis/Nexis, MEDLINE, and PubMed academic journal articles and Google searches that included media sources, transplant tourism Web sites, renal and transplant registries, and reports from health authorities. Shimazono reported that at least 100 nationals from countries such as Saudi Arabia (700 in 2005), Taiwan (450 in 2005), Malaysia (131 in 2004), and South Korea (124 in the first 8 months of 2004) went abroad annually for a commercial kidney transplant. At least 20 nationals from other countries such as the Australia, Japan, Oman, Morocco, India, Canada, and the United States traveled as transplant tourists for trafficked organs (Shimazono, 2007).

Shimazono's analysis of destination sites for organ sales also identified countries that provided 50 or more transplants and the organ source in 2005 and 2006. This included China, where approximately 11,000 transplants (8,000 kidney, 3,000 liver, 200 lung and or heart) were performed (Budiani-Saberi & Delmonico, 2008). China's recently adopted Human Transplantation Act has reduced the number of liver transplants in 2007 to 785 (Budiani-Saberi & Delmonico, 2008). Because the legislation that bans commercialism was adopted on May 1, 2007, there has been a shift from China to the Philippines to purchase organs. For example, at the Asian Task Force on Organ Trafficking held July 20, 2007 in Taipei, Taiwan, it was reported that approximately 400 South Koreans are anticipated to purchase a kidney out of the country by the end of the year. Approximately 1,000 South Korean patients undergo kidney transplantation annually.

Merion and colleagues (2007) reported the initial U.S. experience that includes some patients whose transplants were not obtained from CLDs. One hundred nineteen U.S citizens and resident aliens from 55 transplant centers in 26 states were recorded as having received kidney transplants in 18 foreign countries after a median of 1.5 years (range 21 days to 8.5 years) on the U.S. waiting list.

At least 2,000 kidney transplants have been performed in Pakistan to transplant tourists. In the Philippines, a February 2007 newspaper account of the number of kidney sales reveals over 3,000 have been performed ("RP Admits 'Rampant' Traffic in Human Organs," 2007). The Cebu Province of the Philippines is now reported to be seeking transplant tourists to enlarge Philippine trafficking ("Medical Tourism Plans for Cebu Pushed," 2007). It is estimated by Egyptian nephrologists (Egyptian Society of Nephrology, unpublished meeting notes, Cairo, 2007) that Egypt performs 300–500 kidney transplants annually. Doctors estimate that 90% of these transplants are performed from CLDs, as national legislation on transplants is largely absent (Budiani, 2007). Multiple media sources report that, despite India's strict legislation to prohibit organ sales, organ trafficking still thrives in several urban centers in India (Jha, 2004). No kidney transplants are performed in the medically advanced Persian Gulf country of the United Arab Emirates (UAE) despite their capability; thus, patients have gone out of country to China, India, the Philippines, and Egypt to undergo transplantation. There are no recorded numbers of these patients, but interviews with physicians and patients within the UAE reveal this pattern (Coalition for Organ-Failure Solutions [COFS] Field Research; Budiani & Punekar, 2006). Similar trends are reported for the other Persian Gulf countries.

Indicators such as falling prices and increases in identified numbers of transplant tourists annually suggest that the black market for commercial transplants is expanding. CLDs thus serve as a significant source of organ supplies globally and mainly consist of poor and vulnerable individuals in desperate need of money.

CONSEQUENCES

ORGAN TRAFFICKING FOR commercial transplants entails little regard for the well-being of the recipient or donor. Recipients from commercial transplants often return from a transplant with inadequate reports of operative events and unknown risks of donor-transmitted infection (such as hepatitis or tuberculosis) or a donor-transmitted malignancy. However, CLDs categorically bear among the heaviest consequences of the organ trade. Reports from various countries on health, economic, social, and psychological consequences as a result of the organ procurement indicate similar findings.

In Pakistan, the Sindh Institute of Urology and Transplantation (SIUT) group has detailed a sample cohort of 239 vendors (Naqvi, 2007). The majority of these CLDs (93%) sold a kidney to repay a debt, and 85% said there was no economic improvement in their lives, as they were either still in debt or were unable to achieve their objectives.

Egypt, like Pakistan, is one of the few countries that prohibits organ donation from deceased donors. In the absence of an entity to govern allocation or standards for transplants, the market has become the distribution mechanism. Egypt is also one of the countries in which COFS has conducted extensive field research and long-term outreach service programs for victims of the organ trade (Budiani, 2006). In-depth longitudinal interviews of 50 CLDs reveal that 78% reported a deterioration in their health condition. A kidney sale does not provide a permanent solution to a CLD's financial problems; 81% spent the money within 5 months of the nephrectomy, mostly to pay off current debts rather than investing in quality-of-life enhancements. CLDs are not eager to reveal their identity; 91% expressed social isolation about their donation, and 85% were unwilling to be known publicly as an organ vendor. Ninety-four percent regretted their donation.

The studies in Pakistan and Egypt are consistent with findings in India (Goyal et al., 2002), Iran (Zargooshi, 2001), and the Philippines (Shimazono, 2006). In each of these countries, studies revealed a deterioration in the health condition of the CLDs who received little or no follow-up care—86% in India, 60% in Iran, and 48% in the Philippines. A long-term financial disadvantage is evident following nephrectomy from a compromised ability to generate a prior income level—75% reported in India, 65% in Iran, and 93% in the Philippines. Finally, the common experience also entails a social rejection and regret about their commercial donation—70% in Iran (this data was not reported in the studies in India and the Philippines). These reports are consistent in indicating that a cash payment does not solve the destitution of the vendor.

RESPONSES

IN RESPONSE TO the global illicit market for organs, several transplant professionals and academics have suggested that a regulated market in human organs would reduce or remedy the patient waiting list for organs and would, in turn, work to ameliorate conditions of poverty for organ vendors (Hippen, 2005; Matas, 2007; Radcliffe-Richards, 2003; Veatch, 2003). However, a reliance on financial or material incentives for donation (in a black or a regulated market such as that of Iran) entails various faults. First, this method necessarily targets the poor by providing inducements for their so-called donation. A cash or material payment for an organ most appeals to those individuals with insufficient opportunity to employment, health care, housing, or education. It may even be coercive in a situation where a compensated organ donation is the only alternative for a destitute individual or family.

Second, such incentives undermine altruistic living and deceased donation. This can be seen in countries such as Malaysia and Oman where nationals seek organs abroad relatively easily rather than rely on relatives or a deceased donation. Thus, most transplants of patients from these countries are done via tourism.

Third, it is not possible to regulate a market in organs when, as with other commodities, global prices would vary. Prices would be adjusted by a donor's health and social status such as age, gender, and ethnicity/race. Patients in need would go where prices were affordable.

Finally, financial or material incentives would not secure the best health outcomes for recipients or donors. Such incentives lure potential donors (and their profiting parties) to deny that they may have been exposed to HIV/AIDS, hepatitis, or tuberculosis. Transplant professionals in the North American and Persian Gulf countries share horror stories of recipients who return from Pakistan, China, or the Philippines with illnesses transmitted from the donor.

Efforts to combat organ trafficking, transplant tourism, and transplant commercialism have gained momentum in recent years. Significant attention has been paid to establishing protective policies and guidelines. The WHO Resolution WHA 57.18 on Human Organ and Tissue Transplantation (2004) outlines guidelines on allogeneic and xenogeneic transplants, including urging member states to take measures to protect the poorest and most vulnerable groups from transplant tourism and the sale of tissues and organs.

The Amsterdam Forum on the Care of the Live Kidney Donor (Ethics Committee of the Transplantation Society, 2005) and the Vancouver Forum on the Care of the Live Organ Donor: Lung, Liver, Pancreas, and Intestine (Barr et al., 2006) are deliberations from the Ethics Committee of the Transplantation Society that outline responsibilities of the transplant team performing live donation and call for independent oversight and transparency in transplant practices. Further, numerous declarations have been made against organ trafficking and transplant tourism including those by the World Medical Association (2006) and UNOS (2007). Organs Watch (an academic research organization on organ trafficking) and COFS (a health and human rights nongovernmental organization that combats organ trafficking and provides prevention, policy advocacy, and survivor support) have emerged to advocate this cause beyond just a policy level via field-based work.

CONCLUSION

RECOMMENDATIONS TO COMBAT organ trafficking include:

- The development of national legal frameworks and self-sufficiency in organ donation and transplantation that protect the live donor and assure socially just allocation principles.
- Transparency of transplantation practices that is accountable to the health authorities according to national legislation.
- The prohibition of citizens or insurance and pharmaceutical companies from participating in or supporting commercial transplants such that profits are prioritized over the well-being of the donor or recipient.

While official guidelines and policies have reduced exploitative transplant practices, they have not been sufficient to combat the international organ trade. For example, the establishment of detailed laws to end organ trafficking in India resulted in a shift of transplant tourists from India to Pakistan and the persistence of clandestine transplant centers within India where the organ market still thrives. Thus, civil society–level efforts must also be initiated to combat organ trafficking via public and target group campaigns to raise awareness about altruistic and deceased donation as alternatives to the reliance on the poor as an organs source.

The transplant community must rebuild public trust in transplants. Care for the live donor (altruistic and commercial) that assures safety and addresses donor needs is an essential component of redemption from the exploitative practices via transplant technology. These needs are the legitimate consequences of living organ donation and must be addressed in each country with national oversight, authorized by national legislation and guided by the World Health Organization's resolution on organ transplants.

NOTE

1. Other terms used in the literature on organ trafficking have included *organ vendor* and *organ seller*. However, those terms suggest that the act might be repeated as with other forms of vending. I use the term *commercial living donor* (CLD) as a parallel to the term *commercial sex worker* to demonstrate the act as an economic resort of an organ donor.

REFERENCES

Abouna, G. (1993). Negative impact of trading in human organs on the development of transplantation in the Middle East. *Transplant Proceedings, 25,* 2310–2313.

Abouna, G. (2003). Ethical issues in organ and tissue transplantation. *Experimental and Clinical Transplantation, 1,* 125–138.

Barr, M. L., Belghiti, J., Villamil, F. G., Pomfret, E. A., Sutherland, D. S., Gruessner, R. W., et al. (2006). A Report of the Vancouver Forum on the Care of the Live Organ Donor: Lung, liver, pancreas, and intestine data and medical guidelines. *Transplantation, 81,* 1373–1385.

Budiani, D. (2006, November). *Consequences of living kidney donors in Egypt.* Presentation at the Middle East Society on Organ Transplants (MESOT) Meetings, Kuwait City, Kuwait.

Budiani, D. (2007). Facilitating organ transplants in Egypt: An analysis of doctors' discourse. *Body and Society, 13,* 125–149.

Budiani, D., & Punekar, I. (2006). Organ transplants in the UAE: A COFS report. Retrieved April 13, 2008, from http://www.cofs.org

Budiani-Saberi, D., & Delmonico, F. (2008). Organ trafficking and transplant tourism: A commentary on global realities. *American Journal of Transplantation, 8,* 925–929.

Ethics Committee of the Transplantation Society. (2005). A report of the Amsterdam Forum on the Care of the Live Kidney Donor: Data and medical guidelines. *Transplantation, 79*(6), S53–S66.

Fox, R., & Swazey, J. (1992). *Spare parts: Organ replacement in American society.* New York: Oxford University Press.

Goyal, M., Mehta, R., Schneiderman, L., & Sehgal, A. (2002). Economic and health consequences of selling a kidney in India. *Journal of the American Medical Association, 288,* 1589–1593.

Hippen, B. (2005). In defense of a regulated market in kidneys from living vendors. *Journal of Medicine and Philosophy, 6,* 593–626.

Jha, V. (2004). Paid transplants in India: The grim reality. *Nephrology Dialysis Transplant, 19,* 541–543.

Matas, A. (2007). A gift of life deserves compensation: How to increase living kidney donation with realistic incentives. *Cato Institute Policy Analysis, 604.* Retrieved May 12, 2008, from http://www.cato.org/pub_display.php?pub_id=8780

Medical tourism plans for Cebu pushed. (2007, August 6). *Global Nation,* Retrieved April 13, 2008 from, http://globalnation.inquirer.net/cebudaily news/news/view_article.php?article_id=80868

Merion, R. M., Lin, M., McBride, V., Ortiz-Rios, E., Welch, J. C., Levine, G. N., et al. (2007). *Transplant tourism among patients removed from the U.S. kidney transplant waiting list.* San Francisco: American Transplant Congress.

Naqvi, A. (2007). A socio-economic survey of kidney vendors in Pakistan. *Transplant International, 20*(11), 909–992.

Radcliffe-Richards, J. (2003). Commentary: An ethical market in human organs. *Journal of Medical Ethics, 29,* 139–140.

RP admits "rampant" traffic in human organs. (2007, February 7). *Manila Times.* Retrieved April 13, 2008, from http://www.manilatimes.net/national/2007/feb/07/yehey/top_stories/20070207top1.html

Scheper-Hughes, N. (2000). The global traffic in human organs. *Current Anthropology, 41,* 191–224.

Shimazono, Y. (2006, May). *What is left behind?* Presentation at an Informal Consultation on Transplantations at the World Health Organization, Geneva.

Shimazono, Y. (2007). *Mapping transplant tourism.* Presentation at the World Health Organization's Second Global Consultation on Human Transplantation, March 28–30, Geneva.

Transplanation Society. (2008). *Istanbul declaration.* Retrieved October 27, 2008, from http://www.prnewswire.com/mnr/transplantationsocicty/33914/docs/33914-Declaration_of_Istanbul-Lancet.pdf

United Nations Office on Drugs and Crime. (2000). *Protocol to prevent, suppress, and punish trafficking in persons.* Retrieved April 10, 2008, from http://www.uncjin.org/Documents/Conventions/dcatoc/final_documents_2/convention_%20traff_eng.pdf

United Network for Organ Sharing (UNOS). (2007). *UNOS board further addresses transplant tourism.* Retrieved April 10, 2008, from http://www.unos.org/news/newsDetail.asp?id=891

Veatch, R. (2003). Why liberals should accept financial incentives for organ procurement. *Kennedy Institute of Ethics Journal, 13,* 19–36.

World Health Organization (2004). WHA57.18 Human Organ and Tissue Transplantation. Retrieved October 27, from http://www.who.int/transplantation/en/A57_R18-en.pdf

World Health Organization (2008). WHO Guiding Principles on Human Cell, Tissue, and Organ Transplantation. Retrieved October 27, 2008, from http://www.who.int/transplantation/TxGP08-en.pdf

World Health Organization. (n.d.). *GKT1 activity and practices.* Retrieved April 10, 2008, from http://www.who.int/transplantation/gkt/statistics/en/

World Medical Association. (2006). *World Medical Association statement on human organ donation and transplantation.* Retrieved April 10, 2008, from http://www.wma.net/e/policy/wma.htm

Zargooshi, J. (2001). Quality of life of Iranian kidney "donors." *Journal of Urology, 166*(5), 1790–1799.

61

Ethical Dilemmas in the Management of the Potential Organ Donor After Circulatory Determination of Death

Scott D. Halpern

WITH THE CHASM between the supply and demand for transplantable organs continuing to grow, more than 7,000 Americans are now dying each year while waiting for organs (United Network for Organ Sharing, 2006). The total life-years lost annually because of insufficient organ donation is comparable to the life-years lost annually to stroke or liver disease (Schnitzler, Whiting, et al., 2005). Improving organ donation is a critical public health goal, as each additional deceased donor provides roughly 30 extra life-years to the pool of patients on transplant waiting lists (Schnitzler, Whiting, et al., 2005). Furthermore, the increases in quality-adjusted life expectancy obtained through organ donation are cost-effective by conventional standards (Mendeloff, Ko, Roberts, Byrne, & Dew, 2004) and in the case of kidney transplantation are substantially cost-saving (Schnitzler, Lentine, & Burroughs, 2005).

Despite the promise of increasing organ donation, there are limits to traditional strategies for expanding the organ supply. Most organs come from donation after neurologic determination of death (DNDD, formerly called brain-dead donors), in whom death is declared on the basis of neurologic criteria and the circulatory and respiratory systems are artificially supported through the time of organ procurement. However, even in the unlikely event that all viable organs from DNDD donors were transplanted, there would still be too few organs to meet the growing demand (Guadagnoli, Christiansen, & Beasley, 2003; Sheehy et al., 2003). Other modalities are therefore needed to expand the donor pool.

A recent committee convened by the Institute of Medicine (IOM) suggested that of the several potential pools of extra donors—including living donors, extended-criteria donors (i.e., DNDD donors who do not meet traditional clinical criteria for donation), and donation after circulatory determination of death (DCDD) donors (formerly referred to as non-heart-beating donors)—the optimal way to expand the donor pool would be to increase DCDD (Committee on Increasing Rates of Organ Donation, 2006). DCDD donors are typically patients with devastating neurologic injuries (e.g., stroke or anoxic brain injury) who do not fulfill neurologic criteria for death but who choose (or whose surrogate decision-makers choose) to withdraw life-sustaining therapies, leading to cardiac arrest. Because the timing and location of the withdrawal of life support can be controlled for these patients, organ procurement can be temporally linked, thereby minimizing organ ischemia.

In promoting DCDD, the IOM committee joined the American Medical Association (n.d.), Canadian Medical Association (Shemie, Baker, Knoll, et al., 2006), American College of Critical Care Medicine/Society of Critical Care Medicine (2001), and a recent U.S. Consensus Conference with representation from most transplant policy groups (Bernat, D'Alessandro, Port, et al., 2006) in supporting the ethics of DCDD. Following publication of the IOM committee's conclusions, DCDD rates have increased in the United States, the Joint Commission on Accreditation of Healthcare Organizations (2007) and the United Network for Organ Sharing have required hospitals to produce protocols for DCDD, and organ donation advocates have aggressively promoted DCDD within hospitals and before Congress.

711

*Ethical
Dilemmas in the
Management
of the Potential
Organ Donor
After Circulatory
Determination
of Death*

However, despite this broad support and momentum, ethical challenges to DCDD remain. Early concerns that DCDD involves procuring organs before patients are truly dead persist (Menikoff, 1998; Rady, Verheijde, & McGregor, 2006; Youngner, Arnold, & DeVita, 1999). Furthermore, there are increasing concerns that DCDD presents inextricable conflicts for the critical care clinicians who manage potential donors. Such practitioners are simultaneously asked to provide compassionate end-of-life care—serving as guardians of dignified deaths for the 20% of Americans who die during or shortly following an ICU stay (Angus, Barnato, Linde-Zwirble, et al., 2004)—while also furthering the interests of potential organ recipients by using interventions that promote successful organ procurement.

How effectively critical care physicians and nurses manage such competing interests is unknown, but a highly publicized case of potential misconduct in San Luis Obispo, California, in 2006 has raised public awareness of such conflicts, threatening DCDD acceptability to practitioners and patients (Stein, 2007). The possibility that physicians might use excessive sedation to expedite death and preserve organ viability, as the defendant in this case is charged, raises both ethical concerns and public fears about DCDD.

In this chapter, I consider the ethical challenges to DCDD and the sources of these concerns. I argue that older views that DCDD is unethical because it entails procuring organs prior to death are unfounded. Instead, the most substantive challenge to DCDD regards the potential for conflict between promoting the dying patient's interests at the end of life and the interests of potential organ recipients. I conclude that not only can this potential conflict be avoided through appropriate safeguards but that the promotion of dying patients' donation preferences represents a legitimate component of high-quality end-of-life care.

BACKGROUND

THE GREATEST POTENTIAL for DCDD is among patients with devastating neurologic or pulmonary conditions who have chosen (or whose surrogate decision-makers have chosen) to withdraw life-sustaining therapies. This form of DCDD has been termed *controlled,* in contrast to uncontrolled DCDD, which occurs when a patient who has sustained a spontaneous, unanticipated cardiac arrest goes on to organ procurement after emergently mobilizing the transplant team.

As with candidates for traditional DNDD, the overwhelming majority of controlled DCDD candidates are cared for in intensive care units (ICUs). Thus, as was learned with DNDD (Prottas & Batten, 1988; Siminoff, Arnold, & Caplan, 1995), the success of DCDD requires that intensivists and critical care nurses support and promote DCDD. The ICU team is responsible for identifying potential donors, working collaboratively with representatives of the local organ procurement organization (OPO) to obtain informed consent for donation, providing compassionate end-of-life care, and declaring death. It is widely agreed that, to minimize conflicts, the patient must remain under the care of the ICU team up through the pronouncement of death, and that the provision of palliative care to such patients must not be influenced by the prospect for donation. Only after the pronouncement of death, which requires a waiting period of 2–5 minutes following the cessation of circulation (Committee on Increasing Rates of Organ Donation, 2006), may the transplant surgeons enter the room and begin organ procurement.

ARE DCDD DONORS DEAD?

AN OVERRIDING PRINCIPLE of transplantation ethics is the so-called dead donor rule (Robertson, 1999), which states that the procurement of organs cannot precede or be causally related to the onset of death. Many commentators have posited that DCDD may violate the dead donor rule by questioning the timing of death in such patients (Youngner & Arnold, 2001; Youngner et al., 1999). This view is plausible, though not provable, because there exist neither clear physiologic data nor broad national consensus to determine the precise timing of death. Indeed, death is perhaps most accurately construed as a process that occurs over time rather than as a discrete, instantaneous event.

Given the obscure nature of when death occurs, some are concerned that procuring organs after 2, 5, or even 10 minutes of absent circulation risks removing organs before there is certainty that life cannot be restored. On the other hand, as Youngner and colleagues argue, "if donors were seen by the public as persons who are seriously injured and whose families desperately want to donate organs to give meaning to the death and to respect the patient's final wishes, the number of minutes needed to declare death might well be ignored as a theoretical issue of little magnitude" (Youngner et al., 1999, p. 18). Indeed, legal definitions of death do not require a precise understanding of biology, because the law often ignores or misconstrues biological facts to achieve a public purpose (Charo, 1999) such as organ donation. Thus, so long as DCDD promotes both the donor's and the recipient's interests, and there is no intrinsic unfairness in the process, the ambiguity of the timing of death may safely be ignored (Youngner et al., 1999).

There are still other reasons to assert, as Fost has, that the dead donor rule is not a rule at all, but merely a guideline (Fost, 2004). Fost argues that such a rule may violate modern conceptions of autonomy, which

713

*Ethical
Dilemmas in the
Management
of the Potential
Organ Donor
After Circulatory
Determination
of Death*

dictate that people's interests in what becomes of their bodies—even after death—ought to be respected (Fost, 2004). Indeed, as patients are increasingly allowed to take control of many aspects of their dying process, why should we prohibit patients from violating the dead donor rule if they so choose? When such patients (or their surrogates) choose to have life-sustaining therapies withdrawn, rarely do they do so based on a belief that all cardiopulmonary function will cease within a certain time frame, but rather they do so based on the recognition that the chances for meaningful recovery are unacceptably small. The precise timing of the declaration of death is of no consequence to patients who are choosing to forgo continued interventions that they do not consider consistent with their values and goals. If one of these goals is to be an organ donor, then it does such patients a disservice to deny them this option because of ambiguity about the timing or final cause of death. Indeed, while scholars might continue this debate, empirical research suggests that most members of the public do not consider the timing of death to be an important factor influencing the propriety of organ procurement (Keenan, Hoffmaster, Eberhard, Chen, & Sibbald, 2002; Siminoff, Burant, & Youngner, 2004).

BARRIERS TO PROMOTING DCDD IN THE ICU

Perhaps more salient than concerns about the timing of death are concerns about how ICU clinicians can incorporate DCDD management into their practices (Mandell, Zamudio, Seem, et al., 2006). Some of these concerns are similar to those raised with regard to DNDD (Pearson & Zurynski, 1995; Prottas & Batten, 1988; Siminoff et al., 1995), but others are unique to DCDD. Some or all of the following barriers may help explain why only limited progress (DuBois & DeVita, 2006) has been made in the number of organs procured through DCDD in the 10 years since the IOM first published its support of the practice (IOM, 1997).

Time and Resource Barriers

In an era in which the growth in demand for critical care services is markedly outpacing the growth in supply of these services (Angus et al., 2000; Angus, Shorr, White, et al., 2007; Barnato, Kahn, Rubenfeld, et al., 2007), intensivists may be increasingly unable to expend the time and energy required to manage DCDD patients after the withdrawal of life support. Similar concerns about time constraints were noted in a survey of intensivists regarding DNDD (Prottas & Batten, 1988), but the demands of DCDD may be even greater because, ideally, critical care physicians and nurses leave the ICU to care for patients in the operating room, where life-sustaining therapies are withdrawn and comfort care is provided. Given these requirements, clear evidence of the benefit from DCDD—in terms of improved quality of end-of-life care and clear expansion of the supply of viable organs—may be needed before intensivists can justify the expenditure of limited personal resources on bringing dying patients to transplant.

EDUCATIONAL BARRIERS

INTENSIVISTS MAY NOT be willing to devote time and energy to DCDD because, traditionally, the organs obtained through this practice were considered suboptimal. Many intensivists are likely unfamiliar with recent evidence that transplantation outcomes after DCDD are comparable to those obtained after DNDD for kidneys (D'Alessandro, Fernandez, Chin, et al., 2004; Tojimbara, Fuchinoue, Iwadoh, et al., 2007; Weber, Dindo, Demartines, Ambuhl, & Clavien, 2002; Wijnen et al., 1995) and pancreata (D'Alessandro et al., 2004); that only slight decreases in long-term survival are observed using DCDD livers (D'Alessandro, Hoffmann, Knechtle, et al., 2000; Gomez, Garcia-Buitron, Fernandez-Garcia, et al., 1997; Reich et al., 2007); and that limited early experience suggests the promise of transplanting hearts (Campbell, 2007) and lungs (Love, 2007; Oto, Levvey, McEgan, et al., 2007) following DCDD.

Another educational barrier is that intensivists may not understand the types of patients who are suitable for DCDD and what interventions are required to maximize the viability of their organs. Such deficiencies in donor identification have limited DNDD (Siminoff et al., 1995), and may be even more pervasive in the case of DCDD because the range of neurologic and pulmonary injuries that may make patients optimal controlled DCDD candidates is not widely appreciated and because tools for predicting death shortly after withdrawal of life-sustaining therapies are in their infancy (Lewis, Peltier, Nelson, et al., 2003).

Finally, intensivists may be ill-prepared to broach the issue of donation with families. Such shortcomings have prevented many intensivists from discussing organ donation with families of potential DNDD candidates (Pearson & Zurynski, 1995). And, again, such discussions may be more complex in the case of DCDD. Whereas consideration of donation typically follows a pronouncement of death or impending death in DNDD, in DCDD discussions of donation must closely follow consideration of the withdrawal of life-sustaining therapies from patients who are currently alive. Indeed, such conversations may occasionally happen with the patients themselves because some potential DCDD candidates will be sufficiently alert to participate in their own

715

*Ethical
Dilemmas in the
Management
of the Potential
Organ Donor
After Circulatory
Determination
of Death*

end-of-life decision-making. Without proper training or adequate experience in coordinating such discussions, intensivists may shy away from having them, thereby limiting opportunities for donation.

Given these concerns, both guidelines for how to handle these discussions and evidence that such linked conversations do not exacerbate family members' grieving processes may be needed before critical care practitioners will embrace DCDD. There are presently few guidelines and limited data to guide intensivists in the proper selection and management of DCDD candidates, though the development of such guidelines has been urged by several groups (American Medical Association, n.d.; Committee on Increasing Rates of Organ Donation, 2006; The Joint Commission on Accreditation of Healthcare Organizations, 2007).

ETHICAL BARRIERS

THE CULTURE AND orientation of the ICU has always been to save the lives of critically ill patients (Curtis & Rubenfeld, 2005; Nelson, 1999). Most intensivists now acknowledge their simultaneous roles as guardians of dignity and comfort at the end of life for the many patients who cannot be saved (Curtis & Rubenfeld, 2005; Nelson, 1999). However, for many intensivists, the promotion of organ donation and management of the potential donor seems to represent yet a third role, oriented toward improving public health by increasing the organ supply.

Not only does this apparent third duty seem to add to the already substantive onus of critical care medicine, but it may seem to conflict with the second duty to promote quality end-of-life care for dying patients. For some, even seemingly benign interventions, such as administering heparin prior to death to preserve organ perfusion will be unacceptable because it may seem inconsistent with the patient's wishes to forgo further therapies lacking a clear palliative role. More invasive interventions, such as arterial and venous cannulation, bronchoscopy, or even cardiopulmonary resuscitation in the event of an unanticipated cardiac arrest prior to the withdrawal of mechanical ventilation might therefore seem to be outside the boundaries of palliative care.

PRESERVING OPPORTUNITIES TO DONATE AS PART OF END-OF-LIFE CARE

LOST IN THIS conceptualization of organ donor management as a separate third duty for intensivists is the possibility that dying patients may be greatly comforted by knowing that their wishes to become organ donors will be respected and promoted at the end of

life. There is presently no direct evidence that patients consider the opportunity for organ donation to be an important component of their
dying process. However, evidence that patients with living wills are
more likely to favor organ donation (Thornton, Curtis, & Allen, 2006)
suggests that those who want to control some of the circumstances
that will surround their eventual deaths consider organ donation to be
an important part of this process. The anecdotal experiences of many
seasoned intensivists also suggest that both patients and their family
members may be comforted by knowing that the patient's interests
in becoming an organ donor are being honored. For many, the ability
to save lives through organ donation represents an important part of
their life's legacy.

These observations suggest an alternate frame from which ICU clinicians might view interventions intended to preserve organ function:
that such interventions, albeit potentially life-sustaining for brief periods, serve to promote the patient's donation preferences. If so, they
should be considered a part of compassionate end-of-life care. From
this vantage point, even invasive interventions ought to provided,
with the goal of preserving the patient's opportunity to donate, as long
as they do not clearly cause distress for the donor. With the provision of
adequate sedation, even cardiopulmonary resuscitation might be consistent with the patient's goals of dying peacefully, with dignity, and as
an organ donor.

Even within this framework, however, interventions that do not
clearly serve a palliative role will only be acceptable if the patient (or his
or her surrogate) understands that they might be required to preserve
the opportunity to donate and agrees to their use for this specific goal.
An important research direction, therefore, is to determine whether
this requirement for full disclosure is currently being fulfilled when
ICU clinicians and OPO representatives obtain consent for donation.

CONFLICTS BETWEEN DONATION PREFERENCES AND ADVANCED DIRECTIVES

RECENT REVISIONS TO the Uniform Anatomical Gift Act (National Conference of Commissioners on Uniform State Laws,
2006) imply that for patients who have both designated themselves as
organ donors and stated preferences to forgo life-sustaining therapies
(e.g., in an advanced directive), donation wishes should be prioritized
(Caplan & DeVita, 2007). Although these revisions are presently being
reconsidered, and have not been enacted in all states, the fact that they
ever materialized reflects a misguided perspective that at times a patient's desire to be an organ donor might conflict with the desire not

717

*Ethical
Dilemmas in the
Management
of the Potential
Organ Donor
After Circulatory
Determination
of Death*

to have invasive interventions at the end of life. Such a conflict should never arise—a holistic appraisal of each patient's goals and priorities should provide clear guidance for that patient's care.

Patients' stated wishes to avoid life-prolonging therapies when they are no longer serving desired purposes must never be violated. However, it would be wrong to assume that the presence of such preferences might necessarily prevent organ donation from occurring. For the severely neurologically injured but non-brain-dead donor, maintaining unwanted life support to allow time for the patient to progress to neurologic death is unacceptable. However, DCDD may offer such patients the opportunity to donate following the timely termination of unwanted life support, at least at centers with established DCDD protocols and transplant teams. Indeed, striving to preserve the opportunity for donation through DCDD in this circumstance may maximize the quality of the end-of-life care provided because it simultaneously respects patients' wishes both to avoid life-sustaining interventions and to donate.

CONCLUSION

A LTHOUGH WE LACK evidence regarding the extent to which people value organ donation, observations that many living patients will go to great lengths to provide organs to others—even when these others are unrelated—suggests that donating organs after death may be an important goal for many people. Because the cornerstone of excellent end-of-life care is promotion of the patients' interests and goals, preserving the opportunity to donate is a legitimate goal for critical care clinicians. Thus, with appropriate safeguards in place to ensure the separation of end-of-life care and organ procurement, efforts to promote donation after circulatory determination of death may represent manifestations of a confluence, rather than a conflict, of interests.

REFERENCES

American College of Critical Care Medicine/Society of Critical Care Medicine Ethics Committee. (2001). Recommendations for nonheartbeating organ donation. A position paper by the Ethics Committee, American College of Critical Care Medicine, Society of Critical Care Medicine. *Critical Care Medicine, 29,* 1826–1831.

American Medical Association. (n.d.). *H-370.975 ethical issues in the procurement of organs following cardiac death.* Retrieved August 19, 2008, from http://www.ama-assn.org/ama1/pub/upload/mm/369/ceja_3i94.pdf

Angus, D. C., Barnato, A. E., Linde-Zwirble, W. T., et al. (2004). Use of intensive care at the end of life in the United States: An epidemiologic study. *Critical Care Medicine, 32*, 638–643.

Angus, D. C., Kelley, M. A., Schmitz, R. J., White, A., & Popovich, J., Jr., for the Committee on Manpower for Pulmonary and Critical Care (2000). Caring for the critically ill patient. Current and projected workforce requirements for care of the critically ill and patients with pulmonary disease: Can we meet the requirements of an aging population? *Journal of the American Medical Association, 284*, 2762–2770.

Angus, D. C., Shorr, A. F., White, A., et al. (2007). Critical care delivery in the United States: Distribution of services and compliance with Leapfrog recommendations. *Critical Care Medicine, 34*, 1016–1024.

Barnato, A. E., Kahn, J. M., Rubenfeld, G. D., et al. (2007). Prioritizing the organization and management of intensive care services in the United States: The PrOMIS Conference. *Critical Care Medicine, 35*, 1003–1011.

Bernat, J. L., D'Alessandro, A. M., Port, F. K., et al. (2006). Report of a National Conference on Donation after cardiac death. *American Journal of Transplantation, 6*, 281–291.

Campbell, D. (2007, November 13). *Successful transplantation of pediatric DCD hearts.* Paper presented at Organ and Tissue Donation Conference, Philadelphia, PA.

Caplan, A., & DeVita, M. A. (2007, March 16). Law must do right by dying patients, not their organs. *San Jose Mercury News,* 16A. Retrieved March 16, 2007, from http://www.washingtonspeakers.com/prod_images/pdfs/CaplanArt.LawforDyingPatientsNotOrgans.03.16.07.pdf

Charo, A. R. (1999). Dusk, dawn, and defining death. In S. J. Youngner, R. M. Arnold, & R. Schapiro (Eds.), *The definition of death: Contemporary controversies* (pp. 277–292). Baltimore, MD: Johns Hopkins University Press.

Committee on Increasing Rates of Organ Donation. (2006). *Organ donation: Opportunities for action.* Washington, DC: National Academy Press.

Curtis, J. R., & Rubenfeld, G. D. (2005). Improving palliative care for patients in the intensive care unit. *Journal of Palliative Medicine, 8*, 840–854.

D'Alessandro, A. M., Fernandez, L. A., Chin, L. T., et al. (2004). Donation after cardiac death: The University of Wisconsin experience. *Annals of Transplantation, 9*, 68–71.

D'Alessandro, A. M, Hoffmann, R. M., Knechtle, S. J., et al. (2000). Liver transplantation from controlled non-heart-beating donors. *Surgery, 128*, 579–588.

DuBois, J. M., & DeVita, M. (2006). Donation after cardiac death in the United States: How to move forward. *Critical Care Medicine, 34*, 3045–3047.

Fost, N. (2004). Reconsidering the dead donor rule: Is it important that organ donors be dead? *Kennedy Institute of Ethics Journal, 14*, 249–260.

Gomez, M., Garcia-Buitron J. M., Fernandez-Garcia A., et al. (1997). Liver transplantation with organs from non-heart-beating donors. *Transplantation Proceedings, 29*, 3478–3479.

719

*Ethical
Dilemmas in the
Management
of the Potential
Organ Donor
After Circulatory
Determination
of Death*

Guadagnoli, E., Christiansen, C. L., & Beasley, C. L. (2003). Potential organ-donor supply and efficiency of organ procurement organizations. *Health Care Financing Review, 24,* 101–110.

Institute of Medicine. (1997). *Non-heart-beating organ transplantation: Medical and ethical issues in procurement.* Washington, DC: National Academy Press.

Keenan, S. P., Hoffmaster, B., Eberhard, J., Chen, L. M., & Sibbald, W. J. (2002). Attitudes regarding organ donation from non-heart-beating donors. *Journal of Critical Care, 17,* 29–38.

Lewis, J., Peltier, J., Nelson, H., et al. (2003). Development of the University of Wisconsin donation after cardiac death evaluation tool. *Progress in Transplantation, 13,* 265–273.

Love, R. (2007, November 13). *DCD lungs.* Paper presented at Organ and Tissue Donation Conference, Philadelphia, PA.

Mandell, M. S., Zamudio, S., Seem, D., et al. (2006). National evaluation of healthcare provider attitudes toward organ donation after cardiac death. *Critical Care Medicine, 34,* 2952–2958.

Mendeloff, J., Ko, K., Roberts, M. S., Byrne, M., Dew, M. A. (2004). Procuring organ donors as a health investment: How much should we be willing to spend? *Transplantation, 78,* 1704–1710.

Menikoff, J. (1998). Doubts about death: The silence of the Institute of Medicine. *Journal of Law, Medicine & Ethics, 26,* 157–165.

National Conference of Commissioners on Uniform State Laws. (2006). *Revised Uniform Anatomical Gift Act.* Chicago: Author.

Nelson, J. E. (1999). Saving lives and saving deaths. *Annals of Internal Medicine, 130,* 776–777.

Oto, T., Levvey, B., McEgan, R., et al. (2007). A practical approach to clinical lung transplantation from a Maastricht Category III donor with cardiac death. *Journal of Heart & Lung Transplantation, 26,* 196–199.

Pearson, I. Y., & Zurynski, Y. (1995). A survey of personal and professional attitudes of intensivists to organ donation and transplantation. *Anaesthesia and Intensive Care, 23,* 68–74.

Prottas, J., & Batten, H. L. (1988). Health professionals and hospital administrators in organ procurement: Attitudes, reservations, and their resolutions. *American Journal of Public Health, 78,* 642–645.

Rady, M. Y., Verheijde, J. L., & McGregor, J. (2006). Organ donation after circulatory death: The forgotten donor? *Critical Care, 10,* 166.

Reich, D. J., Manzarbeitia, C., Aguilar, B., Osband, A., Zaki, R., et al. (2007, November 13). *A successful decade of controlled donation after cardiac death donor (DCD) liver transplantation.* Paper presented at Organ and Tissue Donation Conference, Philadelphia, PA.

Robertson, J. A. (1999). The dead donor rule. *Hastings Center Report, 29,* 6–14.

Schnitzler, M. A., Lentine, K. L., & Burroughs, T. E. (2005). The cost effectiveness of deceased organ donation. *Transplantation, 80,* 1636–1637.

Schnitzler, M. A., Whiting, J. F., Brennan, D. C., et al. (2005). The life-years saved by a deceased organ donor. *American Journal of Transplantation, 5,* 2289–2296.

Sheehy, E., Conrad, S. L., Brigham, L. E., et al. (2003). Estimating the number of potential organ donors in the United States. *New England journal of Medicine, 349,* 667–674.

Shemie, S. D., Baker, A. J., Knoll, G., et al. (2006). National recommendations for donation after cardiocirculatory death in Canada: Donation after cardiocirculatory death in Canada. *Canadian Medical Association Journal, 175,* 10.

Siminoff, L. A., Arnold, R. M., & Caplan, A. L. (1995). Health-care professional attitudes toward donation—Effect on practice and procurement. *Journal of Trauma-Injury Infection and Critical Care, 39,* 553–559.

Siminoff, L. A., Burant, C., & Youngner, S. J. (2004). Death and organ procurement: Public beliefs and attitudes. *Kennedy Institute of Ethics Journal, 14,* 217–234.

Stein, R. (2007, September 13). New zeal in organ procurement raises fears. *Washington Post,* A1.

Thornton, J. D., Curtis, J. R., & Allen, M. D. (2006). Completion of advanced care directives is associated with willingness to donate. *Journal of the National Medical Association, 98,* 897–904.

Tojimbara, T., Fuchinoue, S., Iwadoh, K., et al. (2007). Improved outcomes of renal transplantation from cardiac death donors: A 30-year single center experience. *American Journal of Transplantation, 7,* 609–617.

United Network for Organ Sharing. (2006). *Annual report.* Retrieved January 10, 2008, from http://www.optn.org/AR2006/waitlist_outcomes.htm

Weber, M., Dindo, D., Demartines, N., Ambuhl, P. M., & Clavien, P. A. (2002). Kidney transplantation from donors without a heartbeat. *New England Journal of Medicine, 347,* 248–255.

Wijnen, R. M., Booster, M. H., Stubenitsky, B. M., de Boer, J., Heineman, E., & Kootstra, G. (1995). Outcome of transplantation of non-heart-beating donor kidneys. *Lancet, 345,* 1067–1070.

Youngner, S. J., & Arnold, R. M. (2001). Philosophical debates about the definition of death: Who cares? *Journal of Medicine and Philosophy, 26,* 527–537.

Youngner, S. J., Arnold, R. M., & DeVita, M. A. (1999). When is "dead"? *Hastings Center Report, 29,* 14–21.

62

Protecting Live Kidney and Liver Donors

PETER P. REESE, PETER L. ABT,
AND ROY D. BLOOM

LONG WAIT-TIMES FOR deceased donor organ transplantation and the high mortality of patients on the wait-list have increased interest in live donor transplantation (Davis & Delmonico, 2005; Delmonico et al., 2005). Compared to using organs from deceased donors, live donor transplantation creates the ability to avoid wait-listing, and for patients with end-stage renal disease, live donor transplantation offers superior clinical outcomes (Gaston & Wadstrom, 2005). However, live donor transplantation involves a unique ethical scenario in which the donor is subjected to harm in order to benefit another person. Transplant professionals who evaluate live donors must balance the ethical principle of nonmaleficence against that of donor autonomy (Beauchamp & Childress, 2001; Truog, 2005). An ethical challenge of live donor transplantation is ensuring adequate informed consent when the magnitude of short- and long-term risk to the live donor is unknown (Steiner, 2004). In this chapter, we focus in particular on clinical uncertainties and ethical safeguards for live kidney and liver donors.

Recognition of the dire health consequences for patients wait-listed for kidney and liver allografts has generated a sense of urgency about finding ways to increase the number of transplants (Gaston & Wadstrom,

2005; *Organ Donation,* 2006). As shown in Figure 62.1, the number of patients on the kidney transplant waiting list has grown much faster than the number of kidney transplants performed in the United States. For patients with end-stage renal disease (ESRD), wait-list time depends on blood type and geographic region, but the median wait-time for a kidney transplant in the United States is approximately 3 years and 3 months (*Program and Organ Specific Report,* 2008). As waiting times continue to escalate, many patients die while waiting for an organ (Baigent, Burbury, & Wheeler, 2000). Although ESRD patients have the option of chronic dialysis (blood cleansing or purification) while awaiting a kidney transplant, dialysis is physically and emotionally taxing and has an exceptionally high mortality rate (Baigent et al., 2000). Dialysis typically requires thrice-weekly sessions spent in a chair in a dialysis center for 4 hours per session. All patients have major fluid and nutritional restrictions, many are unable to maintain a job, and because of the required commitment to dialysis, most lack flexibility and control over their lives. The unadjusted mortality rate for dialysis approaches 20% per year (U.S. Renal Data System, 2005). Numerous studies have demonstrated that although most patients adjust to the rigors of chronic dialysis, quality of life suffers (Tengs & Wallace, 2000; Unruh & Hess, 2007).

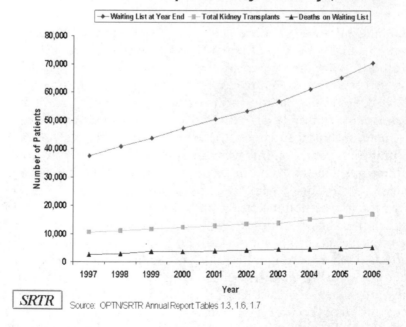

FIGURE 62.1   Widening gap between the number of patients wait-listed for a kidney transplant versus kidney transplants performed.

Average wait-list times for deceased donor liver allografts are also long, and the mortality rate is greatest for liver disease patients with the highest priority for organs. Priority for liver transplantation is determined by the Model for End-Stage Liver Disease (MELD) score, a formula calculated on the basis of labs that reflect the severity of patients' liver and kidney dysfunction (Austin et al., 2007). Patients with the peak scores are offered organs first, but these patients are also the most likely to die of complications of liver disease before an organ becomes available.

The wait-lists for both kidney and liver transplants have not decreased despite increasing willingness by transplant centers and patients to accept organs from deceased donors that are older and that have chronic diseases that may adversely affect the allograft quality and reduce patient and graft survival after transplantation (Keitel et al., 2004; Nickkholgh et al., 2007). As a result of the burgeoning wait-lists, many medical centers have invested efforts in facilitating live donor organ transplantation. Live donor transplantation, however, requires careful attention to ethical guidelines that protect the health and well-being of the donor.

THE SOCIAL CONTEXT OF TRANSPLANTATION: PRESSURE TO ACCEPT LIVE DONORS FROM TRANSPLANT CENTERS, DONORS, AND RECIPIENTS

A NUANCED EXAMINATION OF the decision to accept a live organ donor requires acknowledgment that diverse pressures may influence the judgment of the transplant-center staff. Commitment to shared ethical standards should enable transplant centers to identify these pressures and develop protocols that place the interests of donors first.

Organ transplantation is a high-visibility enterprise that can generate prestige and needed revenue for a transplant center. Despite the fact that the first successful kidney transplant took place over 50 years ago, stories about organ transplantation continue to attract public interest and garner media attention (Parker, 2004; Shelton, 2006). Hospitals often tout their organ transplant programs as evidence of technological sophistication and ability to deliver life-saving surgical procedures (Howard, 2007). Additionally, centers must maintain adequate surgical volume to justify expensive infrastructure and because volume is a quality benchmark by which centers are compared (Axelrod et al., 2004; Howard, 2007). In the United States, for instance, the annual number of transplants and other key clinical outcomes (such as patient survival) are published for each center on a publicly available Web site (the Organ Procurement and Transplantation Network). There is also some evidence in the area of liver transplantation that transplant volume is correlated with both superior patient and graft outcomes. Therefore, transplant staff may feel pressure to accept live donors in order to maintain volume in the center.

Potential recipients, referring physicians, or live donors themselves may also encourage physicians to accept the donor. As noted earlier, for recipients and their families, live organ transplantation may be life-saving and enables avoidance of the wait-list (Davis & Delmonico, 2005). Referring physicians may advocate for recipients but may not have an accurate view of the risk of donation, the donor's health status or medical history, or willingness to donate. Lastly, potential donors often feel a strong obligation to donate. This sense of obligation may stem from profound relationships, such as in the case of a parent donating to a child (Lennerling, Forsberg, Meyer, & Nyberg, 2004). Some studies suggest that the decision to donate does not rely primarily on accurate assessment of risks but rather on a sense of duty (Boulware et al., 2005; Lennerling et al., 2004). These potential donors may feel that the decision to undergo surgery should belong to them.

ETHICAL FRAMEWORK FOR EVALUATION AND ACCEPTANCE OF A LIVE ORGAN DONOR

THE USE OF live organ donors requires transplant centers to weigh ethical principles of nonmaleficence toward the donor and the autonomy of the motivated donor (Beauchamp & Childress, 2001). Medicine poses no other scenario in which a patient volunteers for an invasive procedure with substantial risks, including death or disability, in order to improve the health of another individual. The tension between nonmaleficence and autonomy is usually resolved through the processes of informed consent as well as the medical judgment of the transplant staff regarding the magnitude of risk to the donor (Abecassis et al., 2000). These ethical principles are shown in Table 62.1.

When live organ donation takes place, transplant staff act on the principle of beneficence toward the recipient but defy the standard of nonmaleficence toward the donor. In order to minimize risks, donors undergo a multidisciplinary evaluation to identify those who are healthy enough to endure the procedure (Davis, 2004; Mandelbrot et al., 2007). This testing aims to reveal short-term health risks that might jeopardize immediate postoperative recovery (such as active cardiovascular disease), in addition to longer-term health risks to the remaining organ function (such as hypertension, which might harm

TABLE 62.1   Ethical Principles That Guide Live Donor Transplantation

1. Beneficence toward the recipient
2. Nonmaleficence toward the donor
3. Autonomy of the donor
4. Autonomy of the health care professional

residual kidney function after kidney donation). Notably, studies of live donors after donation have shown that most donors derive emotional satisfaction and indirect benefits from donation, for instance fulfillment from having relieved the suffering of a loved one (Johnson et al., 1999; Lennerling et al., 2004). Nonetheless, the focus of the donor's medical evaluation remains the appraisal of the donor's physical health and ability to make a sustainable recovery from the surgery.

When the medical risk to the potential donor is perceived to be unreasonably high, transplant staff should refuse to accept that patient as a donor; in this situation, the autonomy of the transplant professional may supersede the potential donor's autonomy. Even if a potential donor understands and is willing to accept the risks of donation, the conscience of each member of the transplant-center staff must ultimately prevail if a potential donor's risks are deemed unreasonable. Admittedly, assessment of the magnitude of acceptable clinical risk requires judgment that may be fallible (Steiner, 2004). But transplant professionals who expose patients to possible harm through donation must feel comfortable that the procedure is consistent with their ethical standards. When a donor dies or has a bad outcome, the event is devastating to all involved: the transplant staff, the donor's loved ones, and the recipient.

Another important reason why transplant staff should refuse a potential live donor whose risks are unreasonably high is that a donor with a bad health outcome can jeopardize the public trust in transplantation generally. Stories of vulnerable live donors who sustain serious or enduring health problems as a result of the donation procedure not uncommonly find their way into the media. The vital enterprise of organ donation relies on public trust in the sound ethical foundation of transplantation; organ donation (from deceased or live donors) is considered a gift (Zink, Weinreib, Sparling, & Caplan, 2005). Without public trust, organ donation might decrease—with devastating consequences for recipients (Spital, 2004).

Informed consent also protects live donors, and recent policy proposals by the United Network of Organ Sharing (UNOS) are intended to reinforce the integrity of the consent process (UNOS, 2007). Donors undergo psychosocial evaluation, typically by a social worker or psychiatrist, to formally attest to the donor's capacity and to confirm that the donor does not face coercion from the recipient or others. Additionally, UNOS and other transplant organizations have emphasized the need for donors to be assigned a physician who represents only their interests and does not work with the recipient (UNOS, 2007). Some authors have also argued for instituting a donor advocate into the donor evaluation process. A donor advocate is a medical professional with knowledge of transplantation who ideally does not work directly for the transplant center and who would independently attest that the donor is not coerced (UNOS, 2007). Thus, the informed consent process for potential live donors involves iterative encounters with numerous members of the medical staff over a period of weeks to months; the donor can decline at any step in the process. Some centers also offer to protect a reluctant donor by reporting to the recipient or the family that the donor had an unspecified medical contraindication, even if no such contraindication existed. Such willingness by transplant staff to misrepresent a medical assessment demonstrates the extent to which transplant staff are committed to protecting reluctant donors from social harm.

MEDICALLY COMPLEX DONORS

Medically Complex Kidney Donors

ALTHOUGH MOST LIVE donors are unlikely to develop ESRD, transplant professionals have raised particular concern about acceptance of live donors with risk factors for future kidney disease such as hypertension. We refer to this group as "medically complex donors" (Reese, Caplan, Kesselheim, & Bloom, 2006). The dearth of data about long-term outcomes for medically complex donors threatens the integrity of informed consent.

Numerous studies have demonstrated that live kidney donation is safe, with a risk of death during surgery <0.1% and a risk of ESRD of <1% (Ellison, McBride, Taranto, Delmonico, & Kauffman, 2002; Fehrman-Ekholm, Duner, Brink, Tyden, & Elinder, 2001; Fehrman-Ekholm, Elinder, Stenbeck, Tyden, & Groth, 1997; Gaston & Wadstrom, 2005; Gossmann et al., 2005; Narkun-Burgess et al., 1993), but long-term studies of the subset of complex live kidney donors have not been performed. Our group has proposed criteria for medical complexity at the time of donor nephrectomy, including hypertension, obesity, and evidence of renal dysfunction (Reese et al., 2006). Hypertension is a well-established risk factor for chronic kidney disease (CKD) and ESRD (Chobanian et al., 2003). Obesity has been shown to increase

TABLE 62.2 Examples of Risk Factors for Future Kidney Disease in
Live Kidney Donors That May Threaten the Integrity of
Informed Consent

1. Hypertension
2. Obesity
3. Reduced baseline kidney function (low glomerular filtration rate)

risk for diabetes, glomerular disease, CKD, and ESRD (Chertow, Hsu, &
Johansen, 2006). The prevalence of obesity and related comorbidities
is rising rapidly in Western nations, raising the troubling possibility
that donors will become obese later in life (World Health Organization,
2007). Evidence of kidney dysfunction at the time of nephrectomy includes low glomerular filtration rate (GFR), hematuria, or proteinuria
(Davis & Delmonico, 2005). Although controversy exists regarding acceptance of donors with hypertension, obesity, or low estimated GFR,
a recent preliminary analysis of registry data from UNOS suggests that
a quarter of live kidney donors have one or more of these potential
risk factors for kidney disease later in life (Reese, McBride, Andersen, &
Bloom, 2007). Table 62.2 lists risk factors for chronic kidney disease
that are commonly found in potential live kidney donors.

The processes of informed consent help transplant staff to resolve
the tension between nonmaleficence and donor autonomy, but in the
case of medically complex donors, sparse data about long-term risk
makes adequate informed consent challenging (Reese et al., 2006). For
these donors, in addition to the steps outlined earlier, the informed
consent process should include disclosure of these clinical uncertainties about risk. Postnephrectomy, we believe that these donors should
also commit to periodic assessment of their kidney function and risk
factors for kidney disease. Risk factors such as hypertension should
be assiduously treated (Gaston & Wadstrom, 2005). Additionally, transplant professionals should advocate for funding of high-quality studies
of long-term outcomes for live donors, particularly medically complex
donors (Delmonico, 2005).

MEDICALLY COMPLEX LIVER DONORS

LESS CLINICAL EXPERIENCE exists with adult-to-adult living donor
liver transplantation (AALDLT) than with live donor kidney transplantation, and the procedures differ in that perioperative risks to donor
health are substantially higher with AALDLT. Uncertainty exists about
acceptance of older donors and donors with evidence of liver steatosis. For these donors, informed consent should include admission that
long-term risks are unknown.

AALDLT has been performed in the United States since the late 1990s, for which reason limited data are available regarding long-term donor health outcomes. AALDLT involves resection of the right liver lobe, is a more protracted procedure than kidney donation, and involves challenging vascular and biliary reconstruction. This procedure has a mortality rate of 0.3%–0.5%, an overall complication rate of 29.1%, and a rate of major complications, such as infection, of 3% (Middleton et al., 2006; Patel et al., 2007; Pomfret, 2003). A nationwide survey of outcomes from liver transplant centers reported that 9% of donors required readmission after surgery (Brown et al., 2003). Recovery to full activity including employment takes months for most donors. Small studies of quality of life outcomes for liver donors suggest that a substantial minority experience worse pain and longer recovery than they had anticipated, although the majority report that they did not regret the decision to donate (Chan et al., 2006; Erim et al., 2006; Trotter et al., 2001).

Concerns have been raised by transplant professionals about the safety of accepting older liver donors and those with evidence of liver steatosis (fat infiltration of the liver). Some transplant centers set an upper age limit on live donors of 50 or 55 years old because of concerns about donor ability to survive surgery as well as the ability of the donor liver to regenerate. An analysis of administrative data from New York State and academic medical centers showed that donor age over 50 conferred a substantially higher risk of major complications (Patel et al., 2007). A Japanese study of live donors over 60 showed longer hospital stays compared to younger donors but no difference in short-term health outcomes for these older donors (Kuramitsu et al., 2007). Additionally, analyses of the initial national experience with AALDLT suggest that survival for these recipients is shorter compared to survival after deceased donor liver transplantation (Abt et al., 2004). Therefore, some authors have argued that AALDLT is best suited to recipients who are deemed unlikely to receive an offer for a deceased donor liver in a short time frame (Thuluvath & Yoo, 2004).

Donor liver steatosis has also been identified as a potential risk factor for poor recovery from liver donation (Fan et al., 2000). In studies of nonliver donors, steatohepatitis is associated with obesity, diabetes, hyperlipidemia, and metabolic syndrome. A small proportion of patients with steatohepatitis will develop fibrosis and liver cirrhosis, usually over the course of years (Adams et al., 2005). A small retrospective study of liver donors suggested that liver steatosis was associated with postoperative liver dysfunction (Fan et al., 2000).

The processes of informed consent for live liver donors should highlight that data about long-term outcomes for donors are limited. For older donors and those with liver steatosis, in particular, the possibility of increased risk to donor health should be emphasized. Additionally, the decreased survival for recipients with AALDLT is another factor that potential donors may consider when making a decision to donate.

FINANCIAL INCENTIVES FOR LIVE ORGAN DONATION

STRONG INTEREST IN increasing the volume of live organ donation has led a number of prominent transplant professionals to advocate payment of live donors, although payment remains illegal in the United States. Financial reward for organ donation could relieve the well-documented financial burden that many donors face but could also amplify the likelihood that poor patients would volunteer to donate despite fear of harm.

Organ donation carries financial as well as physical risk. Despite the fact that most donor testing and procedures are covered by recipient health insurance in the United States, donors are often subject to expenses including copayment for procedures, transportation, and unpaid leave from work. A study of living liver donors, for instance, estimated that the average out-of-pocket cost to these donors was $3,600 (Middleton et al., 2006). In order to relieve this burden, some leaders in transplantation have proposed modest monetary payments to donors (Gaston et al., 2006). Other authors, such as Friedman and Friedman (2006) or Matas (2006), have proposed a regulated market of organ sales by live donors. Friedman and Friedman (2006), for example, suggested payment of $40,000 for a live kidney donation. These advocates for payment point to donor autonomy as a suitable ethical rationale to allow sales to proceed. Matas (2006) argues that oversight and regulation by the federal government could effectively prevent acceptance of donors currently considered unacceptable risks.

The ethical objections to payment for live organ donation are based on concerns that human dignity and autonomy are threatened when a part of the body is sold. The threat to human dignity posed by commodification of a person's body has roots in the Christian, Judaic, and Muslim faith; organ sales would likely face strong objections from religious leaders (Stempsey, 2000). Those who object to organ sales also cite reports of illegal organ trafficking, in which impoverished organ donors are recruited from developing countries, paid small sums, and provided with minimal follow-up care (Shepard-Hughes, 2003). The main ethical concern, therefore, is that the judgment of poor patients would be compromised by large monetary rewards, with no safeguards to their future health (Harmon & Delmonico, 2006). This compromised judgment could lead to donor harm, as noted earlier, but also to recipient harm if a donor withheld information about health history or behaviors (such as intravenous drug use) that could lead to transmission of infection or other complications.

Currently, payment for live organ donation remains illegal in the United States and most Western countries and is also opposed by prominent transplantation professional organizations (Harmon & Delmonico, 2006). Advocates for a regulated market for live donor organs have not surmounted strong ethical objections that donor autonomy could be compromised and the health of vulnerable patients exploited.

CONCLUSION

THE DEVASTATING MEDICAL consequences of ESRD and advanced liver disease have caused transplant professionals to focus efforts on maximizing live donor organ transplantation. Live organ donation requires transplant staff to resolve the tension between key ethical principles of donor autonomy and nonmaleficence. Appropriate evaluation of a live donor must involve detailed clinical evaluation that demonstrates minimal risk to the donor and iterative psychosocial assessment that shows that a donor is not coerced. Given sparse data about outcomes for medically complex live donors, the processes of informed consent should include frank admission by transplant staff when accurate assessment of risk is not possible. Additionally, debates about proposed innovations in transplantation, such as payment for live donation, should give considerable voice to patients and other interested members of the public. The continued success of organ transplantation depends on the public's faith that transplant professionals will adhere to transparent ethical standards that place donor interests first.

REFERENCES

Abecassis, M., Adams, M., Adams, P., Arnold, R. M., Atkins, C. R., Barr, M. L., et al. (2000). Consensus statement on the live organ donor. *Journal of the American Medical Association, 284*(22), 2919–2926.

Abt, P. L., Mange, K. C., Olthoff, K. M., Markmann, J. F., Reddy, K. R., & Shaked, A. (2004). Allograft survival following adult-to-adult living donor liver transplantation. *American Journal of Transplantation, 4*(8), 1302–1307.

Adams, L. A., Lymp, J. F., St. Sauver, J., Sanderson, S. O., Lindor, K. D., Feldstein, A., et al. (2005). The natural history of nonalcoholic fatty liver disease: A population-based cohort study. *Gastroenterology, 129*(1), 113–121.

Austin, M. T., Poulose, B. K., Ray, W. A., Arbogast, P. G., Feurer, I. D., & Pinson, C. W. (2007). Model for end-stage liver disease: Did the new liver allocation policy affect waiting list mortality? *Archives of Surgery, 142*(11), 1079–1085.

Axelrod, D. A., Guidinger, M. K., McCullough, K. P., Leichtman, A. B., Punch, J. D., & Merion, R. M. (2004). Association of center volume with outcome after liver and kidney transplantation. *American Journal of Transplantation, 4*(6), 920–927.

Baigent, C., Burbury, K., & Wheeler, D. (2000). Premature cardiovascular disease in chronic renal failure. *Lancet, 356*(9224), 147–152.

Beauchamp, T. L., & Childress, J. F. (2001). *Principles of biomedical ethics* (5th ed.). New York: Oxford University Press.

Boulware, L. E., Meoni, L. A., Fink, N. E., Parekh, R. S., Kao, W. H., Klag, M. J., et al. (2005). Preferences, knowledge, communication and patient-physician discussion of living kidney transplantation in African American families. *American Journal of Transplantation, 5*(6), 1503–1512.

Brown, R. S., Jr., Russo, M. W., Lai, M., Shiffman, M. L., Richardson, M. C., Everhart, J. E., et al. (2003). A survey of liver transplantation from living adult donors in the United States. *New England Journal of Medicine, 348*(9), 818–825.

Chan, S. C., Liu, C. L., Lo, C. M., Lam, B. K., Lee, E. W., & Fan, S. T. (2006). Donor quality of life before and after adult-to-adult right liver live donor transplantation. *Liver Transplantation, 12*(10), 1529–1536.

Chertow, G. M., Hsu, C. Y., & Johansen, K. L. (2006). The enlarging body of evidence: Obesity and chronic kidney disease. *Journal of the American Society of Nephrology, 17*(6), 1501–1502.

Chobanian, A. V., Bakris, G. L., Black, H. R., Cushman, W. C., Green, L. A., Izzo, J. L., Jr., et al. (2003). The seventh report of the Joint National Committee on Prevention, Detection, Evaluation, and Treatment of High Blood Pressure: The JNC 7 report. *Journal of the American Medical Association, 289*(19), 2560–2572.

Davis, C. L. (2004). Evaluation of the living kidney donor: Current perspectives. *American Journal of Kidney Diseases, 43*(3), 508–530.

Davis, C. L., & Delmonico, F. L. (2005). Living-donor kidney transplantation: A review of the current practices for the live donor. *Journal of the American Society of Nephrology, 16*(7), 2098–2110.

Delmonico, F. (2005). A report of the Amsterdam forum on the care of the live kidney donor: Data and medical guidelines. *Transplantation, 79*(6 Suppl.), S53–S66.

Delmonico, F. L., Sheehy, E., Marks, W. H., Baliga, P., McGowan, J. J., & Magee, J. C. (2005). Organ donation and utilization in the United States, 2004. *American Journal of Transplantation, 5*(4 Pt. 2), 862–873.

Ellison, M. D., McBride, M. A., Taranto, S. E., Delmonico, F. L., & Kauffman, H. M. (2002). Living kidney donors in need of kidney transplants: A report from the organ procurement and transplantation network. *Transplantation, 74*(9), 1349–1351.

Erim, Y., Beckmann, M., Valentin-Gamazo, C., Malago, M., Frilling, A., Schlaak, J. F., et al. (2006). Quality of life and psychiatric complications after adult living donor liver transplantation. *Liver Transplantation, 12*(12), 1782–1790.

Fan, S. T., Lo, C. M., Liu, C. L., Yong, B. H., Chan, J. K., & Ng, I. O. (2000). Safety of donors in live donor liver transplantation using right lobe grafts. *Archives of Surgery, 135*(3), 336–340.

Fehrman-Ekholm, I., Duner, F., Brink, B., Tyden, G., & Elinder, C. G. (2001). No evidence of accelerated loss of kidney function in living kidney donors: Results from a cross-sectional follow-up. *Transplantation, 72*(3), 444–449.

Fehrman-Ekholm, I., Elinder, C. G., Stenbeck, M., Tyden, G., & Groth, C. G. (1997). Kidney donors live longer. *Transplantation, 64*(7), 976–978.

Friedman, E. A., & Friedman, A. L. (2006). Payment for donor kidneys: Pros and cons. *Kidney International, 69*(6), 960–962.

Gaston, R. S., Danovitch, G. M., Epstein, R. A., Kahn, J. P., Matas, A. J., & Schnitzler, M. A. (2006). Limiting financial disincentives in live organ donation: A rational solution to the kidney shortage. *American Journal of Transplantation, 6*(11), 2548–2555.

Gaston, R. S., & Wadstrom, J. (2005). *Living donor kidney transplantation*. Oxford, UK: Taylor and Francis.

Gossmann, J., Wilhelm, A., Kachel, H. G., Jordan, J., Sann, U., Geiger, H., et al. (2005). Long-term consequences of live kidney donation follow-up in 93% of living kidney donors in a single transplant center. *American Journal of Transplantation, 5*(10), 2417–2424.

Harmon, W., & Delmonico, F. (2006). Payment for kidneys: A government-regulated system is not ethically achievable. *Clinical Journal of the American Society of Nephrology, 1*(6), 1146–1147.

Howard, R. J. (2007). The challenging triangle: Balancing outcomes, transplant numbers and costs. *American Journal of Transplantation, 7*(11), 2443–2445.

Johnson, E. M., Anderson, J. K., Jacobs, C., Suh, G., Humar, A., Suhr, B. D., et al. (1999). Long-term follow-up of living kidney donors: Quality of life after donation. *Transplantation, 67*(5), 717–721.

Keitel, E., Michelon, T., dos Santos, A. F., Bittar, A. E., Goldani, J. C., D'Almeida Bianco, P., et al. (2004). Renal transplants using expanded cadaver donor criteria. *Annals of Transplantation, 9*(2), 23–24.

Kuramitsu, K., Egawa, H., Keeffe, E. B., Kasahara, M., Ito, T., Sakamoto, S., et al. (2007). Impact of age older than 60 years in living donor liver transplantation. *Transplantation, 84*(2), 166–172.

Lennerling, A., Forsberg, A., Meyer, K., & Nyberg, G. (2004). Motives for becoming a living kidney donor. *Nephrology Dialysis Transplantation, 19*(6), 1600–1605.

Mandelbrot, D. A., Pavlakis, M., Danovitch, G. M., Johnson, S. R., Karp, S. J., Khwaja, K., et al. (2007). The medical evaluation of living kidney donors: A survey of US transplant centers. *American Journal of Transplantation, 7*(10), 2333–2343.

Matas, A. J. (2006). Why we should develop a regulated system of kidney sales: A call for action! *Clinical Journal of the American Society of Nephrology, 1*(6), 1129–1132.

Middleton, P. F., Duffield, M., Lynch, S. V., Padbury, R. T., House, T., Stanton, P., et al. (2006). Living donor liver transplantation—adult donor outcomes: A systematic review. *Liver Transplantation, 12*(1), 24–30.

Narkun-Burgess, D. M., Nolan, C. R., Norman, J. E., Page, W. F., Miller, P. L., & Meyer, T. W. (1993). Forty-five-year follow-up after uninephrectomy. *Kidney International, 43*(5), 1110–1115.

Nickkholgh, A., Weitz, J., Encke, J., Sauer, P., Mehrabi, A., Buchler, M. W., et al. (2007). Utilization of extended donor criteria in liver transplantation: A comprehensive review of the literature. *Nephrology Dialysis Transplantation, 22*(Suppl. 8), viii29–viii36.

Organ donation: Opportunities for action. (2006). Washington, DC: Institute of Medicine, National Academy Press.

Parker, I. (2004, August 2). The gift: Zell Kravinsky gave away millions, but somehow it wasn't enough. *The New Yorker,* 54–63.

Patel, S., Orloff, M., Tsoulfas, G., Kashyap, R., Jain, A., Bozorgzadeh, A., et al. (2007). Living-donor liver transplantation in the United States: Identifying donors at risk for perioperative complications. *American Journal of Transplantation, 7*(10), 2344–2349.

Pomfret, E. A. (2003). Early and late complications in the right-lobe adult living donor. *Liver Transplantation, 9*(10 Suppl. 2), S45–S49.

Program and organ specific report: Time to transplant. (2008). Retrieved February 25, 2008, from http://www.ustransplant.org/csr/current/publicData.aspx?facilityID=PADVOP1XX&t=07&r=pennsylvania

Reese, P., Caplan, A., Kesselheim, A., & Bloom, R. (2006). Creating a medical, ethical and legal framework for complex living kidney donors. *Clinical Journal of the American Society of Nephrology, 1*(6), 1148–1153.

Reese, P., McBride, M. A., Andersen, K., & Bloom, R. D. (2007, May). *Substantial variation in acceptance of complex living kidney donors across renal transplant centers in the USA.* Paper presented at the American Transplant Congress, San Francisco, CA.

Shelton, D. (2006, June 2). Would you give your kidney to a stranger? CNN.com. Retrieved September 1, 2006, from http://www.cnn.com/2006/HEALTH/06/01/living.donors/index.html

Shepard-Hughes, N. (2003). Rotten trade: Millennial capitalism, human values, and global justice in organ trafficking. *Journal of Human Rights, 2*(2), 197–226.

Spital, A. (2004). Rejecting heroic kidney donors protects more than the public's trust. *American Journal of Transplantation, 4,* 1727.

Steiner, R. W. (2004). Risk appreciation for living kidney donors: Another new subspecialty? *American Journal of Transplantation, 4*(5), 694–697.

Stempsey, W. E. (2000). Organ markets and human dignity: On selling your body and soul. *Christian Bioethics, 6*(2), 195–204.

Tengs, T. O., & Wallace, A. (2000). One thousand health-related quality-of-life estimates. *Medical Care, 38*(6), 583–637.

Thuluvath, P. J., & Yoo, H. Y. (2004). Graft and patient survival after adult live donor liver transplantation compared to a matched cohort who received a deceased donor transplantation. *Liver Transplantation, 10*(10), 1263–1268.

Trotter, J. F., Talamantes, M., McClure, M., Wachs, M., Bak, T., Trouillot, T., et al. (2001). Right hepatic lobe donation for living donor liver transplantation: Impact on donor quality of life. *Liver Transplantation, 7*(6), 485–493.

Truog, R. D. (2005). The ethics of organ donation by living donors. *New England Journal of Medicine, 353*(5), 444–446.

United Network of Organ Sharing (UNOS). (2007). *Guidelines for the medical evaluation of living kidney donors (Living Donor Committee).* Retrieved July 25, 2007, from http://www.unos.org/PublicComment/pubcomment PropSub_208.pdf

Unruh, M. L., & Hess, R. (2007). Assessment of health-related quality of life among patients with chronic kidney disease. *Advances in Chronic Kidney Disease, 14*(4), 345–352.

U.S. Renal Data System. (2005). Reference table: Patient survival. *Annual Data Report: Atlas of End-Stage Renal Disease in the United States.* Retrieved November 12, 2008, from http://www.usrds.org/adr_2005.htm

World Health Organization. (2007). *Obesity.* Retrieved September 29, 2007, from http://www.who.int/topics/obesity/en/

Zink, S., Weinreib, R., Sparling, T., & Caplan, A. L. (2005). Living donation: Focus on public concerns. *Clinical Transplantation, 19*(5), 581–585.

63

Organ Transplantation and Retransplantation: Medical and Ethical Considerations

RALUCA VRABIE, VARDIT RAVITSKY,
AND THOMAS W. FAUST

TRANSPLANTATION IS A medically and ethically acceptable treatment for patients with organ failure that does not respond to less-aggressive therapies. For most transplants, 1- and 5-year patient and graft survival is excellent because of advances in surgery, immunosuppression, and organ preservation. Moreover, the quality of life is improved for most patients who undergo transplantation. Unfortunately, the success of organ transplants has increased demand for organs and waiting times in the setting of a relatively static deceased donor organ supply. Retransplantation is a viable option for patients who suffer from life-threatening graft failure. Even though retransplantation can be medically justified, its outcomes are generally inferior to those of primary transplants. Ethical issues around the allocation of these scarce resources arise because an organ used for retransplantation cannot be used for potential recipients waiting for their first graft.

This chapter will address medical and ethical issues pertaining to transplantation and retransplantation of patients with life-threatening organ failure. First, pertinent medical issues pertaining to transplantation and retransplantation of patients with hepatic, renal, cardiac, and pulmonary diseases will be discussed. Second, the ethical arguments pertaining to the allocation of scarce organs for transplantation and retransplantation will be considered.

MEDICAL OVERVIEW OF TRANSPLANTATION AND RETRANSPLANTATION

LIVER TRANSPLANTATION

ORTHOTOPIC LIVER TRANSPLANTATION (OLT) is a widely accepted treatment for patients with life-threatening acute and chronic liver diseases refractory to less-aggressive medical and surgical therapies. Indications for OLT include decompensated cirrhosis, primary hepatic malignancies, and acute liver failure (Keeffe, 2001). Hepatitis C virus (HCV) and alcoholic liver disease are the most common indications for liver replacement in patients with cirrhosis. With the rise in obesity in the United States, cryptogenic cirrhosis ranks third as an indication for OLT. Hepatitis B (HBV) is another appropriate indication for transplantation worldwide. Other less common but equally important indications for liver replacement include autoimmune liver diseases, metabolic liver diseases, and, rarely, patients with the Budd-Chiari syndrome who present with either acute or chronic liver failure from hepatic outflow obstruction.

Additionally, drug- or toxin-induced liver injury is a commonly accepted indication for transplantation. Acetaminophen overdose is the most common cause of drug-induced hepatic failure necessitating OLT in the United States. Finally, patients with hepatocellular carcinoma (HCC) may be appropriate candidates for transplantation. In carefully selected patients with HCC who undergo OLT, patient survival is comparable to that of patients who are transplanted for nonmalignant indications.

The United Network for Organ Sharing (UNOS) administers the Organ Procurement and Transplantation Network (OPTN) and is responsible for allocation policy and compliance with regulations regardless of the type of organ transplanted. A new system of allocation for patients with chronic liver disease or HCC was instituted in 2002: the model for end-stage liver disease (MELD) scoring system (Kamath et al., 2001). Patients with fulminant hepatic failure are listed as status 1 and are not part of the MELD system. Patients with higher MELD scores have a higher risk of dying while on the list. Therefore, UNOS endorses allocation to patients with higher MELD scores, an urgency-based metric. Even though the so-called sickest first policy is in effect, transplant programs need to also consider outcomes when making allocation decisions (Gilbert et al., 1999; Showstack et al., 1999). Since the institution of MELD, there has been a 12% reduction in new listings, a 3.5% reduction in waiting-list deaths, and a 10.2% increase in deceased donor transplants (Freeman et al., 2004). Moreover, there has been no difference in early posttransplant survival in the pre- and post-MELD eras (Freeman et al., 2004). Patient and graft survival is generally good for patients who receive primary liver transplants (Organ Procurement and Transplantation Network [OPTN], 2007).

Retransplantation accounts for 8%–10% of all liver transplants in the United States per year (OPTN, 2007). Depending on the transplant center, rates may vary between 8% and 23% (De Carlis et al., 2001; Wong, Devlin, Rolando, Heaton, & Williams, 1997). HCV accounts for the largest proportion of recurrent diseases necessitating consideration for retransplantation. Retransplant candidates tend to be sicker than primary transplant candidates. Hence, hospital stays are longer, charges are higher, and outcomes are generally inferior following retransplantation (Azoulay et al., 2002; OPTN, 2007). Indications for retransplantation, type of graft, and medical urgency are important predictors of posttransplant outcome. The use of extended donors (non-heart-beating donors, older donors, and donors with fatty livers) is associated with a higher rate of graft loss. Notwithstanding, in carefully selected, low-risk retransplant candidates, outcomes may be comparable to primary transplantation (Biggins, Beldecos, Rabkin, & Rosen, 2002; Ghobrial et al., 1999). Timing of retransplantation is an important determinant of patient and graft survival following retransplantation. Patients retransplanted within the first week and after 30 days did better than those retransplanted between 8 and 30 days after primary transplantation (Markmann et al., 1997).

KIDNEY TRANSPLANTATION

KIDNEY TRANSPLANTATION IS a viable option for patients with renal failure. With restoration of renal function following transplantation, there is improvement in metabolic abnormalities, volume status, and anemia. In contrast to other organ transplants, kidney transplantation can be delayed because of dialysis. Nevertheless, patients who receive kidney transplants have better quality of life and longer survival when compared to patients on dialysis (Hariharan, 2000; Pascual, Theruvath,

Kawai, Tolkoff-Rubin, & Cosimi, 2002). Most programs recommend live donor transplantation whenever possible. As with liver transplantation, allocation of deceased donor organs is based on urgency and ABO blood typing; however, antigen matching and waiting time are also important.

Indications for kidney transplantation include irreversible renal failure and no evidence of active infection, malignancy, decompensated liver disease, or severe cardiovascular disorders. Suitable candidates for either a live or deceased donor kidney should be expected to live for at least 5 years following transplantation. Recreational drug use, psychosis, alcohol abuse, and a history of noncompliance should be excluding criteria during the evaluation.

The demand for cadaveric kidneys far exceeds supply. The current waiting time for deceased donor kidneys approaches 3–4 years for all blood type groups. Hence, living related or unrelated donors account for more than 50% of kidney transplants. Overall, outcomes for recipients of live donor grafts are better than those of recipients who receive deceased donor organs. The most common indications for renal retransplantation are acute and chronic rejection, graft thrombosis, and recurrent disease.

The 1-, 3-, and 5-year graft survival rates for repeat living donor transplants were significantly lower than for primary transplants using living donors. The same trend was observed for deceased donor transplants. Even though retransplantation was associated with inferior graft survival rates when compared to primary transplants, there was no difference in 1-, 3-, and 5-year patient survival for retransplants when compared to 1-, 3-, and 5-year patient survival for primary transplants (OPTN, 2007; Pour-Reza-Gholi et al., 2005).

HEART TRANSPLANTATION

HEART TRANSPLANTATION IS an appropriate treatment for patients with life-threatening irremediable heart disease with an estimated mortality of more than 25%–30% in 1 year without organ replacement. Potential heart recipients are usually 65 years old or younger. Indications for transplantation include ischemic heart disease, idiopathic dilated cardiomyopathy, valvular heart disease, uncontrollable ventricular arrhythmias, restrictive and hypertrophic cardiomyopathies, and congenital heart disease not amenable to surgical correction (Costanzo et al., 1995; Deng, 2002). As with other organ transplants, the benefit of transplantation must exceed the risk and patients must have adequate social support. Major contraindications to cardiac transplantation include significant psychological diseases, substance abuse, advanced physiological age, other systemic illnesses with a poor prognosis, irreversible pulmonary hypertension, acute pulmonary embolism, severe peripheral or cerebrovascular disease, and significant renal or hepatic diseases (Costanzo et al., 1995). Other contraindications include active peptic ulcer disease, diabetes with significant end organ disease, severe obesity or osteoporosis, HIV, HBV, cytomegalovirus, active bacterial or fungal infections, smoking, and malignancy (Costanzo et al., 1995).

Allocation of deceased donor hearts is based on location of the donor, ABO blood type, body size of recipient, size of the organ, and, occasionally, the need for specialized immunologic testing. As with liver and kidney transplants, priority is given to patients with more severe disease. Even though approximately 2,500 to 3,500 heart transplants are performed annually, 10%–30% of patients listed for transplantation die waiting for an organ.

Most retransplants were done for graft failure. By the end of 2005, 5.3% of potential recipients on the transplant waiting list were retransplant candidates. Cardiac retransplantation accounted for 4.7% of transplants. Furthermore, there has been a 66% increase in cardiac retransplant activity from 1996 to 2005 (Magee et al., 2007; OPTN, 2007). The 1-, 3-, and 5-year graft survival for retransplants were all significantly lower than for primary transplants. Moreover, the risk of death was significantly higher for retransplant recipients than for recipients of primary grafts (Shuhaiber et al., 2007). Patient survival following retransplantation is generally inferior to that of primary transplant recipients (OPTN, 2007). Prolonged ischemic time, older donor and recipient age, emergent retransplantation, and ventilator dependency were important predictors of a poor outcome following retransplantation.

LUNG TRANSPLANTATION

PATIENTS WHO HAVE severe pulmonary insufficiency refractory to standard medical therapy and limited life expectancy are candidates for lung transplantation. In general, patients benefit in terms of improved quality and quantity of life. Candidates should be in otherwise good health with the exception of the underlying pulmonary disease. In general, potential recipients for single lung transplants should be younger than 65, whereas those who are candidates for double lung grafts should be younger than 60. At the present time, approximately 16% of patients with severe pulmonary disease die on the list annually waiting for an organ. Transplant options include single lung, bilateral lung, heart lung, and living donor lobar grafts depending on the age of the potential candidate and the underlying disease. Major indications for transplantation include chronic obstructive pulmonary disease (COPD), idiopathic pulmonary fibrosis, alpha-1-antitrypsin deficiency, primary pulmonary hypertension, and cystic fibrosis (ASTP, ATS, ERS, & ISHLT, 1998; Steinman et al., 2001).

Combined heart-lung transplantation is a viable option for patients with advanced lung disease and cor pulmonale or end-stage lung disease with left ventricular dysfunction from ischemic heart disease. Transplantation is not appropriate for candidates with major nonpulmonary organ dysfunction, recent active malignancy, and infection with HIV, HBV, or HCV. Active substance abuse including cigarettes, noncompliance, and severe musculoskeletal disease affecting the thorax are also absolute contraindications. Relative contraindications include poor nutritional status, symptomatic osteoporosis, opportunistic infections, invasive ventilation, psychosocial disorders, diabetes, hypertension, severe obesity, and high-dose steroid use. Lung allocation is based on medical urgency, ABO blood type, and size of the organ and potential recipient.

The 1- and 5-year patient survival after lung transplantation varies between 65%–80% and 38%–52%, respectively. Survival is comparable for patients who received deceased donor and live donor grafts. At the end of 2005, 3.3% of candidates on the waiting list were those waiting for retransplantation (Magee et al., 2007). Additionally, retransplants represented 3.3% of transplants performed during the same time period (Magee et al., 2007). As with cardiac transplants, retransplantation for graft failure has increased significantly from 1996 to 2005 (Magee et al., 2007). The 1-, 3-, and 5-year graft survival for deceased donor retransplants was significantly worse than for primary transplants. The major indications for retransplantation include chronic graft failure from bronchiolitis obliterans, acute graft failure, and airway complications. Retransplantation may be considered for stable intermediate to long-term survivors with progressive loss of lung function secondary to bronchiolitis obliterans with acceptable 1- and 5-year patient survival; however, patient survival following retransplantation is generally worse than that of primary transplantation for patients with acute graft failure or airway complications and for those on ventilator support (Strueber et al., 2006).

ALLOCATION IN ORGAN TRANSPLANTATION AND RETRANSPLANTATION

THE NUMBER OF patients on the waiting list for livers, kidneys, hearts, and lungs far surpasses the number of deceased donor organs available each year. Hence, some form of allocation strategy is required to distribute organs, and decision-making should be based on sound ethical principles.

Allocation of scarce resources can be based on social, sociomedical, medical, and personal criteria (Kilner, 1990). Current UNOS allocation policy is based on medical criteria alone and takes into consideration urgency, not outcomes. In simple words, the right act according to UNOS would be to distribute organs to those in greatest need. However, we argue that the consideration of urgency should to be balanced against the consideration of best outcomes, because both urgency and outcomes are important when making medically and ethically acceptable allocation decisions. These considerations are relevant when decisions are made regarding allocation of an organ both to a first-time, naïve candidate and to a retransplant candidate.

SOCIAL STATUS

THE SOCIAL STATUS criterion means that preference is given to those considered most valuable to society. However, this criterion is impossible to implement. How would we define *value* and who is qualified to make such determinations? For example, should only major contributors to the community be given preference? Even though the social value criterion would appeal to some consequentialists, it would be impossible to rank patients with organ failure using this criterion. Additional knowledge about patients' lives would be required that is either difficult to obtain or overly intrusive. Moreover, applying this criterion would potentially discriminate against minorities, elderly patients, or the disabled.

SCIENTIFIC PROGRESS

ALLOCATION BASED ON scientific progress means that preference in transplantation and retransplantation would be given to those most likely to yield scientifically useful information. For transplantation to advance, basic and clinical research is required. This is applicable to primary and repeat transplants. As most transplant programs are found within academic institutions, all patients who are being evaluated for a transplant could be considered potential research subjects. But how do we determine which patient will be most useful in advancing scientific knowledge, and who should make this determination? Will patients feel obligated to participate in a research protocol against their better judgment? Will investigators find themselves in a conflict of interest at the patients' expense? Should a graft be given preferentially to a patient who has already received an organ rather than to a primary transplant candidate, in order to generate data on retransplantation? These questions make this utilitarian criterion impractical as well.

AGE

SOME ARGUE THAT when allocating scarce resources, the age of the patient should be considered because it is related to the likelihood, length, and quality of the potential benefit and because younger candidates have not had the opportunity to enjoy a full life span. Others, however, argue that people should be entitled to receive care that restores them to an adequate level of functioning regardless of their age. For transplantation and retransplantation, physiological age is more important than chronological age. Healthier, older patients with organ failure should not necessarily be denied a graft in favor of younger, sicker patients. Regardless of age, sicker patients may have worse outcomes when compared to those who are healthier. Consequently, rejecting a primary or retransplant candidate based on age alone would be discriminatory, if that individual has a reasonable chance of a good outcome when compared to a younger, sicker candidate.

PSYCHOLOGICAL APTITUDE

WHEN ALLOCATING SCARCE resources, the patient's psychological profile comes into play. Does the patient have the emotional and intellectual aptitude to understand different therapeutic options? Does the patient truly understand the complexities of transplantation and retransplantation? Will the patient understand and comply with the medical regimen? Most programs are hesitant to allocate organs to patients when their psychological aptitude is uncertain. However, the evaluation of psychological aptitude is sometimes subject to bias, and the determination of psychological fitness for transplantation and retransplantation can be extremely difficult. Transplant candidates should not be categorically denied a graft based on psychological ability alone. For those who lack decision-making capacity, treatment options must be discussed with their proxies. Transplant teams must work with patients or their proxies and mobilize necessary resources in order to improve outcomes.

SUPPORTIVE SURROUNDINGS

UNDER THE SUPPORTIVE surroundings criterion, priority is given to those who have stable social relationships with their family or with members of the community. The transplant team usually recommends that an adequate infrastructure be in place prior to transplantation and retransplantation. If potential recipients are found to lack social support, social workers are frequently able to mobilize the necessary resources. Potential recipients should not be denied access to transplantation because of lack of adequate support. Even though it is commonly believed that supportive environments are necessary for good outcomes, no data conclusively proves that patient and graft survival are compromised if a social network is not in place.

RESPONSIBILITY

IS IT FAIR to allocate organs to patients who engage in unhealthy behaviors? Should alcoholics, smokers, and obese patients be offered transplantation or retransplantation? Should patients with self-abusive histories be denied a graft in favor of patients who develop organ failure through no fault of their own? In general, transplant programs do not list patients who are actively engaging in alcohol or recreational substance abuse, or those who are smoking or morbidly obese, because these behaviors potentially impact medical outcomes. Nonetheless, transplantation is appropriate for patients who comply with recommendations to undergo rehabilitation, stop smoking, and lose weight. Patients should not be categorically denied transplantation and retransplantation because they have a *history* of the aforementioned issues.

MEDICAL SUCCESS

ALLOCATION DECISIONS ARE frequently made based on the likelihood of success. For utilitarian reasons, organs are distributed to those who have a reasonable chance for prolonged survival. As stated previously, patient and graft survival following primary transplantation is generally excellent; however, the outcomes following retransplantation are usually worse, and are particularly poor if retransplant candidates are not chosen carefully. Should patients with graft failure be offered another organ? We argue that they should, under strict selection criteria.

At the present time, allocation of organs is based on urgency of need. Even though it is ethically appropriate to consider treatment of those in greatest need, futile transplants on terminally ill patients should be avoided. From a consequentialist perspective, more lives could be saved if organs are allocated to those sick enough to warrant transplantation or retransplantation but healthy enough to survive the procedure and have a good outcome. In general, retransplantation should not be offered to patients with multisystem organ failure because of uniformly poor outcomes. For carefully selected patients who are reasonably healthy, retransplantation can yield acceptable long-term patient and graft survival.

CONCLUSION

THE ALLOCATION OF a resource as scarce as an organ should be carefully considered and all relevant ethical aspects should be assessed before a decision is made. Physicians are obligated to protect the interests of individual patients, but ethical considerations should guide allocation strategies. Therefore, based on the preceding review, we conclude that carefully selected patients with graft failure following primary liver, kidney, cardiac, and pulmonary transplantation should compete equally with naïve transplant candidates for an organ, assuming that there is a reasonable chance of a favorable outcome following retransplantation.

REFERENCES

The American Society for Transplant Physicians (ASTP), American Thoracic Society (ATS), European Respiratory Society (ERS), & International Society for Heart and Lung Transplantation (ISHLT). (1998). International guidelines for the selection of lung transplant candidates. *American Journal of Respiratory and Critical Care Medicine, 158*(1), 335–339.

Azoulay, D., Linhares, M. M., Huguet, E., Delvart, V., Castaing, D., Adam, R., et al. (2002). Decision for retransplantation of the liver: An experience- and cost-based analysis. *Annals of Surgery, 236*(6), 713–721.

Biggins, S. W., Beldecos, A., Rabkin, J. M., Rosen, H. R. (2002). Retransplantation for hepatic allograft failure: Prognostic modeling and ethical considerations. *Liver Transplantation, 8*(4), 313–322.

Costanzo, M. R., Augustine S., Bourge, R., Bristow, M., O'Connell, J. B., Driscoll, D., et al. (1995). Selection and treatment of candidates for heart transplantation. A statement for health professionals from the Committee on Heart Failure and Cardiac Transplantation of the Council on Clinical Cardiology, American Heart Association. *Circulation, 92*(12), 3593–3612.

De Carlis, L., Slim, A. O., Giacomoni, A., DiBenedetto, F., Pirotta, V., Lauterio, A., et al. (2001). Liver retransplantation: Indications and results over a 15-year experience. *Transplantation Proceedings, 33*(1–2), 1411–1413.

Deng, M. C. (2002). Cardiac transplantation. *Heart, 87*(2), 177–184.

Freeman, R. B., Wiesner, R. H., Edwards, E., Harper, A., Merion, R., Wolfe, R. (2004). Results of the first year of the new liver allocation plan. *Liver Transplantation, 10*(1), 7–15.

Ghobrial, R. M., Farmer, D. G., Baquerizo, A., Colquhoun, S., Rosen, H. R., Yer-siz, H., et al. (1999). Orthotopic liver transplantation for hepatitis C: Outcome, effect of immunosuppression, and causes of retransplantation during an 8-year single-center experience. *Annals of Surgery, 229*(6), 824–831.

Gilbert, J. R., Pascual, M., Schoenfeld, D. A., Rubin, R. H., Delmonico, F. L., & Cosimi, A. B. (1999). Evolving trends in liver transplantation: An outcome and charge analysis. *Transplantation, 67*(2), 246–253.

Hariharan, S., Johnson, C. P., Bresnahan, B. A., Taranto, S. E., McIntosh, M. J., & Stablein, D. (2000). Improved graft survival after renal transplantation in the United States, 1988 to 1996. *New England Journal of Medicine, 342*(9), 605–612.

Kamath, P. S., Wiesner, R. H., Malinchoc, M., Kremers, W., Therneau, T. M., Kosberg, C. L., et al. (2001). A model to predict survival in patients with end-stage liver disease. *Hepatology, 33*(2), 464–470.

Keeffe, E. B. (2001). Liver transplantation: Current status and novel approaches to liver replacement. *Gastroenterology, 120*(3), 749–762.

Kilner, J. F. (1990). *Who lives? Who dies?: Ethical criteria in patient selection.* New Haven, CT: Yale University Press.

Magee, J. C., Barr, M. L., Basadonna, G. P., Johnson, M. R., Mahadevan, S., McBride, M. A., et al. (2007). Repeat organ transplantation in the United States, 1996–2005. *American Journal of Transplantation, 7*(5 Pt 2), 1424–1433.

Markmann, J. F., Markowitz, J. S., Yersiz, H., Morrisey, M., Farmer, D. G., Farmer, D. A., et al. (1997). Long-term survival after retransplantation of the liver. *Annals of Surgery, 226*(4), 408–418.

Organ Procurement and Transplantation Network. (2007). *Database online.* Retrieved August 30, 2008, from http://www.ustransplant.org/csr/current/nationalViewer.aspx?o=LI

Pascual, M., Theruvath, T., Kawai, T., Tolkoff-Rubin, N., & Cosimi, A. B. (2002). Strategies to improve long-term outcomes after renal transplantation. *New England Journal of Medicine, 346*(8), 580–590.

Pour-Reza-Gholi, F., Nafar, M., Saeedinia, A., Farrokhi, F., Firouzan, A., Simforoosh, N., et al. (2005). Kidney retransplantation in comparison with first kidney transplantation. *Transplantation Proceedings, 37*(7), 2962–2964.

Showstack, J., Katz, P. P., Lake, J. R., Brown, R. S. Jr., Dudley, R. A., Belle, S., et al. (1999). Resource utilization in liver transplantation: Effects of patient characteristics and clinical practice. NIDDK Liver Transplantation Database Group. *Journal of the American Medical Association, 281*(15), 1381–1386.

Shuhaiber, J. H., Kim, J. B., Hur, K., Gibbons, R. D., Nemeh, H. W., Schwartz, J. P., et al. (2007). Comparison of survival in primary and repeat heart transplantation from 1987 through 2004 in the United States. *The Annals of Thoracic Surgery, 83*(6), 2135–2141.

Steinman, T. I., Becker, B. N., Frost, A. E., Olthoff, K. M., Smart, F. W., Suki, W. N., et al. (2001). Guidelines for the referral and management of patients eligible for solid organ transplantation. *Transplantation, 71*(9), 1189–1204.

Strueber, M., Fischer, S., Gottlieb, J., Simon, A. R., Goerler, H., Gohrbandt, B., et al. (2006). Long-term outcome after pulmonary retransplantation. *The Journal of Thoracic and Cardiovascular Surgery, 132*(2), 407–412.

Wong, T., Devlin, J., Rolando, N., Heaton, N., & Williams, R. (1997). Clinical characteristics affecting the outcome of liver retransplantation. *Transplantation, 64*(6), 878–882.

Part XII

End of Life

64

Advance Directives

STEPHEN S. HANSON AND DAVID J. DOUKAS

ADVANCE DIRECTIVES, DOCUMENTS written by patients to help direct their care if they become incapable of making their own health care decisions, are a relatively recent development in the practice of medicine. Though living wills began as a grassroots effort in the 1960s (Kutner, 1969), the full extent of what they could encompass, and how they might be limited, was not clearly delineated until the *Cruzan* case (discussed later in this chapter) was decided in 1990 (*Cruzan v. Director, Missouri Department of Health,* 1990). It was only after *Cruzan* that the Patient Self-Determination Act (*Omnibus Budget Reconciliation Act,* 1990) went into effect, making advance directives legally acceptable by statute in all 50 states (Doukas & Reichel, 2007). Furthermore, advance directives not only include legal documents such as the living will, durable powers of attorney for health care, and out-of-hospital do not resuscitate (DNR) orders, but also less formal documentations such as values histories (Doukas & Gorenflo, 1993; Doukas & McCullough, 1991), family covenants (Doukas & Hardwig, 2003) and variants of these (Aging With Dignity, n.d.; Emanuel & Emanuel, 1989; Gunter-Hunt, Mahoney, & Seiger, 2002). It is consequently unsurprising that there remains some confusion about what advance directives can mean and how they are to be followed—the U.S. health care system is still working through the details (Shapiro & Bowles, 2002; Toller & Budge, 2006).

The practice of informed consent has a healthy legal and conceptual background that lends itself well to the recent legal history of advance directives. This background provides much of the clarity necessary for understanding the role of various forms of advance directives in guiding care for patients unable to make their own decisions, because the motivating moral idea behind advance directives is the same as that behind informed consent. Advance directives are, in essence, a proactive informed refusal of those therapies one rejects, and conversely an informed consent to those one would accept, in a future state of incapacity.

LEGAL BACKGROUND

ONE OF THE clearest statements of the motivation for the roots of informed consent comes from *Schloendorff v. Society of New York Hospital* (1914), in which the plaintiff consented to a laparotomy for pelvic pain but explicitly refused surgical removal of anything during the examination. Nevertheless, the surgeon removed a pelvic fibroid (leiomyoma) when found, for which the patient sued the hospital. In his ruling, Judge Benjamin Cardozo held that the additional surgical intervention, however well intended by the surgeon, could not be sustained legally when specifically refused in advance

> Every human being of adult years and sound mind has a right to determine what shall be done with his own body; and a surgeon who performs an operation without his patient's consent commits an assault for which he is liable in damages. (*Schloendorff v. Society of New York Hospital*, 1914, par. 4)

This decision laid the legal foundation for informed consent law, but it also gives a clear description of an advance directive, long before the concept had come into use. Informed consent doctrine was later expanded by other formative cases, including *Canterbury v. Spence* (1972). In this case, Jerry Canterbury sued his physician, Dr. William Spence, for insufficiently informing him of the potential risks of a laminectomy performed on him. In its decision, the court concluded that

> The [relevant] context...is invariably the occasion for decision as to whether a particular treatment procedure [sic] is to be undertaken....[I]t is the prerogative of the patient, not the physician, to determine for himself the direction in which his interests seem to lie. (*Canterbury v. Spence*, 1972, p. 781)

This foundational statement of informed consent law can also be seen as a clear statement of the circumstances surrounding decision-making in the case of an incompetent patient, where an advance directive might come into play. Consider the following statement in the case of Karen Ann Quinlan, who was irreversibly comatose and mechanically ventilated months after an anoxic brain injury, at which point her parents (as guardians) sought to have her ventilator removed:

> The interests of the patient, as seen by her surrogate, the guardian, must be evaluated by the court as predominant, even in the face of an opinion contra by the present attending physicians. (*In re Quinlan*, 1976, p. 664)

Even though Ms. Quinlan was not capable of stating her interpretation of her interests at this time, the appropriate basis for the decision is what treatment best serves her understanding of her interests, even though she could no longer state that understanding. The court explicitly noted:

> We have no doubt, in these unhappy circumstances, that if Karen were herself miraculously lucid for an interval (not altering the existing prognosis of the condition to which she would soon return) and perceptive of her irreversible condition, she could effectively decide upon discontinuance of the life-support apparatus…We perceive no thread of logic distinguishing between such a choice on Karen's part and a similar choice which, under the evidence in this case, could be made by a competent patient. (*In re Quinlan*, 1976, p. 663)

Though the court in the *Quinlan* case ruled that the evidence of Ms. Quinlan's wishes through testimony regarding her prior statements was not specific enough to count as advance informed refusal, it was clear that the court was perfectly willing to extend the rights of a patient to choose the course of her treatment to times after that patient had lost the capacity for decision-making. In addition, this judgment laid the groundwork for health care proxies/surrogates by allowing Ms. Quinlan's father to judge her *best interests* regarding what therapies should intrude upon her body (*In re Quinlan*, 1976).

So, there is no difference, in principle, between a competent patient choosing her own treatment and a noncompetent patient's choice. In practice, of course, the lack of competence makes a great deal of difference, as persons must choose while competent with regard to their care in the future. Living will statutes and durable powers of attorney for health care, which permit a named other to make one's health care decisions upon one's loss of decision-making capacity, even when one's condition is not terminal, were developed in response to this need. This was spurred along by the pivotal case of *Cruzan v. Director, Missouri Department of Health,* in 1990. Because it was a U.S. Supreme Court case, it was decided more narrowly on constitutional grounds than was *Quinlan;* however, a number of important developments arose from it.

Nancy Cruzan was in a persistent vegetative state after a period of anoxia perhaps 12–14 minutes long, following an automobile accident. She was sustained by gastrostomy tube feedings. After several years, her parents requested that her artificial feeding be discontinued to allow her death, based on prior lucid statements by Ms. Cruzan about not wanting life-sustaining dependency on medical technology (*Cruzan*, 1990). A lengthy legal process was eventually resolved in June 1990, when the U.S. Supreme Court held that patients with capacity have a liberty interest under the due process clause to refuse all medical therapy and, further, that refusal of artificially delivered food and water is encompassed within that liberty interest. Though the Court did hold that a state has an interest in preserving life, it also held that the right to refuse therapy takes precedence over the state's interest, though each state is allowed to determine the standard of evidence that must be met before allowing refusal of life-prolonging treatment on the patient's behalf. As the Court noted that by definition "an incompetent person is not able to make an informed and voluntary choice to exercise a hypothetical right to refuse treatment or any other right" (*Cruzan*, 1990, p. 280), in her concurring opinion, Justice O'Connor emphasized the importance of clear oral and written instructions prior to incapacity, as well as clear appointment of durable powers of attorney, as means for the incompetent individual to exercise her choice (*Cruzan*, 1990, pp. 289–292).

The *Cruzan* case was one of the primary motivating factors behind the PSDA of 1990, which aims to reduce the number of situations in which patients do not have written advance directives. It requires institutions, health agencies, and HMOs that receive Medicare and Medicaid funds to notify their patients on admission (or enrollment in the case of HMOs) about their relevant rights under relevant state law to execute an advance directive.

ETHICAL PERSPECTIVES

THIS LEGAL HISTORY helps clarify that the moral basis for advance directives is comparable to that for informed consent. It is well recognized that one of the moral bases for informed consent is respect for patients' autonomous wishes, and so it is also for advance directives. Self-determination in advance directives is exercised by an individual through his making, and then projecting into the future, decisions regarding medical interventions. The living will, then, is an expression of informed consent or refusal in advance of the time in which the patient is terminally ill (or persistently vegetative) and has lost decision-making capacity. Durable power of attorney for health care (DPAHC) determinations empower a named person to choose according to her best understanding of the patient's values and preferences prior to the onset of incapacity and transcend the narrow confines of clinical situations in living wills such as terminal illness or a persistent vegetative state. Both the living will and DPAHC are autonomous statements of self-determination, albeit in circumstances where direct self-determination is not possible.

However, patient autonomy is not the sole moral basis for advance directives. A too-exclusive focus on autonomy leads one to miss the true relevance of that choice: patient wishes are crucial for understanding what is best for a patient. Patient benefit is therefore at the ethical center of advance directives, as these directives allow the patient to determine and guide treatments toward what is best for her. Despite the fact that most persons have focused on self-determination as the central feature of the privacy and/or liberty rights deriving from these cases, the language in the *Canterbury* and *Quinlan* cases shows how critical it is to know the patient's values and interests in order to understand what truly benefits the patient. The decision to be made should promote the patient's interests, and it is the patient's prerogative "to determine for himself the direction in which his interests seem to lie," even in the face of an opposing view by physicians. Though physicians surely know better than virtually all patients what can be accomplished by medicine, that is not all that drives an informed treatment decision. A competent patient must determine which of the available options best promotes his interests; and these he knows better than any other. A decision made by an advance directive is meant, as best as possible, to accomplish the same goals; so, in the same way, the patient is best suited to choose his treatment or name his surrogate.

This shows that a perceived moral dilemma of advance directives—the conflict between a patient's request and what is best for her—is rarely such a conflict at all.[1] The dilemma ostensibly occurs because the *parens patriae* responsibility of a state to protect its dependent citizens, as well as medical ethical obligations to patients, would seem to require directing treatments so as to benefit and avoid harm to an incompetent patient, regardless of any prior request (Dresser, 2003). Yet it is the patient's informed request that determines what is actually best for her, which can differ from person to person depending on different value sets and worldviews. Without the patient's understanding of where her interests lie, as expressed through one or more forms of advance directives, a physician cannot know how to provide benefit and avoid harm for her.

Unfortunately, physicians are known to be reticent about discussing advance directives with their patients, due to concerns about patient upset or worry; yet these same patients are very likely waiting on their physicians to initiate these conversations (Doukas & McCullough, 1991; Emanuel, Barry, Stoeckle, Ettelson, & Emanuel, 1991). As a result, when there is no advance directive or proxy decision-maker, the general preference is to preserve life when possible, but this is at least as much due to the reversibility of providing life-sustaining treatments and the irreversibility of withholding or withdrawing them.[2] The power imbalance between physicians and patients' families, then, clearly favors the medical side of the health care relationship, such that the patient's family and loved ones must then reconstruct what the patient would have wanted in such circumstances—a difficult endeavor, indeed.

A greater focus on the relevance of advance directives to proper patient benefit, rather than exclusively on patient autonomy, will tend to help resolve ethical concerns with advance directives, such as the difficulty in applying specific requests to similar, but not identical, factual circumstances; the overgenerality of other requests preventing them from giving helpful information; or lack of comprehension of particular treatment modalities (Dresser, 2003). If an autonomous request does not directly apply to the given case, then respect for autonomy alone gives little assistance to knowing what to do; a focus on values, interests, and the moral concepts that underlie them does. This focus will not give simple answers to these problems, but it does provide tools to help address them.

Yet here the standard living will often fails patients. In some states, the living will forms lack detail, sometimes referring only to the withdrawal of mechanical or other artificial means of sustaining life. Other forms are more thorough and detailed, but most address only desired treatments, not interests and the values and worldview that underlie those interests. The goal of the advance directive and the forms often used to exercise it are not ideally suited to each other.

PRACTICAL MATTERS

GIVEN THIS INADEQUACY of many living wills to fully and clearly guide decision-making in accordance with the incompetent patient's interests, some critics have counseled dispensing with them altogether in favor of DPAHCs (Fagerlin & Schneider, 2004). But DPAHCs have their own difficulties: while proxy decision-makers are certainly more able to be responsive to novel or changing conditions, they can also have difficulty knowing the patient's interests, particularly in cases where there has been poor communication between patient and proxy (Ditto et al., 2001; Perkins, 2007). They can also find it difficult to make life-ending decisions for loved ones, even when they do know the interests of the patient. These difficulties with the various formal advance directives can help guide practitioners to some simple, but vitally important, steps toward improving the utility of advance directives.

TALK EARLY, TALK OFTEN

FIRST, HEALTH CARE providers (physicians and others) in the primary and tertiary care settings should speak with patients about the role of, and usefulness of, advance directives. Though the PSDA has increased patient awareness of advance health care planning, in practice it is significantly hindered in enabling patients to utilize their values to guide future treatment through poor execution except in simple queries on patient admission regarding signing advance directive forms. The PSDA is not commonly carried out by health care professionals but instead by nonclinical admissions personnel or by a form in a stack of documents sent upon joining an HMO. It takes time, discussion, and patient education for effective advance directives to be created (Bailly & DePoy, 1995; Hoffman & Gill, 2000). Therefore, conversations should take place between every patient of age and their health care providers, not just patients near the end of life or those heading into a risky procedure—though they, too, should be spoken with. Providers should consider these as conversations that continue over time, over multiple visits, aimed not merely at guiding patients to fill out the state's legal form but rather at evaluating and expressing the interests and values that could help guide a decision-maker were the patient unable to make her own decisions.

Such an extended conversation is best engaged in on an outpatient setting, in the practice of regular continuing care of a patient over time, such as in family or general internal medicine offices (Emanuel et al., 1991). Conversely, such a discussion is less optimally suited for the stressful and urgent circumstances in which advance directives are frequently discussed and considered—namely, the ER and ICU. For this reason, discussions of advance directives should be thought of as an essential part of a standard of care for continuing well-patient care for all competent patients over the age of 18.

Discussing advance directives in this context allows for a gradual discussion of the moral issues involved in these decisions, and gives plenty of time for the patient to consider her responses to them carefully (Anonymous, 1991). This also allows time to address at least one obvious difficulty: patients, being human beings, do not like to discuss their own mortality, especially at the young adult ages suggested herein. A gradual and continual conversation over time will help to advance the discussion past such hurdles. Also, physicians can point out that accidents and acute illness can be a cause of unexpected incapacity—such as with Ms. Cruzan—which makes the selection of, and discussions with, a health care proxy an extremely prudent choice by all adults. The conversation ought also to continue after patients have filled out any forms, as the goal of the discussion is not an artificial endpoint of the completion of a form but elaboration and development of a moral worldview regarding future medical care by the patient. People will grow and change over time, and their advance directives should as well.

Engage Potential Proxies

IT IS ALSO prudent to engage family and friends, to the extent the patient desires, in such a discussion, in particular those who may be named as proxies. Proxy decision-makers can only guide treatments according to one's interests as far as they know them; it is crucial to educate them as to the interests they may be asked to protect (Sulmasy et al., 1998). One way to further this process is through the use of a family covenant (Doukas, 1991). The family covenant is an open health care agreement that can facilitate proactive discourse on advance care planning. The family covenant provides a framework for the patient, family, loved ones, and physician to define their roles in an interactive conversation. An initial health care agreement delineates information sharing and proxy consent boundaries, with the physician serving as facilitator in potential future times of conflict (Doukas & Hardwig, 2003). This process-based approach is intended to provide a richer context of values and preferences, and a fuller understanding of them among all. The family covenant also articulates the role of loved ones and encourages discourse among them in forging an ongoing health agreement.

Clarify and Document Values

SINCE INDIVIDUAL VALUES and beliefs are the relevant features of an advance directive, making those values clear and explicit can greatly assist family and physicians in understanding the interests that will promote both self-determination and patient benefit. The "Values History," first authored by Doukas and McCullough in 1988, elicits value-based discourse tethered to preferences of future health care that can then be utilized in unanticipated future medical scenarios that cannot readily be addressed solely by means of a standard advance directive, and this discourse can thereby be a valuable addition to formal legal documents (Doukas & McCullough, 1991; Doukas & Reichel, 2007). Discussions encouraged by the "Values History" can help a patient's family and physician better understand how to invoke the patient's specific directive preferences in unforeseen medical circumstances by heightening awareness of the specific reasons why patients would prefer or not prefer treatment modalities.

CONCLUSION

THE LEGAL AND moral history of advance directives seen in the evolution of informed consent helps inform physicians, patients, and families of the role that such directives are meant to play. Understanding the role of an advance directive as helping a patient to "determine for himself the direction in which his interests seem to lie" and to enact those interests after the loss of decision-making competence allows for a much richer appreciation of the role and importance of these directives than is suggested by a model focused on respect for autonomy. This recognition also suggests methods for physicians to better enable such directives.

NOTES

1. See, for example, *In re Browning* (1990, p. 11), which contrasts the two: "The issue [at hand] involves a patient's right of self-determination and does not involve what is thought to be in the patient's best interests."

2. "An erroneous decision not to terminate results in a maintenance of the status quo; the possibility of subsequent developments such as advancements in medical science, the discovery of new evidence regarding the patient's intent, changes in the law, or simply the unexpected death of the patient despite the administration of life-sustaining treatment, at least create the potential that a wrong decision will eventually be corrected or its impact mitigated. An erroneous decision to withdraw life-sustaining treatment, however, is not susceptible of correction" (*Cruzan,* 1990, p. 283).

REFERENCES

Aging With Dignity. (n.d.). *Five Wishes.* Retrieved July 31, 2007, from http://www.agingwithdignity.org/5wishes.html

Anonymous. (1991). Advance directives for medical care. *New England Journal of Medicine, 325,* 1254–1256.

Bailly, D., & DePoy, E. (1995). Older people's responses to education about advance directives. *Health and Social Work, 20,* 223–228.

Canterbury v. Spence, 464 F.2d 772 (D.C. Cir. 1972) (cert. denied 1972).

Cruzan v. Director, Missouri Department of Health, 497 U.S. 261 (1990).

Ditto, P. H., Danks, J. H., Smucker, W. D., Bookwala, J., Coppola, K. M., Dresser, R., et al. (2001). Advance directives as acts of communication: A randomized controlled trial. *Archives of Internal Medicine, 161,* 421–430.

Doukas, D. J. (1991). Autonomy and beneficence in the family: Describing the family covenant. *Journal of Clinical Ethics, 2,* 145–148.

Doukas, D. J., & Gorenflo, D. W. (1993). Analyzing the values history: An evaluation of patient medical values and advance directives. *Journal of Clinical Ethics, 4,* 41–45.

Doukas, D. J., & Hardwig, J. (2003). Using the family covenant in planning end-of-life care: Obligations and promises of patients, families, and physicians. *Journal of the American Geriatric Society, 51,* 1155–1158.

Doukas D. J., & McCullough L. B. (1988). Assessing the Values History of the aged patient regarding critical and chronic care. In J. J. Gallo, W. Reichel, & L. M. Andersen (Eds.), *The handbook of geriatric assessment* (pp. 111–124). Rockville, MD: Aspen Press.

Doukas, D. J., & McCullough, L. B. (1991). The values history: The evaluation of the patient's values and advance directives. *Journal of Family Practice, 32,* 145–153.

Doukas, D. J., & Reichel, W. (2007). *Planning for uncertainty: Living wills and other advance directives for you and your family* (2nd ed.). Baltimore, MD: Johns Hopkins University Press.

Dresser, R. (2003). Precommitment: A misguided strategy for securing death with dignity. *Texas Law Review, 81,* 1823–1847.

Emanuel, L. L., Barry, M. J., Stoeckle, J. D., Ettelson, L. M., Emanuel, E. J. (1991). Advance directives for medical care—a case for greater use. *New England Journal of Medicine, 324,* 889–895.

Emanuel, L. L., & Emanuel, E. J. (1989). The medical directive: A new comprehensive advance care document. *Journal of the American Medical Association, 261,* 3288–3293.

Fagerlin, A., & Schneider, C. E. (2004). Enough. The failure of the living will. *Hastings Center Report, 34,* 30–42.

Gunter-Hunt, G., Mahoney, J. E., & Sieger, C. E. (2002). A comparison of state advance directive documents. *Gerontologist, 42,* 51–60.

Hoffman, L. J., & Gill, B. (2000). Beginning with the end in mind. *American Journal of Nursing, 5*(Suppl.), 38–41.

In re Browning, 568 So. 2d 4, 13 (Fla. 1990).

In re Quinlan, 70 N.J. 10, 355 A. 2d 647 (cert. denied *sub nom.*) (1976).

Kutner, L. (1969). Due process of euthanasia: The living will, a proposal. *Indiana Law Journal. 44,* 539–554.

Omnibus Budget Reconciliation Act of 1990. Pub L. No. 101-508 (1990).

Perkins, H. S. (2007). Controlling death: The false promise of advance directives. *Annals of Internal Medicine, 147,* 51–57.

Schloendorff v. Society of New York Hospital, 211 N.Y. 125, 105 N.E. 92, 93 (1914).

Shapiro, J. D., & Bowles, K. (2002). Nurses' and consumers' understanding of and comfort with the Patient Self-determination Act. *Journal of Nursing Administration, 32,* 503–508.

Sulmasy, D. P., Terry, P. B., Weisman, C. S., Miller, D. J., Stallings, R. Y., Vettese, M. A., et al. (1998). The accuracy of substituted judgments in patients with terminal diagnoses. *Annals of Internal Medicine, 128,* 621–629.

Toller, C. A., & Budge, M. M. (2006). Compliance with and understanding of advance directives among trainee doctors in the United Kingdom. *Journal of Palliative Care, 22,* 141–146.

65

Medical Futility

Horace M. DeLisser

THE PRACTICE OF medicine has long included the notion that in certain settings an established medical treatment may be nonbeneficial, ineffective, or inappropriate—that is, medically futile—and thus should not be offered or undertaken. Notwithstanding any demands by the patient, bacterial antibiotics are not used to treat viral infections; cancer screening in patients in a vegetative state is not done; and surgical resection of the primary tumor is not offered to patients with stage IV lung cancer with brain metastases. The major exception appears to be the use of life-sustaining interventions for critically ill patients who are dying despite receiving full intensive care or patients with end-stage disease who are close to death.

In these settings the use of medical futility as a basis for decision-making has been vigorously resisted. Despite these challenges there continue to be efforts to incorporate concepts of futility into modern medical practice. After reviewing the rise of the modern futility movement, and the challenges to it, this chapter will present a clinically focused reformulation of medical futility that aims to balance the tension between maintaining professional integrity and affirming the autonomy of patients.

THE RISE OF THE MODERN FUTILITY MOVEMENT

ALTHOUGH ITS LEGITIMACY has been the subject of intense debate in recent years (Trotter, 2007), the concept of medical futility has in fact long been a feature that has defined the practice of medicine. In the Hippocratic writings (third century B.C.), for example, the science of medicine is described as involving "the complete removal of the distress of the sick, the alleviation of the more violent diseases and the refusal to undertake to cure cases in which the disease has already won the mastery, knowing that everything is not possible to medicine" ("The Science of Medicine," 1978, p. 140). Such notions of medical futility went largely unchallenged throughout much of the history of medicine.

Two trends, however, converged in the latter half of the 20th century to bring the issue of futility into the open for debate. The first was a series of major advances in biomedical sciences that lead to treatments capable of sustaining life in ways not previously thought imaginable. Unfortunately, these interventions also had the potential to increase patient suffering and/or merely delay death without returning the patient to consciousness or promoting recovery. The other trend involved the rise of patient autonomy as a dominant principle of modern medical ethics. By the 1980s, autonomy had moved from not only a right to *choose* among medically established or appropriate treatment options (including the right to refuse) but also came to be understood by many as a right to *demand* certain life-sustaining interventions regardless of benefit, effectiveness, or appropriateness. This was particularly the case for cardiopulmonary resuscitation (CPR), where this intervention evolved to an entitlement for all hospitalized patients, even if the likelihood of success or a meaningful outcome was low.

As a result, by the mid-1980s physicians found themselves in a clinical environment in which they were required to provide certain interventions, such as CPR, that in their professional judgment were medically nonbeneficial, ineffective, or inappropriate, at the demands of patients or their families or mandated by institutional policies. This was not only different from how physicians operated in other areas of medicine (e.g., surgery, cancer therapy, or resuscitation of previable fetuses) but seemed to be very inconsistent with long-established, core features of physician professionalism. The reaction to this was a vigorous reassertion of the concept of medical futility as a valid basis for guiding physician practice (Blackhall, 1987; Miles, 1992; Murphy, 1988; Schneiderman, Jecker, & Jonsen, 1990; Tomlinson & Brody, 1988, 1990). Specifically, it was proposed that if an intervention was determined to be futile, the physician was under no ethical obligation to offer, provide, or continue that therapy. Further, the physician could withhold or withdraw futile treatments without the approval of the patient or the patient's surrogates.

Much of the initial efforts involved attempts to provide clinically relevant and workable definitions of medical futility (Brody & Halevy, 1995; Schneiderman et al., 1990; Waisel & Truog, 1995). The various definitions fell into five main categories: (a) *physiological futility,* in which an intervention fails to result in a predictable physiological effect; (b) *quantitative futility,* arising when the physicians conclude (either through scientific reasoning, empirical data, or personal or colleague experiences) that in the last 100 cases, a medical treatment has been useless; (c) *qualitative futility,* where a medical intervention only has the effect of preserving permanent unconsciousness or fails to end dependence on intensive medical care; (d) *imminent demise futility,* in which the patient will die in the hospital before discharge regardless of the treatment; and (e) *lethal condition futility,* which describes circumstances in which the patient may be able to survive to be discharged, but the patient's underlying disease is incompatible with a long-term survival and would not be altered by the treatment(s) in question.

During this time a number of professional organizations also promulgated policy statements on futility (American College of Chest Physicians, Society for Critical Care Medicine Consensus Panel, 1990; American Thoracic Society, 1991; Council on Ethical and Judicial Affairs, American Medical Association, 1991, 1999; Ethics Committee of the Society of Critical Care Medicine, 1997). As a group, these statements evolved to permit the removal of life-sustaining interventions over the objections of surrogate decision-makers if good faith efforts at conflict resolution or transfer to another facility were unsuccessful. There were also efforts to establish regional futility policies (Bay Area Network of Ethics Committees, Nonbeneficial Treatment Working Group, 1999; Halevy & Brody, 1996), and in Texas the updated, 1999 advanced directive law recognized the concept of medically futile treatments and provided a legally sanctioned extrajudicial process for resolving disagreements over end-of-life care that allowed physicians to unilaterally withhold or withdraw futile interventions (Fine, 2001; Fine & Mayo, 2003; Zientek, 2005).

As debates raged in the medical and philosophical literatures, the issue of futility was also fought in the courts during the 1990s through a trio of high profile cases. There were many nuances to these cases, and in the end the results were mixed. In the case of Helen Wanglie, an 86-year-old ventilator-dependent woman in a vegetative state, her physicians went to court to have someone other than her husband decide whether continued ventilator treatment was appropriate. The Minnesota courts, however, rejected these efforts and reaffirmed Mr. Wanglie as his wife's decision-maker (Ackerman, 1991; Blake, Maldonado, & Meinhardt, 1993). This was followed by the case of Baby K, an anencephalic baby girl, who intermittently required ventilatory support. When recommendations to withhold mechanical ventilation were not accepted by the baby's mother, the physicians sought a judgment that would specify their rights and obligations in providing medical care to Baby K.

Viewing Baby K as a disabled, handicapped child, the court concluded that federal antidiscrimination law prevented the hospital from withholding treatments, such as mechanical ventilation, particularly in an emergency setting, without the consent of the baby's mother (Annas, 1994; Bonanno, 1995; *In re Baby "K,"* 1994). In the third case, despite objections by the family, ventilator support had been withdrawn from Catherine Gilgunn, a chronically ill, elderly woman who had sustained a series of devastating seizures that resulted in severe brain injury and ventilator dependence. After she died, the patient's daughter sued, seeking damages for mental anguish, but the jury found that the physicians had not been negligent in their actions and that the extended medical care the patient might have desired was futile (Capron, 1995; *Gilgunn v. Massachusetts General Hospital,* 1995).

OBJECTIONS TO THE FUTILITY MOVEMENT

Fʀᴏᴍ ᴛʜᴇ ᴏᴜᴛꜱᴇᴛ of the futility movement the usefulness and legitimacy of medical futility as a basis for making medical decisions has been strongly challenged (Lantos et al., 1989; Rubin, 1999, 2007; Slosar, 2007; Tomlinson, 2007; Tonelli, 2007; Truog, Brett, & Frader, 1992; Wreen, 2004; Youngner, 1988). The major objections can be summarized as follows:

- Definitions of futility are too vague, arbitrary, and impractical in the clinical setting and require physicians to make prognostic determinations that are beyond their capabilities (Tonelli, 2007).
- Assessments of futility are value laden, and typically involve some consideration of the meaning, significance, worth, or quality of a patient's life. This raises the question of why the physician (and medicine in general) should be the one to determine the value and quality of a person's existence. Should not the meaning and significance of a patient's life be based on the patient's wishes, values, and goals? As asserted by Helft, Siegler, and Lantos (2000), "No one is better able to make judgments about what is beneficial to patients than patients themselves" (p. 294).
- Futility policies, by allowing physicians to make unilateral decisions, cede too much power to the physicians and thus undermine patient autonomy. As stated by Susan Rubin (2007), "Unilateral decision making in any form—from the earlier suggestion of nondisclosure to the more recent suggestions in futility policies that treatment can ultimately be withdrawn over the objections of patients and families after all the specified procedural steps have been followed—is ethically problematic and should give us pause.

It is a violation of patient autonomy, an example of unwarranted generalization of expertise, and an instance of unjustified paternalism" (pp. 57–58).

- Institutionalization of futility will lead to the marginalization of minority individuals or of individuals with minority viewpoints (Rubin, 2007; Truog, 2007). In commenting on Emilio Gonzales, an 18-month-old Texas boy with a progressive neurometabolic disorder who had been on life support for 5 months and whose mother had resisted the efforts of the child's physicians to withdraw life-sustaining interventions, Robert Truog offered: "Rather than jeopardize the respect we hold for diversity and minority viewpoints, I believe that in cases like that of Emilio Gonzales, we should seek to enhance our capacity to tolerate the choices of others, even when we believe they are wrong" (Truog, 2007, p. 3).
- Medicine is not only a moral enterprise defined by its own values and traditions, but a social practice that is also accountable to the broader society (Rubin, 1999). As a result it is asserted that a social consensus, developed through a formal process of public reflection and resolution is required to establish the legitimacy of futility, regardless of how it is defined (Rubin, 1999, 2007; Shelton, 1998; Tomlinson, 2007).

REFORMULATING MEDICAL FUTILITY

DESPITE THESE VERY serious challenges to the concept of medical futility, and articles heralding the demise of the futility movement (Helft et al., 2000), there continue to be efforts to describe workable and defensible formulations of futility (Committee on Ethics, American College of Obstetricians and Gynecologists, 2007; Jecker, 2007; Mohindra, 2007). As a practicing intensive care physician, I would like to offer another approach for conceptualizing futility, one that is clinically focused rather than merely philosophical or theoretical. It attempts to uphold professional integrity while being respectful of patient autonomy and sensitive to wider societal concerns, such as wariness over physician power and protection of vulnerable patients. I begin by highlighting several of the rationales for this approach.

First, much of the debate about futility actually revolves around the use of a limited number of life-sustaining interventions, such as CPR, mechanical ventilation and dialysis, in a few clinical settings, typically critically ill patients or patients dying of advanced disease or cancer. Yet in other areas of medicine, physicians have been given wide latitude to make unilateral decisions based on reasoned and informed medical judgment, such as the use of chemotherapy for cancer patients. As an example consider the patient with end-stage metastatic cancer who is no longer receiving treatment, for whom a cardiac arrest is likely to be a terminal event because CPR will not be effective in restarting the heart. Although in this setting physicians are typically required to get consent from the family to not employ CPR, there is no expectation that physicians would obtain consent to withhold ineffective chemotherapy. There is no logical reason for treating the two therapies differently, if reasoned and informed medical judgment has concluded that they will be ineffective.

Second, for clinicians, futility does exist and is still very real (Tonelli, 2007). Adapting a comment about pornography by a supreme court justice (*Jacobellis v. Ohio,* 1964), most physicians and nurses would say that while they may not be able to define futility, they certainly know it when they see it. During the course of a patient's illness there may sadly come a time when despite the best efforts of the caregivers, it becomes clear that treatments are no longer effective or beneficial and are merely delaying death. For example, to insist that the default should always be CPR, even for an 85-year-old patient with end-stage dementia who is actively dying of a urinary tract infection despite appropriate antibiotics and full intensive care, is both confusing and bewildering to clinicians. Providing such care can be a source of great emotional distress, particularly for nurses and physicians in training.

Third, there is no question that some of the early futility polices emphasized the physician's prerogatives and paid relatively little attention to understanding and respecting the patient's perspective. Although some of the more recent iterations of policy statements do a much better job of considering the rights of patients, there is still the sense among critics that futility is really a reactionary effort to reintroduce a paternalistic model into medicine. While these fears may be somewhat overstated, any reformulation of futility must explicitly incorporate the values of the patient to address these concerns.

Last, even the strongest critics of futility will acknowledge that on some level there are truly ineffective or nonbeneficial treatments that physicians should not offer or provide. As noted by Tonelli: "Even if we continue to quibble over definitions, we can all agree that there must be some cases (even if only absurd or irrelevant to actual clinical practice) where a particular intervention is clearly and utterly ineffective, devoid of any possible benefit.... Once we can agree that there is at least a class of such cases we can say that in some circumstances clinicians can unilaterally decide to withhold an intervention" (Tonelli, 2007, p. 88).

In proposing another approach for conceptualizing futility, I would begin by framing the discussion in terms of the patient–physician relationship. In any relationship each party has fundamental needs that must to be addressed. In the context of the patient–physician relationship, physicians need to be healers and relievers rather than causes of suffering, while patients need to be heard and to have their values respected and considered. Sometimes the various needs may conflict, but in thriving relationships each party will at times accede to the needs of the other(s), knowing that the same will be done for them. Certainly, relationships are dysfunctional when one side always wins and the other is always marginalized. This is also true for the patient–physician relationship. Specifically, a relationship in which the physicians always knows best and his or her values are determinant (paternalism), and a view of autonomy where the patients or their surrogates can demand and expect to receive any desired treatment (consumerism), are both equally corrosive to the relationship between patients and physicians. A concept of futility can thus be viewed as a means of restoring and maintaining a balance to the patient–physician relationship that prevents the destructive extremes of physician paternalism or patient consumerism.

Next, we need to ask what patients seek from their physicians and what physicians strive to provide to their patients. In other words, what is the primary goal of medicine? I would argue that there is a societal consensus, reflected in the way physicians are trained and licensed, that the primary goal of medicine is to restore, maintain, or enhance a life that the patient can sense and be aware of, and then value and cherish. That is, the first goal of medicine is to provide a benefit that patients perceive and believe is meaningful to them. This is what patients hope to receive from their doctor and this is why individuals (ideally) choose to become physicians. Is the pursuit of this goal constrained at times by other wider community goals such as our desire to promote a respect for life, accommodate minority perspectives, or protect vulnerable individuals? The fact that the answer is yes does not in any way diminish this as the goal of medicine.

Such an understanding of the goal of medicine provides a basis for defining futility. That is, an intervention is futile if, based on reasoned and informed medical judgment, it is unlikely to restore, maintain, or enhance a life that the patient can sense and be aware of, and then value and cherish. From this, three sequential questions can be asked to determine whether a particular treatment is futile:

- Question 1: Will the treatment restore, maintain, or enhance biological life? That is, will the treatment have a reproducible, predictable, and clinically relevant physiological effect? (*Biological Futility*)
- Question 2: Will the treatment restore, maintain, or enhance cognitive life? That is, will the intervention directly and ultimately contribute to an outcome in which the patient has some level

of cognition that will allow the patient to interact purposely, even if only very modestly, with their environment? (*Cognitive Futility*)

- Question 3: Will the treatment restore, maintain, or enhance a life that is desired by the patient? That is, will the treatment directly and ultimately contribute to a life that the patient believes is meaningful, significant, and valuable to him or her? (*Desired Life Futility*)

If the answer to any of these questions, asked in the order above, is no (meaning very unlikely), then the intervention should be considered medically futile. Within this framework, futility is a medical determination made by the physician that involves not only obtaining laboratory and physiological information but also acquiring data on the goals and values of the patient.

Once a particular intervention has been determined to be futile, who then gets to make the decision on whether the treatment should be withheld or withdrawn? With respect to biological futility, the patient defers to the physician. This is consistent with how medicine operates in general, with historical notions of physician obligations, and with long-established legal norms. For cognitive futility, the physician negotiates with the surrogates to arrive at a consensus about the appropriate level of care and does not take unilateral actions. The aim of these negotiations is to develop a plan of care, consistent with the goal of medicine, which is focused on patient dignity. This would include simplification of care as medically appropriate; turning of the patient and skin care to prevent bed sores; meticulous attention to the hygiene and grooming of the patient; and interventions to prevent contractures of the extremities. This approach reflects the fact that although most individuals would not want to exist without consciousness and cognition, there is still debate in the wider society about these issues. In the setting of desired life futility, the physician defers to the patient. The physicians can make recommendations, even very strong ones, based on their professional knowledge of the risks and burdens of a particular intervention. In the end, however, the patient's values and goals, and not those of the individual physician, drive futility determinations around desired life, as well as the actual decision to withhold or withdraw treatments based on these determinations. A prospectively defined, efficient process of conflict resolution should be in place to deal with disagreements over intended physician actions based on biological futility.

How certain must the physician be that the treatment in question is unlikely to have its desired effect? In the clinical setting, the vast majority of physicians and patients would agree that if the intervention has a less than a 1 in 100 chance of accomplishing the desired effect, then it is very unlikely to be effective or beneficial. A less than 1% chance is admittedly arbitrary but is not an unreasonable cut-off for saying that an event is unlikely to occur. Importantly, if the physician is unable to conclude, to a reasonable degree of medical certainty, that the treatment has a less than a 1 in 100 chance of being effective, then a determination of futility cannot be made. However, it is important to note that while the physician may be unsure initially about a patient's prognosis, with the passage of time the physician may become much more certain about the outcome. This speaks to the value of time-limited, therapeutic trials in helping to establish clarity about the prognosis of a patient.

MEDICAL FUTILITY REFORMULATED: IMPLICATIONS AND SIGNIFICANCE

A SIGNIFICANT STRENGTH OF this proposal is that while it does constrain the instances in which physicians can make unilateral decisions based on a determination of futility, and thus goes a long way toward affirming autonomy, it still does permit actions without consent in those relatively few situations that cause the most angst for clinicians, that is, biological futility. I believe that allowing physicians to make unilateral decisions based on biological futility would actually assuage the demands for the application of futility to other more problematic, value-laden, quality-of-life settings and would enable many physicians to more enthusiastically embrace the importance of communication and relationship building. To permit physicians to make unilateral decisions based on biological futility in no way dismisses the need to, and value of, respectfully engaging patients or their decision-makers in dialogue about physician actions.

It was previously noted that one of the criticisms of futility is the potential limitation in the ability of physicians to determine prognosis. Such a concern could also certainly be raised regarding the approach that has been proposed here. The reality, however, is that physicians are in the business of determining prognosis. Consequently, those who challenge futility because of the imprecision of prognostic determinations by physicians must also dismiss the prognostic determinations of physicians in other settings, such as when informed consent is obtained. Yet it is clear that we have collectively found a way to tolerate the lack of precision in establishing prognosis in other medical contexts. Given this, there is no reason why we cannot also acquire the ability to do the same for possible instances of ineffective or nonbeneficial treatments in critically ill or dying patients. Further, as emphasized above, with time, the precision of prognostic determinations can and does increase.

In this reformulated approach, futility is a determination made by the physician. However, the patient or the patient's surrogates are unlikely to accept this determination, and the actions that should follow, unless and until the physician has gained their trust (Caplan, 1996). Patients or their loved ones are even less likely to accept physicians' recommendations if they have been dismissed, disrespected, or discounted by them. This in turn increases the likelihood of conflict over physician actions. Thus the successful application of this or any other agreed-on formulation of futility must occur against a backdrop of continuous physician efforts at establishing and maintaining the trust of the patient and his or her loved ones. In the context of the patient–physician relationship, real trust is first built by time and patience. The physician does not assume that he or she should be trusted but instead diligently and compassionately goes about providing the best care possible and in so doing demonstrates over time that the physician is deserving of the patient's or family's trust. Trust also flourishes when the communication from the physician to the patient or family is goal-oriented and patient-centered, timely and consistent, understandable and jargon-free, and truthful and honest. Communicating effectively in this way, and intentionally soliciting, listening to, and understanding the story of the patient and the family will go a long way toward building the kind of trust that helps to prevent conflicts over futile treatments.

CONCLUSION

WITH THE PATIENT–PHYSICIAN interaction, and the goals of that relationship as the foundation, an approach to futility has been presented that provides a clinically relevant tool that can be used to determine the appropriateness of the life-sustaining treatments a patient is receiving. Once a determination of futility has been made, decision-making is assigned in a way that addresses essential needs of patients and physicians and thus strengthens the patient–physician relationship. It does not claim to be value-free, and it is not denied that there are aspects of this formulation that could be argued as somewhat arbitrary. The same, however, can also be said for the rest of medicine. To be successful, particularly in preventing physician frustration or patient/family resentment and resistance, this process must occur in the context of ongoing effective communication and trust-building. While it is unclear if there will ever be a public reflection and resolution to establish the legitimacy of futility, should such a formal process ever get launched, this kind of balanced approach could help to frame that discussion.

REFERENCES

Ackerman, F. (1991). The significance of a wish. *Hastings Center Report, 21,* 27–29.

American College of Chest Physicians, Society for Critical Care Medicine Consensus Panel. (1990). Ethical and moral guidelines for the initiation, continuation, and withdrawal of intensive care. *Chest, 97,* 949–958.

American Thoracic Society. (1991). Withholding and withdrawing life sustaining therapy. *American Review of Respiratory Disease, 144,* 726–731.

Annas, G. J. (1994). Asking the courts to set the standard of emergency care—the case of Baby K. *New England Journal of Medicine, 330,* 1542–1545.

Bay Area Network of Ethics Committees, Nonbeneficial Treatment Working Group. (1999). Nonbeneficial or futile medical treatment: Conflict resolution guidelines for the San Francisco Bay Area. *Western Journal of Medicine, 170,* 287–290.

Blackhall, L. J. (1987). Must we always use CPR? *New England Journal of Medicine, 317,* 1281–1285.

Blake, D. C., Maldonado, L., & Meinhardt, R. A. (1993). Bioethics and the law: The case of Helga Wanglie: A clash at the bedside—medically futile treatment v. patient autonomy. *Whittier Law Review, 14,* 119–144.

Bonanno, M. A. (1995). The case of Baby K: Exploring the concept of medical futility. *Annals of Health Law, 4,* 151–172.

Brody, B. A., & Halevy, A. (1995). Is futility a futile concept? *Journal of Medicine and Philosophy, 20,* 123–144.

Caplan A. (1996). Odds and ends: Trust and the debate over medical futility. *Annals of Internal Medicine, 125,* 688–689.

Capron, A. M. (1995). Abandoning a waning life. *Hastings Center Report, 25,* 24–26.

Committee on Ethics, American College of Obstetricians and Gynecologists. (2007). ACOG committee opinion no. 362: Medical futility. *Obstetrics and Gynecology, 109,* 791–794.

Council on Ethical and Judicial Affairs, American Medical Association. (1991). Guidelines for the appropriate use of do-not-resuscitate orders. *Journal of the American Medical Association, 265,* 1868–1871.

Council on Ethical and Judicial Affairs, American Medical Association. (1999). Medical futility in end-of-life care: Report of the *Journal of the American Medical Association, 281,* 937–941.

Ethics Committee of the Society of Critical Care Medicine. (1997). Consensus statement of the Society of Critical Care Medicine's Ethics Committee regarding futile and other possibly inadvisable treatments. *Critical Care Medicine, 25,* 887–891.

Fine, R. L. (2001). The Texas Advance Directives Act of 1999: Politics and reality. *HEC Forum, 13*, 59–81.

Fine, R. L., & Mayo, T. W. (2003). Resolution of futility by due process: Early experience with the Texas Advance Directives Act. *Annals of Internal Medicine, 138*, 743–746.

Gilgunn v. Massachusetts General Hospital, SUCV92–4820 (Mass Super Ct, Suffolk Co, April 21, 1995).

Halevy, A., & Brody, B. A. (1996). A multi-institution collaborative policy on medical futility. *Journal of the American Medical Association, 276*, 571–574.

Helft, P. R., Siegler, M., & Lantos, J. (2000). The rise and fall of the futility movement. *New England Journal of Medicine, 343*, 293–296.

In re Baby "K," 832 F3d 590 (4th Cir), cert. denied, 513 US 825 (1994).

Jacobellis v. Ohio, 378 U.S. 184, 197 (1964).

Jecker, N. S. (2007). Medical futility: A paradigm analysis. *HEC Forum, 19*, 13–32.

Lantos, J. D., Singer, P. A., Walker, R. M., Gramelspacher, G. P., Shapiro, G. R., Sanchez-Gonzalez, M. A., et al. (1989). The illusion of futility in clinical practice. *American Journal of Medicine, 87*, 81–84.

Miles, S. H. (1992). Medical futility. *Law Medicine Health Care, 20*, 310–315.

Mohindra, R. K. (2007). Medical futility: A conceptual model. *Journal Medical Ethics, 33*, 71–75.

Murphy, D. J. (1988). Do-not-resuscitate orders. Time for reappraisal in long-term-care institutions. *Journal of the American Medical Association, 260*, 2098–2101.

Rubin, S. B. (1999). Why futility policies are not the answer. *Western Journal of Medicine, 170*, 291.

Rubin, S. B. (2007). If we think it's futile, can't we just say no? *HEC Forum, 19*, 45–65.

Schneiderman, L. J., Jecker, N. S., & Jonsen, A. R. (1990). Medical futility: Its meaning and ethical implications. *Annals of Internal Medicine, 112*, 949–954.

The science of medicine. (1978). In G. E. R. Lloyd (Ed.), *Hippocratic writings* (pp. 139–147). London: Penguin Books.

Shelton, W. (1998). A broader look at medical futility. *Theoretical Medicine and Bioethics, 19*, 383–400.

Slosar, J. P. (2007). Medical futility in the post-modern context. *HEC Forum, 19*, 67–82.

Tomlinson, T. (2007). Futility beyond CPR: The case of dialysis. *HEC Forum, 19*, 33–43.

Tomlinson, T., & Brody, H. (1988). Ethics and communication in do-not-resuscitate orders. *New England Journal of Medicine, 318*, 43–46.

Tomlinson, T., & Brody, H. (1990). Futility and the ethics of resuscitation. *Journal of the American Medical Association, 264*, 1276–1280.

Tonelli, M. R. (2007). What medical futility means to clinicians. *HEC Forum, 19*, 83–93.

Trotter, G. (2007). Futility in the 21st century. *HEC Forum, 19*, 1–12.

Truog, R. D. (2007). Tackling medical futility in Texas. *New England Journal of Medicine, 357,* 1–3.

Truog, R. D., Brett, A. S., & Frader, J. (1992). The problem with futility. *New England Journal of Medicine, 326,* 1560–1564.

Waisel, D. B., & Truog, R. D. (1995). The cardiopulmonary resuscitation-not-indicated order: Futility revisited. *Annals of Internal Medicine, 122,* 304–308.

Wreen, M. (2004). Medical futility and physician discretion. *Journal of Medical Ethics, 30,* 275–278.

Youngner, S. J. (1988). Who defines futility? *Journal of the American Medical Association, 260,* 2094–2095.

Zientek, D. M. (2005). The Texas Advance Directives Act of 1999: An exercise in futility? *HEC Forum, 17,* 245–259.

66

Hospice: Past, Future, and Ethical Considerations

AMY M. CORCORAN AND JENNIFER M. KAPO

THE MEDICARE HOSPICE Benefit has allowed many U.S. citizens access to comprehensive end-of-life care in a variety of settings. Unfortunately, the hospice benefit is underutilized. Admission criteria defined by limited prognosis, perceptions of hospice, and a forced transition to a noncurative model of care contribute to the barriers to enrollment and likely to the underutilization of this benefit.

In this chapter, we will trace the evolution of the modern hospice movement from its historical beginning in Europe to its more recent history in the United States. We will then explore the benefits and restrictions with the current Medicare Hospice Benefit as well as consider ethical concerns regarding these restrictions.

EVOLUTION OF THE DEFINITION OF HOSPICE

THE CONCEPT OF hospice care has evolved over centuries. The Latin root word for *hospice* is *hospitium*, which the Romans used to describe as a place where guests were received with lodging and hospitality. Europe has a long, rich history of providing hospice care to dying persons. The first record of an organization devoted to caring for the sick and dying is the nursing order of the Sisters of Charity, which was founded in the 1600s by Vincent de Paul, a French priest and former slave (Campbell, 1986). The first use of the word *hospice* applied to the care of the dying was by Madame Jeanne Garnier in Lyons, France, in 1842 (Saunders, 2005).

In 1879, Our Lady's Hospice of Dublin was founded by Sister Mary Aikenhead, Irish Sisters of Charity. Then in 1905, another hospice named St. Joseph's Hospice in the East End of London was opened. Meanwhile, there were three Protestant homes that opened to welcome dying patients: (a) Friedensheim Home of Rest in 1885 (later St. Columba's Hospital), (b) The Anglican Sisters of the Society of St. Margaret founded the Hostel of God in London, England, in 1891, and (c) St. Luke's Home for the Dying Poor in 1893 (Kerr, 1993; Saunders, 1993, 2005).

PIONEERS OF THE MODERN HOSPICE MOVEMENT

THE MOVEMENT OF the modern hospice had many supporters; however, Dr. Cicely Saunders is often given credit for being a major pioneer of the modern movement. In addition to providing comprehensive end-of-life care, she advocated for education and research in a field that was poorly understood. In 1948, Dr. Saunders, who was initially trained as a nurse then worked as a social worker, cared for a young Polish man dying of rectal cancer. When this young man died, he left £500 to pay for a window in the building Dr. Saunders would build to provide the holistic and compassionate care that meant so much to him as he was dying. Encouraged by a physician with whom she was working, Dr. Saunders returned to school to become a physician. In 1967, she led the establishment of St. Christopher's Hospice (St. Christopher's Hospice, 1967). She developed innovative clinical care, teaching, and research programs. Here, she developed the concept of *total pain* to describe the all-encompassing physical, emotional, spiritual, and social distress experienced by the dying. Drawing from her own unique multidisciplinary background, she used the team approach in caring for her patients, pulling from the expertise of nurses, social workers, chaplains, and physicians (Clark, 2000; St. Christopher's Hospice, 1967; Storey, 1990).

The history of the modern hospice movement in the United States is more recent. In 1963, Dr. Florence Wald was the dean of the Yale School of Nursing when she was inspired by a lecture that Dr. Saunders gave on campus. This prompted her to leave her position at Yale in 1974 to join a group that championed the formation of Hospice, Inc. of New Haven, Connecticut, the first hospice in the United States (*The Hospice Experiment*, n.d.; Wald, 1999).

HOSPICE MEDICARE BENEFIT: ENROLLMENT CRITERIA, PAYMENT STRUCTURE, SERVICES, AND TYPES

THE MODERN DEFINITION of a *hospice* in the United States is a program that provides care to those with terminal illnesses and their families. This is a noncurative approach to pain and symptom management as well as addressing psychological and spiritual needs. By Medicare law, the standard hospice interdisciplinary team includes a visiting nurse, physician, social worker; chaplain, home health aide, and community volunteer needed to address the physical, spiritual, and psychosocial aspects of suffering that may accompany the end of life experience. Patients are eligible to receive respite care and short-term inpatient care, as well as medications, medical equipment, and medical supplies that are related to their admitting hospice diagnosis. Bereavement services following a patient's death are also offered to surviving family members.

In 1982, the U.S. Congress responded to concerns of increasing health care costs in the setting of advancing medical technology by passing the Medicare Hospice Benefit. The benefit aimed to provide comprehensive end-of-life care to Medicare beneficiaries who forfeited curative treatments. Medicare beneficiaries entitled to hospital insurance (Part A) who have terminal illnesses with a life expectancy of 6 months or less have the option of electing hospice benefits in lieu of standard Medicare coverage for curative treatment and management of their terminal condition. The prognosis of 6 months or less must be certified by two physicians and be applied to the specific disease process as it were to follow its natural course. Only care provided by a Medicare certified hospice is covered under the hospice benefit provisions (*Centers for Medicare and Medicaid Services,* n.d.).

The Medicare hospice reimbursement structure is a capitated, per diem system. The rest of hospice payments may be self-pay, insurance, charity, Medicaid, or other government programs (e.g., Veterans Affairs, county-run). Of note, Medicaid pays for hospice in all states except Connecticut and New Hampshire. Of the over 4,500 hospice programs in the United States today, most are certified by Medicare. In the past a majority of the programs were nonprofit; however, the for-profits have been growing and accounted for 46% in 2006 (The National Hospice and Palliative Care Organization, 2007).

Over 1.3 million patients benefited from hospice enrollment in 2006 (The National Hospice and Palliative Care Organization, 2007). There is evidence to support the hypothesis that patients are more satisfied with their care when enrolled in hospice programs at the end-of-life (Kane, Wales, Bernstein, Leibowitz, & Kaplan, 1984). Studies have also demonstrated that improved pain assessment and management, improved bereavement outcomes, and greater family satisfaction occur when utilizing the Medicare Hospice Benefit (Miller, Mor, & Teno, 2003; Miller, Mor, Wu, Gozalo, & Lapane, 2002; Seamark, Williams, Hall, Lawrence, & Gilbert, 1998; Teno et al., 2004).

Given this evidence of the benefit of hospice care, one could argue that the majority of U.S. citizens should be given the opportunity to have the care of a comprehensive hospice team at the end-of-life. Although many U.S. citizens benefit from the previously described hospice care, the majority die without enrolling. The National Hospice and Palliative Care Organization estimates that approximately 36% of all deaths in the United States in 2006 were under the care of a hospice program (The National Hospice and Palliative Care Organization, 2007). In addition, patients were enrolled at the very end of life rather than closer to the 6-month length of stay suggested by the enrollment criteria. The length of stay in hospice in 2006 was 61 days, with a median of 21 days (The National Hospice and Palliative Care Organization, 2007). Theoretically, with such a short time under hospice care, many patients, especially those who die within 24 hours of enrollment, do not benefit from the full scope of care hospice can provide. A shorter length of stay is usually interpreted as a late referral; however, this is not always the case—some people could not have been referred earlier (e.g., late diagnosis of a terminal illness). This suggests that there are significant restrictions or barriers to hospice enrollment.

HOSPICE RESTRICTIONS

THERE ARE SEVERAL proposed reasons for the underutilization of hospice. As noted above, to meet Medicare requirements for hospice enrollment, a physician must certify that he or she believes that a patient has less than 6 months to live if the disease were to take its natural course. Physicians struggle with prognostication in chronic disease, leading to a failure to identify terminally ill patients who are appropriate for hospice enrollment. The benefit also requires that all hospice enrollees forfeit all curative treatments to receive hospice care. For many patients this decision may be too difficult for a multitude of reasons discussed later in this chapter.

THE CHALLENGE OF PROGNOSTICATION

HOSPICE IS THE only Medicare benefit that requires an assignment of poor prognosis to receive the benefit. A national survey of internists revealed that the majority felt that they were inadequately trained in prognostication (Christakis & Iwashyna, 1998). Illness trajectories vary substantially from individual to individual, and there is little empirical evidence to guide assessments, making it difficult to predict how long the patient has to live.

Prognostication in noncancer diseases such as end-stage renal disease and heart failure is particularly difficult. Data suggests that on average, physicians tend to overestimate prognosis of patients (Christakis & Iwashyna, 1998; Forster & Lynn, 1988; Parkes, 1972), leading them to delay referring patients to hospice. In response to this challenge, the National Hospice and Palliative Care Organization created guidelines to help physicians identify patients who are likely to have a prognosis of less than 6 months. These guidelines are primarily based on specialist consensus and a limited number of empirical data. Although these were meant to be guidelines, some hospice organizations use them as hospice enrollment criteria. In reality, data suggests that these guidelines are not useful in identifying patients who are eligible for hospice (Fox et al., 1999).

NONCURATIVE FOCUS

To ENROLL IN hospice, the patient and family must agree to forgo curative treatments. In other words, the goals of care change from curative and life-sustaining therapies to goals of improving quality of life with comprehensive treatment of pain and other forms of suffering. For some, this may be a significant barrier to care, particularly if they have lasting hope for a cure. Others may desire expensive therapies such as radiation and chemotherapy that may have both palliative and curative treatment benefits. While these treatments may be considered palliative in nature and not given with the intent of cure, they are expensive and a cost-burden to many hospice programs. In the capitated system of hospice under Medicare, individual hospices must make treatment decisions based not only on medical indications but also on financial considerations. Wealthier hospices (those with considerable outside funding from private foundations or larger in size, for example) may be able to offer treatments that hospices who rely solely on Medicare funds cannot. Many patients are forced to choose between expensive palliative care treatments that may not be curative (e.g., chemotherapy in advanced lung cancer to alleviate symptoms of troubled breathing and pain), and hospice care, which is limited to a noncurative approach. Patients are forced to choose between curative treatments, comprehensive palliative care, and full hospice benefits under Medicare. Once enrolled in the Medicare Hospice Benefit, curative therapies for the hospice diagnosis are no longer covered, and most programs will not cover palliative chemotherapy or other expensive palliative therapies. This is the dilemma faced by many patients and families, and the fact that the health care system makes them choose is, arguably, unethical. As more innovative medical procedures are developed to provide better palliative care, it would be unfortunate if those who are at the end of life were not able to obtain access to aggressive symptom or pain management.

ETHNIC DISPARITIES

BARRIERS TO HOSPICE are created by prognostic uncertainty and a potential forced choice between curative and hospice care that affect the general population. Almost simultaneously, there may be important ethnic disparities that result in reduced access to hospice care under the Medicare Hospice Benefit. In 2005, approximately one-third of all deaths in the United States were under the care of a hospice program; however, less than 20% of hospice enrollees were non-White ethnic minorities. Although there was an increase in hospice-enrolled minority patients from 16.5% in 2004 to 17.8% in 2005, this still defines an underrepresentation of ethnic minorities for a federally funded program (The National Hospice and Palliative Care Organization, 2007). Proposed barriers to hospice enrollment for non-White patients include lack of knowledge of hospice, cultural beliefs and attitudes, language obstacles, and limited access to a diverse workforce of hospice providers (Born, Greiner, Sylvia, Butler, & Ahluwalia, 2004; Reese, Melton, & Ciaravino, 2004; Rhodes, Teno, & Welch, 2006). At the end of life, racial disparities also persist. Most significantly, racial disparities in perceptions of families and surrogates regarding communication and family needs of those at the end of life existed in a study looking at family perceptions (Welch, Teno, & Mor, 2005).

However, a recent study, suggests that though disparities in perceptions of care at the end-of-life persist, when patients enroll in hospice these disparities may decrease. Researchers found no differences (through quality ratings scores) or less of a disparity in perceptions of concerns with the quality of end-of-life care when compared to the results of a previously reported national mortality survey. There was improvement in the domains examining emotional and spiritual support for the family, adequate communication about what to expect when the patient died, and overall satisfaction with end-of-life care (Rhodes, Teno, & Connor, 2007). Again, this points out the benefit of hospice, but the concern remains that ethnic minorities may face significant barriers to hospice enrollment leading to their underrepresentation in hospice care. Given that this is a federally funded program, access should be equal to all U.S. citizens.

LENGTH OF HOSPICE STAY

NEITHER AMONG PHYSICIANS nor among families is there a consensus regarding the ideal length of stay in hospice. In one study, surprisingly most felt that they enrolled at the correct time even with shorter lengths of stays (Kapo, Harrold, Carroll, Rickerson, & Casarett, 2005). The reluctance of physicians to identify patients with a prognosis of 6 months augmented by the lack of accurate clinical markers for poor prognosis certainly limit patients' access to hospice care. However, bridge programs that offer a greater prognosis interval may not solve this dilemma. A study that looked at one of these programs, where patients with a less than 1-year prognosis were placed in a bridge program, found that those with the longer prognosis lived longer than those in the hospice program (Casarett & Abrahm, 2001).

CONCLUSION

IN THE UNITED States, the Medicare Hospice Benefit has allowed for many patients and families to benefit from comprehensive end-of-life care in a variety of settings. Unfortunately, the hospice benefit may be underutilized because of restrictions in prognostication and focus on a noncurative model of care. In addition, there may be populations of patients, such as ethnic minorities, who may be less likely to enroll because of the previously described barriers. As we move forward and the population ages, with concomitant increases in the prevalence of chronic disease, we will need to constantly evaluate the delivery of end-of-life care and improve access to hospice care for all U.S. citizens.

Change is needed to make the hospice benefit available for more dying U.S. citizens. In addition, more studies to look at ways to improve or modify the hospice benefit are necessary to ensure successful changes in the benefit. Possible future options could involve

- The need to certify that a patient has less than 6 months to live could be eliminated. This will help overcome the barriers created by prognostic uncertainty and alleviate the struggles that physicians face with this task.
- An open-access hospice system could be created that reimburses hospice programs to provide complete palliative care that addresses all forms of suffering, including psychosocial, physical, and spiritual, while at the same time providing aggressive, possibly curative, medical treatment. This eliminates the need for patients to choose between palliative care and curative care. Of

note, several private insurance companies such as Aetna and United Health have piloted open access with the hope that the seriously ill patients will take advantage of hospice benefits sooner to avoid frequent hospitalizations.

⁌ A concerted effort is needed to further define the reasons for minority hospice underutilization through careful research. Once these reasons are defined, a targeted overhaul of the current systems to address these reasons may increase minority utilization of hospice care. For example, if research finds that ethnic minorities are less likely to enroll in hospice because of trust concerns due to lack of diversity of hospice workers, a national effort to increase the diversity of the workforce through incentives may overcome this barrier. Increasing hospice enrollment of a diverse population is of utmost importance so that all U.S. citizens have equal access to comprehensive end-of-life care that hospice provides, regardless of race or ethnicity.

REFERENCES

Born, W., Greiner, K. A., Sylvia, E., Butler, J., & Ahluwalia, J. S. (2004). Knowledge, attitudes, and beliefs about end-of-life care among inner-city African Americans and Latinos. *Journal of Palliative Medicine, 7*(2), 247–256.

Campbell, L. (1986). History of the hospice movement. *Cancer Nursing, 9*(6), 333–338.

Casarett, D., & Abrahm, J. L. (2001). Patients with cancer referred to hospice versus a bridge program: Patient characteristics, needs for care, and survival. *Journal of Clinical Oncology, 19*(7), 2057–2063.

Centers for Medicare and Medicaid services. (n.d.). Retrieved February 22, 2008, from http://www.cms.hhs.gov/

Christakis, N. A., & Iwashyna, T. J. (1998). Attitude and self-reported practice regarding prognostication in a national sample of internists. *Archives of Internal Medicine, 158*(21), 2389–2395.

Clark, D. (2000). Total pain: The work of Cicely Saunders and the hospice movement. *American Pain Society Bulletin, 10*(4). Retrieved December 27, 2007, from http://www.ampainsoc.org/pub/bulletin/jul00/hist1.htm

Forster, L. E., & Lynn, J. (1988). Predicting life span for applicants to inpatient hospice. *Archives of Internal Medicine, 148*(12), 2540–2543.

Fox, E., Landrum-McNiff, K., Zhong, Z., Dawson, N. V., Wu, A. W., & Lynn, J. (1999). Evaluation of prognostic criteria for determining hospice eligibility in patients with advanced lung, heart, or liver disease. SUPPORT investigators. Study to understand prognoses and preferences for outcomes and risks of treatments. *Journal of the American Medical Association, 282*(17), 1638–1645.

The hospice experiment: The revolution in dying. Florence Wald (part 4). (n.d.). Retrieved February 22, 2008, from http://americanradioworks.publicradio.org/features/hospice/a4.html

Kane, R. L., Wales, J., Bernstein, L., Leibowitz, A., & Kaplan, S. (1984). A randomised controlled trial of hospice care. *Lancet, 1*(8382), 890–894.

Kapo, J., Harrold, J., Carroll, J. T., Rickerson, E., & Casarett, D. (2005). Are we referring patients to hospice too late? Patients' and families' opinions. *Journal of Palliative Medicine, 8*(3), 521–527.

Kerr, D. (1993). Mother Mary Aikenhead, the Irish sisters of charity and our lady's hospice for the dying. *American Journal of Hospice and Palliative Care, 10*(3), 13–20.

Miller, S. C., Mor, V., & Teno, J. (2003). Hospice enrollment and pain assessment and management in nursing homes. *Journal of Pain and Symptom Management, 26*(3), 791–799.

Miller, S. C., Mor, V., Wu, N., Gozalo, P., & Lapane, K. (2002). Does receipt of hospice care in nursing homes improve the management of pain at the end of life? *Journal of the American Geriatrics Society, 50*(3), 507–515.

National Hospice and Palliative Care Organization. (2007). *NHPCO facts and figures: Hospice care in America* (No. 2008). Retrieved December 27, 2007, from http://www.nhpco.org/files/public/Statistics_Research/NHPCO_facts-and-figures_Nov2007.pdf

Parkes, C. M. (1972). Accuracy of predictions of survival in later stages of cancer. *British Medical Journal, 2*(5804), 29–31.

Reese, D. J., Melton, E., & Ciaravino, K. (2004). Programmatic barriers to providing culturally competent end-of-life care. *American Journal of Hospice and Palliative Care, 21*(5), 357–364.

Rhodes, R. L., Teno, J. M., & Connor, S. R. (2007). African American bereaved family members' perceptions of the quality of hospice care: Lessened disparities, but opportunities to improve remain. *Journal of Pain and Symptom Management, 34*(5), 472–479.

Rhodes, R. L., Teno, J. M., & Welch, L. C. (2006). Access to hospice for African Americans: Are they informed about the option of hospice? *Journal of Palliative Medicine, 9*(2), 268–272.

Saunders, C. (1993). Mother Mary Aikenhead, the Irish sisters of charity and our lady's hospice for the dying. *American Journal of Hospice and Palliative Care, 10*(5), 3.

Saunders, C. (2005). Foreword. In D. Doyle, G. Hanks, N. Cherny, & K. Calman (Eds.), *Oxford textbook of palliative medicine* (3rd ed., pp. xvii). New York: Oxford University Press.

Seamark, D. A., Williams, S., Hall, M., Lawrence, C. J., & Gilbert, J. (1998). Dying from cancer in community hospitals or a hospice: Closest lay carers' perceptions. *British Journal of General Practice, 48*(431), 1317–1321.

St. Christopher's Hospice. (1967). *British Medical Journal, 3*(5558), 169–170.

Storey, P. (1990). Goals of hospice care. *Texas Medicine, 86*(2), 50–54.

Storey, P., & Knight, C. (2003). *UNIPAC one: The hospice/palliative approach to end-of-life care* (2nd ed.). Larchmont, NY: Mary Ann Liebert.

Teno, J. M., Clarridge, B. R., Casey, V., Welch, L. C., Wetle, T., Shield, R., et al. (2004). Family perspectives on end-of-life care at the last place of care. *Journal of the American Medical Association, 291*(1), 88–93.

Wald, F. S. (1999). Hospice care in the United States: A conversation with Florence S. Wald [Interview by M. J. Friedrich]. *Journal of the American Medical Association, 281*(18), 1683–1685.

Welch, L. C., Teno, J. M., & Mor, V. (2005). End-of-life care in black and white: Race matters for medical care of dying patients and their families. *Journal of the American Geriatrics Society, 53*(7), 1145–1153.

67

Palliative Care

Debra Wiegand

PALLIATIVE CARE CAN be integrated along with traditional medical therapies throughout one's life. The main goal of palliative care is to prevent and relieve suffering and to support the best possible quality of life for patients and their families, regardless of the stage of the disease or the need for other therapies (National Consensus Project for Palliative Care, 2004). Palliative care interventions are used to prevent and relieve distressing symptoms and facilitate decision-making, while supporting patients and families. Palliative care may play a smaller role in the initial illness course but may play a larger role as one's illness progresses and aggressive treatment options become fewer or less effective (see Figure 67.1).

Good, open, and honest communication is essential among the interdisciplinary health care teams and between patients, families, and the health care team (Lilly et al., 2000; Lilly, Sonna, Haley, & Massaro, 2003; Norton, Tilden, Tolle, Nelson, & Eggman, 2003; O'Callahan, Fink, Pitts, & Luce, 1995; Tilden, Tolle, Nelson, Thompson, & Eggman, 1999; Wiegand., 2006). The President's Commission for the Study of Ethical Problems in Medicine and Biomedical and Behavioral Research (1983) identifies patients' families as their best advocates. This is of utmost importance when a patient is unable to speak on his or her own behalf. Patients and families need information and support throughout the illness trajectory. Families are better able to cope when knowledge is shared with them and when active support is given by health care providers (Woods, Beaver, & Luker, 2000).

Creating an ethical environment is essential in the provision of quality palliative care. Ethical considerations related to palliative care include a patient's right to self-determination, family advocacy and decision-making, utility or benefit versus burden of therapy, withholding and

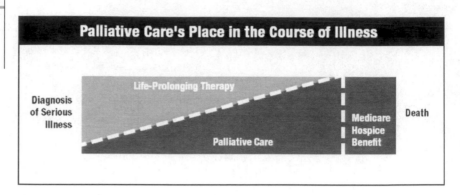

FIGURE 67.1   Palliative care integrated with life-prolonging therapy.

withdrawing life-sustaining therapy, medical futility, management of distressing symptoms, and the principle of double effect related to the administration of analgesia.

SELF-DETERMINATION

AUTONOMY IS KEY to palliative care decisions. As defined by Beauchamp and Childress (2001), the principle of autonomy means that an individual has the right to determine a course of action in accordance with a plan chosen by him or herself. In order to choose palliative care, patients need to be aware of this option. If a patient desires, not only will aggressive interventions be offered but palliative interventions will also be offered to manage the patient's symptoms and illness. Autonomy allows individuals to drive their care and keeps care focused on what the individual wants. Autonomy is threatened when the medical care provider (physician, advance practice nurse, or other health care provider) takes a paternalistic approach and provides care that he or she thinks the patient should have.

The voluntary choice of a competent and informed patient determines whether medical treatments, including life-sustaining therapy, will be initiated, continued, or withdrawn (President's Commission for the Study of Ethical Problems in Medicine and Biomedical and Behavioral Research, 1983). Individuals with decision-making capacity decide on their treatment options. Criteria have been suggested to guide health care providers in determining if an individual has decision-making capacity. Sulmasy, FitzGerald, and Jaffin (1993) recommend that the following criteria be used to determine decision-making capacity:

- The patient's judgment is intact.
- The patient can understand the nature of the procedure under consideration, its risks, benefits, and the consequences of deciding to accept or to forgo the procedure.

⟨ The patient can communicate a decision.

⟨ The patient can explain the reasons for a decision in a way that is consistent with his or her life history and previously held values.

⟨ The patient's decision remains relatively stable over time.

Important information needs to be ascertained to determine if patients have made their treatment preferences known. The Patient Self-Determination Act (1990) was passed in an effort to encourage Americans to consider what they would and would not want toward life's end. It is estimated that 15%–25% of Americans have an advance directive (Braun, Onaka, & Horiuchi, 2001; Hanson & Rodgman, 1996; Jezewski, Meeker, & Schrader, 2003; McKinley, Gareeth, Evans, & Danis, 1996). The advance directive may be in the form of a living will, a document that identifies specific treatments that a patient would or would not want, or in the form of a durable power of attorney for health care or health care proxy, which designates the individual who will make decisions on the patient's behalf if he or she is unable to do so (see chapter 64 of this volume).

Each patient's advance directive should be reviewed as an initial step to palliative care. If patients have advance directives, it is important to confirm with each individual that the advance directive is current and accurate. Individuals without advance directives should be encouraged to develop advance directives and to communicate their health care preferences verbally and in writing.

FAMILY ADVOCACY AND DECISION-MAKING

PALLIATIVE CARE INVOLVES patients and their families. Families need support and guidance throughout a family member's illness trajectory. Patients should be encouraged to share information with family members and to include family members in health care visits. Ethical issues can arise when family members do not support goals of care determined by patients.

If conflict occurs within a patient's family, family–health care provider discussions can be helpful. To avoid or mitigate conflict, family members should be involved in discussions related to goals of care. When everyone is together it is important to have the patient articulate his or her wishes and preferences. The patient, family, and health care providers can determine a plan of care that will best meet the patient's needs. Palliative care experts can help patients and families with difficult situations.

If a patient is unable to communicate his or her wishes, families are often asked to make important decisions on the patient's behalf. Families or individual family members may not follow patients' wishes. If this occurs, it is important that health care providers reinforce with families that treatment decisions should be made based on prior goals determined by the patient and shared with his or her health care proxy or other surrogate decision-makers. Families of patients dying in the acute care setting have found advance directives helpful when making end-of-life decisions related to life-sustaining therapies (Jacob, 1998; Mayer & Kossoff, 1999; O'Callahan et al., 1995; Swigart, Lidz, Butterworth, & Robert, 1996; Tilden, Tolle, Nelson, & Fields, 2001; Tilden et al., 1999). In the acute care setting, family meetings held within 72 hours of patient admission to critical care increased consensus related to goals of care and early access to palliative care (Lilly et al., 2000).

BENEFIT VERSUS BURDEN OF THERAPY

ETHICAL ISSUES CAN arise when the burdens of treatment outweigh the benefits of treatment. Treatments should be determined based on the potential benefits versus burdens to the patient (Hastings Center, 1987; President's Commission for the Study of Ethical Problems in Medicine and Biomedical and Behavioral Research, 1983). Thus, all treatments should be considered individually and collectively as to their potential benefits versus burdens to the patient.

Instrumental to palliative care and end-of-life decisions are patient values, advance directives, and choices. Distinguishing between benefit and effectiveness of interventions is also a consideration (Sulmasy et al., 1993). Effectiveness relates to the impact of the intervention on the biomedical good of the patient and is an objective determination made by the health care team, whereas benefit is much broader, encompasses any positive change in the patient condition (as the patient perceives it), and is a subjective determination (Sulmasy et al., 1993).

WITHHOLDING AND WITHDRAWING LIFE-SUSTAINING THERAPY

IN 1983 THE President's Commission for the Study of Ethical Problems in Medicine and Biomedical and Behavioral Research clearly stated that there is no moral difference between withholding and withdrawing treatments, even life-sustaining treatment. The fundamental issue is the efficacious use of the treatment and the patient's desire for the treatment. Each individual has the right to accept or refuse any treatment. Of utmost importance is the right to start a treatment and then choose to stop the treatment if desired. There is no moral difference between starting and stopping.

Time-limited interventions can be trialed, in conjunction with palliative care interventions. From an ethical perspective, erring on the side of aggressive treatments is a greater good than erring on the side of too little treatment or treatment that is withdrawn too quickly (Schneiderman & Spragg, 1988). Life-sustaining therapy can be initiated with the knowledge that if it proves to be nonbeneficial or disproportionately burdensome, it can later be stopped (Schneiderman & Spragg, 1988).

MEDICAL FUTILITY

ETHICAL CHALLENGES OFTEN arise in cases of medical futility. Medical futility is "any clinical circumstance in which physicians and their consultants, consistent with the available medical literature, conclude that further treatment (except comfort care) cannot, within a reasonable possibility, cure, ameliorate, improve or restore a quality of life that would be satisfactory to the patient" (Hudson, 1994, p. 26). Luce (1997) suggests that treatment is futile when a patient cannot benefit from treatment, the patient's acute disorder is not reversible, it is projected that the patient will not survive the current hospitalization, or the quality of the patient's life following discharge will be poor.

Recognizing futility is fraught with complexity (see chapter 65 in this volume). Futility decisions often face patients and families as goals of care become unobtainable. An intervention that once worked does not work or is not as effective the next time it is used. Realizing that a treatment is futile is not easy and is usually a process that becomes clear over time. The patient, family, or health care provider(s) may determine that an intervention is futile. Conflicts arise when the patient, family, and health care providers do not agree about whether further treatment is futile. Family disagreements with the medical team's determination of futility and recommendations regarding patient care have been reported (Jacobs & Taylor, 2005).

Health care providers are not obligated to provide futile care. Yet this creates a dilemma as health care providers need to balance their unwillingness to provide futile care with their unwillingness to abandon vulnerable patients. Futility guidelines may help to resolve issues (Tomlinson & Czlonka, 1995), to work through conflict, and to facilitate compromise.

Early identification of patient goals may limit the incidence of medical futility. For example, if patients are clear that they want certain therapies and not others, futile treatments may not be initiated or may be stopped as soon as it is determined that the treatments will not contribute to achievement of personal goals and improved health. As stated by Jecker (1995), "Refraining from medically futile interventions is often the best way to care humanely for patients at the end of life" (p. 287).

MANAGEMENT OF DISTRESSING SYMPTOMS

PATIENTS MAY EXPERIENCE a multiplicity of symptoms and syndromes that vary based on their underlying medical conditions. Varying types of pain may occur with the possibility of other symptoms such as dyspnea, anxiety, agitation, confusion, and delirium. If symptoms are not effectively managed they can add to patient suffering and family distress. Assessment of symptoms, early detection, and treatment are key to promoting patient comfort and minimizing distress.

Palliative sedation can be used as a last resort to reduce patient suffering (Truog et al., 2001). Palliative sedation is defined as the intentional administration of sedatives in such dosages and combinations as required to reduce the terminal patient's consciousness as much as needed to adequately control one or more refractory symptoms (Broeckaert, 2000). Palliative sedation is used when a patient has distressing symptoms that do not respond to traditional pharmacological agents. Palliative sedation can be achieved by a continuous infusion of benzodiazepines, accompanied by analgesic and sedative infusions. "Heavy sedation should be reserved for when all reasonable measures to treat the symptoms directly with conventional therapies have been exhausted" (Woods, 2004, p. 245).

THE PRINCIPLE OF DOUBLE EFFECT

THE PRINCIPLE OF double effect "is invoked to justify claims that a single act having two foreseen effects, one good and one harmful (such as death), is not always morally prohibited if the harmful effect is not intended" (Beauchamp & Childress, 2001, p. 206). For example, pain medication may be titrated to promote comfort, yet a secondary effect may be a decrease in blood pressure or respiratory rate. In such cases, the context of care is of importance. If patients are aggressively seeking treatments and are not at the end of life, then pain needs to be managed carefully, minimizing the potential secondary effects. If, however, the patient is at the end of his or her life and the primary focus is palliative care, with little to no focus on aggressive life-sustaining therapy, then the secondary effects do not necessarily raise ethical concerns. The administration of analgesics to decrease discomfort is a beneficent act, even though death may be hastened. This double effect is recognized as ethically justified (Hastings Center, 1987). The principle of double effect has been upheld by the U.S. Supreme Court, who has determined that dying patients have the right to receive palliative care even if palliative care might hasten death (*Vacco v. Quill*, 1997).

CONCLUSION

THE LAST PHASE of life varies based on one's illness trajectory and clinical course (Lunney, Lynn, Foley, Lipson, & Guralnik, 2003; Lunney, Lynn, & Hogan, 2002). Hope is a complex process that is central to the provision of palliative care (Woods et al., 2000). Although hope for a cure is important, health care providers can help patients and their families by supporting this hope while preparing them for other outcomes as well. Hope for a cure may need to be redirected toward hope for prevention and relief of distressing symptoms or toward hope for comfort.

Palliative care is essential as illness progresses. Ethical palliative care can be achieved when patients' wishes are honored, comfort and dignity are maintained, families are included and supported, and the family decision-making process is facilitated.

REFERENCES

Beauchamp, T. L., & Childress, J. F. (2001). *Principles of biomedical ethics*. New York: Oxford University.

Braun, K. L., Onaka, A. T., & Horiuchi, B. Y. (2001). Advance directive completion rates and end-of-life preferences in Hawaii. *Journal of the American Geriatrics Society, 49*(21), 1708–1713.

Broeckaert, B. (2000). Palliative sedation defined or why and when terminal sedation is not euthanasia. Abstract 1st Congress RDPC, December 2000, Berlin. *Journal of Pain and Symptom Management, 20*(6), S58.

Hanson, L. C., & Rodgman, E. (1996). The use of living wills at the end of life. A national study. *Archives of Internal Medicine, 156*(9), 1018–1022.

The Hastings Center. (1987). Guidelines on the termination of life-sustaining treatment and the care of the dying. Briarcliff Manor, NY: Author.

Hudson T. (1994, February 20). Are futile-care policies the answer? *Hospitals and Health Networks*, 26–32.

Jacob, D. A. (1998). Family members' experiences with decision making for incompetent patients in the ICU: A qualitative study. *American Journal of Critical Care, 7*, 30–36.

Jacobs, B. B., & Taylor, C. (2005). Medical futility in the natural attitude. *Advances in Nursing Science, 28*(4), 288–305.

Jecker, N. S. (1995). Medical futility and care of dying patient. *Western Journal of Medicine, 163,* 287–291.

Jezewski, M. A., Meeker, M. A., & Schrader, M. (2003). Voices of oncology nurses: What is needed to assist patients with advance directives. *Cancer Nursing, 26*(2), 105–112.

Lilly, C. M., De Meo, D. L., Sonna, L. A., Haley, K. J., Masaro, A. F., Wallace, R. F., et al. (2000). An intensive communication intervention for the critically ill. *American Journal of Medicine, 109,* 469–475.

Lilly, C. M., Sonna, L. A., Haley, K. J., & Massaro, A. F. (2003). Intensive communication: Four-year follow-up from a clinical practice study. *Critical Care Medicine, 31*(5 Suppl.), S394–S399.

Luce, J. M. (1997). Withholding and withdrawal of life support from critically ill patients. *Western Journal of Medicine, 167,* 411–416.

Lunney, J. R., Lynn, J., Foley, D. J., Lipson, S., & Guralnik, J. M. (2003). Patterns of functional decline at the end of life. *Journal of the American Medical Association, 289*(18), 2387–2392.

Lunney, J. R., Lynn, J., & Hogan, C. (2002). Profiles of older Medicare decedents. *Journal of the American Geriatric Society, 50,* 1108–1112.

Mayer, S. A., & Kossoff, S. B. (1999). Withdrawal of life support in the neurological intensive care unit. *Neurology, 52,* 1602–1609.

McKinley, E. D., Gareeth, J. M., Evans, A. T., & Danis, M. (1996). Differences in end-of-life decision making among black and white ambulatory cancer patients. *Journal of General Internal Medicine, 11,* 651–656.

National Consensus Project for Palliative Care. (2004). *Clinical practice guidelines for quality palliative care.* Brooklyn, NY: Author.

Norton, S. A., Tilden, V. P., Tolle, S. W., Nelson, C. A., & Eggman, S. T. (2003). Life support withdrawal: Communication and conflict. *American Journal of Critical Care, 12*(6), 548–555.

O'Callahan, J. G., Fink, C., Pitts, L. H., & Luce, J. M. (1995). Withholding and withdrawing of life support from patients with severe head injury. *Critical Care Medicine, 23,* 1567–1575.

Patient Self-Determination Act 4206-4751, Pub L No. 101-508 (1990).

President's Commission for the Study of Ethical Problems in Medicine and Biomedical and Behavioral Research. (1983). *Deciding to forgo life-sustaining treatment: A report on ethical, medical and legal issues in treatment decisions.* Washington, DC: U.S. Government Printing Office.

Schneiderman, L. J., & Spragg, R. G. (1988). Ethical decisions in discontinuing mechanical ventilation. *The New England Journal of Medicine, 318,* 984–988.

Sulmasy, D. P., FitzGerald, D., & Jaffin, J. H. (1993). Ethical considerations. *Critical Care Clinics, 9,* 775–789.

Swigart, V., Lidz, C., Butterworth, V., & Robert, A. (1996). Letting go: Family willingness to forgo life support. *Heart and Lung: The Journal of Acute & Critical Care, 25*(6), 483–494.

Tilden, V. P., Tolle, S. W., Nelson, C. A., & Fields, J. (2001). Family decision-making to withdraw life-sustaining treatments from hospitalized patients. *Nursing Research, 50*(2), 105–115.

Tilden, V. P., Tolle, S. W., Nelson, C. A., Thompson, M., Eggman, S. C. (1999). Family decision making in foregoing life-extending treatments. *Journal of Family Nursing, 5*(1), 126–112.

Tomlinson, T., & Czlonka, D. (1995). Futility and hospital policy. *Hastings Center Report, 25,* 28–35.

Truog, R. D., Cist, A. F. M., Brackett, S. E., Burns, J. P., Curley, M. A. Q., Danis, M., et al. (2001). Recommendations for end-of-life care in the intensive care unit: The Ethics Committee of the Society of Critical Care Medicine. *Critical Care Medicine, 29*(12), 2332–2348.

Vacco v. Quill, 521 U.S. 793 (1997).

Wiegand, D. L. (2006). Withdrawal of life-sustaining therapy after sudden, unexpected life-threatening illness or injury: Interactions between patients' families, healthcare providers, and the healthcare system. *American Journal of Critical Care, 15*(2), 178–187.

Woods, S. (2004). Is terminal sedation compatible with good nursing care at the end of life? *International Journal of Palliative Nursing, 10*(5), 244–247.

Woods, S., Beaver, K., & Luker, K. (2000). Users' views of palliative care services: Ethical implications. *Nursing Ethics, 7*(4), 314–326.

Index